Primary Care
for the

PHYSICAL
THERAPIST
Examination and Triage

http://evolve.elsevier.com/Boissonnault/primary/

Instructor (only)

- **Image Collection**
  Search, view, and download the large selection of images from the textbook.

- **Supplemental Image Collection**
  Additional images to supplement chapters 10 and 11 in the textbook.

- **Skin Lesion Slides**
  Additional images to supplement chapter 8 in the textbook.

- **Part 1: PowerPoint Presentation on Medical Screening Principles**
  This presentation includes additional text, images, and tables to accompany Chapters 5 to 11.

- **Part 2: PowerPoint Presentation on Principles of Diagnostic Imaging**
  This presentation relates to Chapter 17.

- **Part 3: PowerPoint Presentation on Pharmacologic Principles**
  This presentation relates to Chapter 16.

- **Part 4: Patient Cases**
  These four patient cases supplement the textbook.

- **Examinations**
  The examinations, which include Answer Keys, contain multiple choice questions, true/false questions, and matching type questions that are useful for PT and transitional DPT students and people in residency programs.

- **WebLinks**
  An exciting resource that lets you link to hundreds of websites carefully chosen to supplement the content of the textbook. The WebLinks are regularly updated, with new ones added as they develop.

Student (and Instructor)

- **Supplemental Image Collection**
  Additional images to supplement chapters 10 and 11 in the textbook.

- **Skin Lesion Slides**
  Additional images to supplement chapter 8 in the textbook.

- **WebLinks**
  An exciting resource that lets you link to hundreds of websites carefully chosen to supplement the content of the textbook. The WebLinks are regularly updated, with new ones added as they develop.

Primary Care
for the
PHYSICAL
THERAPIST
Examination and Triage

William G. Boissonnault, PT, DHSc, FAAOMPT

Assistant Professor
University of Wisconsin–Madison
Program in Physical Therapy
Madison, Wisconsin

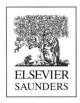

ELSEVIER
SAUNDERS

ELSEVIER
SAUNDERS

11830 Westline Industrial Drive
St. Louis, Missouri 63146

PRIMARY CARE FOR THE PHYSICAL THERAPIST: EXAMINATION AND TRIAGE
Copyright © 2005 Elsevier Inc. All rights reserved.

Notice

Physical Therapy is an ever-changing field. Standard safety precautions must be followed, but as new research and clinical experience broaden our knowledge, changes in treatment and drug therapy may become necessary or appropriate. Readers are advised to check the most current product information provided by the manufacturer of each drug to be administered to verify the recommended dose, the method and duration of administration, and contraindications. It is the responsibility of the licensed prescriber, relying on experience and knowledge of the patient, to determine dosages and the best treatment for each individual patient. Neither the publisher nor the editor assumes any liability for any injury and/or damage to persons or property from this publication.

The Publisher

Acquisitions Editor: *Marion Waldman*
Developmental Editor: *Marjory I. Fraser*
Publishing Services Manager: *Linda McKinley*
Project Managers: *Judy Ahlers*
Designer: *Julia Dummitt*

ISBN-13: 978-0-7216-9659-1
ISBN-10: 0-7216-9659-7

Printed in the United States of America

Last digit is the print number: 9 8 7 6 5 4

REVIEWERS

Sharon Dunn, BSPT, MHS
Program Director
Louisiana State University
Shreveport, Louisiana

Lee Grinonneau, MS, PT
Chairman
Owens State Community College
Toledo, Ohio

Matthew Hyland, BS, MPT
Part-Time Faculty
Mercy College
Dobbs Ferry, New York

Ed Maher, PT, MS, OCS
Faculty
Carroll College
Waukesha, Wisconsin

Corrie Mancinelli, MPT
Assistant Professor
Rutgers University–University of Medicine and Dentistry of
 New Jersey
Stratford, New Jersey

CONTRIBUTORS

Jill Schiff Boissonnault, PT, PhD
Faculty Associate
Program in Physical Therapy
Department of Orthopedics and Rehabilitation
University of Wisconsin-Madison
Madison, Wisconsin

William G. Boissonnault, PT, DHSc, FAAOMPT
Assistant Professor
Program in Physical Therapy
University of Wisconsin-Madison
Senior Physical Therapist
University of Wisconsin Hospital/Clinics
Madison, Wisconsin

Adjunct Faculty
University of St. Augustine Center of Health Sciences
St. Augustine, Florida
College of Allied Health Sciences
University of Tennessee-Memphis
Memphis, Tennessee
Massachusetts General Hospital Institute
  of Health Professions
Boston, Massachusetts
Krannert Graduate School of Physical Therapy
University of Indianapolis
Indianapolis, Indiana
Physical Therapy Program
University of Medicine and Dentistry of New Jersey
Newark, New Jersey

Jennifer M. Bottomley, PT, MS, PhD
Independent Geriatric Rehabilitation Program Consultant
Boston, Massachusetts
President, Section on Geriatrics-APTA

William P. Brookfield, RPH, MSc
Global Product Safety Consultant
Eli Lilly and Company
Indianapolis, Indiana
Adjunct Faculty
Purdue University School of Pharmaceutical Sciences
Lafayette, Indiana
Butler University School of Pharmacy
Indianapolis, Indiana

Joe Daly, PT, MA, MHS
Industrial Consultant
NovaCare Rehabilitation
Columbus, Ohio

Gail Deyle, PT, DPT, OCS, FAAOMPT
Graduate Program Director
Rocky Mountain University of Health Professions
Provo, Utah
Assistant Professor
US Army-Baylor University Postprofessional Doctoral
  Program in Orthopaedic Manual Physical Therapy
Brooke Army Medical Center
Fort Sam Houston, Texas

Sherry Fadel, PT, MS
Total Rehabilitation Services
Columbia, South Carolina

Julie M. Fritz, PT, PhD
Assistant Professor
Division of Physical Therapy
College of Health
University of Utah
Salt Lake City, Utah
Clinical Outcomes Research Scientist
Intermountain Health Care
Salt Lake City, Utah

Matthew B. Garber, PT, DSc, OCS, FAAOMPT
Assistant Chief, Physical Therapy
Assistant Professor
US Army-Baylor University Postprofessional Doctoral
  Program in Orthopaedic Manual Physical Therapy
Brooke Army Medical Center
Fort Sam Houston, Texas

Joseph J. Godges, DPT, MA, OCS
Coordinator
Kaiser Permanente Southern California
Physical Therapy Residency and
  Fellowship Programs
Los Angeles, California
Assistant Professor
Department of Physical Therapy
School of Allied Health Professions
Loma Linda University
Loma Linda, California

David Greathouse, PT, PhD
Professor and Chairman
School of Physical Therapy
Belmont University
Nashville, Tennessee

Kristine M. Hallisy, PT, MS, OCS
Faculty Associate
Physical Therapy Program
Department of Orthopedics and Rehabilitation Medicine
University of Wisconsin–Madison
Madison, Wisconsin

Steven C. Janos, PT, MS, OCS
Orthopedic Clinical Specialist
Sports and Orthopedic Rehabilitation Services
Tampa, Florida

Ronnie Leavitt, PT, MPH, PhD
Associate Clinical Professor
School of Allied Health
University of Connecticut
Storrs, Connecticut

Deborah Lechner, PT, MS
President, Ergoscience, Inc.
Birmingham, Alabama

Kathryn Maltchev, OTR/L
Hand Therapist
Concentra Medical Center
San Antonio, Texas

Ivan Matsui, PT, FAAOMPT
Faculty
Kaiser Permanente Hayward Physical Therapy
  Fellowship in Advanced Orthopedic
  Manual Therapy
Clinical Specialist and Supervisor
Department of Rehabilitation Services Kaiser Hayward
  Medical Center
Clinical Specialist
Adult Primary Care
Department of Medicine, Kaiser Hayward
  Medical Center
Hayward, California

Barbara McKelvy, PT
President
Strategic Rehabilitation Options
Columbus, Ohio

Michael McKeough, PT, EdD
Associate Professor
Physical Therapy Program
Shenendoah University
Winchester, Virgina

Brian P. Murphy, MPT
Chair, Veterans' Health Administration Physical Therapy
  Advisory Council
Washington, District of Columbia
Clinical Manager, Rehabilitation
Veterans Administration Salt Lake City Healthcare System
Adjunct Faculty and Clinical Instructor
Division of Physical Therapy
University of Utah
Salt Lake City, Utah
Adjunct Faculty and Clinical Instructor
University of Montana
Missoula, Montana
President, Section on Veterans Affairs
American Physical Therapy Association
Alexandria, Virginia

Gerald G. Ryan, MD
Associate Professor
University of Wisconsin-Madison Medical School
Madison, Wisconsin

Rebecca Gourley Stephenson, PT
Principal, Stephenson Physical Therapy
Medfield, Massachusetts
Instructor
Education Resources Inc. Massachusetts
Medfield, Massachusetts

Steven H. Tepper, PT, PhD
Professor and Program Director
Physical Therapy Program
Shenendoah University
Winchester, Virginia

Lucy J. Wall, MT (ASCP), MA
Advisor, Physical Therapy Program
Department of Orthopedics and Rehabilitation
Assistant Dean for Admissions
University of Wisconsin Medical School
Madison, Wisconsin

To: My parents, Greg and Geneva Boissonnault, for their unwavering and unconditional support.

To: My partners throughout life's travels, Jill, Josh, Jacob, and Eliya.

To: Dr. Michael Koopmeiners, a personal friend and mentor who has championed physical therapist participation in the collaborative medical model.

To: The students and patients who have taught me so much over the years. I am indebted to them for their insight, their passion for knowledge, and their zest for life. Work has rarely felt like work.

To: The American Physical Therapy Association's Vision 2020. May it guide us and push us all, as we strive to help meet society's health care needs.

Take care!

FOREWORD

Early in the 1990s, the Pew Health Professions Commission produced a report designed to assist health care professions in the process of economic reform and listed several recommendations for streamlining care. One of those recommendations was reported to be a suggestion that outpatient facilities should "cross-train" personnel so that one person could handle the responsibilities of both nurse and physical therapist. This just did not make good sense to me, and therefore I asked a colleague who served on the Pew Commission (not a physical therapist) what in the world this recommendation was intended to accomplish. She explained to me (actually to a group of us at a meeting) that this recommendation was being misinterpreted. She offered that the Pew Commission envisioned an ideal outpatient or walk-in clinic that would be staffed professionally by a family nurse practitioner *and* a physical therapist. These two professionals could perform the primary care screening and examination of organ systems and movement systems and then make appropriate referrals to other practitioners as needed. I could see the cost-saving aspects of this idea immediately, and I hoped that this suggestion was meant to propel direct access legislation in all 50 states for physical therapists. Surely it was meant to take full advantage of the generalist skills of nurse practitioners and physical therapists. However, physical therapists were more commonly known as rehabilitation professionals and rehabilitation was not traditionally associated with primary care.

About that same time, the term *primary care* began to emerge more frequently in the American Physical Therapy Association (APTA) House of Delegates motions, and I was asked by the Section for Education to give a 2-hour presentation on "Translating the Role of the Physical Therapist in Primary Care into Student Expectations" at the Combined Sections meeting in Dallas in 1997. To prepare for this presentation, I wondered what the APTA meant by "primary care" and so my graduate assistant, Neva Kirk-Sanchez, and I began a search of the APTA Policies, the Standards of Practice, the Department of Education Normative Model for Physical Therapy Education, the Code of Ethics and Guide to Professional Conduct and, finally, the Standards for Accreditation from the Commission on Accreditation in Physical Therapy Education (CAPTE). We were looking for mention of the term *primary care* or descriptions of practice that seemed to indicate responsibility in direct access situations, plus skills in interdisciplinary communication, holistic screening and referral to others as appropriate, community health and education skills, and the ability to perform a thorough patient interview and history that would lead to a physical therapy diagnosis and treatment plan, with or without a referral to another health professional.

We found many statements indicating that the role of primary care practitioner was totally consistent with the expectations of education and practice as stated in the official documents of the APTA and of CAPTE. Most specifically and to the point is the APTA Position on Primary Care as captured in RC 23-95

Physical therapists are primary providers who, as individuals or members of primary care teams, make unique contributions to people with neuromusculoskeletal dysfunction. Through the process of screening, triage, examination, evaluation, referral, intervention, coordination of care, education and prevention, physical therapists prevent or reduce impairments, functional limitations and disabilities, and achieve cost-effective clinical outcomes.

Thus, what does primary care practice in physical therapy look like, how does it compare with primary care medicine and nursing, and why don't we hear more educational programs describing this as a goal? The military programs, particularly the Army and the U.S. Public Health Service, have always excelled in interview and triage functions. In the early 1990s, when Florida succeeded in passing direct access legislation, the University of Miami sponsored continuing education for the community on screening and diagnosis, and Colonel David Greathouse taught us how the process of screening and diagnosis was carried out in the Army. Goodman and Snyder's textbook, *Differential Diagnosis in Physical Therapy*, was published in 1990. This text by an army physical therapist (Catherine Goodman) and an army nurse (Teresa Snyder) made great strides in helping us feel more knowledgeable about screening for organ system disease and referred pain patterns. Then Bill Boissonnault published his *Examination in Physical Therapy Practice*, which was oriented toward screening for specific organ diseases and added important content on radiologic assessment and psychological disorders. As helpful as these texts were, none of these efforts represented what seemed to be the physical therapist equivalent of the *total* of primary care practice as performed, for example, by nurses and physicians. At this stage of our professional development, beyond the APTA Policy on Primary Care and the myriad evaluative criteria that fall within CAPTE's expectations and the Normative Model criteria, physical therapy has yet to provide, in one place, a complete and coherent description of the role and responsibilities of the physical therapist as a primary care practitioner and, more important, the context of that role in the management of movement disorders and in rehabilitation in general.

Vision 2020, the vision statement adopted by the APTA for future practice in the year 2000, states that:

> By 2020 physical therapy will be provided by physical therapists who are doctors of physical therapy, recognized by consumers and other health care professionals as the practitioners of choice to whom consumers have the direct access for the diagnosis of, interventions for, and prevention of impairments, functional limitations, and disabilities related to movement, function and health.

Now that seems to be reaching more toward a description of primary care responsibility, and it specifically links this level of expectation to the clinical doctorate. At this writing, 67 of the 213 physical therapy programs offer the DPT as the entering degree into clinical practice, and many more are making the transition from master's to clinical doctorate. In the United States, a clinical doctoral degree indicates education at the maximum level to be able to carry out interdisciplinary autonomous practice. Physical therapists, step by step, seem to be taking rightful responsibility for being in charge of disorders of movement in four systems: musculoskeletal, neuromuscular, cardiopulmonary, and integumentary, as outlined in the *Guide to Physical Therapist Practice*. However, on the whole, I have not seen a significant difference in the attitudes, confidence, and assertiveness of new DPT graduates, compared with master's degree graduates, in stepping up to the plate and taking charge of patient care in an assertive way. I recognize that for new graduates to be able to practice with new skills and attitudes, the environment in health care must make at least a tiny space for this to occur, and at times, I believe that clinicians with years of practice are not as aware as they need to be to help that space to open up. This speaks to the extreme importance of the success of the tDPT, or transitional DPT degree being offered by educational programs (many online) to "upgrade" the knowledge and skills of those practitioners with baccalaureate and master's degree knowledge and outdated clinical expectations. However, I have to wonder how many DPT programs are truly preparing a generalist practitioner capable of primary care practice? First, I wonder how many DPT programs offer the coursework required to screen patients adequately at first entry into the health care system? How many transitional DPT programs are taking responsibility in upgrading their postgraduate students in the knowledge of medical pathology, pharmacology, comprehensive diagnostic imaging, and tests? And how many entry-level and postprofessional-level curricula offer coursework in effective communication, assertiveness training, interviewing skills, negotiation, and referral practices and cultural awareness and sensitivity? Surely this would represent minimum knowledge, attitudes, and skills to upgrade professional knowledge to the level implied by the clinical doctorate in physical therapy. We educators and clinicians both seem to lack a cohesive and universal vision of whom we are educating to do what at the DPT level.

In summary, I believe that it is the vision of the great leaders in physical therapy, such as Catherine Worthingham, Geneva R. Johnson, Helen J. Hislop, Steve Rose, Marilyn Gossman, Eugene Michels, Marilyn Moffat, and Shirley Sahrmann that physical therapists should take their rightful place alongside physicians and nurse practitioners as colleagues in direct access patient care, specifically in charge of disorders in movement. I believe that for us to be successful in this endeavor, *we must embrace an identity as a primary care practitioner*, and we must use not only accurate interviewing and evidence-based diagnostic testing and treatment skills, but also must embody the identity of a mature healing professional with well-developed communication skills, negotiation and assertiveness skills, knowledge and appreciation of culturally diverse behaviors, and confidence in our ability to develop rapport with patients and their families and with our colleagues in the professions.

This textbook represents a major contribution in moving our profession forward toward this goal. Dr. Boissonnault is the most competent physical therapist educator and clinician possible to write and edit this text. His entire career has led to the creation of this work. He grasps the importance not only of the necessary knowledge needed for primary care but also of the importance of the affective behaviors and the art of this process, and he has injected this awareness into this text. A cursory look at the table of contents reveals the inclusion of material reflective of the necessary intricate balance of the knowledge of the art and science of primary care. I predict that this textbook will take its place alongside the great texts in our profession that have helped move all of us forward, especially educators, as well as clinicians, in taking our rightful place as health care professionals in charge of the examination, diagnosis, and treatment of movement disorders. And if you were fortunate enough to hear Dr. Boissonnault's Maley lecture at the APTA Annual Conference of 2000, you know that he would include the important content on knowing when and how to confidently refer to our colleagues those patients whose disorders fall outside our scope of practice. When we begin educating our students and practicing in the ways that this text instructs us, we will be living up to the expectations of our patients and clients, who believe in us as primary care providers. And we will be going a long way to actualize the dreams of our great leaders in physical therapy and the APTA vision of future practice.

Carol M. Davis, PT, EdD, MS, FAPTA
Division of Physical Therapy
University of Miami School of Medicine

PREFACE

Primary Care for the Physical Therapist: Examination and Triage is written in the spirit of the American Physical Therapy Association's (APTA) long-term goals expressed in the APTA Vision Sentence for Physical Therapy 2020 (HOD 06-00-24-35):

> By 2020 physical therapy will be provided by physical therapists who are doctors of physical therapy, recognized by consumers and other health care professionals as the practitioners of choice to whom consumers have direct access for the diagnosis of, intervention for, and for the prevention of impairments, functional limitations, and disabilities related to movement, function and health.

Tremendous opportunities await physical therapist practitioners as the profession moves toward *Vision 2020*, including unlimited potential in the area of primary care. Primary care has been described by the Institute of Medicine (IOM) as "the provision of integrated, accessible health care services by clinicians who are accountable for addressing a large majority of personal health care needs, developing a sustained partnership with patients, and practicing within the context of family and community." The APTA has endorsed the concepts of primary care set forth by the IOM, including that "Primary care can encompass myriad needs that go well beyond the capabilities and competencies of individual caregivers and that require the involvement and interaction of varied practitioners." The 2002 APTA *Interactive Guide to Physical Therapist Practice* describes that "for acute musculoskeletal and neuromuscular conditions, triage and initial examination are appropriate physical therapist responsibilities, and for certain chronic conditions physical therapists should be recognized as principal providers of care within a collaborative Primary Care Team." Key words and phrases from these statements include examination, triage, principal providers of care for certain conditions, and collaborative team.

Examination and triage are two valuable functions that physical therapists can provide in a primary care setting. Primary care models are already in place where physical therapists are the entry point for selected patient populations (Chapter 1). The goals of these patient encounters include (1) deciding whether certain imaging modalities are warranted to assist in the diagnostic process, (2) deciding if a physician consultation is indicated, (3) determining whether a referral to a physical therapist certified clinical specialist is warranted, and (4) implementing a physical therapy plan of care when appropriate. Considering that hypertension, diabetes mellitus, and low back pain are among the most frequently reported reasons for patient visits to a physician clinic, there is tremendous opportunity for physical therapists, not only as examiners and those who perform triage but also as principal providers of care. Interestingly, much of the impetus for including physical therapists in the primary care models described in Chapter 1 came from physician groups within the described health care systems.

The APTA's "collaborative team" emphasis is an important message for those within and outside our profession. When I envision the delivery of primary care, I do not envision individuals (of any discipline), but I do picture a cohesive interdisciplinary health care delivery system. Such a cohesive system requires team building and communication skills, a solid understanding of the background and potential roles of the various providers, and defined roles for the various providers. With the appropriate training, physical therapists can be active participants and leaders in the development of primary care delivery models; training commensurate with the professional doctoral degree (DPT).

Written for the student, resident, fellow, and the experienced clinician new to the primary care environment, *Primary Care for the Physical Therapist: Examination and Triage* provides information designed to help prepare physical therapists to assume a significant role in the primary care delivery model. The major emphasis of this textbook is the examination and triage and interdisciplinary health care components related to the physical therapist's potential role. The book is divided into five sections: (1) Introduction, (2) Examination/Evaluation: The Patient Interview, (3) Examination/Evaluation: The Physical Examination, (4) Special Populations, and (5) Clinical Medicine. The Introduction section begins with an overview of primary care from a physician and physical therapist perspective. G. Ryan, MD, provides an overview of events leading to the current status of primary care in the United States, as well as a physician's perspective of potential roles for physical therapists and challenges facing all disciplines involved in primary care. Each of the three physical therapist contributors provides an in-depth description of an existing primary care model where physical therapists play a significant role. The hope would be that this information would facilitate the development of additional similar models with physical therapists taking a lead role in the planning and implementation phases. The second chapter, *Evidence-Based Examination of Diagnostic Information*, provides physical therapists with the tools necessary to practice in an evidence-based practice environment; with the focus on screening and diagnostic processes. The third chapter, *Cultural Competence*, provides essential information related to effective patient care in the ever-diversifying U.S. patient population. Chapter 4, *The Patient Interview: The Science Behind the Art*, provides the art and science behind effective patient-therapist interchange.

Sections II and III of the textbook (Chapters 5 to 11)—Examination and Evaluation—focus on the physical therapist's examination and triage skills vital to a primary care environment. Central to these skills is the data evaluation process that leads to a differential diagnosis and establishment of the appropriate plan of care. An important part of the triage responsibilities is the recognition by physical therapists of those patients who need to be referred to other members of the primary care team, as well as recognition of those patients who should be seen by a certified clinical specialist (physical therapists). Effective and efficient means to collect the necessary patient data during the history and physical examination are presented along with important follow-up questions and tests to help identify patient health care and wellness issues.

In an effort to promote efficient and effective practice, this section is organized as a PT might collect the patient data. The desired outcome is that the therapist understands all of the potential items that could make up an examination, but equally important is understanding what is most relevant for a particular patient during the initial visit. Not every question needs to be asked of every patient; and not every examination technique needs to be used, especially during the initial visit. The therapist must be comfortable with the fact that there is a risk of missing something significant during the visit with leaving something out of the examination. The therapist also should appreciate that portions of the examination will and should overlap with those of other practitioners, helping to minimize the risk of overlooking an important health issue. The information in this section, along with the detailed regional examination skills therapists possess, should provide the foundation necessary for making the essential clinical decisions.

Section IV, Special Populations, describes client groups (adolescents, obstetric patients, injured workers, and geriatric patients) with unique issues and challenges commonly served by physical therapists. Understanding the distinctive anatomical, physiological, psychosocial, and pathological factors associated with each group will help prepare the therapist to quickly establish an accurate and effective plan of care. Experts in our field present recommended examination modifications for these groups with an overview of diseases and disorders commonly noted in these populations. Although the pediatric population is not addressed specifically, important developmental issues are covered in the chapter on the adolescent population. Considering that infants and toddlers are much more than "little adults," an entire text is probably a more appropriate vehicle to address this very unique population. Finally, another objective of this section is to present potential practice niches where physical therapist involvement would greatly enhance the delivery of care.

Section V, Clinical Medicine, includes chapters on pharmacology, diagnostic imaging, and laboratory tests and values. The information contained in these chapters is designed to enhance therapists' abilities related to professional communication, functioning effectively within an interdisciplinary health care delivery model, and clinical decision making associated with all of the elements listed in the patient management model in the *Guide to Physical Therapist Practice*. Primary care models (see Chapter 1) already are in place within which therapists refer patients for selected diagnostic imaging modalities and prescribe specific medications. Understanding the evidence to guide this type of decision making is essential. This section also provides background information describing other health professionals participating in the delivery of primary care.

The intent of this book is to complement therapists' knowledge and other published texts and articles related to specific regional examination and intervention approaches. The information provided should facilitate therapists' role as active participants in the shaping of the future of health care delivery in the United States and international communities. The challenge that faces us is whether we can put into action the charges described in the APTA *Vision 2020*, a challenge that must be met. I believe that maintaining the status quo of our practice is not a viable option. Two choices are available—either we regress back to the era when we were functioning more as aides and we join the ranks of the numerous recently developed groups of "supportive" practitioners, or we join the ranks of the decision makers. I am confident that you will agree that there is really only one option.

William G. Boissonnault, PT, DHSc, FAAOMPT

ACKNOWLEDGMENTS

I would like to acknowledge the physical therapist visionaries who forged *Vision 2020*, and the doctors of physical therapy who will lead the way. I also applaud colleagues such as Catherine Goodman for providing a vision as to what differential diagnosis means from a physical therapist's perspective.

I am forever indebted to the contributing authors who invested valuable time and energy in this project. I learned a great deal from them. My thanks also goes to Ed Maher, a key manuscript reviewer, and the others who provided valuable input regarding the book content and organization.

CONTENTS

SECTION ONE

Introduction

Introduction to Primary Care Medicine

Gerald G. Ryan, MD
David Greathouse, PT, PhD
Ivan Matsui, PT, FAAOMPT
Brian P. Murphy, MPT

Objectives

After reading this chapter, the reader will be able to:

1. Describe the historic events that have helped shape the current practice of primary care medicine.
2. Provide an overview of primary care medicine from a physician perspective.
3. Describe examples of current physical therapy primary care practice models.
4. Provide strategies for facilitating a patient consult or referral to another health care provider.

The National Academy of Sciences defines primary care as "the provision of integrated, accessible health care services by clinicians who are accountable for addressing a large majority of personal health care needs, developing a sustained partnership with patients, and practicing in the context of family and community." Family physicians, general internists, and pediatricians provide the majority of primary care medicine in the United States (Table 1-1). Primary care services are provided on a much smaller scale by a broad range of specialists, most notably obstetrician-gynecologists. Nonphysician specialists such as physician assistants (PAs) and nurse practitioners (NPs) also serve as primary care providers. The level of physician supervision for nonphysician providers can vary greatly. Despite the variety of practitioners functioning as primary care providers, the demands placed on these providers are remarkably similar. Providers must continuously balance the needs of their patients with the time constraints and fiscal realities of modern medical practice. Physical therapists (PTs), collaborating with members of the primary care team, can help balance these seemingly disparate realities of modern medical practice.

The role of the PT in a primary care environment is rapidly evolving. The overall goals of this chapter are to familiarize PTs with primary care medicine to facilitate collaboration with other members of an interdisciplinary health care team and to identify potential roles for the PT within this model.

Modern Health Care in the United States

An awareness of the dynamics that have shaped our current health care system will help PTs appreciate the various demands placed on the primary care provider. The first major change in the delivery of health care in the United States occurred in 1965 with the establishment of Medicare and Medicaid. Before this, health care services in the United States were delivered almost exclusively by individual health care providers on a fee-for-service basis. With the passage of the Medicare and Medicaid Acts the U.S. government for the first time guaranteed availability of health care services for the elderly and the poor.

Medicare and Medicaid were cornerstones of President Johnson's "great society." The Johnson administration envisioned subsequently offering similar programs to the entire population as a way of providing universal health care access. Much to the chagrin of the framers of the original Medicare legislation, health care expenditures for Medicare recipients increased dramatically in the decade that followed. This rapid increase in health care costs put a halt to any plans to expand government-guaranteed health care coverage further and spawned several pieces of legislation that shaped later changes for health care delivery within the United States.[16]

In response to the rapid rise in health care costs in both the private sector and Medicare, Congress passed the Health Maintenance Organization Act in 1973. This provided financing and other legislative support for the development of health maintenance organizations (HMOs). However, not until the 1980s did HMOs begin to exert a major influence on the delivery of health care in the United States. Enrollment in HMOs and preferred provider organizations (PPOs) rose from 10 million in the early 1980s to 55 million by the start of the 1990s.[4] In the face of rapidly rising Medicare costs, the Tax Equity and Fiscal Responsibility Act established diagnosis-related groups (DRGs) as the method of payment for inpatient services rendered to Medicare recipients. With the passage of this legislation physician and hospital services were no longer reimbursed on the basis of charges for services rendered to the patient during the hospital stay. Hospitals were instead reimbursed a

TABLE 1-1

Patient Visits to Physician Specialty

Physician Specialty and Professional Identity	No. of Visits (in Thousands)	Percent
All visits	756,734	100.0
PHYSICIAN SPECIALTY		
General and family practice	170,571	22.5
Internal medicine*	135,607	17.9
Pediatrics	74,045	9.8
Obstetrics and gynecology	59,518	7.9
Ophthalmology	51,165	6.8
Orthopedic surgery	40,516	5.4
Dermatology	32,704	4.3
Psychiatry	23,346	3.0
General surgery	21,174	2.8
Urology	17,415	2.3
Cardiovascular disease	16,566	2.2
Otolaryngology	16,369	2.2
Neurology	8298	1.1
All other specialties	90,440	12.0

Sources: U.S. Department of Health and Human Services, Public Health Service, Centers for Disease Control and Prevention, National Center for Health Statistics, 1999 data. Accessed at www.aafp.org/facts.
*Includes only general internal medicine.

flat rate determined by the patients' diagnoses. Institutions with extensive lengths of stay or high utilization of expensive services received the same reimbursement as those with shorter lengths of stay and more conservative use of medical services. The establishment of DRGs resulted in the first reduction of utilization of Medicare services since the program's inception. Resource-based relative value scales (RBRVS) were developed in 1989 to quantify outpatient Medicare services in much the same way as DRGs were being used to define payment for inpatient services. RBRVSs were fully implemented in 1997.[15]

Although DRGs and RBRVSs were effective in controlling the rise in Medicare expenditures in the 1980s, health care expenditures for the remainder of the population rose at an alarming rate during this period. By the close of the 1980s health care costs made up 14% of the gross national product (GNP). High health care costs were of particular concern to major manufacturers and industries. Health care costs for American workers were significantly higher than for workers in Western Europe. This added cost to the manufacturing industry made it difficult for American goods to be cost competitive in the world market. The rising cost of health care was a central issue in the 1992 presidential election. Bill Clinton made the National Health Care Initiative (NHCI) a major element of his campaign platform. After the elections President Clinton appointed his wife, Hillary Rodham Clinton, to head a task force charged with the reform of health care in the United States. Many health care reformers of the time believed that the United States would follow the lead of most Western European nations and establish a national health care system. Clinton's NHCI collapsed in 1994 under intense lobbying by the insurance and hospital industries as well as the sheer complexity of the task force's final recommendations.

With the demise of the NHCI, HMOs were aggressively promoted as the free market system's answer to controlling health care costs. The most common HMO model includes a physician gatekeeper. With this model all services are directly provided by the patient's primary care provider or, if specialty services are required, authorized by the primary care provider. HMO plans assumed that requiring everyone to see a primary physician first would result in significant savings. Studies have consistently shown that patients with primary care physicians consume fewer services, have lower overall health care costs, and have better health outcomes than patients without primary care providers. Primary care physicians were also given further incentives to conserve medical resources by receiving bonuses based on health care expenditures. Physicians using fewer health care resources would be paid bonuses based on the amount of money the insurance plan was able to save over expected costs.

Changing Attitudes Toward Gatekeepers

The rapid rise of gatekeeper HMOs thrust primary care physicians—primarily family physicians, general internists, and pediatricians—into a pivotal role in the delivery of health care services. This proved to be a precarious position. The shift to HMOs by a large portion of the American public initially did slow the increase in health care costs. Concurrent with the increase in HMO enrollment, the number of patient complaints also began to rise. Patients accustomed to unlimited access to health care services began to voice their discontent when denied medical services by their primary care gatekeeper. Patients initially directed these complaints at the insurance carriers. When denied reconsideration by the HMOs, increasing numbers of patients turned to their political representatives for redress of their grievances. Financial arrangements that rewarded gatekeeper physicians for holding down costs came under increased scrutiny. Patients and politicians accused primary care providers of sacrificing patient well-being for personal financial gain. For most health care providers, this was the first time they were viewed by the public as an agent of the insurance industry and not as a patient advocate. The initial cost savings experienced during the rapid rise of HMOs was most likely attributable to a preferential enrollment of a young, healthy population in the HMOs. As HMOs competed for an older and more chronically ill population, the initial financial success of many health care plans began to erode. Insurance carriers subsequently placed greater and greater pressure on primary care physicians to further limit access to services. Services frequently targeted for strict cost constraints included mental health services, physical therapy, radiology services such as MRIs, and alcohol and drug rehabilitation programs.

As the 1990s came to a close, the gatekeeper model for the delivery of health care services began to unravel. Insurance carriers came under pressure from the public and politicians as well as from the primary care providers themselves. Patients wanted a primary care provider involved in their health care decisions but did not want access to health care services dependent on the approval of these providers. Primary care providers no longer wanted to be in an adversarial role with their patients. More and more HMOs have abandoned the gatekeeper model. Double-digit increases in health care costs have once again caused alarm in the business community as well as in the federal government. Primary care providers will closely watch how the most recent rises in health care costs will affect their role in the delivery of health care services in the near future.[5,20]

Primary Care Providers in the United States

Family physicians, general internists, and pediatricians constitute the bulk of primary care physicians in the United States. PAs and NPs are increasingly being used to improve patient access to primary care services. Although all these groups are considered primary health care professionals, there are significant differences in training and patient populations served between groups.

Family physicians receive 3 years of training after graduation from medical school. The care of patients in an outpatient setting is the cornerstone of family practice residency training programs; the typical family physician spends 90% or more of his or her time in the outpatient setting. The first year of residency consists primarily of inpatient rotations of specialty services including, but not limited to, pediatrics, obstetrics/gynecology, surgery, adult medicine, emergency medicine, and intensive care. The family medicine resident maintains an outpatient continuity practice even during this first year of intensive inpatient training. During the second and third year of residency training, the amount of time spent in the outpatient setting increases. Further specialty training is received in a variety of outpatient specialty clinics such as otolaryngology, dermatology, urology, and rheumatology. A minimum of 1 month is spent concentrating on musculoskeletal conditions. This time may be spent with either an orthopedist or a sports medicine physician.

A heavy emphasis throughout the training is placed on the psychosocial model of medical care. This model emphasizes the influence the patient's social situation, family dynamics, and emotional well-being may have on his or her total health. All family medicine training facilities have full-time mental health specialists involved in the daily education and supervision of the residents. Family physicians potentially treat patients from "the cradle to the grave," although in reality many family physicians develop practices that are more limited in scope.

General internists also spend 3 years in postgraduate training. In contrast to family medicine residency training, the emphasis of general internal medicine is the caring for hospitalized patients. Internal medicine residents do spend a limited amount of time providing outpatient services, but outpatient services always represent a small portion of the total time spent in the training programs. Internal medicine residents spend a significant amount of time in settings such as cardiac and medical intensive care units. Little, if any, time is spent under the supervision of mental health educators, and there are no requirements for training with either orthopedists or sports medicine physicians to develop an understanding about musculoskeletal problems. On completion of their training, general internists tend to limit their practice to the care of adults, and many general internists do not provide women's health services. On completion of the residency training, internists generally spend as much, if not more, time caring for hospitalized patients as they do patients in the outpatient setting. A current trend is for in-patient care within hospitals to be provided by internal medicine physicians serving as "hospitalists." These individuals are responsible for caring for all patients admitted to the hospital by referring physicians. They do not maintain any outpatient practice. Hospitalists are not considered primary care providers even if they were trained in a general internal medicine residency program.

General pediatricians also spend 3 years in postgraduate training. Pediatric residents train in neonatal intensive care units, pediatric intensive care units, and general pediatric inpatient services. They also spend time in both general and specialty pediatric outpatient clinics. The first year of most pediatric training programs is primarily spent in the hospital setting, with the subsequent 2 years more evenly split between the inpatient and outpatient settings. Pediatric training programs place great emphasis on childhood developmental stages. Recognition of congenital malformations, including orthopedic conditions, is part of the formal pediatric training. Training in the care of musculoskeletal illness in the older child is less formalized but has received greater emphasis in recent years. Pediatricians typically limit their scope of practice to patients younger than 18 years but can provide care for patients of any age.

An increasing number of nonphysician health care providers are delivering primary care services in the United States. NPs and PAs make up the bulk of these nonphysician providers. The focus and training of these two disciplines have important distinctions.

Enrollees in NP training programs are graduates of a registered nurse training program. The length and focus of an NP training program can vary dramatically depending on the focus of the particular program. Much of this variation in training programs is from the number of accrediting agencies involved in NP education. Many NP training programs will focus on a particular field of practice, such as geriatrics or pediatrics. A separate accrediting body determines the educational requirements for each of the areas of interest. Even within a particular area of interest there may be more than one recognized accrediting body for that field. Because of this variety it is hard to describe a typical NP training program. The various accrediting bodies are reviewed by a national agency to ensure that accrediting agencies comply with legislative requirements, but individual program educational content is not the focus of these reviews. Instructors within an NP training program are also typically nursing professionals and not physicians. NP programs award a Master of Science or a professional doctorate degree to their graduates. Each state has a defined certification process for NPs that varies greatly from state to state. Depending on these regulations NPs may function as independent practitioners or practice only under the direction of a physician supervisor. NPs have prescriptive authority in all states, but the level of supervision required varies. The local certification and review of NPs are functions of state boards of nursing and not local medical boards.

PAs were originally Army medics returning from the Vietnam War. These medics received an additional year of training to adapt what they had learned in the service and in the field to the needs of the civilian population. The training programs were then expanded to include other individuals with prior health care experience, such as nurses or paramedics. Over time, PA programs grew in length and offered a broader level of health care training. Although prior health care experience is encouraged for those applying to PA programs, most programs no longer require prior experience as a prerequisite for enrollment. Most programs are 2 years in length with 1 year spent in a classroom setting and 1 year involved in various inpatient and outpatient clinical experiences. Unlike NP training programs, all PA training programs must meet the educational requirements established by a single national accrediting body. The organization is composed of both PAs and representatives of various medical organizations. PA graduates are certified to practice after successfully completing an accredited training program and passing a national certification test. Graduates typically are awarded a Bachelor of Science or a professional Master of Science degree, but the certification process does not depend on the degree received. PAs never practice as independent practitioners, working solely in collaboration with a supervising physician. Each state sets the required level of physician supervision. Most states allow PAs prescriptive authority; however, as with NPs, the level of physician supervision varies. Supervising physicians are held liable for the scope of practice and the quality of care a PA renders. As such, medical oversight of PA practices is the responsibility of state medical boards. The type of patients seen by a PA depend on the supervising physician's expertise. PAs involved in primary care are typically supervised by family physicians, general internists, and emergency medicine physicians.

Primary Care Providers' Dilemma

The variety of medical problems seen by primary care physicians frequently leads to scheduling difficulties. Patients with ongoing medical illnesses may require extended appointments, limiting the time available to care for acutely ill patients. Setting aside time for the treatment of acutely ill patients is a delicate balance. If a large portion of the daily schedule is reserved for the treatment of patients with acute illnesses, then the amount of time available for the treatment of patients with chronic illnesses will be limited (Table 1-2). If an inadequate amount of time is set aside for acute care patients, then patients must be worked into the schedule. Work-in appointments can infringe on the time of scheduled patients and usually result in a significant increase in the waiting time for all patients seen that day.

The balance between urgent and chronic care needs may vary daily during times of endemic or epidemic community illnesses. Appropriate scheduling of patients is a constant struggle for most primary care provider networks.

Primary care physicians must also balance the need to see an adequate number of patients in a day to maintain financial viability while spending enough time with each patient to provide adequate evaluation and treatment. Primary care providers spend an average of 20 minutes per patient. This average is misleading, however; actual time spent with each patient varies greatly (Table 1-3). Complete physical examinations and office procedures may require 45 minutes to 1 hour. The additional time spent providing more involved services limits the time providers can spend with patients with more limited problems. Physicians will often have 10 minutes or less to evaluate and treat individuals with acute illnesses and injuries. In addition, most primary care physicians care for patients in hospital, nursing home, and emergency department settings, placing further demands on their time.

The treatment of musculoskeletal conditions, both traumatic and nontraumatic in origin, constitutes a major portion of the primary care physician's daily practice. Sprains and strains of the lower back are consistently in the top 20 diagnoses seen by primary care physicians (Table 1-4). Nontraumatic orthopedic problems as a group are the second most common presenting symptom for patients of all ages and represent 10% of the practice of large multiclinic family physician networks. As surprising at it may seem to some, orthopedic surgeons do not provide the majority of musculoskeletal care in the United States. Data compiled by the National Center for Health Statistics indicate that orthopedic surgeons see only 6% of the total number of patients with musculoskeletal disorders.[12] Most patients with these disorders are seen by a variety of other health care providers (Table 1-5).

Role of Physical Therapy in Primary Care (Physicians' Perspective)

PTs can play an important role in a variety of ways working in a primary care setting to help meet the numerous needs of patients with neuromusculoskeletal symptoms. Patients with

---

TABLE 1-2

Reason for Patient Visit to Physician

Reason for Visit	All Physicians	General and Family Practice	Pediatrics	Internal Medicine*	Obstetrics and Gynecology
Total visits	100.0	100.0	100.0	100.0	100.0
Acute problem	35.3	49.5	53.8	39.5	17.8
Chronic problem, routine	29.6	23.0	7.6	34.4	10.0
Chronic problem, flare-up	7.7	7.6	2.9	8.3	4.3
Before or after surgery or injury follow-up	9.3	3.0	1.7	3.3	7.1
Nonillness care	15.9	15.0	31.4	10.8	59.8
Unknown or not reported	2.2	1.9	2.6	3.7	1.0

Sources: U.S. Department of Health and Human Services, Public Health Service, Centers for Disease Control and Prevention, National Center for Health Statistics, 1999 data. Accessed at www.aafp.org/facts.
*Includes only general internal medicine.

TABLE 1-3

Length of Patient Visit

Length of Visit	All Physicians	General and Family Practice	Pediatrics	Internal Medicine*	Obstetrics and Gynecology
Total visits	100.0	100.0	100.0	100.0	100.0
0 min†	4.3	5.6	3.4	4.9	3.7
1-5 min	3.5	2.8	6.6	0.8	3.5
6-10 min	20.9	27.0	29.8	11.3	23.0
11-15 min	32.0	30.3	35.1	39.5	34.4
16-30 min	31.3	30.3	23.0	35.1	29.9
31-60 min	7.5	3.6	1.5	8.0	5.6
≥61 min	0.5	0.4	0.6	0.4	0.0

Sources: U.S. Department of Health and Human Services, Centers for Disease Control and Prevention, National Center for Health Statistics, 1999. Accessed at www.aafp.org/facts.
*Includes only general internal medicine.
†There was no face-to-face patient-provider interaction.

acute soft tissue injuries often are "work-in" or "add-on" patients in a physician's schedule. Scheduled visits for musculoskeletal conditions are usually limited in time and scope. Because of these time constraints, a physician may not be able to take a detailed history or perform a detailed examination. In addition, academic instruction and training in the evaluation of musculoskeletal problems are very limited for most primary care physicians. Despite the frequency of musculoskeletal disorders, family practice training programs typical have only 1 to 2 months of required orthopedic instruction, and most pediatric and internal medicine programs have no required orthopedic training. Because of this limited training in the evaluation of musculoskeletal injuries, many physicians will rely on the PT to perform a more detailed examination of a patient's injury and symptoms and participate in the diagnostic process. Most physicians welcome the additional insight the PT can provide regarding potential causes of a patient's condition and will also rely on the therapist to report any additional health issues of concern.

Most primary care physicians have no formal exposure to the practice of physical therapy during their training programs and have very little, if any, exposure to advancements that occur in the field. Despite a lack of formal training or continuing medical education in rehabilitation methods, primary care physicians are often expected to oversee the physical therapy services provided to their patients. The physicians often must function under significant restrictions regarding those services placed under responsibility by insurance carriers.

TABLE 1-4

Number of Office Visits in the United States in 1999 (in Thousands)

Principal Diagnosis by Physician (All Ages)	All Specialties	General and Family Practice	Pediatrics	Internal Medicine*
Total visits	756,734	170,571	74,045	135,607
Essential hypertension	31,962	12,598	116	14,075
Acute upper respiratory infections of multiple or unspecified sites	17,691	8105	6794	1999
General medical examination	13,405	5495	302	2460
Diabetes mellitus	19,585	5061	98	8537
Chronic sinusitis	10,797	4924	1498	2538
Health supervision of infant or child	22,626	3807	18,000	679
Bronchitis, not specified as acute or chronic	8083	3179	1295	2861
General symptoms	9008	3178	614	2421
Disorders of lipid metabolism	7788	2851	21	4015
Special investigations or examinations	14,609	2777	139	1215
Acute pharyngitis	7835	2740	2303	1776
Contact dermatitis and other eczema	7590	2651	881	896
Suppurative unspecified otitis media	11,843	2600	7427	1068
Sprains and strains of other and unspecified parts of back	5624	2456	0	260
Other and unspecified disorders of back	8627	2419	127	2349
Other disorders of urethra and urinary tract	7111	2350	409	1615
Influenza	4027	2322	237	840
Allergic rhinitis	16,662	1866	833	2923
Depressive disorder, not elsewhere classified	6461	1844	136	1552
Normal pregnancy	16,402	1838	57	0

Sources: U.S. Department of Health and Human Services, Public Health Service, Centers for Disease Control and Prevention, National Center for Health Statistics, 1999 data. Accessed at www.aafp.org/facts.
*Includes only general internal medicine.

TABLE 1-5

Delivery of Services to Patients with Musculoskeletal Conditions in the United States

Provider Type	Total Services Delivered
Physical therapists	27%
Family physicians	23%
Chiropractors	23%
Osteopathic physicians	15%
Orthopedic surgeons	6%
Other	6%

Sources: U.S. Department of Health and Human Services, Public Health Service, Centers for Disease Control and Prevention, National Center for Health Statistics, 1999 data. Accessed at www.aafp.org/facts.

Few physicians will provide detailed rehabilitation plans but will instead simply send a patient for "shoulder rehabilitation" or "treatment of ankle sprain." A referral may simply consist of the phrase "evaluate and treat." The PT should not become frustrated with the lack of clarity of the request but instead consider the referral as an opportunity to suggest the most cost-effective approach to the patient's problem. To better prepare the physician to respond to questions and concerns the patient or third-party payer might voice, therapists should provide the physician with a detailed treatment plan and prognosis and keep the physician apprised of progress and problems in a timely fashion.

Cost Containment

As outlined earlier in the chapter, physical therapy services are frequently the focus of intense cost-control measures for many insurance providers. Physicians are often caught in the middle of providing needed services while also exercising fiscal restraints. Rehabilitation plans that entail extensive use of hospital or office visits or require the use of expensive therapeutic modalities will quickly exhaust the medical benefits of many patients. Rehabilitation plans that emphasize patient empowerment and self-management, including home exercise programs, and entail the judicious use of expensive treatment modalities are much less likely to place the primary care provider in a difficult position with either the patient or the patient's insurance carrier.

The following sections include descriptions of three physical therapy primary care practice models. These models do not represent the entire current scope of such models, but do include one of the original models and encompass three very different practice and health care environments: the military, a large HMO structure (Kaiser Permanente), and a large hospital system (Veterans Affairs). The historic perspective (including the original impetus for the inclusion of physical therapy), the encountered barriers, and resultant benefits will provide PTs with a better understanding of roles therapy can play in the primary care arena. Ideally, the outcome will be the involvement of physical therapy in the creation of new primary care initiatives, with the PT taking a lead role.

Primary Care Physical Therapy

U.S. Army Model

The mission of U.S. Army PTs is to provide physical therapy evaluation and treatment to correct or prevent physical impairments resulting from injury, disease, or preexisting problems. Army PTs also serve as independent practitioners in a nonphysician health care provider or physician extender role when performing primary care or evaluation and treatment for patients with neuromusculoskeletal (neuromuscular) conditions.[6,7] In addition, Army PTs serve as technical advisors to commanders of troop units, providing guidance in the areas of physical fitness and wellness, physical training, and injury prevention. In the event of a mass casualty situation, Army physical therapy personnel assist in managing patients categorized as "delayed" or "minor" and augment the orthopedic section of the military hospital or clinic.[6-8,22]

HISTORY. Before the Vietnam conflict, Army PTs had a variety of wartime experiences but worked primarily in a prescriptive environment. In support of the military mission in South Vietnam between 1962 and 1973, the Surgeon General of the Army deployed 24 hospitals, which were established as fixed medical installations with area support missions. These installations included surgical, evacuation, and field hospitals as well as a 3000-bed convalescent center.[6,7,18] The primary factor behind the assignment of Army PTs to Vietnam was the direct request for physical therapy services by hospital commanders. The primary goal of physical therapy services in Vietnam was the rehabilitation of patients who were capable of being returned to duty. For patients requiring evacuation out of the war zone, treatment focused on basic rehabilitation procedures that would be continued at each evacuation stage.[6,7]

During the war, orthopedic surgeons assigned to Army hospitals in Vietnam found that most of their time was consumed with evaluating and treating patients requiring surgical intervention. This resulted in a large number of patients with nonsurgical musculoskeletal problems who had to wait until physicians became available to evaluate and treat them. Because of this delay in the evaluation, treatment, and subsequent redeployment for patients with neuromuscular conditions, Army PTs assigned to the combat zone acquired a new and expanded role: nonphysician health care providers.[6-8] The newly designated function for Army PTs was the timely evaluation and treatment of patients with nonsurgical neuromuscular conditions—under physician supervision but without physician referral.[6-8,18] The resultant protocol and program outcomes included decreased hospitalization rates, decreased patient waiting and treatment times, and facilitation of soldiers' rapid return to duty.[6-8]

The need for Army PTs to assume the role of a primary nonphysician health care provider for patients with neuromuscular disorders was a direct result of the evolving practice of physical therapy in a wartime environment and then continued because of the shortage of Army physicians, especially orthopedic surgeons, after the Vietnam War. After the draft ended in 1972, the Army Medical Department was faced with vast numbers of patients with neuromuscular conditions and a shortage of orthopedic surgeons to manage these patients.

This shortage, combined with the increasing emphasis on physical fitness in the military and the injuries associated with the rigors of military training, resulted in long delays in the administration of health care to patients with neuromuscular conditions.[6,7] The result was a continuation of the PTs' wartime role as a physician extender.

Since the mid-1980s, United States Army PTs and enlisted specialists have been deployed with Army Medical Department units in humanitarian missions in countries such as El Salvador, Russia, Turkey, Romania, and Croatia. In addition to the general practice of physical therapy, this type of assignment enables the therapists to serve as consultants and educators for the local community.[6,7] Wartime deployments for Army physical therapy personnel have included missions to Bosnia, the Persian Gulf region, and Afghanistan.[7]

In August 1990, the United Nations (UN) quickly responded to the Iraqi invasion of Kuwait by mobilizing UN forces. As a part of this mobilization of American forces, 6 Army PTs and 12 physical therapy enlisted specialists were deployed to Saudi Arabia, Kuwait, Iraq, and the communications zone in Europe during the Persian Gulf War. U.S. Navy and Air Force PTs were also deployed to the war zone during the Persian Gulf War.[6,7] In addition, Army PTs were used in military hospitals in the United States in support of this operation. The role of Army PTs in the Persian Gulf War was similar to that assumed during the Vietnam War. PTs served as independent practitioners and nonphysician health care providers performing primary evaluation and treatment of patients with neuromuscular complaints. U.S. Army PTs also treated prisoners of war and supplemented the staff in host nation hospitals, which required a shift from standard practice models to community health models with cultural integration. As a result of these experiences in the Persian Gulf War, a significant "lesson learned" by the Army Medical Department regarding Army physical therapy services was that an insufficient number of physical therapy personnel were deployed to the war zone. A complete description of the Army physical therapy personnel and their use during the Persian Gulf War can be found in the *Textbook of Military Medicine: Rehabilitation of the Injured Combatant*, volume 1.[7]

ARMY PHYSICAL THERAPY TRIAGE MODEL. The traditional Army triage system for patients with neuromuscular conditions included initial evaluation and diagnosis by a primary care physician, PA, or NP, followed by referral to an orthopedic surgeon, followed by a referral for physical therapy services. The modified system of triage for patients with neuromuscular problems was entry-point triage followed by evaluation, diagnosis, and treatment by a PT with appropriate referral to orthopedic surgery or other medical specialties as required. Entry-point personnel are often enlisted corpsmen comparable in skill levels to nurses' aides and licensed practical nurses. These personnel record vital signs, record the area of complaint(s), and triage patients with neuromuscular problems to physical therapy. In the military system patients could also receive physical therapy services though the traditional route of referral from physicians, PAs, podiatrists, dentists, and nurse clinicians. A major concern for practitioners working in both patient-directed access and referral environments is that

patients with serious pathologic conditions that mimic neuromuscular symptoms might be overlooked. As in the public sector, the physical therapy responsibilities regarding initiating a consult/referral for patients with health concerns are the same in both practice environments within the military system.[6,7]

Experienced PTs, both civilian and military, can easily recall patients with occult disease or misdiagnosed conditions being sent to them. A strength of the Army physical therapy program is the efficiency with which patients with nonmusculoskeletal conditions are identified and subsequently referred to the appropriate medical specialty. The training system in place that provides this safety net includes three components: a series of progressive educational experiences, expanded clinical privileges, and the use of a physician supervisor.

TRIAGE MODEL: THERAPIST EDUCATION AND CREDENTIALING. Implementation of the primary care role for Army PTs required formalized training and privileging protocols. Army regulations 40-48 and 40-68 document the Army PT nonphysician health care provider role.[23,24] Army PTs who serve as nonphysician primary health care providers must be credentialed at the Army Medical Department Activity where they practice. This credentialing process includes a review by the commander of all educational and professional experiences both as a physical therapy and neuromuscular evaluator. These credentials are periodically updated and reviewed, and when PTs are assigned to a new Army health care facility the practitioner's credentials are reviewed by the new command.[6,23,24] At each Army Medical Department Activity where PTs serve as nonphysician health care providers, continuous quality improvement programs are implemented as a part of the total improvement process.[23,24]

The U.S. Army physical therapy educational program prepares clinicians for their role as physician extenders. The U.S. Army-Baylor University Graduate Program in Physical Therapy, located at Fort Sam Houston, Texas, is a professional (entry level) masters degree program accredited by the Commission on Accreditation for Physical Therapy Education (CAPTE). The Army Physical Therapy Program is currently in the process of transitioning their curriculum to a professional Doctorate of Physical Therapy (DPT) degree. The Army-Baylor Physical Therapy Program has a quad-service mission to prepare PTs for active duty service in the Army, Navy, Air Force, and Public Health Service. The faculty is composed of representatives from the three military services; however, the Army remains the lead agent.[6]

The Army-Baylor program meets the accreditation requirements of CAPTE for an entry-level, generalist PT, but the evaluation and treatment of patients with neuromuscular problems are emphasized. Students learn that their first task is to swiftly identify patients who fall outside the scope of physical therapy practice. Army PTs are neither qualified nor expected to diagnose nonmusculoskeletal pathologic conditions, but they are expected to refer patients to someone who can make the appropriate diagnosis.[1] PT students in the Army-Baylor program understand the history and physical examination "red flags" that suggest pathologic origins of symptoms. The principle of being able to alter (provoke or alleviate) symptoms to help identify mechanical versus nonmechanical origins of symptoms is emphasized in the physical examination (see Chapters 10 and 11). In addition, these students learn the principles associated with ordering diagnostic imaging tests and prescribing nonsteroidal anti-inflammatory medications. Postprofessionally, the Army-Baylor Physical Therapy Program graduates and other Army PTs, gained either through the Reserve Officer Training Program (ROTC) or by direct accession, receive training that follows specific credentialing protocols. These therapists are then credentialed, leading to their role of nonphysician health care providers in the evaluation and treatment of patients with neuromuscular dysfunction.[6,7,23,24]

A 2-week, postprofessional neuromuscular evaluation course, offered annually at the Army Medical Department Center and School, Fort Sam Houston, Texas, has been designed to enhance the training of all military PTs who will serve as physician extenders. The neuromuscular evaluation course is a required course for all Army PTs who will serve in this role. The goal is to have these officers attend the course during the first 3 years of their initial assignments in the military. The 2-week neuromuscular evaluation course consists of lecture, laboratory, and seminar experiences with an emphasis on primary care physical therapy, including decision-making regarding ordering diagnostic imaging tests and prescribing nonsteroidal antiinflammatory medications. The course instructors include PTs, physicians, pharmacists, and other health care providers, with the focus being current trends in primary care relevant to physical therapy practice in this setting. On completion of the training the students do not immediately take written or practical examinations, but are subsequently evaluated by the physical therapy neuromuscular clinical preceptor, the physical therapy clinic chief, and the neuromuscular evaluation physician supervisor. Additional continuing health care education courses and in-services on these topics are also offered at each local Army medical treatment facility.

PRIMARY CARE PHYSICAL THERAPIST: PRIVILEGES. Expanded privileges beyond the traditional scope of physical therapy practice are mandatory if PTs are to serve in a primary care setting safely and effectively. In addition to the standard privileges included in the scope of physical therapy practice, Army PTs refer patients to radiology for diagnostic imaging evaluations (radiographs, magnetic resonance, computed tomography, and bone scans), can restrict patients to quarters for up to 72 hours, restrict work and training for up to 30 days, and refer patients to all medical specialty clinics. In some medical treatment facilities, PTs may be credentialed to prescribe specified analgesic and nonsteroidal antiinflammatory medication.[2,6,23]

With the aforementioned privileges comes a formal support system. Army regulation 40-48 requires that a physician supervisor be assigned to PTs serving in nonphysician health care provider roles.[23] This requirement is similar to one used for PAs and NPs serving in expanded roles. The physician supervisor is appointed by the medical facility commander and must be available for consultation in person or by telephone and, if absent, must have an alternate. From the medical commander's point of view, the physician supervisor ensures that the PT's practice remains within the privileges granted and provides

periodic written evaluation addressing diagnostic techniques, therapeutic practice, and patient care documentation. Orthopedic surgeons and family practice physicians are excellent choices to serve as physician supervisors for the PT.[1]

PRIMARY CARE PHYSICAL THERAPY MODEL: OUTCOMES. The use of PTs as nonphysician health care providers in the Army has been an overwhelming success. There is no record of any legal action being brought against Army PTs or the U.S. government as a result of care provided by PTs serving in the physician extender role. This is remarkable testimony, considering the literally millions of neuromuscular evaluations performed by Army PTs.[2,6,7] The advantages of having PTs perform in their role as nonphysician health care providers include (1) prompt evaluation and treatment for patients with neuromuscular conditions, (2) promotion of quality health care, (3) decrease in sick call visits, (4) more appropriate use of physician services, and (5) more appropriate use of PT education, training, and experience.[2,6,7]

The peacetime use of Army PTs as primary neuromuscular screeners was first studied by James and Stuart in 1973.[10] Two Army hospitals and 2117 patients with low back pain participated in the study. Data collected in a baseline phase under the traditional prescriptive patient access system were compared with data collected during the direct access phase. The investigation concluded that patients received more expeditious care in the direct access sample; use of radiographic examinations was reduced by 50%; PTs' job satisfaction increased; patient acceptance was high; 14 of 14 orthopedic surgeons believed that the program should be permanently adapted, with the exception of certain patient categories (e.g., pediatric patients younger than 12 years); and the appropriate use of orthopedic physicians' skills and expertise was enhanced.[10]

James and Abshier[11] assessed the neuromuscular evaluation program at Darnall Army Hospital, Fort Hood, Texas, in 1981. The study confirmed the program's efficiency, effectiveness, and acceptability. PTs preferred the expanded role, and all preferred to intersperse the screening/primary care role with their general practice. The time required for direct access evaluations was noted to be twice that for the prescriptive visits; the direct access initial visit generally took 30 to 45 minutes, with intervention usually following the evaluation process. Less than 4% of active duty patients screened by PTs in this study required orthopedic consultation.[11]

Kaiser Permanente Model

Another physical therapy model found in a primary care environment is currently being practiced within the largest nonmilitary setting in the United States—at Kaiser Permanente (KP). This practice model includes patient management responsibilities found in traditional physical therapy outpatient departments and involves a multitude of additional responsibilities. In spite of the inherent challenges, the primary care setting that includes PTs affords significant service improvement for patients, professional growth opportunities for the PTs, growth for the physical therapy profession in line with the American Physical Therapy Association's Vision 2020, and a potential cost savings for health care organizations. The following is a description of the primary care model developed at KP in Northern California, with key elements to consider when contemplating the inclusion of physical therapy services in other primary care settings.

KP, the nation's largest not-for-profit HMO, was founded in 1945 and currently operates in five states serving 8.9 million members (6.3 million members are in California). The prepayment system used in today's HMO was born from the concept adopted by Dr. Sydney Garfield and Henry J. Kaiser, who formulated the health plan for workers and families at Kaiser-managed shipyards and steel mills in 1942. KP became a federally qualified HMO in 1977. The Northern California region of KP is where physical therapy services have been integrated into primary care. This region covers California from the Sacramento Valley southward through the San Francisco Bay Area and into Fresno and currently includes more than 3.2 million members.[1]

The medical practice model developed at KP allows PTs to be in close proximity to other medical providers through shared clinic space and an integrated referral and medical record system. Internal medicine departments, where primary care clinics are located, are generally in close proximity to emergency departments, radiology, pharmacy, neurology, and other specialty clinics such as orthopedics. In addition to the physical layout, the long-term philosophy of the organization provides support to its practitioners for making patient management decisions on the basis of medical necessity. Clinicians are responsible for medical management of their patients. The organization provides a mission, such as goals of improved quality, accessibility, affordability, and patient satisfaction, but the health plan does not issue mandates regarding clinical care (e.g., number of visits, length of stay, limits on tests). The clinicians practice autonomously within the context of the organization's mission based on the medical needs of each patient.

The organizational structure and philosophy of KP facilitated the ease with which PTs were included on the primary care team. Clinicians working together under one umbrella are more likely to have a clear idea of what each other's strengths, needs, and capabilities are, which enhances communication and ultimately effective and efficient patient care.

EVOLUTION OF THE PRIMARY CARE MODEL. In an increasingly competitive market for health care organizations, KP undertook a redesign using an interrdisciplinary team approach with several objectives in mind, including:

- Increase quality of health care
- Increase patient satisfaction and accessibility to services
- Provide a more sustainable practice for physicians

Part of the impetus behind the adult primary care clinic (APC) redesign (Figure 1-1) at KP derived from a concern regarding the numerous practice demands on physicians in primary care. A consensus within the medical group that PTs possess the expertise to manage patients with musculoskeletal conditions and impairments led to a decision to include PTs on the APC team.[1] After piloting physical therapy services in several primary care clinics for more than 2 years, in 1997 PTs were placed in roughly half of the approximately 100 APCs located throughout the Northern California region. See Table-1-6 for a summary of the APC teams with integrated PTs.

At these clinics, instead of having the patient initially see a physician and then return on a later date to see another professional such as a health educator or PT, KP developed referral processes and algorithms that enabled the patient to be triaged when the patient called in for care. In addition to the usual primary care members, such as physicians, NPs, medical assistants, and nurses, the KP model incorporates services from behavioral medicine specialists, clinical health educators, PTs, and, in some cases, pharmacists.

Behavioral medicine is provided by psychologists and social workers (both licensed professionals). Psychologists have a

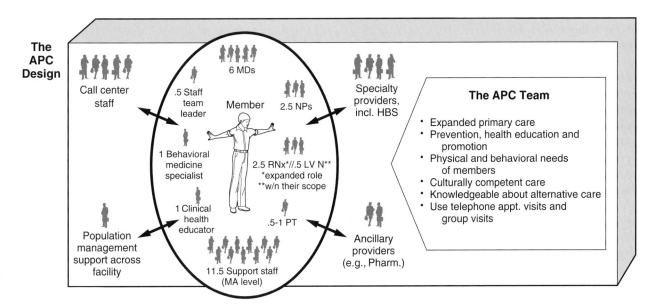

FIGURE 1-1 Various members of the adult primary care (APC) team.

Summary of APC Teams Including Physical Therapists

Data Collected in the First Quarter of	No. of Teams with PTs	Total No. of APC Teams
1999	51	99
2000	65	99
2001	61	101
2002	56	101

APC, Adult primary care.

doctorate in health psychology[7] or clinical psychology, and social workers possess Masters degrees in clinical social work. Their purpose on the APC team is to improve clinical outcomes by providing behavioral medicine interventions to patients with mental disorders or behavioral problems that affect their health status or are a consequence of their medical condition.

The professional training of the *clinical health educator* in the KP system varies, but all have expertise in the areas of educating patients, negotiating health behavioral changes, enhancing compliance with treatment plans, and building confidence in self-care skills. To carry out their varied roles the interventions often include both individual sessions as well as group encounters with patients. They also serve as a resource for the APC team regarding existing educational opportunities such as classes, patient education materials, and community resources.[1]

The inclusion of physical therapy services was partly because between 20% and 25% of visits to primary care clinics are for musculoskeletal conditions. The organization recognized the diagnostic and treatment expertise of PTs in managing patients with musculoskeletal conditions and impairments and the potential cost savings of freeing physician and NP time to focus on the management of patients with nonmusculoskeletal conditions. Data from the first quarter of 1999 to the first quarter of 2002 revealed that musculoskeletal diagnoses account for 20% to 25% of all KP primary care visits. APC PTs account for 3500 to 4200 visits per year, approximately 10% of all primary care visits.[9]

PATHWAYS AND WORK FLOWS. Generally, members can access physical therapy services in APCs through one of four pathways:
1. Health plan members see the PT after seeing their physician. This member may have had a visit with his or her physician specifically for the musculoskeletal disorder, or the patient may be referred to the PT after the physician addressed only the nonmusculoskeletal concerns. In the latter case, the physician relies on the PT to evaluate the musculoskeletal condition and screen for red flags (problem areas that require further medical examination or screening).
2. The physician and PT may jointly consult on a patient during the clinic visit. The physician will frequently call on the expertise of the PT while conducting his or her routine medical examination. The PT's role during these joint consults can include determining the cause of a musculoskeletal problem, providing input on work modifications, instructing the patient in one or two exercises, and discussing additional examinations or referrals to other departments.

3. The member might access primary care physical therapy services by calling or arriving at the medical station without an appointment. In this case, the physician triages the patient's case by reviewing the patient's actual or electronic chart. In cases in which it appears the condition is likely of musculoskeletal origin, of recent onset, and not work related, the physician will have the nurse or medical assistant recommend an appointment with the primary care PT.
4. A member may also contact a "medical advice" call center staffed with specially trained medical assistants and nurses. The call staff uses a protocol list of questions developed by a therapist and physician joint panel. The purpose of these questions is to determine whether it is appropriate for the member to see a primary care PT directly or if he or she should be seen by another provider. To date, through the facilities with APC physical therapy, the median percentage of patients seen as direct appointments to the PT in the APC is approximately 30%.

The region-wide guidelines for eligible populations that can be seen directly by a PT include:
- Age 18 to 65 years
- Nonindustrial injury
- Non–third-party liability of any type
- Afebrile
- No chest pain
- No abdominal pain
- Not seeking medication intervention
- Willing to see a PT instead of a physician or NP

Each facility and each primary care team have the ability to customize any of the pathways to best address their patient population.

Regardless of the avenue by which the patient is scheduled to see the APC PT, there are several components to the primary care PT visit:
- A screen for signs and symptoms that may require referral to or consult with a physician
- Efficient history and physical examination of the patient's primary problem area
- Consultation and discussion with the physician on the scope of the patient's problem areas to obtain a medical diagnosis and physician signature
- Hands-on treatment if indicated
- Detailed instruction in home exercise and self-management strategies
- Discussion with the physician on specialty referrals, work readiness, and other patient health issues

Of the many experiences that are a priority in the primary care setting, six are discussed.

Medical Screening. Medical screening for red flag conditions is important for all patients seen in primary care, especially for "direct book" patients. Many primary care PTs use a medical screening form to assist in screening for warning signs. These questionnaires prompt the patient to reveal the presence of potential constitutional symptoms, upper motor neuron lesions, history of cancer, and other medical diagnoses and to identify current medications and whether they have a history of anticoagulant or steroid use or smoking. See Chapter 5 for examples of such forms.

Physical Proximity of Health Care Providers. PTs have always been included as part of the interdisciplinary medical team, although in the typical outpatient setting PTs, physicians, and NPs have rarely worked in the same space, sharing the same rooms. A closer degree of proximity affords several benefits:

- Provides an avenue for the medical oversight of PTs obtaining medical diagnoses and signatures, as required by the state practice act. This avenue provides a smoother path for patients seen by direct access as well as those referred for same-day appointments
- Enables a more thorough knowledge of each other's scope of practice, challenges, limitations, and capabilities
- Offers opportunities for physicians to learn from PTs, such as building skills in (1) examining musculoskeletal dysfunction, (2) broadening knowledge of conservative management of musculoskeletal disease, and (3) learning what is appropriate and inappropriate use of rehabilitation services for these patients
- Offers opportunities for the PTs to learn from the physicians on a case-specific basis, such as interpreting laboratory data, learning what warrants concern in palpating an abdomen, observing unfamiliar deformity, or interpreting a confusing history
- Helps the various clinicians to know each other better personally, which inevitably results in enhanced communication

Patient Types, Acuity, and Prognosis. As mentioned, increasing patient accessibility to services was one of the goals of the KP primary care redesign. In general, protocols or algorithms facilitate referrals that direct patients with chronic and stable orthopedic or neurologic problems or those requiring postoperative management into the non-APC physical therapy departments. Within KP, physical therapy services provided in the primary care clinic are, for the most part, *additional services* provided to patients. It is not a matter of shifting patients that were previously seen in the physical therapy department into the primary care clinic. Many of the patients seen by the primary care PT are those who in the past were seen only by the physician without subsequent referral to physical therapy, unless the problem did not respond to the first line of intervention. These patients generally have more acute peripheral or spinal conditions and are often younger than patients typically seen in the physical therapy department. This difference in the acuity of the patient population may be a relevant factor when interpreting literature that compares costs of patients seen by direct access versus physician referral because of differences in prognosis for the two populations.[9,17] Earlier physical therapy intervention could also suggest a better prognosis because the patient is involved sooner. Many therapists working in APC are trained in the use of manual therapy, and there is evidence in the literature supporting the use of this intervention in patients with low back pain in this more acute population.[3,14,16,19,21] The hope is that earlier intervention could minimize the development of chronic conditions that may require protracted services.

Patient Concerns and Goals. Another important difference between the APC and non-APC physical therapy settings is the type of goals or concerns that the patient might express to the PT. When a patient with a musculoskeletal condition is first seen by a physician, concerns such as "Will this lead to an amputation?" or "Is this related to diabetes?" may be expressed. In a more traditional outpatient physical therapy setting, the physician may have already addressed these issues before the patient is referred to the therapist. The aforementioned concerns are more commonly expressed by patients in APC, yet for various personal or cultural reasons may not be not clearly articulated or heard. Patient concerns of this magnitude are often only uncovered when the clinician observes subtle clues from the patient's voice or body language. Communication skills are very important for effective, patient-oriented practice in the primary care setting (see Chapter 4). The timeliness in which the PT hears and addresses the patient's reasons for seeking medical care can directly affect the course of treatment.

Intervention. The difference in acuity and prognosis for this patient population also dictates a difference in treatment intervention. The course of APC physical therapy treatment is generally shorter than in a typical outpatient physical therapy department and largely addresses primary sources of symptoms as opposed to focusing on various contributing factors (e.g., addressing an inflammatory component as opposed to addressing muscle lengths or weaknesses that may have brought about the symptomatic condition). The scope of PT interventions can be similar to that provided within the regular outpatient physical therapy department (e.g., joint mobilization, exercise, education), but the patient population in primary care clinics is typically less willing or able to return for as much follow-up care as that seen in the physical therapy department. With this in mind, the initial goals of physical therapy are to select the intervention(s) that most quickly reduce the symptoms and degree of disability to a level that the patient can self-manage and to select interventions that will minimize recurrence. Therefore the interventions are heavy on guidance in self-treatment, including patient education and self-administered modalities such as ice/heat, body mechanics, and exercise instruction. For much of the primary care population, their initial mindset or expectations for care are quite different from patients typically seen in outpatient physical therapy departments. Once the primary condition is reduced to a satisfactory level, their willingness and ability to invest more time for additional physical therapy are often limited. Most patients receive one or two therapy visits in the primary care clinic. Skilled orthopedic manual PTs with good teaching skills are ideally matched for this setting because there is typically limited equipment available.

Scheduling. Besides the overall course of physical therapy being shorter, other time frames are different compared with the standard physical therapy department. The therapist has to be able to function more like other members of the primary care team. In any given day, the PT performs more new evaluations, the majority of which are for same-day bookings, has shorter appointment times, sees additional new "work-in" patients, and must be prepared to consult on the spot when another team member seeks assistance. The ability of the therapist to respond to the needs of patients and primary care team members promotes respect for the therapist's skills and knowledge and helps determine the amount of decision-making autonomy.

Therapist Preparation for the Primary Care Clinic. Is it possible for a therapist to flourish in a setting that has such a fast pace, imposes greater practice responsibilities, and demands high-level diagnostic and management skills? This is not a setting in which to thrive without appropriate training and experience. The first prerequisite to working in an APC is a strong foundation in orthopedic physical therapy. The therapist must be able to recognize and differentiate a broad range of clinical patterns quickly, establish a prognosis, and determine whether a patient is an appropriate candidate for physical therapy or should be referred to the primary care physician or other medical specialties. The efficiency of the PT in making these decisions governs the appropriate use of other resources throughout the health care organization.

KP developed competencies (e.g., continuing education tests, manager performance evaluations) for the primary care therapists and established a guideline that those functioning in this role should have a minimum of 4 to 6 years of outpatient orthopedic experience, demonstrate broad-based continuing education experience in orthopedic physical therapy, and demonstrate excellent team communication skills. To prepare therapists for this role, KP has provided various forms of continuing education in selected areas. Each of the following courses, whether given as self-study or in the form of a weekend course, is competency based as determined by written examination:

- Differential diagnosis of musculoskeletal versus nonmusculoskeletal conditions
- Acute musculoskeletal injuries of peripheral joints
- Radiologic review of plain films and magnetic resonance images
- Laboratory values relevant to primary care practices
- Pharmacology

The organization has also produced clinical library modules for specific areas (e.g., shoulder, knee, elbow, and ankle/foot) that focus on educating the therapist in how to examine and efficiently manage the common problems applicable to the primary care setting. The last element, and perhaps the most valuable, is a mentoring program in which seasoned APC therapists travel to various sites to facilitate the advancement of the necessary skills.

KP of Northern California made a region-wide commitment to change a delivery system, as did the military, when they chose to move PTs into primary care. The move toward primary care requires leadership from PTs to envision, advocate, and choreograph their services within the medical group. The road toward change met many challenges and barriers along the way, but the autonomy of practice and expansion of skills and knowledge of PTs continue to move in a positive direction.

Department of Veterans Affairs Model

A pilot program is underway within the U.S. Department of Veterans Affairs (VA) that emphasizes the role of PTs as integral members of the primary care team. The development of this program, the professional opportunities and implications for physical therapy practice, and the evolution into a training program for PT interns are discussed.

DESCRIPTION OF THE VA SYSTEM. The VA health care system is the largest in the United States, with 163 hospitals in the 48 contiguous states, Puerto Rico, and the District of Columbia. The VA also operates 850 ambulatory care clinics and 137 nursing homes. This system exists primarily to deliver health care to America's 25 million living veterans; it also has a significant role in health care education, research, and support of the Department of Defense during times of war. The medical profile of the veteran patient is complex but consistent with the typical Medicare patient that therapists outside the VA may see. The veteran patient frequently has multiple medical problems such as heart disease, hypertension, diabetes, and arthritis that make providing comprehensive health care a complex undertaking. The patient population's relatively advanced age—35% are 65 years or older, compared with 17% of the general population—increases the likelihood for multiple medical problems. In addition to their medical needs, there are often social circumstances that further complicate their care. The VA has chosen to address this issue of complexity through a primary care management model that emphasizes the use of an interdisciplinary, interdependent health care team. This team is usually composed of a physician, NP, pharmacist, dietitian, and social worker. Traditionally, PTs have been looked on as specialty care providers who are used for the rehabilitation of injuries rather than as members of the primary care team.

VA MODEL PROGRAM DEVELOPMENT. In February 2000, a group of PTs at the VA Salt Lake City Healthcare System began discussion on how to integrate physical therapy practice with primary care. A few members of this group had a relatively thorough understanding of the U.S. Army model described earlier and used this model as a starting point. However, as they looked at the applicability of this model to the VA population, it became apparent that the role of a PT on an interdisciplinary primary care team was broader than just neuromuscular care and really encompassed the entire domain of mobility. When delivering primary care in a team setting, each provider has responsibility for a specific domain, with the physician having responsibility for the overall coordination of care (Figure 1-2).

As this model is typically implemented, the domain of activity, mobility, and exercise is often neglected or addressed simply by admonishing the patient to "walk more" or "be more active." In a complex patient population, this is neither reasonable nor appropriate and led to the idea that PTs had a significant role to play on this team. In the VA model, exercise prescription is analogous to medication prescription, in that "one size does not fit all." The PT who serves on, or consults with, the primary care team principally addresses the bodily systems that affect the patient's mobility, including the integumentary, musculoskeletal, neurologic, and cardiovascular/pulmonary systems as outlined in the American Physical Therapy Association's *Guide to Physical*

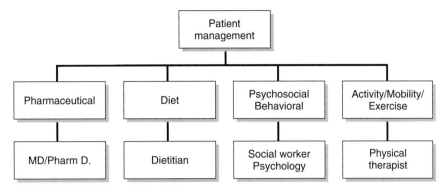

FIGURE 1-2 Primary care management of chronic conditions and the providers of choice for each area. The physician is responsible for coordination of care delivery through a multidisciplinary, interdependent health care team.

Therapist Practice. Functioning well in this capacity with a complex patient population imposes significant burdens of responsibility and competency on a PT wishing to serve on this team.

COMPETENCIES REQUIRED FOR PRIMARY CARE PHYSICAL THERAPISTS. Before implementing the program, the physical therapy department looked at what knowledge, skills, and abilities were necessary to safely and effectively function as the main provider in the domain of mobility for a complex patient population. These competencies included some relatively obvious areas such as differential diagnosis and orthopedic screening and evaluation but also include a thorough understanding of primary and secondary disease prevention and what systems affect mobility. This understanding is necessary to ensure consistent communication with the patient from all members of the primary care team, to assist in identifying and managing emerging health problems, and to appropriately risk-stratify patients for intervention. If a patient's ability to ambulate is affected by cardiovascular disease or diabetes, the primary care PT must understand how to safely provide the necessary interventions for these patients. Necessary skills in the affective domain were also identified, including confidence, excellent communication abilities, a desire for personal and professional growth, and solid teaching abilities. The degree of competency that a primary care PT, considering the complex VA (or Medicare) patient population, would need led to the belief that few, if any, new graduates from professional physical therapy education programs would be adequately equipped to function in this capacity. This conclusion and the potential future expansion of this program to other VA sites, and eventually outside the VA system to the private sector, led to the development of a primary care physical therapy internship program.

INTERNSHIP PROGRAM. The primary care internship program was specifically designed to prepare new graduates to function as principal providers for mobility issues on a multidisciplinary primary care team and to address the related areas previously mentioned. Interns who participate in this program come from a small group of affiliated universities who were willing to send students for a minimum of 4 months. Selection of interns is competitive, and those selected are paid a small stipend during their tenure. The program includes both clinical and didactic educational sessions that emphasize the skills necessary for autonomous practice with a complex patient population as well as leadership and communication skills. The mission statement of the program is:

> We provide a challenging clinical internship program that produces leaders in the field of physical therapy who can thrive both as primary care providers and as members of an interdependent health care team. We capitalize on the many unique opportunities the VA provides to develop the clinical, affective, and administrative skills necessary for our interns to excel in today's dynamic health care environment.

A multiple-mentoring model of clinical education is used in place of the more traditional 1:1 clinical instructor/student model. This model closely mimics the traditional medical education model in which an attending physician may have teaching responsibilities for two or more interns in a given clinic. These attending responsibilities rotate among the staff so the interns benefit from the collective knowledge and experience of everyone. Similarly, the rotating responsibility for interns reduces the burden on individual staff members and allows the program to run throughout the year. The goal of the internship program is to produce new graduates who will have the skills necessary to practice in primary care safely and effectively, the affective skills to successfully integrate their practice with others, and the desire to do so. As of November 2002 more than 20 interns have completed the program, with several working at VA sites around the country.

PATIENT ACCESS TO PHYSICAL THERAPIST SERVICES. Patients use three primary methods to access physical therapy services:
1. Emergency departments (EDs)
2. Primary care clinics
3. Telephone triage systems staffed by registered nurses

Patients are frequently seen in the ED with acute musculoskeletal injuries or exacerbations of chronic conditions. When this happens the intake nurse or examining physician pages the on-call PT. Responsibility for being on call rotates on a daily basis among an attending staff PT and intern. The therapist will go to the ED and screen the patient, resulting in one of three things:
1. The patient is deemed appropriate for physical therapy services
2. The patient is deemed appropriate for physical therapy services and also needs referral for further work-up
3. The patient is not appropriate for physical therapy services

These examinations are frequently performed collaboratively with the ED physicians. If appropriate, the patient is provided needed physical therapy interventions while in the ED or transported to the outpatient physical therapy clinic for treatment. Often these interventions are single occurrences because of the large geographic area served by the medical center. The abilities to screen and examine quickly, yet thoroughly, and develop and teach a home exercise program are critical skills in this environment.

Patients may also access physical therapy services through their established primary care clinic. If a patient is seen with what appears to be a mobility disorder, whether of a single joint or the entire body, the provider may page the on-call PT for assistance. The therapist and an intern will examine the patient, screen as appropriate, and provide any needed intervention while in the primary care clinic. These consultations have proven to be valuable teaching opportunities both for the PT interns and the primary care residents and attending physician. Most of these providers are internal medicine physicians who do not receive a great deal of training in musculoskeletal evaluation. This leads many of them to order imaging studies and other specialty consults when physical therapy intervention would be more appropriate. The integration of physical therapy practice with primary care has improved this situation tremendously. The primary care provider may also page the on-call PT when a patient is requesting an exercise (mobility) program for weight loss or to improve general health. The PT will screen the patient, identify risk factors for exercise testing with the American College of Sports Medicine criteria, and, if needed, schedule the patient for an exercise test. Formal exercise programs are generated at future appointment dates, but the patient education process begins at the first contact with the PT.

The third way that patients may access PT services is by a nurse-managed telephone triage system. If a patient calls with a symptom that is neuromusculoskeletal in nature but does not appear to require an ED visit, the nurse will page the on-call PT. The PT will speak with the patient and determine the appropriate course of action. The nurse places an electronic consult into the computerized patient record system that the VA uses and flags it for the veteran's primary care provider's signature. All three of these patient access routes to physical therapy services are enhanced and facilitated by the computerized patient record system. This system allows all providers, no matter where they are physically located, to see the patient's medical record. It also helps to ensure that everyone involved in the patient's care knows what the others are doing.

PROGRAM OUTCOMES. Although only in existence for slightly more than 2 years, the program has achieved some striking results at the local level. Veteran patients receive faster access to appropriate care, clinic waiting times for specialty providers such as orthopedics have gone down, fewer imaging studies are ordered, and patient satisfaction with the program is high. A grant application to study these outcomes formally is in process. Ultimately, this program should save money and improve the quality of health care the VA and the private sector are able to deliver. Despite the commitment in time and energy to the development of this program and ongoing teaching of primary care interns, a review of productivity data revealed a 26% increase in the number of patients seen over a similar period before implementation of the program.

FUTURE OF THE PRIMARY CARE PHYSICAL THERAPY PROGRAM. The VA Physical Therapy Advisory Council, made up of a group of PTs, has been charged with providing direction on physical therapy practice within VA. The council has been looking closely at the outcomes associated with the current program and has begun to establish other test sites across the VA system. It is anticipated that over time this model of care will be adapted across the entire VA system. It is hoped that the interns who complete this program will foster and promote that expansion with their skills and energy. As stated earlier, what makes this primary care physical therapy initiative unique is the provision of care to arguably one the most complex patient populations in the United States. Considering that by many estimates more than 70 million Americans will be older than 65 years by the year 2020, this program may become a model for other facilities servicing this population.

Summary

Predicting how the coming years will affect the practice of physical therapy and medicine and the role of primary care is difficult. Recent increases in the cost of medical care have once again focused a spotlight on controlling health care costs. Unlike the early 1990s, however, national health plans of many countries are having similar difficulties controlling rising health care expenditures. In addition, managed health care plans no longer appear to be an effective solution for controlling these costs. The only point most analysts will agree on is that the solutions of the 1990s have not solved the problems and more changes in the system will be needed. Challenges inherent in the primary care setting have been discussed, and central to meeting these challenges is the practice of interdisciplinary medicine. Who should the key players be within such a model? There appear to be preliminary data that suggest these three models may contribute to cost-effective care associated with high levels of patient and health care practitioner satisfaction. It is hoped that additional primary care models will be developed in the future, with PTs being heavily involved in both the planning and the implementation stages.

REFERENCES

1. *APC Learning and Development, Physical Therapist APC Orientation Manual*, Hayward, CA, 1998, Kaiser Permanente.
2. Benson CJ, Schreck RC, Underwood FB, et al: The role of Army physical therapists a nonphysician health care providers who prescribe certain medications: observations and experiences, *Phys Ther* 75:380-386, 1995.
3. Bigos S, Bowyer O, Brown K, et al: *Acute low back pain in adults.* Clinical practice guideline no. 14. AHCPR publication no. 95-0642. Rockville, MD, 1994, Agency for Health Care Policy and Research, U.S. Department of Health and Human Services.
4. Bischof RO, Nash DB: Managed care: past, present and future, *Med Clin North Am* 80:225-244, 1996.
5. Clancy CM, Cooper JK: Approaches to primary care: current realities and future visions, *Am J Med* 104:215-218, 1998.

6. Greathouse DG, Schreck RC, Benson CJ: The United States Army physical therapy experience: evaluation and treatment of patients with neuromusculoskeletal disorders, *J Orthop Sports Phys Ther* 19:261-266, 1994.

7. Greathouse DG, Sweeney JK, Hartwick AM: Physical therapy in a wartime environment. In Dillingham TR, Belandres PV, eds: *Textbook of military medicine: rehabilitation of the injured combatant*, Washington, DC, 1998, Borden Institute, pp 19-30.

8. Hartwick AM: *Army Medical Specialist Corps 45th anniversary commemorative monograph*, Washington, DC, 1993, Center of Military History, US Department of the Army.

9. Hensher M: Improving general practitioner access to physiotherapy: a review of the economic evidence, *Health Serv Manage Res* 10:225-230, 1997.

10. James JJ, Stuart RB: Expanded role of the physical therapist: screening musculoskeletal disorders, *Phys Ther* 55:121-131, 1975.

11. James JJ, Abshier JD: The primary evaluation of musculoskeletal disorders by the physical therapist, *Mil Med* 146:496-499, 1981.

12. Karpman RR: Musculoskeletal disease in the United States: who provides the care? *Clin Orthop Rel Res* 385:52-56, 2001.

13. KP learning works. In *Kaiser orientation handbook*, Hayward, CA, 2001, Kaiser Permanente.

14. Larcombe A: Physical therapy. In Bartley R, Coffey P, eds: *Management of low back pain in primary care*, Oxford, 2001, Butterworth Heinemann.

15. Liberman A, Rotarius T: Managed care evolution—where did it come from and where is it going? *Health Care Manager* 18:50-57, 1999.

16. MacDonald RS, Bell CMJ: An open controlled assessment of osteopathic manipulation in nonspecific low back pain, *Spine* 15:364-370, 1990.

17. Mitchell JM, Lissovoy GA: Comparison of resource use and cost in direct access versus physician referral episodes of physical therapy, *Phys Ther* 77:10-18, 1997.

18. Neel S: *Medical support of the U.S. Army in vietnam*, Washington, DC, 1973, Department of the Army.

19. *RCGP clinical guidelines for the management of acute low back pain*, London, 1996, Royal College of General Practitioners.

20. Starfield B: The future of primary care in a managed care era, *Int J Health Serv* 27:687-696, 1997.

21. Van Tulder MW, Koes BW, Bouter LM: Conservative treatment of acute and chronic nonspecific low back pain. A systematic review of randomized clinical trials of the most common interventions, *Spine* 22:2128-2156, 1997.

22. U.S. Department of the Army: *DEPMEDS policies/guidelines and treatment briefs*, Washington, DC, 1992, Defense Medical Standardization Board.

23. U.S. Department of the Army: *Non-physician health care providers (Army regulation 40-48)*, Washington, DC, 1992, Department of the Army.

24. U.S. Department of the Army: *Quality assurance administration (Army regulation 40-68)*, Washington, DC, 1992, Department of the Army.

Evidence-Based Examination of Diagnostic Information

2

Julie M. Fritz, PhD, PT, ATC

Objectives

After reading this chapter, the reader will be able to:

1. Describe the process physical therapists (PTs) use to identify the most efficient and effective clinical diagnostic tests.
2. Describe the elements of a "best" clinical diagnostic test.
3. Provide an overview of evidence-based practice and diagnosis, including the rules to apply to judge the existing evidence.

The *Guide to Physical Therapist Practice*[20] identifies five elements of patient/client management that must be integrated by PTs in an attempt to optimize the outcome of care (Table 2-1). The examination is the process of obtaining data from the patient. Evaluation requires the therapist to make judgments on the basis of the data. The examination and evaluation lead to a diagnosis, or classification. Diagnosis therefore has a preeminent role in the patient management process because it represents the end result of the examination and evaluation process and is responsible for guiding the selection of interventions and establishing a prognosis.[19,20] Despite its importance, many clinicians are unaware of how to optimize the selection and interpretation of diagnostic tests and integrate this information into patient management decisions.

The *Guide* describes diagnosis as having two aspects: the process of evaluating data obtained from the examination and the end result of that process. The process of evaluating diagnostic data requires the therapist to select and perform the necessary diagnostic tests for a particular patient and then make the appropriate interpretation of the results. The second step, arriving at the end result, requires an integration of the results of all tests performed into a cluster, or classification, that in turn directs the treatment. The classification may differ from the medical diagnosis because it is based on impairments and functional limitations assessed during the examination and not on pathologic origins.[6,28,52] The need for developing classification systems within the profession of physical therapy has been emphasized to facilitate professional communication, improve the outcomes of care, and increase the power of clinical research.[47] Understanding the diagnostic process in physical therapy involves much more than simply memorizing a list of classification labels; it requires the PT to learn how to select the best tests to perform efficiently and effectively and how to integrate the results to arrive at a diagnostic decision.

One of the first steps in examining and interpreting diagnostic tests is to consider why the test is being performed. The tests used by PTs are performed for two basic purposes.[8,55] Some are performed to examine the status of an anatomic structure, exclude or include certain anatomical regions for further examination, or detect conditions not appropriate for physical therapy management. These tests are often used as screening procedures and need to demonstrate diagnostic efficacy; they should have a high level of accuracy in distinguishing between individuals with or without the condition of interest. For example, a PT may use the anterior drawer test during the examination of a patient with knee pain in an attempt to assess the status of the anterior cruciate ligament. Another example is asking questions regarding unexplained weight loss or night pain in a patient with a musculoskeletal disorder to determine if the patient's symptoms may be caused by a previously undiagnosed neoplasm. Tests designed for diagnostic efficacy are used to focus further examination and may be concerned with anatomical considerations instead of selecting specific treatment techniques.

The second reason why PTs perform certain diagnostic tests is because the results, singularly or in combination with other findings, are believed to indicate that a particular type of intervention will be most effective for the patient. Tests used in this manner form the foundation of classification systems and should demonstrate outcome efficacy. For example, the observation of frontal plane displacement of the shoulders relative to the pelvis (i.e., lumbar lateral shift) in a patient with low back pain (LBP) is frequently cited as an important examination finding.[7,30,38,45] Several pathoanatomical hypotheses have been posited in explanation of the phenomenon, including disk herniation,[5,38] muscle spasm,[17] and segmental instability,[7] yet the precise condition resulting in a lateral shift is often unknown.[45] Despite this, the observation of a lateral shift is often an important diagnostic finding because it may indicate a specific intervention (e.g., correction of the lateral shift) that will be most useful in reducing pain and disability.[7,39]

It is possible that one test may have the potential to serve both diagnostic and classification purposes. For example, the neck distraction test is frequently performed during the examination of patients with neck pain. The test is positive when manual distraction of the neck relieves the patient's symptoms. The distraction test has been described as a test for diagnosing

TABLE 2-1

The Elements of Patient Management

Examination	The process of obtaining a history, performing relevant systems reviews, and selecting and administering specific tests and measures to obtain data.
Evaluation	A dynamic process in which the PT makes clinical judgments on the basis of data gathered during the examination.
Diagnosis	Both the process and the end result of evaluating information obtained from the examination, which the PT then organizes into defined clusters, syndromes, or categories to help determine the most appropriate intervention strategies.
Prognosis	Determination of the level of optimal improvement that might be attained through intervention and the amount of time required to reach that level.
Intervention	Purposeful and skilled interaction of the PT with the patient and, if appropriate, with other individuals involved in the care of the patient using various physical therapy methods and techniques to produce changes in the condition that are consistent with the diagnosis and prognosis.

From the Guide to physical therapist practice, ed 2, *Phys Ther* 81:9-746, 2001.

cervical nerve root compression and has been shown to have some validity.[59,60] However, the test may also be used to select an intervention. When the distraction test is positive, some therapists may interpret this finding as indicating a need for cervical traction.[40] Considering the purpose of a test is important for further consideration of the diagnostic process from an evidence-based perspective because the purpose has significant implications for examining the evidence related to its usefulness in clinical practice.

Evidence-Based Practice and Diagnosis

Evidence-based practice can be defined as "the conscientious and judicious use of current best evidence in making decisions about the care of individual patients."[48] To practice in an evidence-based manner, the clinician must be able to determine what constitutes the "best" evidence. Developing proficiency at reading and interpreting the evidence in the literature related to diagnostic tests is an important skill for PTs who want to become efficient and skillful at clinical diagnosis. Many PTs will be familiar with some of the principles for determining the best evidence when examining studies comparing different interventions. Most therapists understand that the best evidence in this area comes from randomized clinical trials with relatively long-term and complete follow-up periods.[9,21,58] When seeking to determine the best evidence on diagnostic tests, the rules governing the evaluation of studies regarding treatment outcomes are no longer applicable.[49] Rules for judging evidence offered by a study of a diagnostic test have been described; however, these rules are not as familiar to most therapists.[1,24,34,41] These rules primarily apply to two important aspects of designing or interpreting a study of a diagnostic test: the study design and data analysis.

Judging the Evidence: Study Design

The optimal design for a study examining a diagnostic test is the one that most effectively reduces susceptibility to bias (a deviation of the results from the truth in a consistent direction).[14,24] The optimal design for examining a diagnostic test is "a prospective, blind comparison of the test and the reference test in a consecutive series of patients from a relevant clinical population."[34] In other words, a study investigating a diagnostic test should use a prospective design in which all subjects are evaluated by the diagnostic test and a reference standard representing the definitive, or best, criteria for the condition of interest. When performed in this manner, the results of the test and the reference standard can be summarized in a 2×2 table (Figure 2-1). Each subject will fit into only one box in this table. The distribution of subjects into these different boxes will then be used to determine the usefulness of the diagnostic test. Other aspects of the study design besides the basic layout are important for determining the strength of evidence offered by the study. These factors include the reference standard, the diagnostic test itself, and the patient population studied.

Reference Standard

When studying a diagnostic test, the test must be compared with a reference standard, or gold standard. The reference standard is the criterion that best defines the condition the test is attempting to detect.[25] It is important to recognize, however, that reference standards are not perfect but should offer the best approximation of the condition.[50] The selection and application of the reference standard are an extremely important considerations in a study of a diagnostic test. If the reference standard cannot be accepted as the best method of determining whether the patient has the condition of interest, the study will not be able to provide meaningful information.[26] The reference standard must be consistent with the purpose of the test. If the test is primarily being used for diagnosing pathology in a certain anatomical structure, then a reference standard related to pathoanatomy, such as a magnetic resonance image or radiograph, would be appropriate. If a test is being used to select an intervention, a reference standard related to pathoanatomy would not be appropriate. Because such tests are attempting to predict which patient will respond to a particular intervention, the reference standard needs to be related to the therapeutic outcome of the intervention.

	Reference Standard Positive	Reference Standard Negative
Diagnostic test positive	True-positive results A	False-positive results B
Diagnostic test negative	False-negative results C	True-negative results D

FIGURE 2-1 Contingency table created by comparing the results of the diagnostic test and the reference standard.

A study investigating tests for carpal tunnel syndrome provides a good example of this distinction in reference standards.[4] One test that was examined in this study was Phalen's test. This test is typically used to diagnose compression of the median nerve in the carpal tunnel. The authors of the study, however, also hypothesized that a positive Phalen's test result may be helpful in determining that a patient may respond to wrist splinting. To assess Phalen's test for both of these purposes, two different reference standards were needed—one to represent the pathoanatomical purpose of the test and the second to represent its role in selecting an intervention. The authors chose to use a nerve conduction velocity study as a pathoanatomical reference standard and the response of symptoms to 2 weeks of splinting as the intervention reference standard. This second reference standard permitted an examination of the usefulness of Phalen's test in determining if splinting should be performed, regardless of its ability to diagnose pathology in the median nerve.

The results of a study that uses a reference standard reflecting one purpose cannot be generalized to other possible uses of the test. For example, Spurling's test is typically described as a test for cervical radiculopathy.[57] One study that examined the validity of Spurling's test compared the results against a reference standard of subject-reported neck pain present during the week preceding the examination.[53] By using this reference standard, the authors conceptualized the tests as essentially screening procedures designed to distinguish between individuals with or without a recent history of neck pain. This is not the reason why most PTs perform Spurling's test during an examination. Therapists typically use the test to help determine if a cervical nerve root lesion is present. Therapists may use the results of Spurling's test to make an intervention decision. For example, some therapists may consider a positive Spurling's test result an indication to perform cervical traction.[40] A reference standard of self-reported neck pain makes the results difficult to interpret because it is inconsistent with what Spurling's test is used for. Examining the reference standard and ensuring its consistency with the purpose of the test are essential for evaluating diagnostic test studies. Although the majority of studies in the literature use pathoanatomical reference standards, physical therapists are often concerned with issues related to classification and outcome efficacy. If the reference standard is inappropriate for the purpose of the test, the study will not provide useful results.

Other factors related to the reference standard are important to consider. The reference standard must be consistently applied to all subjects in the study. For example, a study of screening examinations was performed by nurses with goniometry to detect cerebral palsy in preterm infants.[44] Infants with a high suspicion of cerebral palsy were referred to a neurologist whose evaluation served as the reference standard, whereas a less rigorous reference standard consisting of chart reviews was used for the remaining subjects.[44] The adequacy of chart reviews for diagnosing cerebral palsy with the same accuracy as a clinical examination leaves this study susceptible to bias, which can lead to an overestimation of the diagnostic value of a test.[34,46]

In addition, the reference standard should be judged by an individual who is unaware of, or blinded to, the diagnostic test results and the overall clinical presentation of the subject. If blinding is not maintained, judgments of the reference standard may be influenced by expectations based on knowledge of the test results.[16] Review bias occurs in situations when either the reference standard or the diagnostic test is judged by an individual with knowledge of the other result.[46] For example, in a study by Lauder et al,[32] various clinical diagnostic tests were compared against a reference standard of electrodiagnostic testing to determine their utility in diagnosing lumbar radiculopathy. In the study, it is unclear if the individual performing the diagnostic tests was aware of the results of the electrodiagnostic studies. Clearly, if the examiner was aware of the electrodiagnostic test results, this knowledge could have influenced the judgment of the diagnostic test results.

Diagnostic Tests

The diagnostic tests being studied must be described in sufficient detail to allow the reader to understand and replicate the procedures. The actual physical performance of the test also needs to be described because the same test may be performed differently by different examiners. A study's results can only be generalized to the test as it was performed in the study. For example, Levangie[33] examined the diagnostic usefulness of pelvic asymmetry for detecting the presence of LBP among subjects referred to physical therapy. If asked how to test for the presence of pelvic asymmetry, most PTs would probably describe the palpation of certain bony landmarks, with the patient standing or sitting. In this study, however, pelvic asymmetry was determined by using a pelvic inclinometer to assess iliac crest height. It cannot be assumed that determination of pelvic asymmetry with palpation would yield similar results.

Description of the diagnostic test should cover physical performance and the criteria defining positive and negative results. Many tests commonly used by PTs have variable or unclear grading criteria. Determining the presence of centralization in patients with LBP is an example. What constitutes a positive finding of centralization varies. Some use definitions strictly based on movement of symptoms from distal to proximal.[13,38] Others have defined centralization to include diminishment of pain during testing.[29] Such disagreements point out the need to clarify how positive and negative results are defined within a particular study. Grading the diagnostic test is also susceptible to review bias if the individual judging the test is aware of the results on the reference standard. If this blinding is not maintained, the usefulness of the test is likely to be somewhat overestimated.[34]

Study Population

The subjects of a diagnostic test study are an important consideration. The subjects should be similar to patients that a therapist would consider applying the test to in clinical practice. Some people in the study will end up having the condition of interest, whereas others will not. Furthermore, those who do have the condition should reflect a continuum of severity from mild to severe.[26] Those who do not have the condition should have similar symptoms.[23] Unfortunately, many studies include some healthy subjects. Any diagnostic test will look more useful than it really is when it is used to distinguish between healthy individuals and those with severe conditions.[34] Spectrum bias occurs when study subjects are not representative of the population in whom the test is typically applied in practice.[34] Spectrum bias can profoundly affect the results of a study. The best way to avoid spectrum bias is to use a prospective design in which a consecutive group of subjects from a clinical setting is studied.[1]

Comparing the study by Burke et al[4] with another study examining the value of Phalen's test for diagnosing carpal tunnel syndrome illustrates the concern over spectrum bias. A study by Gellman et al[15] also compared Phalen's test against a reference standard of nerve conduction velocity. The only substantial difference between the two studies was the subjects. All the subjects in the Burke et al study had symptoms consistent with carpal tunnel syndrome.[4] The study by Gellman et al[15] involved subjects with symptoms consistent with carpal tunnel syndrome but also included a group of 50 hands that were asymptomatic. Inclusion of hands without symptoms creates a spectrum bias. Not surprisingly, the results of this study demonstrated much greater diagnostic accuracy for Phalen's test than the study relatively free from spectrum bias.

Using the Data: Analysis

The basic layout of the results from a study of a diagnostic test is shown in Figure 2-1. The result for each subject fits into only one of the four categories on the basis of a comparison of the results of the diagnostic test and the reference standard. The defining characteristics of the four categories are:

- True-positive (a) subjects who are positive on both the reference standard and the diagnostic test
- False-positive (b) subjects who are negative on the reference standard but positive on the diagnostic test
- False-negative (c) subjects who are positive on the reference standard but negative on the diagnostic test
- True-negative (d) subjects who are negative on both the reference standard and the diagnostic test

From this layout several statistics can be calculated that are useful for understanding the value of a diagnostic test (Table 2-2).[16]

Sensitivity, Specificity, and Predictive Values

Sensitivity and specificity values are calculated vertically from the 2×2 table and represent the proportion of correct diagnostic test results among individuals with and without the condition. *Sensitivity* (or true-positive rate) is the proportion of true-positive subjects among all subjects who have the condition of interest. *Specificity* (or true-negative rate) is the proportion of true-negative subjects among all subjects without the condition.[50]

Predictive values are calculated horizontally from the table and represent the proportion of subjects with a positive or negative diagnostic test result that are correct results. The *positive predictive value* is the proportion of true-positive subjects among all subjects with a positive diagnostic test. The *negative predictive value* is the proportion of true-negative subjects among all subjects with a negative diagnostic test.[18] The predictive values are generally of less value in interpreting the

---

TABLE 2-2

Statistics Commonly Used in Studies of Diagnostic Tests

Statistic	Formula	Description
Positive predictive value	$a/(a + b)$	Given a positive test result, the probability that the individual has the condition.
Negative predictive value	$d/(c + d)$	Given a negative test result, the probability that the individual does not have the condition.
Sensitivity	$a/(a + c)$	Given that the individual has the condition, the probability that the test will be positive.
Specificity	$d/(b + d)$	Given that the individual does not have the condition, the probability that the test will be negative.
Positive LR	sensitivity/ $(1 - \text{specificity})$	Given a positive test result, the increase in odds favoring the condition.
Negative LR	$(1 - \text{sensitivity})/$ specificity	Given a negative test result, the decrease in odds favoring the condition.

LR, Likelihood ratio.

---

usefulness of a test because they depend highly on the prevalence of the condition of interest in the study population. Positive predictive values will be lower and negative predictive values higher in study populations with a low prevalence of the condition. If prevalence is high, the trends reverse.[23] Sensitivity and specificity values remain fairly consistent across different prevalence levels[50] and are preferred over predictive values.

Sensitivity and specificity values provide useful information for interpreting diagnostic tests. For example, a test with high sensitivity has relatively few false-negative results. High test sensitivity therefore attests to the value of a negative test result.[51,54] In other words, if a test has high sensitivity, few false-negative results will be found, and therefore the examiner can have some level of trust that the negative result actually represents the absence of the condition. Sackett et al[50] have advocated the acronym *SnNout* (if sensitivity is high, a negative result is useful for ruling out the condition). High sensitivity indicates that a test is useful for excluding, or ruling out, a condition when it is negative but does not address the value of a positive test. A diagnostic test with high specificity has relatively few false-positive results and therefore speaks to the value of a positive test result.[51,54] The acronym advocated is *SpPin* (if specificity is high, a positive result is useful for ruling in the condition).[50]

Unfortunately few diagnostic tests have both high sensitivity and high specificity. Knowledge of sensitivity and specificity of a diagnostic test can improve clinical decision-making by helping clinicians weigh the value of both positive and negative results. A study examining history and physical examination findings in predicting rotator cuff tears in older patients provides an illustration.[35] Numerous diagnostic tests were compared against a reference standard of shoulder arthrogram. No test had high levels of both sensitivity and specificity (Table 2-3). A painful arc

TABLE 2-3

Diagnostic Efficacy of Clinical Tests for Detecting Rotator Cuff Tears

Diagnostic Test	Sensitivity	Specificity	Positive LR	Negative LR
Presence of night pain	87.7	19.7	1.09	0.62
Presence of supraspinatus atrophy	55.6	72.9	2.05	0.61
Shoulder elevation PROM <170°	30.2	78.1	1.38	0.89
Shoulder external rotation PROM <70°	19.0	83.6	1.16	0.97
Neer impingement sign	97.2	9.0	1.07	0.31
Weakness with external rotation strength test	75.9	57.3	1.78	0.75
Painful arc during elevation PROM	97.5	9.9	1.08	0.25

From Likater D, Pioro M, El Bilbeisi H, et al: Returning to the bedside: using the history and physical examination to identify rotator cuff tears, *JAGS* 48:1633-1637, 2000.
PROM, Passive range of motion.

during passive elevation of the arm was the most sensitive, and limited external rotation passive range of motion to less than 70° was the most specific.[35] The high sensitivity (97.5%) of the presence of a painful arc indicates that this finding is useful for ruling out a rotator cuff tear; however, the low specificity (9.9%) indicates that a positive painful arc has little meaning. Few false-negative results are found when testing for a painful arc, and it would be unlikely that the patient actually has a rotator cuff tear if a painful arc is not present. Conversely, limited external rotation was highly specific (83.6%), indicating that a positive test is useful for confirming a rotator cuff tear. The sensitivity of limited external rotation was poor (19%), indicating a lack of value for a negative test result.

Likelihood Ratios

Sensitivity and specificity values provide helpful information; however, they do not provide a complete picture. The actual performance of a diagnostic test is related to sensitivity and specificity values and also depends on the pretest probability that the condition is present. Useful tests should produce large shifts in probability once the result of the test is known.[10,31,36] Sensitivity and specificity values cannot quantify shifts in the probability given a certain test result. The best statistics for quantifying shifts in probability, based on the results of a diagnostic test, are likelihood ratios.[3,27] Likelihood ratios (LRs) combine sensitivity and specificity values into a value that can be used to quantify shifts in probability once the diagnostic test result is known.[56] The positive LR is calculated as sensitivity/(1 − specificity) and indicates the increase in odds favoring the condition given a positive test result. The negative LR is calculated as (1 − sensitivity)/specificity and indicates the change in odds favoring the condition given a negative test result.[24] An LR value of 1 indicates the test result does nothing to change the odds favoring the condition, whereas an LR value greater than 1 increases the odds of the condition and an LR value of less than 1 diminishes the odds of the condition. Table 2-4 provides a guide for interpreting the strength of an LR.[27]

A diagnostic test with a large positive LR (e.g., >5.0) indicates that the shift in odds favoring the condition will be relatively large when the diagnostic test is positive. It is therefore desirable for a test to have a large positive LR value. In general, diagnostic tests with high levels of specificity will also have

TABLE 2-4

A Guide to Interpretation of LR Values

Positive LR	Negative LR	Interpretation
>10	<0.10	Generate large and often conclusive shifts in probability
5-10	0.1-0.2	Generate moderate shifts in probability
2-5	0.2-0.5	Generate small, but sometimes important, shifts in probability
1-2	0.5-1	Alter probability to a small, and rarely important, degree

From Jaeschke R, Guyatt GH, Sackett DL: Users' guides to the medical literature. III. How to use an article about a diagnostic test. B. What are the results and will they help me in caring for my patients? *JAMA* 271:703-707, 1994.

large positive LR values because both attest to the usefulness of the positive test result. The negative LR value indicates the change in odds *favoring* the condition given a negative diagnostic test result. Because a negative test result is supposed to reduce the odds that a condition is present, it is desirable for a test to have a small (e.g., <0.20) negative LR value. A small negative LR indicates a diagnostic test that is useful for ruling out a condition when the result is negative. Tests with high sensitivity values generally have small negative LR values.

Examining the tests for rotator cuff tears discussed earlier provides an example of the importance of combining sensitivity and specificity values (see Table 2-3). The most sensitive test was a painful arc (97.5%), and this test also had the smallest negative LR. The most specific test was external rotation range of motion (83.6%); however, positive LR value was greater for the presence of supraspinatus atrophy (1.78 vs. 2.05). This is because the sensitivity value for the finding of supraspinatus atrophy was much better than the sensitivity for external rotation range of motion limitation.

Using the Data: Interpretation

The diagnostic process requires therapists to think in terms of probability and revision of probabilities. Before performing a diagnostic test, a therapist will have some idea of the likelihood that the patient being evaluated has the condition of interest. Although this probability is rarely articulated or quantified in the therapist's mind, all clinicians develop at least a sense that certain conditions are more likely, and others less likely, for certain patients. The condition of interest in the therapist's mind may be related to pathology or pathoanatomy; for instance, is it likely that this patient has a cervical disk lesion that is causing his arm pain? The condition of interest being considered by the therapist may involve treatment decision making; for instance, will this patient's arm pain be relieved with traction treatments? The therapist also has some threshold level of certainty, at which point he or she will be "sure enough" and ready to act.[36,42] Again, this threshold is typically not quantified, but there is some amount of assurance that any therapist must reach before an action is taken with the patient. The threshold is a factor of the costs associated with making an incorrect decision versus the benefits of being correct.[2,43] For example, a high threshold of certainty would be required if the question involved ruling out metastatic disease in the lung as a source of arm pain. If a therapist had any lingering doubts about such a diagnosis, it would be incumbent to refer the patient for further diagnostic workup before pursuing physical therapy. On the other hand, if the question concerned the application of a treatment with minimal cost and low potential for risk, such as mechanical cervical traction, the threshold for action would be lower. A therapist will likely be willing to initiate traction treatment if he or she is fairly certain the patient may benefit and if there is not greater certainty that the patient would benefit from an alternative treatment. LRs provide the information needed to select the diagnostic test or tests that will most efficiently move the therapist from the uncertainty associated with the pretest probability to a posttest probability that crosses a threshold for action.

The probability that a patient has a particular condition before performing the diagnostic test can come from sources other than the clinical experience and expertise of the examiner. Other sources of pretest probabilities include epidemiologic data on prevalence rates for certain conditions, the prevalence of the condition in studies examining diagnostic test properties, clinical databases, and information already obtained on the patient from the examination.[2] Whatever the source of the pretest probability, LR values quantify the direction and magnitude of change in the pretest probability on the basis of the diagnostic test result.[25] To illustrate the process, consider the case of a 37-year-old male patient with a 1-week history of LBP and right buttock pain that does not extend below the knee. The question is one related to treatment decision-making: "Is this patient likely to respond to a manipulation intervention?"

What is a reasonable pretest probability that the patient will respond to manipulation? On the basis of a randomized trial demonstrating that many patients with LBP will respond to manipulation[22,37] as well as clinical experience, the probability may be fairly high, perhaps 60%. What information should be gathered to alter this probability? To answer this question, the results of a recent study examined the usefulness of various diagnostic tests against a reference standard of success with manipulation (defined as a 50% decrease in self-reported disability occurring over two treatment sessions).[12] The results of this study (Table 2-5) show the best test would be asking the patient how long the symptoms have been present (positive LR = 4.4 for 15 days or less). It is not uncommon that factors from the history prove more useful than those from the physical examination. If the test is positive (i.e., the duration of symptoms is <16 days), what should the new probability of success with manipulation be? Two methods can be used to make this determination. The simpler but somewhat less precise method uses a nomogram (Figure 2-2).[11] A straight edge is anchored along the left side at the point representing the pretest probability. The straight edge is then aligned with the appropriate LR value (4.4 in this example), and the line is then extended through the right side of the nomogram. The point of intersection on the right side indicates the posttest probability.[50] In this example, if the duration of the patient's symptoms was less than 16 days, the posttest probability of success with manipulation appears to be approximately 83%.

The posttest probability can be quantified with greater precision by using a calculation process described by Sackett et al[50] and outlined in Box 2-1.

TABLE 2-5

Diagnostic Usefulness of Various Signs and Symptoms for Determining if a Patient with Low Back Pain Will Respond to a Manipulation Technique

Test	Sensitivity	Specificity	Positive LR	Negative LR
FACTORS FROM THE HISTORY				
Duration of symptoms ≤15 days	0.56	0.87	4.4	0.51
Symptom distribution not distal to the knee	0.88	0.36	1.4	0.33
Episodes of LBP not becoming more frequent	0.75	0.44	1.3	0.59
FACTORS FROM THE PHYSICAL EXAMINATION				
Hypomobility with prone spring testing in at least one lumbar segment	0.97	0.23	1.3	0.13
Hip internal rotation PROM greater than 35° in at least one hip	0.50	0.85	3.3	0.59
No peripheralization during lumbar standing AROM	0.84	0.33	1.3	0.48

Adapted from Flynn T, Fritz J, Whitman J, et al: A clinical prediction rule for classifying patients with low back pain who demonstrate short term improvement with spinal manipulation, *Spine* 27:2835-2843, 2002.
LBP, Low back pain; *PROM,* passive range of motion; *AROM,* active range of motion.

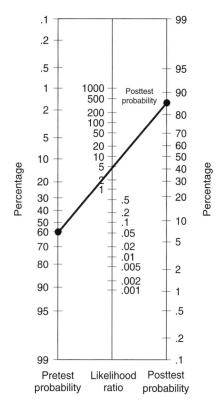

FIGURE 2-2 Nomogram for estimating posttest probability of a diagnosis. (From Fagan TJ: Nomogram for Bayes's theorem, *N Engl J Med* 293:257, 1975.)

By using these calculations, the pretest probability of 60% would correspond to pretest odds of 1.5:1. Multiplying this by the LR value of 4.4, the posttest odds would be 6.6:1. Converting this back to probability results in a posttest probability of 87%. Examples such as this highlight the importance of attending to the most important examination findings for clinical decision-making. If the examiner had instead focused on the lack of symptoms distal to the knee as confirming evidence that this patient was likely to benefit from manipulation, the actual posttest probability would only increase to a 68% probability of success. Without knowledge of the relative unimportance of this finding, the therapist might overinterpret the finding.

If the pretest probability were lower, the therapist may instead want to seek a finding that would confirm that the patient does not need manipulation but instead would benefit

---

BOX 2-1

Calculation of Posttest Probability

Step 1: Convert the pretest probability to pretest odds:

$$\text{Pretest odds} = \frac{\text{Pretest probability}}{1 - \text{Pretest probability}}$$

Step 2: Multiply the pretest odds by the LR value:

Pretest odds × LR = posttest odds

Step 3: Convert the posttest odds to posttest probability:

$$\frac{\text{Posttest odds}}{\text{Posttest odds} + 1} = \text{Posttest probability}$$

---

more from another type of intervention.[6] For example, consider if the patient told the therapist that for previous episodes of LBP, treatment with spinal manipulation had not been successful. In this case, the therapist would likely believe the pretest probability of success with a manipulation technique to be much lower, perhaps as low as 15%. In this circumstance, the finding that the current duration of symptoms was less than 16 days would only increase the probability of success to 44%. The therapist may be better served to use the test with the smallest negative LR value because if this finding is negative, it is likely that the posttest probability will be small enough to exclude manipulation as a treatment option and move on to other considerations. The test with the smallest LR value was prone posterior-to-anterior spring testing over the spinous processes in the lumbar spine (see Table 2-5). If this testing did not reveal any hypomobility, the posttest probability of success with manipulation would be only 2%.

Summary

LRs provide the most powerful tool for quantifying the importance of a particular test within the diagnostic process. Because LR values can be calculated for both positive and negative results, the importance of both positive and negative test results can be examined independently. This is important because few tests provide useful information in both capacities, and understanding the relative strength of evidence provided by a negative or a positive test result helps to refine interpretation of the diagnostic test. Understanding the information contained in statistics, such as sensitivity, specificity, and LRs, can assist therapists in improving their diagnostic and decision-making skills. Developing these skills is paramount for therapists working in primary care settings.

REFERENCES

1. Begg CB: Methodologic standards for diagnostic test assessment studies, *J Gen Intern Med* 3:518-520, 1988
2. Bernstein J: Decision analysis, *J Bone Joint Surg* 79-A:1404-1414, 1997.
3. Boyko EJ: Ruling out or ruling in disease with the most sensitive or specific diagnostic test, *Med Decis Making* 14:175-179, 1994.
4. Burke DT, Burke MA, Bell R, et al: Subjective swelling: a new sign for carpal tunnel syndrome, *Am J Phys Med Rehabil* 78:504-508, 1999.
5. Charnley J: Orthopaedic signs in the diagnosis of disc protrusion, *Lancet* 1:186-192, 1951.
6. Delitto A, Snyder-Mackler L: The diagnostic process: examples in orthopedic physical therapy, *Phys Ther* 75:203-211, 1994.
7. Delitto A, Erhard RE, Bowling RW: A treatment-based classification approach to low back syndrome: identifying and staging patients for conservative management, *Phys Ther* 75:470-489, 1995.
8. Deyo RA, Haselkorn J, Hoffman R, et al: Designing studies of diagnostic tests for low back pain or radiculopathy, *Spine* 19(suppl):2057s-2063s, 1994.
9. Dickersin K, Scherer R, Lefebvre C: Identifying relevant studies for systematic reviews, *BMJ* 309:1286-1291, 1994.
10. Dujardin B, Van den Ende J, Van Gompel A, et al: Likelihood ratios: a real improvement for clinical decision making? *Eur J Epidemiol* 10:29-36, 1994.
11. Fagan TJ: Nomogram for Bayes's theorem, *N Engl J Med* 293:257, 1975.
12. Flynn T, Fritz J, Whitman J, et al: A clinical prediction rule for classifying patients with low back pain who demonstrate short term improvement with spinal manipulation, *Spine* 27:2835-2843, 2002.
13. Fritz JM, Delitto A, Vignovic M, et al: Inter-rater reliability of judgments of the centralization phenomenon and status change during movement

testing in patients with low back pain, *Arch Phys Med Rehabil* 81:57-61, 2000.

14. Geddes JR, Harrison PJ: Closing the gap between research and practice, *Br J Psychiatry* 171:220-225, 1997.
15. Gellman H, Gelberman RH, Tan AM, et al: Carpal tunnel syndrome: an evaluation of the provocative diagnostic tests, *J Bone Joint Surg* 68-A: 735-737, 1986.
16. Greenhalgh T: How to read a paper: papers that report diagnostic or screening tests, *BMJ* 315:540-543, 1997.
17. Grieve GP: Treating backache: a topical comment, *Physiotherapy* 69:316, 1983.
18. Griner PF, Mayewski RJ, Mushlin AI, et al: Selection and interpretation of diagnostic tests and procedures. Principles and applications, *Ann Intern Med* 94:557-592, 1981.
19. Guccione AA: Physical therapy diagnosis and the relationship between impairments and function, *Phys Ther* 71:499-504, 1991.
20. Guide to Physical Therapist Practice, ed 2, *Phys Ther* 81:9-746, 2001.
21. Guyatt GH, Sackett DL, Cook DJ: Users' guide to the medical literature: II. How to use an article about therapy or prevention: A. Are the results of the study valid? *JAMA* 270:2598-2601, 1993.
22. Hadler NM, Curtis P, Gillings DB, et al: A benefit of spinal manipulation as an adjunctive therapy for acute low-back pain: A stratified controlled study, *Spine* 12:703-705, 1987.
23. Hagen MD: Test characteristics: how good is that test? *Med Decis Making* 22:213-233, 1995.
24. Irwig L, Tosteson ANA, Gatsonis C, et al: Guidelines for meta-analyses evaluating diagnostic tests, *Ann Intern Med* 120:667-676, 1994.
25. Jaeschke RZ, Meade MO, Guyatt GH, et al: How to use diagnostic test articles in the intensive care unit: diagnosing weanability using f/Vt, *Crit Care Med* 25:1514-1521, 1997.
26. Jaeschke R, Guyatt G, Sackett DL: Users' guides to the medical literature. III. How to use an article about a diagnostic test. A. Are the results of the study valid? *JAMA* 271:389-391, 1994.
27. Jaeschke R, Guyatt GH, Sackett DL: Users' guides to the medical literature. III. How to use an article about a diagnostic test. B. What are the results and will they help me in caring for my patients? *JAMA* 271:703-707, 1994.
28. Jette AM: Diagnosis and classification by physical therapists: a special communication, *Phys Ther* 69:967-969, 1989.
29. Karas R, McIntosh G, Hall H, et al: The relationship between nonorganic signs and centralization of symptoms in the prediction of return to work for patients with low back pain, *Phys Ther* 77:354-360, 1997.
30. Khuffash B, Porter RW: Cross leg pain and trunk list, *Spine* 14:602-603, 1989.
31. Kortelainen P, Puranen J, Koivisto E, et al: Symptoms and signs of sciatica and their relation to the localization of the lumbar disc herniation, *Spine* 10:88-92, 1985.
32. Lauder T, Dillingham R, Andary M, et al: Effect of history and exam in predicting electrodiagnostic outcome among patients with suspected lumbosacral radiculopathy, *Am J Phys Med Rehabil* 79:60-68, 2000.
33. Levangie PK: The association between static pelvic asymmetry and low back pain, *Spine* 24:1234-1241, 1999.
34. Lijmer JG, Mol BW, Heisterkamp S, et al: Empirical evidence of design-related bias in studies of diagnostic tests, *JAMA* 282:1061-1066, 1999.
35. Likater D, Pioro M, El Bilbeisi H, et al: Returning to the bedside: using the history and physical examination to identify rotator cuff tears, *JAGS* 48:1633-1637, 2000.
36. Lurie JD, Sox HC: Principles of medical decision making: spine update, *Spine* 24:493-498, 1999.
37. Meade TW, Dyer S, Browne W, et al: Randomised comparison of chiropractic and hospital outpatient management for low back pain: results from extended follow up, *BMJ* 311:349-351, 1995.
38. McKenzie RA: *The lumbar spine: mechanical diagnosis and therapy*, Waianae, New Zealand, 1989, Spinal Publications.
39. McKenzie RA: Manual correction of sciatic scoliosis, *NZ Med J* 76: 194-199, 1972.
40. Moeti P, Marchetti G: Clinical outcome from mechanical intermittent cervical traction for the treatment of cervical radiculopathy: a case series, *J Orthop Sports Phys Ther* 31:207-213, 2001.
41. Mulrow CD, Linn WD, Gaul MK, et al: Assessing quality of diagnostic test evaluation, *J Gen Intern Med* 4:288-295, 1989.
42. Pauker SG, Kassirer JP: The threshold approach to clinical decision making, *N Engl J Med* 302:1109-1117, 1980.
43. Pauker SG, Kassirer JP: Therapeutic decision-making: a cost benefit analysis, *N Engl J Med* 293:229-234, 1975.
44. Pinto-Martin JA, Torre C, Zhao H: Nurse screening of low-birth-weight infants for cerebral palsy using goniometry, *Nurs Res* 46:284-287, 1997.
45. Porter RW, Miller CG: Back pain and trunk list, *Spine* 11:596-600, 1986.
46. Reid MC, Lachs MS, Feinstein AR: Use of methodological standards in diagnostic test research: getting better but still not good, *JAMA* 274: 645-651, 1995.
47. Rose SJ: Physical therapy diagnosis: role and function, *Phys Ther* 69: 535-537, 1989.
48. Sackett DL, Richardson WS: Evidence based medicine: what it is and what it isn't, *BMJ* 312:71-72, 1996.
49. Sackett DL, Wennberg JE: Choosing the best research design for each question. It's time to stop squabbling over the "best" methods, *BMJ* 315:1636, 1997.
50. Sackett DL, Haynes RB, Guyatt GH, et al: *Clinical epidemiology: a basic science for clinical medicine*, ed 2, Boston, 1992, Little, Brown.
51. Sackett DL: A primer on the precision and accuracy of the clinical examination, *JAMA* 267:2638-2644, 1992.
52. Sahrmann SA: Diagnosis by the physical therapist—a prerequisite for treatment, *Phys Ther* 68:1703-1706, 1988.
53. Sandmark H, Nisell R: Validity of five common manual neck pain provoking tests, *Scand J Rehab Med* 27:131-136, 1995.
54. Schulzer M: Diagnostic tests: a statistical review, *Muscle Nerve* 17:815-819, 1994.
55. Schwartz JS: Evaluating diagnostic tests—what needs to be done? *J Gen Intern Med* 1:266-276, 1986.
56. Simel DL, Samsa GP, Matchar DB: Likelihood ratios with confidence: sample size estimation for diagnostic test results, *J Clin Epidemiol* 44:763-770, 1991.
57. Spurling RG, Scoville WB: Lateral rupture of the cervical intervertebral discs: a common cause of shoulder and arm pain, *Surg Gynecol Obstet* 78:350-358, 1944.
58. van Tulder MW, Assendelft WJ, Koes BW, et al: Method guidelines for systematic reviews in the Cochrane Collaboration back review group for spinal disorders, *Spine* 22:2323-2330, 1997.
59. Viikari-Juntura E, Porras M, Laasonen EM: Validity of clinical tests in the diagnosis of root compression in cervical disc disease, *Spine* 14:253-257, 1989.
60. Wainner RM, Fritz JM, Irrgang JJ, et al: Reliability and diagnostic accuracy of the clinical examination and patient self-report measures for cervical radiculopathy, *Spine* 28:52-62, 2003.

Cultural Competence: An Essential Element of Primary Health Care

3

Ronnie Leavitt, PT, MPH, PhD

Objectives

After reading this chapter, the reader will be able to:

1. Describe the concept of and the variables associated with a culturally competent practitioner.
2. Describe cultural considerations associated with treating a diverse population.
3. Provide specific strategies that will enhance communication with diverse populations.
4. Describe elements associated with a culturally competent organization.

In today's world, human diversity is the norm rather than the exception. Patients taking part in the health care system are likely to look, think, and act, at least in some ways, differently from the health care professional. People have a wide range of ethnic identifications, religions, material realities, beliefs, and behaviors that lead to rich diversity and cultural complexity. Each patient and each physical therapist (PT) is a unique individual.

The goal of this book is to address the needs of the PT outpatient practitioner in a primary care environment. The concept of primary health care is especially appropriate for the wide range of patient impairments likely to be seen in an outpatient setting. By definition, primary health care by a PT presumes practice to meet the needs of a patient within the context of the individual patient, family, community, and broader cultural milieu. Furthermore, interest is rising in the need to provide health care in a more effective and efficient way to maximize limited resources and meet an ever-expanding array of health concerns. We want to do our job well; we do not want to be ineffective or waste precious resources. The goal of cultural competence, as is the goal of competence in any area, is to maximize the potential for a successful interaction between the clinician and patient. Today and in the foreseeable future, rehabilitation practitioners, organizations, and systems need to be culturally competent.

Cultural competence is a set of behaviors, attitudes, and policies that come together on a continuum to enable a system, agency, or individual to function effectively in transcultural interactions.[12] Cultural competence is an essential element for PT outpatient practitioners to facilitate effective and efficient examination, diagnosis, and development of a plan of care. Developing rapport, collecting and synthesizing patient data, recognizing personal functional concerns, and developing treatment suggestions for a particular patient require cultural competence.

Understanding the concept of culture is key to understanding cultural competence. Lynch and Hanson[32] describe culture as the framework that guides and binds life practices. This definition is in contrast to a rigidly prescribed set of behaviors or characteristics. Individuals do not inherit a culture biologically; they learn it. People may share cultural tendencies and pass them among generations. However, cultural frameworks are constantly evolving, and many factors such as ethnic identification, socioeconomic status, migration history, gender, age, and religion each have a profound impact on one's cultural way of life. On the basis of these variables, individuals may be members of several subcultures, or smaller units within a larger culture. One's culture is closely interrelated to cultural value systems, health beliefs and behaviors, and communication styles. These variables are particularly relevant to the PT working in a cross-cultural environment such as an outpatient orthopedic setting.

A culturally competent practitioner must:

- *Acknowledge the immense influence of culture.* It is essential to understand that each of us is immersed in our own culture, with its associated beliefs, attitudes, and behaviors that guide our personal and professional interactions. However, human nature is such that we all tend to be rather ethnocentric, that is, believing that our own cultural way of life is the norm, the standard by which all others are judged. What we forget is that the next person, from another culture, is also ethnocentric. The relevance of this self-awareness, or lack of it, is especially critical when therapists are working with patients who are different from themselves. It is not merely the "other" who has a unique culture, but each of us.

- *Assess cross-cultural relations* and be vigilant toward the dynamics that result from cultural differences. With cross-cultural interaction comes the possibility of misjudging the other's intentions and actions. Each party to an interaction brings to the encounter a specific set of experiences and styles. One must be vigilant to minimize misperception, misinterpretation, and misjudgment.

- *Expand one's cultural knowledge* and institutionalize it so that it can be accessed and incorporated into the delivery of services. We must attempt to seek out sociocultural information about the individual patient that will then help us have a better feel for how to perform an interview or history—what to ask, how to ask—and how to modify treatment interventions appropriately on the basis of a person's cultural reality. It is impossible, and unnecessary, to learn all there is to know about all cultural subgroups, but clinicians must be aware of the ethnographic information related to the local community and relevant beliefs and behaviors of their patients and the patients' families.

- *Adapt to diversity.* Therapists need to develop culturally sensitive examination and treatment techniques that allow a patient to be culturally comfortable. The clinic should be adapted to create a better fit between the needs of the people requiring services and those meeting their needs. It is important to remember what cultural competence is not. It is not abandoning your own culture and becoming a member of another culture by taking on their attitudes, values, and behaviors.
- Developing cultural competence is a lifelong process and all therapists will not be equally culturally competent. Cross et al[12] describe at least six possibilities along a continuum of cultural competence ranging from cultural destructiveness to cultural proficiency. Many therapists today are moving from stage 3 to 4.
- *Cultural blindness (stage 3)* presumes an unbiased philosophy and that all people are the same. Facility policy and practices do not recognize the need for culturally specific approaches to solve problems.
- *Cultural "pre-competence" (stage 4)* moves toward the more positive end of the continuum. Here therapists recognize weaknesses in the system or their personal cultural knowledge base and explore alternatives. There is a commitment to responding appropriately to differences.
- *Cultural competence (stage 5) and the last stage (stage 6), cultural proficiency* are where one recognizes the need to conduct research, disseminate the results, and develop new approaches that might increase culturally competent practice.

The goal of this chapter is to facilitate the process by which PTs can become culturally competent. Campinha-Bacote[7] has suggested four factors that contribute to a culturally competent model of care:

- Developing cultural awareness (cultural sensitivity). This includes becoming aware of and minimizing your cultural biases.
- Increasing cultural knowledge. Understanding the theoretical and conceptual frameworks for others' worldviews, and some of the details influencing daily life.
- Developing cultural skills. How do we assess and treat individuals appropriately?
- Experiencing cultural encounters. Exposure to people from different cultures and an opportunity to work with them toward achieving shared goals.

This chapter focuses primarily on the second factor of increasing your knowledge base so that cultural awareness and skill development can be facilitated. A cultural encounter is bound to occur in all work environments. Examples are derived from a variety of cultures and patient populations, emphasizing those you are more likely to come into contact with by virtue of national demographic trends or working in an outpatient orthopedic practice setting.

Terminology and Demographics

Terminology identifying individuals and groups of people is often controversial. From a sociocultural perspective, the term *ethnicity* is a better label than race. Ethnic identification is classified by common traits or customs. It is based on one's identity as belonging to a distinct behavioral or ideational group based on presumed shared cultural heritage. Ethnicity may be based on color, religion, one's own or ancestor's place of origin, language, or geographic territory. Race, a concept historically used to divide the world into three biological species, is an increasingly meaningless concept.

Broad categories are often a necessity for expedience but fail to represent subgroups and the presence of *intracultural* diversity and individuality. For example, the category *Asian* encompasses at least 18 subgroups and *Hispanic* or *Latino* encompasses more than 20 subgroups. There are more than 500 American Indian tribal groups in the United States. *Black* may refer to African Americans, Jamaicans, Nigerians, and so forth. There is also an enormous variety of individuality among white cultures. The term *Euro-American* encompasses people whose ancestors come from many European nations, including England, Italy, Greece, Poland, and so forth. Considerable individual differences exist within each of the aforementioned groups, that is, not all people from Mexico are the same. Assessment of the culture and of each patient as an individual is critical. The phrase *people of color* is often the preferred terminology used in the United States today for nonwhite individuals. According to census data, this combined group of people will become the majority over the next generations, and they will require rehabilitation services.[29]

In the year 2000, approximately 75% of the population of the United States was white; 12.5% black or African American; 12.5% Hispanic/Latino; 1% American Indian or Alaska native; 3.7% Asian, Native Hawaiian, or other Pacific Islander; 2.4% identified as two or more ethnic groups; and 5.5% identified as other. Between 1980 and 1990, the total U.S. population increased 9.8%, but the rate of growth varied widely: the Asian/Pacific Island population growth was 107.8%; Hispanic/Latino, 53%; American Indian, 37.9%; black, 13.2%; and white, 6%.[48,49] Between 1990 and 2000, this population trend continued. During the last two decades, there has been a tremendous influx of immigrants from South and Central America and Asia, and this trend is expected to continue. By far the greatest number of immigrants coming to the United States are Mexican. Also, birth rates are generally higher for Hispanics, especially Puerto Ricans.[48,49]

Understanding the 2000 census is somewhat complicated by the fact that, although seen as necessary by many, there were 63 possible ethnic categories from which to choose (to accommodate individuals who identify themselves in ways that are different from the classifications above or as multiracial) instead of the previously used five. Still, the trends are clear and the raw percentages speak for themselves.

By the year 2050, on the basis of immigration patterns and fertility rates, it is projected that white, non-Hispanic

Americans will represent approximately 53% of the total population, demonstrating a continued downward trend. Hispanic Americans will account for 24%, African Americans 15%, and Asian/Pacific Island Americans 9%.[50] Also relevant to the practice of outpatient physical therapy is the great increase in the population older than 65 years expected during the next decades. The relative increase will be greatest for people of color.

An additional consideration is the substantial disparity between the number of individuals from particular ethnic groups enrolled in health professional schools and their representation in the society as a whole. The American Physical Therapy Association estimates that approximately 10% of the membership are people of color.[1] Although moving in the right direction, the profession of physical therapy remains "diversity challenged." It is essential to realize that yes, it is best if professionals are proportionately represented within the treatment setting, but it is equally important for *all* therapists, no matter what their own ethnic background, to be culturally competent. Also, the didactic and clinical educational materials we have historically learned from are generally presented from a Western medical model/Eurocentric point of view with regard to disability, health, and illness. All this contributes to a less-than-ideal delivery of professional service to people from diverse backgrounds and can result in a cultural clash and conflicting expectations between patient and therapist.

A strong word of caution is in order. Broad categories as used above are practical for descriptive purposes, but they can perpetuate culturally biased racial or ethnic stereotyping and prejudices. Clearly, this is not the intent. Rather, the intent is to incorporate knowledge about the patient population, considering the extensive cultural landscape in which they live as well as their individual characteristics, to recognize *interethnic* and *intraethnic* diversity. In an orthopedic outpatient setting, generalization about an ethnic group is as inappropriate as generalizing about a frozen shoulder or torn knee ligament. If a patient came in with an unfamiliar diagnosis, you would obtain information about the problem. Similarly, it is appropriate to obtain information about the patient's cultural ways of life.

Cultural Considerations When Treating a Diverse Patient Population: Developing Cultural Competence

To facilitate the process of becoming culturally competent in physical therapy practice, especially in the primary health care setting, we must, in essence, perform a medical ethnography. Ethnography is the work of describing a culture with the aim of understanding another way of life from the native point of view. The ethnographer seeks to learn from a culture, be taught by the population, and discover the insider's, or emic, point of view rather than the outsider's, or etic, point of view.[45] This chapter introduces several variables that must be considered during the process of ethnography. Assessing each of these domains is critical so that the examination and treatment interventions may be appropriately modified on the basis of a person's cultural reality. The following subheadings never stand alone. Each is intertwined with the others.

This brief introduction to several variables should not be used to stereotype individuals but can be used as a starting point from which to assess further how we and our patients may view the world from different vantage points. We need to sense patterns and variations without overgeneralizing. Diversity and contradictions abound among populations. Clearly, improving our understanding of the many subcultures encountered in practice requires greater research of individual ethnic groups and different geographic regions. Further emphasis needs to be placed on the difficult task of parsing out the relative influence of biological/genetic factors from socioeconomic factors from cultural lifestyle habits.

Socioeconomic Status

Arguably, the most relevant variable affecting someone's worldview is socioeconomic status. Poverty is not randomly distributed through the population. Rather, it is strongly related to race or ethnicity, sex, and age. In the United States approximately 22% of African American families and 21% of Hispanic families live in poverty compared with 10.8% of Asian and Pacific Islanders and 7.5% of white families.[47] Although most poverty in this country is categorized as relative (i.e., people are able to afford basic necessities but are unable to maintain an average standard of living), it is commonly known that people who live in poverty have more health problems than people with higher incomes. Associated with poverty are many frequently cited obstacles to maintaining health, such as poor housing (or even homelessness) and environmental conditions, inadequate nutrition, harmful lifestyle habits, and lack of access to transportation and child care services. Furthermore, poverty is known to influence the use of and interaction with the health care system and the outcomes associated with health care.[9,39]

Specifically, in an outpatient setting hours of operation and available means of transportation if a patient does not have a car should be assessed. For example, hourly workers may not have the flexibility to take off from work during the typical workday, and public transportation may be less available at certain times. Can you assume that your patient has electricity or running water at home? Can resistive weights be bought or do you need to be creative by filling a bag with rocks or cans of food? Availability of resources should not be assumed.

The possibility of domestic violence should be on therapists' radar screens. Although not just a problem among low-income people, it is nevertheless an issue often associated with the stresses of poverty. Therapists working in a primary care environment need to be familiar with the signs and symptoms of abuse and helpful resources related to domestic violence. PTs might be the ones to first notice indications that abuse is present. Sensitivity to these socioeconomic and cultural issues can be tricky. How do you inquire without being insulting or taking away the patient's pride? Level of skill development can be especially important in this area.

Of obvious import to the primary health care outpatient practitioner is the patient's health insurance status and the impact of federal policy on Medicare and Medicaid. The changing economic and political landscape of the early 21st century will likely disproportionately affect low-income and less acculturated people of color because of their considerable reliance on these programs. The ethnic group most likely to be completely uninsured is the Hispanic population (more than one third of the population). Recent immigrants are also less likely to be insured.[46]

Racism

Although a detailed discussion of the effects of racism is outside the scope of this chapter, therapists must be cognizant of the marked effect of racism on health status and health care interactions.[9,42,43] For example, the collective experience of African Americans includes the Tuskegee syphilis study, sterilization initiatives, and sickle cell screening abuses, which have led to distrust of the medical profession by many black Americans.[4] According to a recent article by Schneider et al,[41] after adjustment for potential confounding factors, black Medicare beneficiaries enrolled in managed care plans were less likely than whites to receive eye examinations, beta-blocker medication after myocardial infarction, and follow-up after hospitalization for mental illness.

Degree of Acculturation

Acculturation is a process through which people in subcultures adopt traits of the larger, or normative, culture. Individuals range from being highly assimilated (in which the boundaries between the old and new culture are erased) to bicultural to highly traditional (in which values and behaviors are similar to those found in the country of origin). The degree to which people acculturate to the mainstream North American culture (heretofore the white, Anglo-Saxon, Protestant culture) is influenced by such things as age, level of education, number of years in a new country, and socioeconomic status and will affect a person's health status and interaction with the health care system.

The PT should be aware of the patient's migration history as one means to initiate an assessment of degree of acculturation. For example, Vietnamese who arrived in the United States during the mid-1970s were primarily well educated, upper class, Christian individuals escaping a repressive political regime. In contrast, during the 1980s Vietnamese immigrants were more likely to be escaping economic as well as political deprivation, and they had fewer economic resources, different and more considerable health problems, and a more marginalized social support system. A look at the migration history for the Cuban American population will reveal a similar distinction between the first and second waves of immigrants.[21]

Predictive of more traditional beliefs and behaviors are emigration from a rural area, frequent returns to the country of origin, limited formal education, poor English language skills, low socioeconomic status, recent immigration to the United States or immigration at an older age, and housing segregation. Typical ways to measure the degree of acculturation are based on language used within the home, the language of preferred media sources, and who makes up a primary support system.[21] Although you might not formally measure your patient's acculturation status, a primary care therapist can ask questions of the patient that will give a better understanding of the patient's degree of assimilation.

INCIDENCE AND PREVALENCE OF DISEASE AND DISABILITY. A primary care orthopedic physical therapy practice setting is likely going to treat people with a range of diagnoses, impairments, and functional disabilities. Disease and disability are not randomly distributed among human beings. Many factors, including race, ethnicity, socioeconomic status, geography, and migration history, play a role in determining the incidence and prevalence of disease and disability. Discovering the determinants of disease, that is, risk factors that relate to the development and cause of the condition, is a major aspect of epidemiologic work. Broadly speaking, risk factors can be related to inherited characteristics, environmental factors, or personal behavior and lifestyle.[5,26,36,43]

In the United States people of color have many more health problems than the white population.[9,42,51] They are also more likely to report poor health and more restricted activity than white people. Women are especially disadvantaged and report greater limitation in activities of daily living. People of color have a lower life expectancy, higher infant mortality rates, and higher morbidity and mortality rates for a wide range of diseases. Cardiovascular disease, hypertension, and strokes disproportionately affect African Americans. For example, the death rate for persons having a stroke is 52 per 100,000 for African American men and 39.9 per 100,000 for women (97.7% higher than white American men and 77.3% higher than white American women).[35] Approximately 85% of elderly Hispanics have one or more chronic diseases, such as diabetes (especially among Mexican Americans), arthritis, and depression, resulting in greater rates of morbidity and mortality. Chronic liver disease and AIDS are far more prevalent among blacks and Hispanics.[53]

The incidence of non-insulin-dependent diabetes mellitus (type 2) has shown an alarming increase during the last few years, especially among young and old American Indian, African American, and Hispanic populations. Family history, genetics, obesity, and age are key risk factors. An example of the interaction of both genetic and lifestyle variables is the implication of the so-called thrifty gene theory as it relates to Mexican American and American Indian diabetics. When particular tribes were seminomadic they frequently subsisted on a feast-or-famine diet. The tribes genetically developed an ability to metabolize their food efficiently. Today, when food is more abundant and likely to be high in fat and calories, and when exercise is less a part of daily living, a higher rate of obesity and diabetes occurs. People with more Indian admixture are more inclined to insulin resistance and the inability to break down glucose in the blood. On the positive side, some American Indians have the benefit of a gene that causes their blood sugar levels to respond to moderate exercise more quickly than others.[21,37,54]

Healthy People 2010, a guiding document for the U.S. Public Health Service, has as one of its three major goals the elimination of disparity between people of color and the white population.[52] PTs working in a cross-culture environment need to be knowledgeable about the variables affecting the incidence and prevalence of orthopedic and medical conditions so that they can be better prepared to treat these conditions, answer patient and family questions concerning the condition, and develop special preventive and educational programs targeted to those in need.

Comparative Value Orientations

In contrast to material culture, or the more easily observed and understood parts of culture (clothing, food, music, forms of greeting, ceremonial rites of passage), nonmaterial culture is more difficult to assess. Sometimes similarities in the material culture obscure profound differences in the nonmaterial culture that are relevant to the therapist-patient interaction. These value orientations are as important, or even more important, for the PT to pay attention to.

Many observers have identified recurrent themes and patterns in cultures (Table 3-1). These cultural elements may be the core of one's *worldview*, or values people live by. Typically, cultures that have been most heavily influenced by Euro-American values will match those cultural characteristics listed in the left column of Table 3-1, whereas those influenced by a Latin or Hispanic, Asian, Middle Eastern or African culture, for example, will fit the characteristics listed on the right. However, worldview can be heavily influenced by personality traits and socioeconomic and acculturation status. Also, people do not necessarily fit into a rigid category; some may fall at the far end of one dichotomous scale, in the middle for a second, or at the other end for a third.

If forced to choose one contrasting element for these two columns, it would arguably be an individualist society versus a collectivist society. These adjectives symbolize general social organization and relationships and can be linked to many of the other values listed. There are innumerable ways in which these characteristics can influence the therapeutic encounter. For example, Euro-American values emphasize the importance of the individual and the ability of each person to affect his or her future through hard work. In this type of cultural orientation,

both time and nature are commodities to be used profitably and the success—or lack of success—of each person is credited to that individual. Professionals with this type of cultural value system would emphasize the autonomy and personal responsibility of their patients and expect them to work hard while in therapy. Desires and expectations would be clearly stated in a direct manner.

In contrast, patients may have a cultural value system that emphasizes the importance of the group over the individual. In the Hispanic culture, possibly the most significant value is that of *familismo*. Consistent with a collectivist society, the emphasis is on family commitment and responsibility. The welfare and honor of the family are preeminent concerns. The father is typically the final arbiter of decision making. The mother is central within the household and is responsible for child rearing and cultural and social stability.[40] Kinship bonds across generations are common. Thus a patient may arrive at the clinic with several family members and feel there is little point to working too hard because they will be cared for by the family, and much of what happens to people—including disability—is predetermined by fate. For both of you to save face they might act politely and be accommodating when, in fact, they may not understand your instructions or know that your goals and theirs are not in sync. Other cultural values associated with the Hispanic culture include *personalismo* (friendliness), *simpatia* (kindness, avoid conflict; sympathy), and *fatalismo* (fatalism).

Core cultural values associated with African Americans include community and connection to ancestors and history, religion and spiritualism, oral expressiveness, commitment to family, and intuition and experience.[5] Core cultural values of Asian people are associated with the teachings of Buddhism, Taoism, and Confucianism. Harmony between and among human beings and nature is critical.[44]

Perhaps the most difficult cultural differences to overcome in an outpatient orthopedic clinic, especially for North Americans, relates to pace of life and notion of time.[20] The different views on the importance of an appointment time can have profound psychologic and business impact. Monochronism is the view that events happen in chronologic order, work tasks and socialization are separate, and adherence to schedules is important. Euro-Americans are monochronic: they are action oriented and are often unforgiving about such things as missed appointments and a casual approach to punctuality, "red tape," bureaucratic delays, and the sense that time is an unimportant concept.

Polychronism, on the other hand, is the view that events can happen concurrently and that fixed schedules are insignificant. The focus is on a more personal interaction, with less concern toward completion of the task at hand. With the Hispanic patient as an example, there is the value for *personalismo*, or a more humanistic approach. The attention to a work orientation and the acquisition of material goods may not be present among individuals who more highly value a relaxed, human relationship–oriented lifestyle. Imagine the potential for misunderstanding if a Cuban patient, for example, arrives late for an appointment and expects the therapist to chat for a few minutes about nontherapeutic issues, such as the well-being of

TABLE 3-1	
Comparative Value Orientations	
Euro-American	**Cross-Cultural Comparison**
Individualism/privacy	Collectivism/group welfare
Personal control over environment	Fate
Time dominates	Human interaction dominates
Precise time reckoning	Loose time reckoning
Future orientation	Past orientation
Doing (working, achieving)	Being (personal qualities)
Human equality	Hierarchy/rank/status
Self-help	Birthright inheritance
Competition	Cooperation
Informality	Formality
Directness/openness/honesty	Indirectness/ritual/"face"
Practicality/efficiency	Idealism/theory
Materialism	Spiritualism
Values youth	Values elders
Relative equality of sexes	Relative inequality of sexes

Adapted from Ferraro[16] and Lynch and Hanson.[32]

his family, and the therapist, already annoyed about her schedule being interrupted, immediately launches into a discussion about how to do exercises. In a rehabilitation setting, even the development of group exercise programs may be influenced by comparative value systems. For example, does the patient value competition or cooperation?

The role and status of medical personnel may be different depending on cultural orientation. A patient from a Middle Eastern culture would more naturally defer to the health professional, who is considered an authority figure worthy of high esteem. An interactive conversation about health options is less likely to occur.

Comparative value systems may affect behaviors around a particular age group of patients. For instance, there may be particular expectations of Asian American adolescents that are different from those of a typical Euro-American adolescent. In contrast to how young children are obliged and indulged, older children are expected to be well disciplined and to take on some adult roles. An older, adolescent sibling may be expected to accept personal sacrifice and assume child care for young children in the extended family, while at the same time maintaining a strong academic record. A sense of duty or obligation to the family may be pronounced, and this is learned through proper role modeling. If there is misbehavior by a younger sibling, an older sibling might be rebuked for not setting a good example. High expectations may be a source of stress. Adolescents are likely to be recipients of a parenting style that is somewhat controlling, restrictive, and protective. This may lead to distancing behaviors or distrust of outsiders. Discussions about sensitive topics such as sexuality may be avoided, and the willingness to discuss personal issues related to treatment can be minimal.[32]

Similarly, special considerations may be necessary when working with elder or terminal patients that reflect a particular worldview. Widespread respect for elders is prevalent among many ethnic groups. Signs of respect may include use of the terms "Ma'am" or "Sir" or asking for tales of wisdom. Although the orthopedic primary care PT is not typically faced with discussions regarding end-of-life decisions, this is still a possible topic of conversation, especially with family members. Of note, in Asian and Hispanic cultures disclosure of a terminal disease may take away any hope that the patient may have. Family members have a strong obligation to protect loved ones from emotional distress.

Furthermore, elder adults are likely to have variations in attitudes toward advance directives. For example, Chinese elders may be less likely to write something down because they honor the spoken word. In actuality, Chinese elders commonly do not discuss the likelihood of death at all because it is believed to be a bad omen. The Navajo feel similarly. Negative thoughts would be in conflict with the concept of "hozho," which involves goodness, harmony, and positive attitude. Japanese elders place great faith in family and professional relationships, and it is less likely that individual decision-making would be a norm. Children, particularly the oldest son, feel the duty to maintain a parent's life. For the Navajo as well, major decisions are collaborative, and family and tribespeople would have input into any advance health directives.[4]

African Americans who have been socioeconomically marginalized tend to be more likely to desire life-sustaining treatment and are less likely to desire or receive hospice care. In contrast, white people are more likely to feel empowered and in control, which may account for their greater willingness to forgo life-sustaining treatment.[4] Finally, considering a person's value system may influence whether accepting a gift from a patient or their family is ethically appropriate. In many cultures it would be a great insult to refuse a gift; a person's pride may be at stake.

Communication

Communication, language, cultural value orientations, and culture overall are intertwined and inseparable. Thus communication is an additional exceptionally important variable when working cross culturally or seeking to understand one's cultural value system and explanatory model. In addition to the obvious problems encountered when the provider and patient do not speak the same language, it is imperative to understand that both obvious and subtle differences in the interactive styles of the people exist. For example, verbal communication in individualistic societies is associated with direct, "low-context" communication. It is expected that someone will get right to the point, and it is assumed that surrounding context is not necessary for interpretation. Rather, what is heard in the verbal message is what is being communicated. The notion of privacy is important, and questions of a more personal nature might be considered off-limits.

In contrast, a person from a collectivist culture may speak indirectly, in a more circular fashion, always keeping in mind the need for everyone to "save face." The Hispanic culture, for example, will rely more on *indirectas*. Communication is more high context, or sensitive to situational and contextual features. There is a more spiral logic, more indirect verbal negotiation, and subtle nonverbal nuances. The notion of privacy is less pervasive, but this must take into account the idea of not embarrassing someone or causing either party to "lose face." The focus is more on human relationships. People are especially more reluctant to express negative feelings and unlikely to share concerns about taking medication ordered by a physician or ask questions that may be perceived as stupid.[6]

Another difference in verbal communication is the amount of "wait time," or pace of conversation. American Indians typically have a slower pace of conversation, which requires waiting until the person has finished speaking before interrupting or asking questions. Euro-Americans are typically uncomfortable with silence. Wait time is also increased if patients need to translate the words into their own language in their minds before responding.[28] In some cultures, many people may speak at once.

Many nonverbal, observable differences exist in communication style between different cultural groups. As much as 93% of the total meaning of an encounter is communicated by nonverbal factors.[34] Differences occur regarding eye contact, facial expression, body movement, comfortable distance zones, and overall formality. The PT may believe a patient is acting disinterested if eye contact is not direct, yet the patient may believe it is impolite to look directly at someone perceived as the authority figure. A white therapist may firmly shake the hand of a American Indian or traditional Asian patient on introduction and may presume this is an appropriate, friendly, polite gesture. The patient may consider this aggressive or hostile because he is more used to a subtle, soft, nonthreatening handshake.

What is the preferred distance zone for your patient? How close does the patient like to stand when speaking with you? It is wise to observe your patient's response when you stand closer or further away during a general conversation. During a treatment session, does a person of the opposite sex seem more uncomfortable than you might expect? Have you observed how those from a different culture act with each other compared with how they may act with you? Touch can provide reassurance and kindness or it can be a discomfort and annoyance. Gender and age are important variables influencing distance zones.

The PT who is educating a patient about a diagnosis or a home program must also recognize that methods of teaching and learning differ between cultures. Knowledge transmission in Euro-American cultures, for example, often relies on taking notes and studying written texts, as well as intense discussions with a great deal of interaction between therapist and patient. Other cultures rely more on a straight lecture format with few questions and little discussion. And other cultural groups, such as African Americans, rely almost entirely on oral training and demonstration. A written list of exercises, even with diagrams, may not be as effective as "hearing and feeling" such exercises. Typically, family members should be included in a discussion about a home program and prevention of further problems.[31,32]

It is obviously ideal for the therapist and patient to speak the same language, but it is often not possible. Therapists should learn at least a few key words in the patient's language but realize there are often differences in dialects and accents between and within countries. More typically, family (often children) or friends act as translators. Although this may be the only available alternative, it is fraught with problems. Be aware that you are now dealing with an untrained third party who may be interpreting the information before passing it on to you, or there may be topics that are inappropriate to discuss with the translator because they are more personal or sensitive in nature (e.g., family planning, spousal abuse, terminal illness). Interpretation requires knowledge of medical terminology, a good memory, ability to concentrate, and the ability to know how and when to edit messages so that the true meaning of the interpretation can be accurately transmitted. If possible, a professional translator should be used. A professional interpreter is likely to be bicultural and have a good grasp of the medical and cultural nuances.

Any written materials should be translated in grammatically correct, simple language with appropriate, meaningful vocabulary so that it may be used for its intended purpose and be culturally relevant to the patient. Always translate it back into the original language to verify accuracy.

Because language barriers are such a significant and prevalent obstacle to good health care, the Office of Civil Rights within the U.S. Department of Health and Human Services has developed policies for individuals with limited English proficiency. These include assistance options appropriate to each facility's needs. Massachusetts is the first state to require the services of competent interpreters for those with limited English proficiency, and more states are expected to follow suit.[11]

The key question is how to best develop rapport with patients to enhance the likelihood of both the patient and therapist being satisfied with an encounter. Understanding a range of communication styles—both verbal and nonverbal—and the ability to interpret an interaction properly and engage in good communication will undoubtedly minimize barriers that may otherwise exist.

Health Beliefs and Behaviors

Historically, the available models for the provision of care have generally relied on the values and belief systems of the "majority"; that is, the white, middle-class person. These models have been culturally insensitive by denying the realities of non-Western systems of thinking. Although it is recognized that biomedicine and its professionals have a lot to offer, there is an increased awareness of the limitations of a system based solely on a biological understanding of the human being. In the pluralistic medical systems that exist throughout the world, a range of health care beliefs and behaviors, as well as practitioners, is present.

When working in a multicultural environment, PTs must make an effort to understand how people in different cultures and social groups explain the causes of ill health, the types of treatment they believe in, and to whom they turn if they do get ill. One process of medical ethnography through which local health care systems are analyzed has been developed by Arthur Kleinman, a psychiatrist and medical anthropologist.[25] Specifically, Kleinman has developed the theory of an "explanatory model" (EM) to analyze such things as patterns of belief about the causes of illness, decisions about how to respond to specific episodes of sickness, and actions taken to effect a change. "EMs are the notions about an episode of sickness and its treatment that are employed by all those engaged in the clinical process. The study of patient and family EMs tells us how they make sense of given episodes of illness, and how they choose and evaluate particular treatments."[25]

Open-ended questions should be used to allow patients to explain and expand on their situations based on their own perceptions of a particular illness or condition. The therapist can ask the patient such things as "What do you call your problem?" "What do you think caused your problem?" "What are the greatest problems your illness has caused for you?" "What do you fear most about the consequences of this illness?" "What are the most important results you hope to get from your treatment?" Kleinman's EM is considered an internal, clinical view of the patient's cultural health care system. Because the EM is recognized to depend on many variables—such as societal attitudes toward the sick and disabled, the degree to which the disabled are stigmatized, the material realities of the environment, and the adaptation mechanisms that are available—it is necessary to analyze EMs in a concrete setting.

Presumably, for persons with a disease or disability and their families, there are specific medical care systems and explanatory models that account for the beliefs about the impairment and the cultural patterns of behaviors relating to diagnosis and treatment. Although PTs need to focus on the patient EM, it is essential to explore and understand that we as healers also have an EM and operate within our own distinct culture. Thus to enhance the relationship between interacting parties and to affect the outcome of an interaction positively, the culture of both the patient and practitioner must be taken into account. Patients and their families cannot always completely comply with the practitioner EM, and the health professional cannot always accept the patient EM.

Much variation exists in culturally perceived causes of chronic illness or disability.[17-19,24] Patients may have a naturalistic or supernatural belief system. One naturalistic explanation by a Jamaican mother of a child was "jaundice at birth and she premature. The hospital didn't have the facilities for the jaundice, to burn it out, so the jaundice damage her."[30] A different mother, when asked why she believed her child had a disability, answered "like how I have the children fast, and the food me eat. Maybe I did need more nutritious food . . . . Me had a problem with me big daughter . . . sent her to buy shoes and she run away with a guy and she never come back until long after the baby born. I was very worried." In actuality, this child had Down syndrome, so the explanation is not scientifically feasible.[30]

Although scientific rationales may exist, traditional beliefs are in some patients' cultural backgrounds and may be brought to the forefront during times of stress or uncertainty. In some instances, individuals believe that disability is a form of punishment. A person may have sinned or violated a taboo, either in this life or a previous life, thereby causing the wrath of God or a source of wickedness. Throughout much of the world, there is belief in the evil eye. Generally, the concept implies that an evil spell has been put on a victim, which causes the person to fall ill. The motive is usually envy. As quoted by Mardiros[33] in an article about disability in Mexico, one informant stated "Before we were married my husband had a lot of women. One of them asked this lady to put a hex on us. She's a bruja [sorcerer or witch]. Because of her we always had bad luck. People are so mean these days . . ."

Alternatively, in some cultures an imbalance of elements, or humors, may be responsible for the ailment. In the Asian Indian Ayurvedic system, health is equated with balance. Similarly, traditional Chinese medicine requires a balance of yin and yang. The Navajo believe that their health depends on harmony with family, community, self, and nature; they do not have the concept of communicable disease. The Navajo language does not have a word for *germ*.[4] In some communities, importance is placed on a balance of hot and cold. These mutually complementary forces are required to be in harmony with nature.

Treatment for a disease or disability is also culture specific, although intraethnic variation abounds. Indigenous healers, or practitioners of traditional medicine, are prevalent in every

society. The *espiritismos* may be the preferred source of care for the Puerto Rican. *Espiritismo* involves the belief in the importance of the spiritual world, and "do unto others as you would have them do unto you" is considered the highest ethical principle. The *espiritista*, usually a female medium, helps patients with both physical and emotional problems by connecting with good spirits and exorcising evil spirits.[35] The *curanderos* may be preferred for the Mexican American, the singer for the Navajo, the voodoo priest for the Haitian, and the herbalist for the Chinese. For the Laotian Hmong, the *shaman* may use herbal concoctions and animal sacrifice.[14] For Jamaicans, the *obeah* may use such materials as blood, feathers, parrots' beak, grave dirt, egg shell, and medicinal herbs to treat a person with a disability.[30] For American Indians "talking circles," where stories are shared, are used to demonstrate the interconnectedness of life, the cycle of life and death, and the balance required for good health. They may be used to educate about preventive and treatment measures so that the notion of fatalism can be replaced with the idea of control over one's health.[37]

There are two theoretical explanations for why ritual healing practices may be successful. One is neurobiological. There is increasing evidence that endorphins may play a role in diminishing pain. These neurochemicals produced by the brain may be released by psychological experiences. Alternatively, the placebo effect may help the body to heal itself. A placebo may be word or action, not just a pharmaceutical substance. By engaging the patient's mind and emotions, the healer may aid physiological repair.[35]

Traditional practices may also influence the response of a patient to a suggested Western medical protocol. Many Vietnamese believe that Western medicine is designed to suit the body size of Westerners. Thus the quantity prescribed may be seen as inappropriate for the typical Vietnamese, who is much smaller than the typical American.[27] Likewise, many Hispanic and Asian people classify substances as hot or cold. These categorizations affect the patient's decision regarding what medicines to use and foods to eat. For example, the therapist working in the area of women's health might want to know that there may be special considerations associated with childbirth. Within the traditional Asian culture, a woman who is pregnant or has recently given birth may have a diet with selected hot or cold foods. During the first trimester of pregnancy, a woman may eat "hot" foods such as eggs, meat, black pepper, or ginger. In the second trimester, she eats "cold" foods such as squash, fruits, bean curd, sugar, and herbal tea. During the last trimester, when she is in a "hot period," "hot" foods or medicines are strictly limited. During the entire pregnancy, shellfish, lamb, and rabbit are forbidden. Immediately postpartum, during the "cold" period, there is a specific taboo against some "cold" foods. Different Asian cultures prepare special dishes to assist with the involution of the uterus, chase the "bad blood" away, and regulate menstrual flow. In the Cambodian culture, a postpartum mother may be placed on a slatted bed with a heat source under the bed. The practice is referred to as "mother roasting" and it is meant to replace the heat lost during childbirth. Going out of doors, drinking cold water, washing the hair, and taking a shower are also not advised.[8]

Clinicians should not assume that the father will take part in labor and delivery. Although presence of the father is common among Euro-Americans, in many cultures childbirth is not a "family" matter, but a job for the woman and her female support system. Social roles are separate, and other female family members or women trained specifically to assist with childbearing and child care are deemed more appropriate.[8]

The use of an alternative treatment is often the source of misunderstanding and conflict. Asian practices used to draw evil from the body, such as coin rubbing—in which a coin is rubbed on the skin until a raised red mark appears—or cupping—when a heated glass is placed on the body to create a vacuum, causing the skin to raise and become red—may be perceived as harmful to a child by a Western practitioner. The traditional Hmong harbor superstitions toward American health practitioners. Some Hmong believe that surgeons cut out body parts of the deceased to sell them as food or eat them themselves.[14]

Even when using typical Western physical therapy treatment procedures it is necessary to consider the appropriateness of that treatment within the context of the patient's culture. For example, in many Asian cultures people usually squat rather than sit, thus necessitating greater range of motion even at the expense of stability. Also, eating with hands or chopsticks may require different movement patterns and range than those typically used by Westerners.

Especially relevant to the PT working with patients who have a wide range of orthopedic impairments is the notion that pain means different things to people from various ethnic groups and that their response to pain is guided by cultural rules. Research on the psychosocial and behavioral aspects of pain has found a significant relation between ethnic variation and perception of pain intensity and the responses to pain.

Zborowski[56] in his famous study compared different white populations, including Jewish, Italian, Irish, and "old" or "Yankee" Americans, and determined that in some groups it was permissible to complain about pain whereas other groups were expected to report pain in a dispassionate manner. Members of some groups wanted immediate relief of pain with painkillers, whereas others worried more about the long-term implications of pain and did not want medications for fear that pharmacologic treatment would mask a more serious problem. Societal rules also promote gender or age differences regarding pain tolerance, but these are not cultural universals.

During the late 1980s, Bates and Edwards[3] completed a similar study to determine patient meanings and explanations associated with pain. American-born white (mostly Protestant), Hispanic, Irish, Italian, French Canadians, and Polish people, all of whom were outpatients in a Massachusetts pain treatment facility, were studied. Variation in ethnic identity and locus of control style was consistently associated with differences in pain intensity and response. The Hispanic group demonstrated the highest pain expressiveness, the greatest interference with work and social activities, and the highest degree of emotional and psychological stress. The Italian group was second in each of these categories, and either the Polish or "old" American group was the lowest in each category. The notion of interethnic group variation was supported.

Nevertheless, intragroup variation analysis demonstrates within-group differences on the basis of both generation and degree of heritage consistency. More recent immigrants or first-generation American-born, who have high degrees of heritage consistency and who believe that they have a strong support system, report less severe responses to pain. Thus the notion of intraethnic variation is supported as well.

Looking more closely at one particular group, Santana and Santana[40] cite a 1995 study by Villarruel, who identified the ways in which Mexican Americans experience pain. Beliefs about pain include (1) pain is an accepted and expected part of life; (2) pain does not negate one's responsibilities and duties; (3) pain is predetermined by the gods; (4) pain is a consequence of immoral behavior; (5) pain should be endured with a stoic attitude; and (6) pain may best be alleviated by maintaining balance. PTs need to contemplate the meaning of pain for an individual patient.

PTs serving as primary health care practitioners would also benefit from knowledge about their patients' dietary practices. There is profound social and cultural meaning, as well as nutritional value, in food. Specific foods for the African American community are identified as "soul food." These may be unhealthy from a nutritional perspective but significant to an individual, representing a rich cultural history and memories. It is unlikely that a person will completely alter their eating habits on your suggestion to eat more healthily. Finding a compromise is likely the best solution.

Practices that can appear in pregnant African American women are pica (eating inedible substances such as laundry starch) and geophagy ("earth eating"). Eating clay or dirt is a practice brought from Africa during slavery and was presumed beneficial to both mother and unborn child. In fact, red clay is rich in iron. In more recent times, since working on a farm is less common, laundry starch may be substituted.[44]

Health beliefs and behaviors that are closely intertwined with comparative value systems relate to the role that religion plays in one's EM. Religious beliefs and customs may affect the acceptance and the administration of more orthodox rehabilitation-related practices. This may be an area in which the PT has difficulty accepting someone else's moral and ethical viewpoint and actions. A common point of conflict is the willingness of a practitioner to accept the refusal of a Jehovah's Witness to allow a medical intervention if it involves the need for a blood transfusion. Another common frustration occurs when a patient has a strong faith in the ability of their supreme spiritual being (God, Allah, Brahma, etc.) to cure them, thus avoiding any other treatments. It may be less than ideal from a therapist's perspective if a Lubavitcher orthodox Jew turns to a *rebbe* for healing prayers or an African American to a "tent meeting." From the Mexican study, in which the respondents were Roman Catholic, "the most commonly reported cultural prescription was prayer through which children were given spiritually to either the patron saint or the Lady of Guadeloupe. Through the fulfillment of vows and pilgrimages, by offering the child to God, cutting off one's hair, ceasing drinking, becoming dedicated to the child and family, the child would be ensured a perpetual place next to God."[33]

A fascinating domain unlikely to be familiar to the PT is that of culture-bound syndromes, sometimes referred to as folk illnesses. These culture-specific syndromes exist in most cultures and are associated with unique beliefs about the cause of an illness and specific prescribed treatments. *Susto* is the most studied culture-bound psychosomatic illness within Hispanic cultures. *Susto*, or "shock," refers to a magical fright or soul loss, which happens when a frightening event causes the soul to leave the body. Symptoms include sleepiness, loss of appetite, insomnia, and generalized depression and are considered body metaphors for psychological distress. Other culture-bound syndromes within the Hispanic community include *emphacho* (stomach aches, diarrhea, vomiting, and fever are symptoms of having eaten an inappropriate food, which is said to "stick" to the stomach lining), *envidia* (set off when a person is envious of another), and *mal aire* (bad air caused by an evil wind, with symptoms similar to those of a cold or flu).[35,38]

A culture-bound syndrome from the Haitian culture is "arrested pregnancy syndrome," in which a woman who is expected to be carrying a child and feels as though she is pregnant actually is not. It is often associated with infertility in a culture that highly values the ability to have children.[10] Anorexia nervosa, a psychological disorder with which most PTs are familiar, is considered a North American culture-bound syndrome.[2]

It is expected that most people, to varying degrees, intertwine modern or Western medicine with indigenous or folk medicine. People are more likely to partake in indigenous practices if they are less acculturated, poorer, and more rural based. Family and a hierarchy of lay healers are often the first line of defense. Practical matters such as cost, seriousness of illness, and availability of practitioners often determine the use of traditional practices. This results in medical pluralism, or the existence and use of many different health care alternatives within societies.[13,55]

The PT should learn as much as possible about the relevant traditional practitioners in his or her community. Most patients do not report the use of complementary and alternative medicines to their health provider, so the PT must ask the right questions.[4] To learn more, ask the patient to bring you to a session with a traditional healer or take you to the local *botanica* (store for herbal remedies and religious items in a Hispanic community). Only if the traditional healer prescribes an unhealthy, dangerous remedy should the PT be concerned. Why not think in terms of multiple treatment options—each serving its own purpose? The best scenario, in theory, involves the therapist serving as a "culture broker" between the patient, the traditional healers, and the mainstream health care system.

Expanded information on particular cultural group beliefs and behaviors can be accessed from the resources found in the Suggested Readings.

More Practical Strategies to Facilitate Cultural Competence

The information in this chapter provides the PT with knowledge to enhance cultural competence. The following additional practical strategies are offered to encourage a climate in which multiculturalism is the norm. Multiculturalism encompasses cultures that differ in age, color, ethnicity, sex, national origin, political ideology, race, religion, and sexual orientation and includes the presence and participation of those with disabilities and those from differing socioeconomic backgrounds.

Moving Toward Becoming a Culturally Competent Organization and Workplace
HUMAN/PERSONNEL CONSIDERATIONS

- Does the organization know the patient demographic data?
- What is the ethnic background of the staff and the board of directors?
- If you drew an organizational chart, what would it look like? Who is in a position of power? Who is at the bottom of the hierarchy?
- Who is the "face to the wider world" for the organization? Who travels for the organization?
- Are the employee benefits meeting the needs of individuals with unique circumstances?
- Is there a commitment to ongoing discussion and training on issues of cultural competence on the staff/board level?
- Has the organization established collegial and collaborative relationships with other relevant community groups to improve the health status of patients?
- Are there clear recruitment and retention/affirmative action goals for the organization? Does everyone in the organization understand the meaning of affirmative action and know these goals?
- Do the white people in the organization value working in a diverse setting? How is this evident?
- Is there a safe forum for people to learn how they may have unknowingly excluded or slighted their colleagues?
- Has anyone ever been rewarded in any way for their efforts to become culturally competent? Has anyone in the organization ever been penalized in any way for their inappropriate behavior?
- Is there a specific survey to assess patient and staff satisfaction with the facility and personnel?
- Has the organization hired a bicultural translator as necessary?
- Has the organization become aware of the state, federal, and professional organization standards requiring cultural competence?*

---

*For example, to ensure that the health care system better responds to the needs of an increasingly diverse patient population, the U.S. Department of Health and Human Services Office of Minority Health has developed national standards for culturally and linguistically appropriate services. The 14 standards are organized by themes: Culturally Competent Care (standards 1 to 3), language access services (4 to 7), and organizational supports for cultural competence (8 to 14). Although these standards are intended to be inclusive of all cultures, they are particularly designed to assist in the elimination of racial and ethnic health disparities in the United States by making the health care environment more inviting to those groups who historically have experienced unequal access to health services.[15] Specific ways to put culturally and linguistically appropriate services into action are found in the document. For example, standard 2 states that diversity is a necessary but not sufficient condition to achieve a culturally competent organization. The notion of a diverse staff includes all personnel from maintenance to administrative to medical professionals. The use of proactive incentives, mentoring programs, staff education, and training are all given forethought to avoid the need for resolution of conflict.

ENVIRONMENTAL CONSIDERATIONS

- What images decorate the space?
- What magazines are placed in public meeting spaces and/or in the waiting area? Are publications in more than one language? Do pictures in the literature look like the people who frequent the facility?
- Are the signs around the workplace in more than one language?
- What types of foods are served at group gatherings?
- Does the organization follow the Christian calendar? (Are Christian holidays observed as holidays for everyone?)
- Who considers the "fun" days (group picnics, parties, dinners, etc.) fun?
- Is the workplace fully wheelchair accessible?

Moving From Concern to Action: Personal Inventory

- Have I consciously thought about my own cultural identity and come to realize how much it is a part of who I am? For example, does my name have a relationship to my ancestors' ethnic identity? What belongings in my home are meaningful to me and why? Do my preferences regarding food, music, clothes, and so forth give an indication of who I am? Do I have health beliefs and behaviors that have been passed down to me from my ancestors?
- Have I spent some time reflecting on my own childhood and upbringing and analyzing where, how, and when I was receiving cultural, ethnocentric, and racist messages?
- Have I spent some time recently looking at my own attitudes and behaviors as an adult to determine how I am contributing to or combating ethnocentrism?
- Have I intentionally and aggressively sought to educate myself further on issues of culture, bias, and racism by talking with others, viewing films and videos, finding reading material, attending lectures, or joining a study group?
- Have I evaluated my use of language, light and dark imagery, and other terms or phrases that might be degrading or hurtful to others?
- Have I grown in my awareness of subliminal messages in television programs, advertising, and news coverage?
- Have I supported political candidates or contributed financially to an agency, fund, or program that actively confronts the problems of inequality and discrimination or enhances my patients' likelihood of receiving more culturally competent health care?
- Have I worked directly or indirectly to dispel misconceptions, stereotypes, prejudices, and other adverse feelings that members of one group have against members of another group? For example, have I openly disagreed with an insensitive comment, joke, reference, or action among those around me?
- Have I taken the initiative in dispelling prejudices, stereotypes, and misunderstandings among staff and discouraging or preventing patterns of informal discrimination, segregation, or exclusion of individuals?
- Do I listen with an open mind to staff members of other groups, even if their communications are initially disturbing or divergent from my own thinking?

Moving From Concern to Action: Professional Inventory

- Have I asked my patients appropriate questions about their culture and way of life and let them know I have a lot to learn?
- Have I considered doing research that includes people of diverse backgrounds to enable the profession of physical therapy to become more culturally proficient? For example, have I considered the need for assessment tools that address culture-specific functional tasks such as squatting or eating with chopsticks?
- Have I made overtures toward traditional healers to collaborate and increase my understanding of their ideas and ways?
- Does my clinic conduct inspire patients to respect one another and be open and honest in their communications with others and me?

Culture Shock

When working cross-culturally, "culture shock" can be experienced. The term describes the more pronounced reactions to the psychological disorientation most people have when immersed in a culture markedly different from their own. Culture shock is a cyclical phenomenon in which one moves through four basic phases of adjustment: excitement in a new environment, withdrawal and hostility, adjustment and appreciation of differences, and adaptation.[24]

In a sense, culture shock is an occupational hazard of cross-cultural immersion. There are no easy remedies, but there are some things you can do to help lessen its impact. Admitting your ethnocentrism and understanding your own culture are the first steps. Also, continue to learn about the particular cultures that you work with. Ask questions and be astute in your observations. Have realistic expectations of yourself and others and remember that problems and challenges are inevitable.

What personal characteristics are likely to foster a more successful cross-cultural encounter? High on the list are a sense of adventure, patience, flexibility, tolerance for ambiguity and difference, a sense of humor, and cultural sensitivity. Ironically, many successful professionals have some of the characteristics that are not conducive to working cross-culturally. That is, we are task oriented, overachievers, and fearful of failure. It is important to acknowledge that although almost all PTs are likely to work with patients who are culturally different from themselves, not all are equally suitable for working cross-culturally.

Summary

In the new millennium, national population patterns will continue to shift and practitioners will increasingly be required to share and practice their knowledge and skills in less familiar multicultural settings. The challenges to delivering effective and humanistic care will become even greater than they are today. Do not underestimate the obstacles to achieving the goal of cultural competence. Yet competency in recognizing bias, prejudice, discrimination, and our own discomfort when faced with difference and using cultural resources and overcoming cultural barriers can be learned. PTs must be cognizant of usable strategies to minimize existing barriers between people from different cultural contexts and seek ways to make therapeutic goals and the patients' or families' goals compatible rather than conflicting. An understanding of the macro and micro level sociocultural variables in the health care setting and an individual patient's worldview should lead to an improved clinical encounter. Health professionals increasingly understand that health care interaction that incorporates negotiation and preservation of cultural health-related beliefs and practices will likely increase treatment adherence and self-efficacy for both parties.[23] As Ibrahim[22] proposes, "Each individual in a professional-consumer dyad [should] be viewed as a unique 'cultural entity' with an emphasis on the individual's 'subjective reality' or worldview . . . . [This] can lead to professional-consumer cultural matching."

In essence, the "culture of rehabilitation" needs to change and adapt in response to the environment and conditions present in a particular time and place. So it is that the PT is increasingly becoming skilled as a primary health care practitioner. The path of intercultural learning to cultural proficiency takes a long time and conscious effort. The challenge of embracing diversity and differences, reshaping practice protocols, redefining research priorities, and developing the most appropriate service models and public policy to benefit the patient must be faced.

REFERENCES

1. APTA Office of Minority and International Affairs, *APTA minority membership statistics,* Washington, DC, 2002, American Physical Therapy Association.
2. Basch P: *Textbook of international health,* Oxford, 1999, Oxford University Press.
3. Bates M, Edwards WT: Ethnic variations in the chronic pain experience. In Brown P, ed: *Understanding and applying medical anthropology,* Mountain View, Calif, 1998, Mayfield Publishing.
4. Berger J: Culture and ethnicity in clinical care, *Arch Intern Med* 158: 2085-2090, 1998.
5. Braithwaite R, Taylor S, eds: *Health issues in the black community,* San Francisco, 2001, Jossey Bass.
6. Brice A, Campbell L: Cross-cultural communication. In Leavitt R, ed: *Cross-cultural rehabilitation: An international perspective,* Philadelphia, 1999, WB Saunders.
7. Campinha-Bacote J: *The process of cultural competence: A culturally competent model of care,* Wyoming, Ohio, 1994, Transcultural C.A.R.E Associates.
8. Chan S: Families with Asian roots. In Lynch E, Hanson M, eds: *Developing cross-cultural competence,* Baltimore, Md, 1998, Paul Brookes.
9. Collins K, Hughes D, Doty M, et al: *Diverse communities, common concerns: Assessing health care quality for minority Americans,* New York, 2002, The Commonwealth Fund.
10. Coreil J, Barnes-Josiah D, Augustin A, et al: Arrested pregnancy syndrome in Haiti: Findings from a national survey, *Medical Anthropology Q* 10: 424-436, 1996.
11. *Closing the gap.* Washington, DC, February/March 2001, Office of Minority Health and Science, U.S. Department of Health and Human Services.
12. Cross TL, Bazron BJ, Dennis KW, et al: *Towards a culturally competent system of care,* vol 1, Washington, DC, 1989, National Technical Assistance Center for Children's Mental Health, Georgetown University.
13. Fabrega H: *Disease and social behavior: An interdisciplinary perspective,* Cambridge, Mass, 1974, MIT Press.
14. Fadiman A: *The spirit catches you and you fall down: a Hmong child, and her American doctors, and the collision of two cultures,* New York, 1997, Farrar, Straus & Giroux.
15. Federal Register (vol 65, number 247, pp 80865-80879), Washington, DC, Dec. 22, 2000, Office of Minority Health, Public Health Service, U.S. Department of Health and Human Services.
16. Ferraro G: *The cultural dimension of international business,* ed 2, Englewood Cliffs, NJ, 1994, Prentice-Hall.
17. Foster G: Disease etiologies in non-Western medical systems, *Am Anthropologist* 78:773-782, 1976.
18. Galanti GA: *Caring for patients from different cultures,* Philadelphia, 1991, University of Pennsylvania Press.
19. Groce N, Zola I: Multiculturalism, chronic illness, and disability, *Pediatrics* 91:1048-1055, 1993.
20. Hall ET: *The dance of life,* New York, 1983, Doubleday.
21. Huff R, Kline M: *Promoting health in multicultural populations: A handbook for practitioners,* Thousand Oaks, CA, 1999, Sage Publishing.
22. Ibrahim F: Multicultural influences on rehabilitation training and services: The shift to valuing non-dominant cultures. In Karan O, Greenspan S, eds: *Community rehabilitation services for people with disabilities,* Boston, 1995, Butterworth-Heinemann, pp 187-205.
23. Kavanagh K, Absalom K, Beil W, et al: Connecting and becoming culturally competent: a Lakota example, *Adv Nurs Sci* 21:9-31, 1991.
24. Kohls R: *Survival kit for overseas living,* Chicago, 1979, Intercultural Press.
25. Kleinman A: *Patients and healers in the context of culture,* Berkeley, Calif, 1980, University of California Press.
26. Knutson L, Leavitt R, Sarton B: Race, ethnicity and other factors influencing children's health and disability: implications for pediatric physical therapists, *Pediatr Phys Ther* 7:175-183, 1995.
27. Ladinsky JL, Volk ND, Robinson M: The influence of traditional medicine in shaping medical care practices in Vietnam today, *Soc Sci Med* 25: 1105-1110, 1987.
28. Ladyshewsky R: Cross-cultural supervision of students. In Leavitt R, eds: *Cross-cultural rehabilitation: an international perspective,* Philadelphia, 1999, WB Saunders.
29. Leavitt R, editor: *Cross-cultural rehabilitation: an international perspective,* Philadelphia, 1999, WB Saunders.
30. Leavitt R: *Disability and rehabilitation in rural Jamaica: an ethnographic study,* Madison, NJ, 1992, Fairleigh Dickinson University Press.
31. Levitt S: The collaborative learning approach in community based rehabilitation. In Leavitt R, ed: *Cross-cultural rehabilitation: An international perspective,* Philadelphia, 1999, WB Saunders.
32. Lynch E, Hanson M: *Developing cross-cultural competence,* Baltimore, Md, 1998, Paul Brookes.
33. Mardiros M: Conception of childhood disability among Mexican-American parents, *Medical Anthropology* 12:55-68, 1989.
34. Mehrabian A: *Silent messages,* Belmont, Calif, 1971, Wadsworth.
35. Nakamura R: *Health in America: A multicultural perspective,* Upper Saddle River, NJ, 1999, Allyn & Bacon.
36. Paul T, Thorburn M: Epidemiological considerations in the assessment of disability. In Leavitt R, editor: *Cross-cultural rehabilitation: an international perspective,* Philadelphia, 1999, WB Saunders.
37. Pember M: The Ho-Chunk way, *The Washington Post,* Health section, April 9, 2002.
38. Rebhun LA: Swallowing frogs: Anger and illness in Northeast Brazil, *Medical Anthropology Q* 8:360-382, 1994.
39. Reviere R, Hylton K: Poverty and health: An international overview. In Leavitt R, editor: *Cross-cultural rehabilitation: an international perspective,* Philadelphia, 1999, WB Saunders.
40. Santana S, Santana F: *An introduction to Mexican culture for rehabilitation service providers.* Buffalo, NY, 2001, Center for International Rehabilitation Research Information and Exchange (CIRRIE).
41. Schneider E, Zaslavsky A, Epstein A: Racial disparity in the quality of care for enrollees in Medicare managed care, *JAMA* 287:1288-1294, 2002.
42. Smedley B, Stith A, Nelson A, editors: *Committees on understanding and eliminating racial and ethnic disparities in health care,* Washington, DC, March 2002, Institute of Medicine.
43. Smey J: Understanding racial prejudice, discrimination and racism and their influence on health care delivery. In Leavitt R, ed: *Cross-cultural rehabilitation: an international perspective,* Philadelphia, 1999, WB Saunders.
44. Spector R: *Cultural diversity in health and illness,* East Norwalk, Conn, 1996, Appleton & Lange.
45. Spradley J: *The ethnographic interview,* New York, 1979, Holt, Rinehart & Winston.
46. *Racial and ethnic disparities in access to health insurance and health care,* Los Angeles, CA, 2000, UCLA Center for Health Policy and Kaiser Family foundation.
47. United States Bureau of the Census: *Current population reports,* Washington, DC, 2001, U.S. Bureau of the Census.

48. United States Bureau of the Census: *Current population reports*, Washington, DC, 2000, U.S. Bureau of the Census.
49. United States Bureau of the Census: *Current population reports*, Washington, DC, 1990, U.S. Bureau of the Census.
50. United States Department of Commerce: *Population projections of the United States by age, sex, race, and Hispanic origin, 1995 to 2050*, Washington, DC, February 1996, U.S. Bureau of the Census.
51. *Report of the secretary's task force on black and minority health*, Washington, DC, October 1998, United States Department of Health and Human Services.
52. United States Department of Health and Human Services. Office of Disease Prevention and Health Promotion. *Healthy People 2010*, Washington, DC, 1998.
53. Villa VM, Torres-Gil FM: The health of elderly Latinos. In Aguirre-Molina M, Molina C, Zambrana R, eds: *Health issues in the Latino community*, Washington, DC, 2001, Jossey-Bass.
54. Wasson S: Treatment of the Native American population, *Orthop Phys Ther Clin North Am* 8:215-223, 1999.
55. Young J, Garro L: Variations in the choice of treatment in two Mexican communities, *Soc Sci Med* 16:1453-1465, 1982.
56. Zborowski M: Cultural components in responses to pain, *J Soc Issues* 8:16-30, 1952.

SUGGESTED READINGS
Particular Ethnic Groups

Braithwaite R, Taylor S, eds: *Health issues in the black community*, San Francisco, 2001, Jossey-Bass.
Fadiman A: *The spirit catches you and you fall down: a Hmong child and her American doctors, and the collision of two cultures*, New York, 1997, Farrar, Straus & Giroux.
Galanti GA: *Caring for patients from different cultures*, Philadelphia, 1991, University of Pennsylvania Press.
Huff R, Kline M: *Promoting health in multicultural populations: a handbook for practitioners*, Thousand Oaks, CA, 1999, Sage Publishing.
Leavitt R, editor: *Cross-cultural rehabilitation: an international perspective*, Philadelphia, 1999, WB Saunders.
Leavitt R: *Disability and rehabilitation in rural Jamaica: an ethnographic study*, Madison, NJ, 1992, Fairleigh Dickinson University Press.
Lynch E, Hanson M: *Developing cross-cultural competence*, Baltimore, Md, 1998, Paul Brookes.
Nakamura R: *Health in America: A multicultural perspective*, Upper Saddle River, NJ, 1999, Allyn & Bacon.
Spector R: Cultural diversity in health and illness, East Norwalk, Conn, 1996, Appleton & Lange.

Web Resources

The Commonwealth Fund's 2001 Health Care Quality Survey report
http://www.cmwf.org

Office of Minority Health
http://www.omhrc.gov

http://www.apta.org/Advocacy/minorityaffairs/IncreaseCompetency, resource for physical therapists on enhancing cultural competence

Health Resources and Services Administration resource on providing culturally competent care
http://erc.msh.org/quality&culture

Center for International Rehabilitation Research Information and Exchange
http://cirrie.buffalo.edu/mseries.html

The Patient Interview: The Science Behind the Art   4

Matthew B. Garber, PT, DSc, OCS, FAAOMPT
William G. Boissonnault, PT, DHSc, FAAOMPT

Objectives

After reading this chapter, the reader will be able to:

1. Identify potential impediments to an effective and efficient patient interview.
2. Describe the elements of the patient-centered interview.
3. Describe strategies, including setting the environment and nonverbal and verbal communication skills, PTs can use to enhance the interview process.
4. Provide an overview of strategies designed to enhance the interview process of patients with hearing deficits, patients who angry or combative, and patients who are depressed.

> We have been given two ears and but a single mouth in order that we may hear more and talk less.
> Zeno of Citium

Physical therapy management for patients with neuromusculoskeletal conditions without a physician referral is now a reality in most states. With direct access comes a heightened awareness of the obligation to all patients of providing a comprehensive, evidence-based examination to accurately diagnose the spectrum of conditions likely to respond to physical therapy interventions while promptly recognizing conditions that require referral to other medical providers. The patient interview is a crucial element of this process.

The majority of the essential diagnostic information arises from the patient interview.[15,21,66] Despite the recognized importance of this core clinical skill, many health care providers perform inadequate patient interviews. Platt and McMath[56] observed more than 300 clinical interviews by physicians and found five primary areas of deficiency: (1) interviews with low therapeutic content; (2) inattention to primary data (symptoms); (3) a high control style; (4) an incomplete database, usually omitting patient-centered data and active problems other than the present illness; and (5) thoughtless interviews in which the physician fails to formulate a needed working hypothesis.

The typical length of a physician visit, including the physical examination, ranges from 3 to 74 minutes,[61,63] with the average between 15 and 21 minutes.[43,61,63,80] In primary care the average consultation times for family doctors, internists, and pediatricians are 13, 19, and 13 minutes, respectively.[63] In an informal survey of Army physical therapy clinics, Garber[19] found the average new patient visit length was 35 minutes,

whereas the average follow-up visit was 23 minutes. In two unrelated studies, researchers found that only 23% to 28% of patients are able to complete their opening statement of concerns before being interrupted or redirected.[8,43] In one study only one patient was able to complete his entire opening statement.[43] Patients are interrupted by the physician an average of 18 to 23 seconds into the interview—typically after only one initial concern is stated.[8,43] This is important because if given the opportunity, patients typically express an average of three concerns per visit, and the first concern is not always the primary complaint.[43,80] Furthermore, once interrupted, patients may not mention the information again.[58] Interrupting the patient may hinder the amount and quality of pertinent data gained through the interview.[58] Physicians typically take control of the interview after interrupting and use more closed-ended questions for the remainder of the interview.[8] Patients allowed to complete their initial statements take only 6 seconds longer than those patients who are interrupted.[43] The average time for a patient to disclose main concerns fully is 32 to 90 seconds, with a maximum of approximately 2 minutes.[8,43] An average of 21 interruptions occur in a typical primary care visit.[58] Patients bring up new problems not previously mentioned—commonly referred to as the "Oh, by the way . . ." concerns—during the closing moments of approximately 20% of patient visits.[43,80]

Most studies have focused on the physician-patient relationship, but PTs are certainly not exempt from these same inadequacies. These data should make therapists reflect on their own interview styles and relationships with patients. The majority of these studies were performed in primary care settings. PTs working in a primary care environment will likely face similar challenges.

Considering the importance of the patient interview as described in the current medical literature, why are health care providers so poor at this core clinical skill? Moreover, why is so little time devoted to teaching the skills associated with performing an effective interview? How can we gather these data accurately, efficiently, and in adequate detail and still have time to complete the physical examination, provide an intervention, and educate the patient given the time constraints common in clinical practice?

The primary objective of this chapter is to provide PTs with the communication, technical, and clinical decision-making skills associated with the interview process. The development of these skills will result in the therapist: (1) developing an accurate clinical hypothesis; (2) developing an examination and intervention approach to meet the individual's cultural, communication, anatomical, and physiological needs and abilities; (3) recognizing patient symptoms and signs that necessitate communication with other health care providers; and (4) participating in the decision-making process regarding the selection of appropriate diagnostic testing. Excellent communication skills serve as a vital foundation for all these aspects of patient care. The end result will be the PT providing high-quality patient care and assuming a valuable role on an interdisciplinary health care team.

Communication: An Overview of the Medical Literature

> I know that you believe you understand what you think I said, but I am not sure you realize that what you heard is not what I meant.
>
> Anonymous

In the medical professions, clinicians have a need for routinely using effective and sharply honed communication skills. These critical skills are taught in medical school and entry-level allied health training programs, yet are rarely emphasized.[50,53,66] To make a correct diagnosis and to establish an effective intervention, PTs must have the communication skills that allow them to completely comprehend important details of the patient's problem. Proficiency in communication skills is necessary to collect important patient data efficiently and effectively, provide exercise instruction, explain the diagnosis and prognosis, and teach the details of a treatment program to a patient. Patience and repeated hard work, humility, clarity, and self-criticism are all required to acquire highly effective communication skills.[11,41]

Increased public dissatisfaction with the medical professions is related to deficiencies in clinical communication. Studies in a number of countries have confirmed that serious communication problems are common in clinical practice. These findings led Simpson et al[66] to conclude that there is a "clear and urgent need" for teaching core clinical communication skills to medical students and that this training should be continued in the postgraduate setting and continuing medical education courses. Similarly, PTs could benefit from communication skills training at all levels of their professional and postprofessional education. As far back as 1985, Singleton[67] called for an increased emphasis on written and oral communication skills in physical therapy curricular offerings when direct access was approved in North Carolina. Malpractice claims could possibly increase against PTs as they take on more responsibility for patient management in primary care. Clearly, PTs working in primary care must develop excellent communication skills to try to defuse potentially disgruntled patients.

Clinicians need to understand the many complexities surrounding effective communication. Indeed, successful communication can be difficult to achieve. Wright and Hopkins[83] found that physicians, PTs, and patients disagree about the definition of commonly used medical terms. Physicians and patients showed poor agreement on more than 40% of the

words included in a questionnaire. PTs and patients demonstrated poor agreement for the terms *numbness, ligaments, lumbar, back,* and *sciatic nerve.* What may be even more alarming is that physicians and PTs could not agree on 30% of these commonly used medical terms. Among words with fair to poor agreement were *arthritis, back, weakness of the arm, swelling of a joint,* and *sciatic nerve.* Indeed, it is a travesty that physicians and PTs cannot agree on the definition of *back.* Similar results were found in a study done by neurologists.[27] Perhaps this is one reason Waddell called low back pain "a twentieth century medical disaster."[77]

In a comprehensive review of patient-physician communication, Roter et al[63] found that many different types of communication are used throughout the interview process. They grouped these communication patterns into broad categories of communication process variables: information-giving, information-seeking, partnership-building, social conversation (positive talk), and negative talk. These same authors found that patients provide 40% of the talk in the visit and physicians contribute approximately 60%.[63]

Roter et al[60] later identified a number of distinct communication patterns in primary care visits. Interestingly, patients and physicians prefer different styles.[60] The "narrowly biomedical" pattern occurred in 32% of visits. Closed-ended medical questions and primarily biomedical talk characterize this pattern. Thirty-three percent of visits were "expanded biomedical," similar to the narrow biomedical pattern but included moderate levels of psychosocial discussion. The "biopsychosocial" pattern contained a balance of biomedical and psychosocial topics. This pattern comprised 20% of the visits. High levels of psychosocial interaction characterized "psychosocial" visits. The "consumerist" pattern primarily consisted of patient questions and physician information-giving. The psychosocial and consumerist patterns each comprised 8% of the visits. Physician satisfaction was lowest in the narrowly biomedical pattern and highest in the consumerist pattern, whereas patients preferred the psychosocial pattern.

Jensen et al[29,30] have provided some interesting observations on novice and expert PTs. Clinical experts spend considerable time with patients in hands-on care, seeking information and evaluating and educating the patient. Expert clinicians enter the lives of their patients, listen well, detect confusion, seek clarification, and know when they are being understood—they are patient centered. Whereas novice PTs tend to be more procedural and mechanical when dealing with patients, experts are more responsive, listen intently, and build on what the patient says.

Similar to expert PTs, Marvel et al[44] found that exemplary family physicians with excellent communication skills involve patients more in the medical interview, offer more emotional support, and use a more biopsychosocial approach to patient care. Community physicians serving as control subjects focused more on the biomedical model. Of particular note is the fact that the exemplary physicians used no more time per patient than the control subjects.

In addition to communicating with patients, PTs need to develop expertise in communicating with physicians and insurance companies.[18] In a study of communication between physicians and PTs, Hulme et al[28] found that PTs desire more accessibility to and communication with physicians, whereas physicians want brief communication with clear objective data provided by the therapist. They found that therapists prefer a more autonomous practice in which the physician recognizes the therapist's expertise. Physicians want to communicate with therapists who have high levels of expertise, yet they generally do not facilitate therapist autonomy.[28] The idiosyncratic attitudes of physicians and PTs toward communication, combined with the lack of agreement on definitions of common medical terms,[83] make this one area of communication that still needs to be fostered. This is especially true if PTs are to be successful practitioners in a primary care setting.

Another important aspect of communication relates to patient education and compliance. Increased compliance may occur if the therapist is able to communicate effectively with patients.[78] A PT who speaks highly of all members of the health professions helps to assure patients that they are being cared for by a team of cooperative and knowledgeable providers. Physical therapists need to portray a level of confidence when interacting with patients, never giving the impression of incompetence. This includes demonstrating a willingness to explore multiple health issues or make the appropriate referral when indicated. In addition to confidence, the communicator should provide information in a friendly, sympathetic, and concerned manner, thus increasing the likelihood of compliance.[78] People remember best what they are told first. Moreover, they remember what they believe is important and what has been repeated to them.[78] Providing patients with the most important information first, stressing how important it is, using short words and sentences, repeating key points frequently, and providing specific information may improve compliance.[78] For instance, "Do your exercises regularly" is likely not as effective as telling the patient to do "three 30-second repetitions of each stretch once per day."

As health care professionals we often undervalue or forget the potency of good communication skills.[48] Limiting our communication with patients because of managed care, capitation, and other work pressures could lead to longer recovery times for patients simply because of gaps or errors in patient data collection.[48] Becoming a skilled communicator with patients, physicians, and insurers, among others, should be a high priority for any PT desiring to work in a primary care arena.

Listening: An Active Process

> Listening is itself, of course, an art: that is where it differs from merely hearing. Hearing is passive; listening is active. Hearing is voluntary; listening demands attention. Hearing is natural; listening is an acquired discipline.[41]

The average person spends approximately 45% of their waking hours involved in listening activities, but with an efficiency of 25%.[11] Being a good listener—picking up new lines of thought or inquiry from verbal and nonverbal cues—is vital to the success of the examination and intervention.[48] Grieve[24] stated that

PTs are "in danger of overlooking the simple (psychological) potency of giving patients a good hearing, listening attentively, giving them the benefit of the doubt." This inability to fully examine in a patient-centered format, according to Grieve, "may lead to unnecessary mischief." In fact, a number of authors have reported on the therapeutic effect of the patient interview.[11,16,73]

Listening attentively and allowing patients to provide their perspective regarding their health has many potential benefits. The PT may learn something important about the patient's personality, background, and values, leading to a better understanding of the patient's problem. This in turn may make the patient listen more attentively to the therapist, which improves rapport through more effective communication.[11,57]

Listening becomes effective only when what is said is also heard and understood.[57,78] Whereas hearing connotes attention to sounds and perhaps the interpretation of their literal meanings, listening requires that the listener grasp the true meaning of what is communicated through verbal and nonverbal cues.[11] Effective listening is hindered by a number of factors: (1) the listener being unwilling to listen; (2) the listener attending only to what he or she wishes to hear (i.e., selective listening); (3) the listener's thoughts wandering; and (4) language differences leading to perceptual differences between the listener and the speaker. Controlling these factors is a major determinant of good listening.[11]

Although the content of our verbal communication is important, other factors influence interpretation of what we say. Tone of voice, inflection, and facial expressions affect how a verbal message is perceived.[30]

Several authors have also found that patients commonly offer verbal and nonverbal clues that frequently go unrecognized by physicians.[33,36,74] This has been attributed to the physician being "off in differential-land"[33] rather than focusing on the patients' psychosocial needs. In contrast to commonly held beliefs, visits in which physicians took the time to use active listening and responded to these clues were actually shorter than those in which clues were missed.[36]

Nonverbal Communication

> Looking (observing) is itself a skill: that is where it differs from merely seeing. Seeing is passive; looking is active. Seeing is natural; looking is an acquired discipline.[42]

Of equal importance to listening and verbal communication skills is nonverbal communication. The exchange of verbal messages during the medical encounter may not correlate with nonverbal communication.[76] The impact of nonverbal signals is usually stronger, quicker, and more direct than the impact of verbal signals.[41] Nonverbal communication is a subconscious reflex action and can therefore be expected to be more genuine.[41] Whereas verbal communication is discontinuous, with periods of silence, our body language, facial expressions, and other nonverbal mannerisms are continuous—even when we are not conscious of them.[76] Skillful understanding of nonverbal communication is similar to active listening. It involves conscious effort and discipline. Many messages are conveyed through nonverbal communication. For instance, pain may be expressed by a grimace or wince on the patient's face. Direct eye contact, nodding of the head in agreement, and facing the patient during the interview may convey sincerity and acknowledgment of the patient's problem.

In spite of the perceived importance of nonverbal communication, this topic has received much less systematic research by health professionals than verbal communication. Thornquist[76] reviewed videos of 30 interviews from PTs in three different practice settings. Patients were more likely to look down during the greeting while therapists tended to decide on the spatial relationship between the patient and therapist. Therapists occasionally writing notes had a distancing effect by decreasing eye contact and turning away from the patient. Manual therapists were especially good at active listening, eye contact, posture, and limited writing. This indicates interest, approachability, and attentiveness.[76] In addition, manual therapists made active use of their hands throughout the interaction, remained physically close to the patient, and adapted their tempo and rhythm to match the patient, thereby creating interaction. Thornquist concluded that this communicated a sense of caring and acknowledgment that can create an atmosphere of confidence.[76] This confidence, in addition to credibility of the communicator, is an important aspect of effective communication.[78]

Patient-Centered Interview

> To know what kind of person has a disease is as essential as to know what kind of a disease a person has.[71]

There is a growing body of literature demonstrating that good interpersonal skills of health care providers result in increased patient satisfaction,[69] improved patient outcome,[61] increased provider satisfaction,[4,39,68,70] improved efficiency,[17,72] decreased patient anxiety,[61] and decreased malpractice claims.[37] Despite complaints by many health care providers that interviews that attend to the patient's feelings, ideas, and values take longer, there is clear evidence that these interviews take the same or less time as the biomedical interview.[17,36,43]

The majority of complaints about health care providers are not associated with clinical competency problems but with communication problems.[59] In fact, the majority of malpractice allegations against physicians arise from problems in communication.[65] The difference between sued and never-sued physicians is not explained by negligence, quality of care, or poor documentation. Patients and families are more likely to sue if they believe the physician is not caring or compassionate.[37] Beckman et al[7] found that 70% of malpractice depositions were attributed to communication problems between the patient and the physician. Primary care physicians who use active listening, use more statements of orientation, laugh and use humor, and facilitate patient input are less likely to have malpractice claims than other physicians.[37] It appears that how we communicate with patients—through tone of voice, demeanor, and empathy—is perhaps more important than the context of the message.[37,46]

Although asking for patient input and inquiring about feelings makes sense, this is done in fewer than 50% of patient visits.[16] Many health care providers find it difficult to go beyond the disease-centered or biomedical model of patient care. Others simply do not have the training to investigate adequately the patient's feelings, values, or ideas, leading to interviews focusing only on the patient's disease or diagnosis. Some wish to focus more on the patient but simply "don't know what to say."[54] The patient-centered interview is one method of addressing the patient as a person by incorporating biopsychosocial concepts and encouraging more patient participation during the medical encounter in addition to diagnosing and treating their disorder.[16] The patient-centered interview provides a mechanism for the health care provider to develop a more effective relationship with patients and to ensure that patients are understood and valued.[54]

Within this model are six interactive components[72]: (1) exploring both the patient's disease/diagnosis and its impact on his or her life; (2) understanding the whole person; (3) finding common ground regarding intervention or management; (4) advocating prevention and health promotion; (5) enhancing the patient-provider relationship; and (6) providing realistic expectations. Within this framework, the provider must also explore the dimensions of the illness experience,[54] including:

1. Who is the patient (patient profile)? This consists of information on the patient's hobbies, interests, and professional and personal life.
2. What does the patient want from the provider (patient's goals)? It is important to know whether the patient just wants advice on diagnosis and prognosis, desires only a home exercise program, or expects a full return to prior level of activity. Depending on the scenario, it is important to determine if the patient has realistic expectations based on the nature, stage, and history of the disorder.
3. How does the patient experience illness (functional limitations)? It is important to know how the person deals with being sick, how he or she respond to symptoms and changes in function, as well as how the patient's family, coworkers, and social network deal with illness or disability.
4. What are the patient's perceptions about the disorder? Asking for the patient's opinion about what the source of the symptoms is and what he or she thinks about the diagnosis, prognosis, or intervention.
5. What are the patient's feelings about the disorder? It is important to note whether the patient is sad, depressed, optimistic, or motivated.

In addition to strong evidence that the patient-centered interview improves outcomes and patient and provider satisfaction and decreases malpractice claims, there is clear evidence that these communication skills can be taught and learned by medical students, physical therapy students, and practicing clinicians.* Clearly this dispels the theory that communication skills and good listening are character traits rather than acquired skills.[15] Furthermore, it is important to note that clinical experience alone does not necessarily improve communication skills.[66]

---

* References 15, 22, 26, 32, 35, 45, 49-51, 53, 68, 72.

Interview Process

A health care provider who cannot take a good history, and a patient who cannot provide one, are at risk of giving and receiving poor care.

Author unknown

Up to 80% of the information needed to determine the source of symptoms is obtained from the history.[21] The goals of obtaining the patient history include establishing rapport, identifying any barriers to communication, identifying the patient's preferred learning style, and establishing the patient's goals for physical therapy. In addition, the therapist can use this information to assist in determining the severity, irritability, nature, stage and stability of the patient's condition (Box 4-1).[41] Furthermore, the history enables the therapist to establish an early hypothesis regarding the source(s) of the patient's symptoms, plan an appropriate physical examination, and establish a baseline of symptoms and functional level to measure changes subsequent to any interventions. Early hypothesis formation is one of the characteristics that distinguish expert clinicians from novice clinicians.[29,30]

The patient interview should be conducted in a room with as little noise and distraction as possible. Therapists should control the frequency of interruptions once the patient visit begins, allowing for contact of urgent nature only. What constitutes a contact of urgent nature should be clearly communicated to receptionists and other support staff. Rooms with bright lights and clutter inhibit good eye contact[13] and should be avoided. A recommendation is that patients be offered the choice of where to sit (or lie down) so they can establish the desirable level of eye contact and remain comfortable during the interview.[13] A brief, general discussion of what is about to take place during the initial visit, and confirmation that this is what the patient was expecting, can set the stage for meaningful verbal interchange.

Verbal skills are vital during the patient interview. Starting with open-ended questions and then "funneling" to closed-ended questions that require a "yes" or "no" response to clarify information is recommended (Table 4-1). Open-ended questions allow patients to elaborate on details surrounding their primary concerns, whereas closed-ended questions provide more limited information and therefore should come later in the interview. Also important is avoiding the use of biased questions that lead the patient to the answer the therapist wants to hear.[41] For example, instead of asking "did the treatment make you feel better?," it may be more effective to ask "How did the treatment make you feel?" or "Did the treatment make you any worse?" If the patient truly does feel better, the clinician may have more confidence in the patient's response with answers to the latter two questions.

Other effective verbal communication strategies include asking only one question at a time, speaking slowly and deliberately, and keeping questions brief. This prevents the patient from getting confused and helps the patient answer questions more accurately.[41] Periodically restating or summarizing what the patient has reported can also be beneficial, especially when the clinician is about to change topics or categories of questions. Using the patient's own words whenever possible can facilitate this process.[41] Simple sentences free of medical jargon are also helpful in preventing patient confusion.[41] For example, asking the patient to "flex" or "extend" their arm, or referring to their "signs and symptoms" should be avoided. Likewise, avoid using medical jargon for diagnosis. Terms such as "subacromial" or "retropatellar" typically do not have meaning to patients. Instead, use common terms such as "under your shoulder" or "behind your kneecap." Using the patient's line of thought, or paralleling the patient's mental processes, may also be helpful. In doing so, the therapist is more likely to get an accurate picture of the patient's symptoms and how they are affecting his or her

---

BOX 4-1
SINSS: Operational Definitions/Guidelines

Severity: This is the term used to describe the clinician's assessment of the intensity of the patient's symptoms as they relate to a functional activity. Therapists may consider the patient's perception of the severity and their assessment of the severity.

Irritability: This term is used to describe the clinician's assessment of the ease with which the symptoms can be provoked or stirred up. It has three components: (1) the amount of activity needed to trigger the patient's symptoms, (2) the severity of the symptoms provoked, and (3) what activity and the amount of time before the patient's symptoms subside (duration).

Nature of the Complaint: This is the term that represents the clinician's assessment of:

1. Hypotheses of the structures (if appropriate), syndrome/classification, or pathoanatomic structures or syndromes responsible for producing the pain—nerve root, disk, inflammatory component, lumbar dysfunction versus sacroiliac joint dysfunction, etc.
2. Anything about the problem or overall condition that may warrant caution with the objective examination (trauma, whiplash, etc.).
3. The character of the presenting person or the problem: consider the psychological, personality, ethnic, and socioeconomic factors or the patient's pain tolerance.

Stage of Pathology: This term is used to describe the clinician's assessment of the stage in which the disorder is presenting (acute, subacute, chronic, acute on chronic). It involves a time frame from onset, which depends on the pathoanatomic nature of the problem and phase of tissue healing—fracture versus soft tissue, etc. Stage may be obtained from the history, past and present. It is common to see a chronic symptom pattern with episodic acute aggravation of symptoms.

Stability: Describes the progression of the patient's symptoms over time (the current episode or of all episodes over time). Is the problem getting better, worse, or staying the same?

Adapted from *Orthopaedic manual physical therapy: A description of advanced clinical practice*, Biloxi, Miss, 1998, American Academy of Orthopaedic Manual Physical Therapists.

TABLE 4-1
Open-Ended Versus Closed-Ended Questions

Open-Ended Questions	Closed-Ended Questions
What makes your pain worse?	Does bending increase your pain?
What happens to your pain at night?	Does the pain worsen at night?
How did you feel after our last visit?	Were you any better after our last visit?
Can you describe the pain for me?	Is the pain dull or sharp?
How do you feel upon waking?	Are you still or sore upon waking?

life.[41] Assumptions should be avoided, and any misunderstanding that does occur should be blamed first on the therapist's inability to communicate effectively.[41] Physicians have been found to most often attribute communication problems to the patient rather than their own limitations.[39] Attributing frustration to patient characteristics alone may interfere with building a trusting relationship necessary for an optimal patient-provider relationship.[39] Instead of blaming the patient for the miscommunication, we should instead rephrase the question. "I'm sorry, I wasn't very clear with that question. What I meant was . . ." is a good way to clarify without blaming the patient. These moments of misunderstanding and clarification are excellent opportunities for the therapist to use self-evaluation and reflection to improve verbal skills. Reflecting on various aspects of clinical practice is another characteristic of expert clinicians.[29,30] Periodic self-assessment of the entire examination process, including the interview, with videotapes and audiotapes is a useful tool to critique one's ability to conduct an examination.

Throughout the patient interview, remembering that each question has a specific purpose that will assist in early hypothesis formation and differential diagnosis is important. With each question, therapists must know what they want to know and why, what is the best way to word the question, what possible answers the patient may provide, and how the answer will influence future questions.[41]

Ethics, Empathy, and Humanism

> I have not been critical of the quality of services you deliver; I have been critical of the quality of their delivery.[75]

The complexities of clinical practice coupled with the spectrum of patient needs and personalities pose significant challenges for the PT. With changes in Medicare, capitation, health maintenance organizations, and managed care, clinical practice continues to be even more complex. As a result, clinicians can easily lose sight of the humanistic side of clinical practice. With advanced technology, we often focus more on the pathoanatomical components of the patient rather than the patients themselves. Many of us have caught ourselves referring to "the ACL reconstruction patient" or "the fibromyalgia patient" rather than "Mr. Jones, the plumber with three children who is unable to return to work 6 months after an ACL reconstruction." Clinicians often shift from the human experience of illness or disability to various technologic facts about the disorder.[2] At times we have difficulty understanding human suffering that cannot be explained by specific anatomical or physiological conditions. To help us bridge this gap between the patient's experience with illness or functional limitations and the health care provider's focus on the most appropriate anatomical diagnosis, we need to have a paradigm that incorporates a more complete understanding of the human predicament.[2] We must reconcile scientific understanding with human understanding, using one to guide the other.[2] Although active listening, good eye contact, and open-ended questions are examples of strategies to incorporate empathy and humanism

into the patient encounter, we must also be willing to venture beyond this to fully recognize and understand the concerns of the patient.[47] To make the humanistic aspect of patient care a habit, it is important to identify the multiple health issues present during a patient visit, reflect on possible conflicts, and support the patient's perspective.[47]

The foundation of humanistic patient care is understanding that each patient visit consists of three perspectives: the provider's, the patient's, and the patient's family.[47] Providers must learn to reflect and think critically about their own behavior and skills. True behavioral change only occurs when reflecting new experiences and changing the structure of our own knowledge.[47] This reflective practice is also one of the characteristics of clinical expertise in physical therapy practice identified by Jensen et al.[29] Finally, the provider must choose altruism—supporting the patient's perspective, even if it conflicts with the provider's own agenda.[47]

Like patient-centered interviewing skills, empathy and humanism can also be learned.[55,64,74] This process involves recognizing when the patient is expressing strong feelings or emotions, allowing the patient to express these feelings, acknowledging these feelings make sense, and offering assistance.[55] Many times the complicated and frustrating patient encounters can become productive interactions for both the patient and provider by pausing—doing nothing other than listening to the patient, rather than feeling compelled to "do something."[12,55] Several words and phrases have been identified that build empathy, enabling the provider to connect with the patient (Box 4-2).[12] "Will you tell me more about that," "Is there anything else," and "Let me see if I have this right . . ." are all useful in practicing clinical empathy.[12]

We cannot forget that ethical practice is a hallmark of our profession. If patients or other health care providers perceive, through our verbal and nonverbal communication, our personal values and attributes as deficient, it is likely to have a negative impact on the patient visit. We must use conduct that

---

BOX 4-2
Words That Build Empathy

Queries
Would you tell me more about that?
What has this been like for you?
Is there anything else?
Hmmmm . . .

Clarifications
Let me see if I have this right.
I want to make sure I understand you.
Am I hearing this right?
You let me know if I'm off track, OK?

Responses
That sounds tough.
I imagine you might feel . . .
I can see that you are . . .
That's very good. You should feel good about that.

Adapted from Coulehan JL, Platt FW, Egener B, et al: "Let me see if I have this right . . .": words that help build empathy, *Ann Intern Med* 135:221-227, 2001.

is decent, modest, sensitive, honest, sincere, benevolent, empathetic, courteous, and capable.[20]

Barriers to Communication

Cultural differences, gender-related issues, and sensory impairments must be considered during any patient interaction. Female physicians have been found to conduct longer medical visits than male physicians (22.9 minutes vs 20.3 minutes), with approximately 40% more discussion occurring during the patient interview.[62] Patients of female physicians talk 58% more than patients of male physicians.[62] Female physicians engage in more positive talk, partnership-building, question-asking, and information-giving.[62] On the basis of these statistics, Roter et al concluded that female physicians might be more patient centered in their interviewing than their male counterparts.[62]

White patients tend to receive more information and more positive talk than African Americans or Hispanics.[63] Working class patients are less likely to question the health care provider than those from higher social classes.[63] Although these differences in content were noted, there was no difference in overall length of visits by race,[63] and no differences in outcomes have been reported.

Language barriers and other sources of communication barriers must also be considered.[31] Patients with hearing loss, difficulty reading or seeing, social anxiety disorders, and other cultural issues may hinder effective communication. One must remember that the patient is not the barrier, and either the patient or the provider with these impairments will have to develop strategies to be effective communicators. Sometimes it is unclear if language is the barrier or if cultural practices prevent clear understanding between the patient and therapist.[12] Understanding and respecting any cultural differences that may exist because of ethnic, social, and religious beliefs of the patient is important (see Chapter 3). Likewise, knowing your own cultural values and biases is helpful because these attitudes can influence communication with patients and potentially affect outcome.[13,38,41] Developing a familiarity with the cultural values, health beliefs, and illness behaviors of the ethnic and religious groups commonly served in your clinical practice may help improve communication.[12] Having health screening forms and patient outcome measures translated into several languages may also assist with gathering pertinent information (see Chapter 5).

Patients with Hearing Deficits

For the purposes of this discussion, it is assumed that the patient's hearing deficit does not warrant a physician consult (see Chapter 8 for a discussion of how to determine whether hearing loss should be reported to the physician). Interviewing patients with hearing disturbances has unique challenges for the therapist. The therapist's history-taking goals described earlier are no different for these patients, but the therapist will need to make adjustments for the interview to be judged a success by both the patient and the therapist. The following discussion presents strategies for interviewing patients with partial hearing and for those who are deaf.[9,14]

Finding a quiet area for the interview is paramount when working with a patient who is hearing impaired because excessive background noise can interfere with communication. Patients with hearing aids should be wearing them, and if glasses are necessary for clear vision, they should be worn as well. For the patient to read lips, the therapist should be sitting in a well-lit area and positioned directly facing the patient. An exception to the recommendation of directly facing the patient is if the patient has unilateral hearing loss; then the therapist should sit more toward the patient's "hearing side." Sitting 3 to 6 feet from the patient is recommended as the ideal distance to facilitate the communication process.[14] To facilitate continued visual facial contact, the therapist should avoid covering his or her mouth while speaking and should avoid speaking to the patient while looking away to write down patient responses. Looking away to write down patient responses can also lead to the therapist's voice "trailing off." Speaking deliberately and in a relatively low-pitched voice can also aid communication. Presbycusis, hearing loss associated with aging, is the most common cause of hearing deficits in the elderly and in most cases begins with a reduced capacity to hear higher frequencies.[25,84] To compensate for the patient's hearing impairment, therapists may be prone to speak very loudly, but yelling is not recommended. Speaking at a slightly louder than normal volume is more appropriate, and not allowing the voice to trail off at the end of sentences or questions is also important. Gestures and demonstrations are important strategies designed to reinforce the verbal communication. In certain situations handwritten questions and answers may be necessary (although they are time consuming) to ensure accurate collection of data. Written questionnaires can facilitate the efficiency of collecting these data (see Chapter 5 for an example). Beyond the history-taking process, any oral instructions for these patients should be complemented with written instructions to ensure safe and accurate patient follow-through.

For patients who are deaf, the therapist should determine the patient's preferred mode of communication. If lip reading is the choice, then the aforementioned strategies are appropriate. If using sign language is the patient's preference and the therapist does not have this skill, working with an interpreter is appropriate.[9] First and foremost, the interpreter should have specific qualifications, including familiarity with medical concepts and terminology. A general rule to follow is that the interpreter should not be a family member or a child. Before starting the patient interview the interpreter should be oriented to how the examination will proceed, and time should be provided for the interpreter and the patient to establish some rapport. The therapist should pose all questions directly to the patient, keeping them short and simple and avoiding highly technical jargon. Verifying mutual understanding by periodically asking the patient to restate what has been discussed is important to ensure obtaining accurate information. Lastly, to avoid frustration on the therapist's part, it is important to understand that these visits will take longer than usual and to make plans accordingly.

Patients Who Are Angry

Clinicians will periodically encounter a patient who appears angry. How the clinician reacts and responds to such a patient will determine whether the rehabilitation visit is productive or not and whether the situation escalates into a hostile situation. Recognizing that the patient may be angry is the first step toward resolving the situation. For some patients the anger will be obvious—expressed verbally with direct statements that reflect unreasonable demands, annoyance, and resentment— and that may be a part of an outburst. Other patients may express their anger in a more subtle fashion, such as with statements marked with sarcasm, cynicism, or negativism. Actions that are potentially self-destructive, such as noncompliance with recommended treatment, may also represent angry behavior. Finally, for some patients nonverbal manifestations may be the initial cues that something is awry. The patient who is angry often has clenched fists or jaw, a pronounced frown on the face, or lips tightly compressed, and their gestures may be abrupt or jerky in nature.[3,79] Once the therapist recognizes that anger may be an issue, confirming that observation with the patient and determining why he or she is angry are the next important steps.

If the therapist is not certain but suspects that the patient may be angry, simply asking if the patient is upset or angry about something is appropriate. If the patient asks why the question is being asked, the therapist should describe the observations that led to the inquiry. If the angry behavior is overt, simply stating the obvious is appropriate: "You appear to be upset today, Mr. Jones; are you?" In either scenario, when the manifestations associated with the anger are subtle or obvious, the therapist needs to inquire about the reason for the anger.

Potential reasons for a patient's anger are numerous and many times legitimate: adverse life events, a response to the suffering and disability associated with their illness, or the sense of being helpless or mistreated within the health care system. Other possible reasons for the anger include the patient waiting for an unacceptable period of time because the therapist is behind schedule, the patient being treated in an inconsiderate or insensitive manner by the therapist or other staff, or the patient's behavior reflecting that of the therapist, who appears to be angry.[9] Once the source of anger is identified, the clinician can begin exploring the issues and formulating a specific plan. The clinician should not react to any of the patient's comments with hostility or come across as being judgmental. Maintaining a calm voice and relaxed posture and making it clear that you are there to work with the patient can help prevent the situation from escalating. Actively engaging the patient in addressing the identified issues and possible solutions, and *not* focusing on the patient's behavior, can also facilitate a constructive resolution.[79] Displaying this empathetic attitude does not necessarily mean that the therapist agrees with the patient's sentiments, but it is essential for an open and frank professional discussion to take place. If the anger is present during multiple patient visits, communication with the patient's physician is warranted. Persistent anger may be a manifestation of an organic or psychological disorder, including chemical dependency or withdrawal.[1,3]

Finally, to protect the therapist and the patient, the therapist must be vigilant for signs of potential violence on the patient's part. The following are behavioral clues suggesting potential violent behavior:[34]

- Patient tensely moving to the edge of the chair
- Patient tensely gripping the arm rests
- Loud, forceful speech
- Restless agitation, pacing, and inability to sit still

Besides staying calm, as described earlier, showing respect, maintaining eye contact, listening attentively, maintaining a safe distance from the patient, and avoiding any physical contact can help begin to defuse the situation. Trying to redirect the patient away from the factors contributing to the agitation and appealing to the patient to work with you toward identifying goals and solutions may also help.[79] In addition to these strategies, each facility should have operational procedures established in the event of a hostile interaction. These procedures should be reviewed as frequently as those associated with fire or violent weather.

The Depressed Patient

The patient who is depressed may present the therapist with multiple challenges during the interview. Impaired concentration is often a manifestation of depression[1] and can result in some patients being "poor historians." Strict adherence to the strategies outlined earlier in this chapter may facilitate the transfer of information from the patient to the therapist, but short, delayed, and vague responses to questions can lead to frustration on the therapist's part. This frustration, if unchecked, will only impair the communication process. To complete an adequate examination within the usual time constraints, the therapist may need to prioritize the interview questions even more than usual. Focusing on questions designed to assist in the planning of the physical examination should be emphasized initially. Once the physical examination begins the therapist can continue to ask questions to collect additional information geared toward treatment planning and developing a prognosis. Ultimately in this scenario, the therapist's clinical decision-making may be directed primarily by the physical examination findings and much less so by the data collected during the history.

Beyond the examination process, the impaired concentration can affect the patient's ability to follow through with home instructions. For these patients it is not a matter of purposely disregarding the therapist's advice; the disease interferes with their ability to follow seemingly simple (from the therapist's perspective) instructions. Again, the therapist should prioritize the exercises and the postural or ergonomic instructions to avoid overloading the patient. Providing written materials that are clear and concise may also facilitate compliance, but at times it may be necessary to recruit a caregiver or family member to assist with the home program. Awareness that impaired concentration is a manifestation of this disease, just as chest pain can be a manifestation of ischemic heart disease, may keep this communication challenge in perspective. An understanding of how the often-present impaired concentration can affect the rehabilitation process may help minimize frustration on the therapist's part, which if present will only further impede the communication process. This awareness should direct the therapist to use strategies designed to promote follow-through, other than just scolding the patient for not doing the exercises. Lastly, contacting the attending physician or clinical psychologist for suggestions of strategies may be necessary.

Another potential challenge when working with patients who are depressed is that the depressed behavior or affect may be so intense that a productive visit is prohibitive. Counseling strategies (cognitive, behavioral, and interpersonal therapies) as summarized by Brody et al[10] can be adapted and used by the therapist to help salvage the visit of a patient with mild to moderate major depression. First, simply acknowledging that the patient appears to be depressed or feeling down: "Ms. Jones, you appear to be having a rough day today" or Ms. Jones, you appear to be down in the dumps today" may open the door to a constructive conversation. Exploring the potential reasons for the patient's condition occur next. Sometimes stating the obvious is necessary: "Two weeks ago you were completely independent, but the fall and hip fracture have rendered you reliant on others for most of your daily care." Pointing out that these feelings are common in people who have had such a loss may help patients recognize that their predicament is not necessarily a result of failure or shortcomings on their part. This communication portrays empathy and acknowledgment that you are aware of their feelings, and in some sense these statements give the patient permission to feel as they do. Then, discussing the short-term rehabilitation goals with the patient, and clearly describing the plan of how they will be attained, is very important. The thought of how much the patient needs to overcome to return to the preinjury level of function can seem insurmountable, leading to despondency, or the patient may have unrealistic expectations. This can be an equally important conversation to have with family members and caregivers to promote appropriate support for the patient.

Finally, suicide is a potential risk in patients who are depressed, as evidenced by the estimate that 15% of patients with a major depressive disorder will commit suicide.[1] The expression of hopelessness is considered a risk factor for suicide in patients with major depression.[5,6,40,82] Statements such as "I am not sure how much longer I can stand this" or "I am not sure this therapy is going to help" may be expressions of this sentiment. Follow-up questions related to the expression of hopelessness are important to determine the depth of the patient's despair. If the patient appears to have truly given up, the question "Have things have gotten so bad that you are considering harming yourself or taking your life?" is appropriate. If the answer is affirmative, the therapist should follow with questions regarding the patient's plan and the availability of resources to carry out the plan. Avoiding the topic with a patient is not an appropriate action, and in fact many patients with suicidal ideation are relieved to be asked about their intentions.[82] Once this information is collected, implementing the facility's standing "suicidal patient procedure" is appropriate. Practitioners should not avoid asking patients if they have had thoughts of hurting themselves or taking their lives in the fear of suggesting the idea of suicide to the patient.[81] Acknowledging suicidal ideation must occur first for proper management to take place. Chapters 5 and 7 further describes screening for conditions such as depression and suicidal ideation.

Summary

A painstaking exercise in discernment and a grasp of small detail are infinitely worthwhile because in time they provide a grasp of musculoskeletal problem behavior which no other exercise in education can give.

G.P. Grieve, on the patient interview

It is quite evident that communication between health care providers and patients is more than just an art. The concepts of patient-centered care, empathy, and humanism are not simply acquired skills. These skills can be taught, learned, and retained by aspiring health care providers as well as experienced clinicians. Specific training in psychosocial medicine improves patient and provider satisfaction, patient outcomes, and diagnostic efficiency and decreases malpractice claims. Despite the pressures and time constraints of managed care, patient-centered interviews require no more time to complete than purely biomedical examinations. In light of this convincing evidence, clinicians should strive to improve their communication skills and remember that the patient is the focus of clinical practice. Without the patient we would not have a mechanism to learn, grow, and reflect on why we chose a career in the health sciences.

Perhaps one of the most highly skilled communicators in physical therapy practice is Geoffrey Maitland. He "is prepared to visit carefully and thoughtfully that subjective world of [his] patients to ensure that [he] really does approximate [his] way of thinking to that of the patient."[23] Maitland "enters a close, point-to-point, moment-to-moment feedback loop" with his patients.[23] This is the essence of patient-centered care. Unfortunately, many health care providers remain inadequate at this core clinical skill. The age of paternalistic medicine has passed. Patients will hold us accountable for our attitudes as well as our actions. As a result, clinicians, educators, and students must place more emphasis on this often-neglected science behind the art of clinical practice.

REFERENCES

1. American Psychiatric Association: *Diagnostic and statistical manual of mental disorders*, ed 4, Washington DC, 1994, American Psychiatric Association, pp 196-200, 327, 340.
2. Baron RJ: An introduction to medical phenomenology: I can't hear you while I'm listening, *Ann Intern Med* 103:606-611, 1985.
3. Barsky AJ: Approach to the angry patient. In Goroll AH, Mulley AG, eds: *Primary care medicine*, Philadelphia, 2000, Lippincott Williams & Wilkins, pp 1187-1188.
4. Bates AS, Harris LE, Tierney WM, et al: Dimensions and correlates of physician work satisfaction in a Midwestern city, *Med Care* 36:610-617, 1998.

5. Beck AT, Steer RA, Kovacs M, et al: Hopelessness and eventual suicide: a 10 year prospective study of patients hospitalized with suicidal ideation, *Am J Psychiatry* 142:559-563, 1985.

6. Beck AT, Brown G, Berchick RJ, et al: Relationship between hopelessness and ultimate suicide: a replication with psychiatric outpatients, *Am J Psychiatry* 147:190-195, 1990.

7. Beckman HB, Markakis KM, Suchman AL, et al: The doctor-plaintiff relationship: lessons from plaintiff depositions, *Arch Intern Med* 154:1365-1370, 1994.

8. Beckman HB, Frankel RM: The effect of physician behavior on the collection of data, *Ann Intern Med* 101:692-696, 1984.

9. Bickley LS: *Bates' guide to physical examination and history taking*, ed 7, Philadelphia, 1999, JB Lippincott, pp 30, 33.

10. Brody DS, Thompson TL, Larson DB, et al: Strategies for counseling depressed patients by primary care physicians, *J Gen Intern Med* 9:569-575, 1994.

11. Conine TA: Listening in the helping relationship, *Phys Ther* 56:159-162, 1976.

12. Coulehan JL, Platt FW, Egener B, et al: "Let me see if I have this right. . .": words that help build empathy, *Ann Intern Med* 135:221-227, 2001.

13. Croft JJ: Interviewing in physical therapy, *Phys Ther* 60:1033-1036, 1980.

14. Dwyer B: Detecting hearing loss and improving communication in elderly persons. In *Focus on geriatric care & rehabilitation*, Rockville, Md, 1987, Aspen Publishers, p 6.

15. Duffy DF: Dialogue: a core clinical skill, *Ann Intern Med* 128:139-141, 1998.

16. Epstein RM: The science of patient-centered care, *J Fam Pract* 49:805-807, 2000.

17. Evans BJ, Stanley RO, Mestrovic R, et al: Effects of communication skills training on students' diagnostic efficiency, *Med Educ* 25:517-526, 1991.

18. Farrell JP: In search of clinical excellence, *J Orthop Sports Phys Ther* 24:115-121, 1996.

19. Garber MB: Informal survey (unpublished data), March 2001.

20. Gartland G: Essentials of ethics in clinical practice: a communications perspective, *Physiother Canada* 39:179-182, 1987.

21. Goodman CC, Snyder TE: *Differential diagnosis in physical therapy*, ed 2, Philadelphia, 1995, WB Saunders, p 24.

22. Gordon JH, Walerstein SJ, Pollack S: The advanced clinical skills program in medical interviewing: a block curriculum for residents in medicine. *Intl J Psychiatry Medicine* 26:411-429, 1996.

23. Graham J: Communication. In *Maitland's vertebral manipulation*, ed 6, London, 2001, Butterworth-Heinemann, pp 21-22.

24. Grieve GP: *Mobilization of the spine*, ed 5, London, 1991, Churchill Livingstone, p 43.

25. Gulya AJ: Evaluation of hearing loss. In Goroll AH, Mulley AG, eds: *Primary care medicine*, Philadelphia, 2000, Lippincott Williams & Wilkins, pp 1108-1112.

26. Haber RJ, Lingard LA: Learning oral presentation skills: a rhetorical analysis with pedagogical and professional implications, *J Gen Intern Med* 16:308-314, 2001.

27. Hawkes CM: Communicating with the patient in an example drawn from neurology, *Br J Med Educ* 8:57-63, 1974.

28. Hulme JB, Bach BW, Lewis JW: Communication between physicians and physical therapists, *Phys Ther* 68:26-31, 1988.

29. Jensen GM, Gwyer J, Hack LM, et al: *Expertise in physical therapy practice*, London, 1999, Butterworth-Heinemann, pp 31-33, 174, 240-242.

30. Jensen GM, Shepard KF, Hack LM: The novice versus the experienced clinician: insights into the work of the physical therapist, *Phys Ther* 70:314-323, 1990.

31. *Joint Commission on Accreditation of Hospitals and Organizations handbook*, Chicago, 2001, Joint Commission on Accreditation of Hospitals and Organizations.

32. Ladyshewsky R, Gotjamanos E: Communication skill development in health professional education: the use of standardised patients in combination with a peer assessment strategy, *J Allied Health* 26:177-186, 1997.

33. Lang F, Floyd MR, Beine KL: Clues to patients' explanations and concerns about their illnesses: a call for active listening, *Arch Fam Med* 9:222-227, 2000.

34. Leonard J, Harbst T: Medical emergencies in physical therapy. In Boissonnault WG, ed: *Examination in physical therapy practice: screening for medical disease*, ed 2, New York, 1995, Churchill Livingstone, pp 358-360.

35. Levin MF, Riley EJ: Effectiveness of teaching interviewing and communication skills to physiotherapy students, *Physiother Canada* 36:190-194, 1984.

36. Levinson WL, Bhat RG, Lamb J: A study of patient clues and physician responses in primary care and surgical settings, *JAMA* 284:1021-1027, 2000.

37. Levinson W, Roter DL, Mullooly JP, et al: Physician-patient communication: the relationship with malpractice claims among primary care physicians and surgeons, *JAMA* 277:553-559, 1997.

38. Levinson W, Roter D: Physicians' psychosocial beliefs correlate with their patient communication skills, *J Gen Intern Med* 10:375-379, 1995.

39. Levinson W, Stiles WB, Inui TS, et al: Physician frustration in communicating with patients, *Med Care* 31:285-295, 1993.

40. Lewinsohn PM, Rohde P, Seeley JR: Adolescent suicidal ideation and attempts: prevalence, risk factors, and clinical implications, *Clinical Psychology: Science and Practice*, 3:25-46, 1996.

41. Maitland G, Hengeveld E, Banks K, et al: *Maitland's vertebral manipulation*, ed 6, London, 2001, Butterworth-Heinemann, pp 23-36.

42. Maitland GD: *Peripheral manipulation*, ed 3, London, 1991, Butterworth-Heinemann, pp 15-19.

43. Marvel MK, Epstein RM, Flowers K, et al: Soliciting the patient's agenda: Have we improved? *JAMA* 281:283-287, 1999.

44. Marvel MK, Doherty WJ, Weiner E: Medical interviewing by exemplary physicians, *J Fam Pract* 47:343-348, 1998.

45. Maxwell M, Dickson DA, Saunders C: An evaluation of communication skills training for physiotherapy students, *Medical Teacher* 13:333-338, 1991.

46. May WF: Listening carefully, *Second Opinion* 20:47-49, 1994.

47. Miller SZ, Schmidt HJ: The habit of humanism: a framework for making humanistic care a reflexive clinical skill, *Acad Med* 74:800-803, 1999.

48. Moore A, Jull G: The art of listening, *ManualTtherapy* 6:129, 2001.

49. Novack DH, Volk G, Drossman DA, et al: Medical interviewing and interpersonal skills teaching in US medical schools: progress, problems, and promise, *JAMA* 269:2101-2105, 1993.

50. Novack DH, Dube C, Goldstein MG: Teaching medical interviewing: a basic course on interviewing and the physician-patient relationship, *Arch Intern Med* 152:1814-1820, 1992.

51. Oh J, Segal R, Gordon J, et al: Retention and use of patient-centered interviewing skills after intensive training, *Acad Med* 76:647-650, 2001.

52. *Orthopaedic manual physical therapy: a description of advanced clinical practice*, Biloxi, Miss, 1998, American Academy of Orthopaedic Manual Physical Therapists.

53. Payton OD: Effects of instruction in basic communication skills on physical therapists and physical therapy students, *Phys Ther* 63:1292-1297, 2001.

54. Platt FW, Gaspar DL, Coulehan JL, et al: "Tell me about yourself": the patient-centered interview, *Ann Intern Med* 134:1079-1085, 2001.

55. Platt FW, Keller VF: Empathic communication: a teachable and learnable skill, *J Gen Intern Med* 9:222-226, 1994.

56. Platt FW, McMath JC: Clinical hypocompetence: the interview, *Ann Intern Med* 91:898-902, 1979.

57. Ramsden EL: Interpersonal communication in physical therapy, *Phys Ther* 48:1130-1132, 1968.

58. Realini T, Kalet A, Sparling J: Interruption in the medical interaction, *Arch Fam Med* 4:1028-1033, 1995.

59. Richards T: Chasms in communication, *BMJ* 301:1407-1408, 1990.

60. Roter DL, Stewart M, Putnam SM, et al: Communication patterns of primary care physicians, *JAMA* 277:350-356, 1997.

61. Roter DL, Hall JA, Kern DE, et al: Improving physicians' interviewing skills and reducing patients' emotional distress: a randomized clinical trial, *Arch Intern Med* 155:1877-1884, 1995.

62. Roter D, Lipkin M, Korsgaardt A: Sex differences in patients' and physicians' communication during primary care medical visits, *Med Care* 29:1083-1093, 1991.

63. Roter DL, Hall JA, Katz NR: Patient-physician communication: a descriptive summary of the literature, *Patient Education and Counseling* 12:99-119, 1988.

64. Rubin FL, Judd MM, Conine TA: Empathy: can it be learned and retained? *Phys Ther* 57:644-647, 1977.

65. Shapiro RS, Simpson DE, Lawrence SL, et al: A survey of sued and nonsued physicians and suing parents, *Arch Intern Med* 149:2190-2196, 1989.

66. Simpson M, Buckman R, Stewart M, et al: Doctor-patient communication: the Toronto consensus statement, *BMJ* 303:1385-1387, 1991.

67. Singleton MC: Independent practice—on the horns of a dilemma: a special communication. *Phys Ther* 67:54-57, 1987.

68. Smith RC, Lyles JS, Mettler J, et al: The effectiveness of intensive training for residents in interviewing: a randomized, controlled clinical trial, *Ann Intern Med* 128:118-126, 1998.

69. Smith RC, Lyles JS, Mettler JA, et al: A strategy for improving patient satisfaction by the intensive training of residents in psychosocial medicine: a controlled, randomized study, *Acad Med* 70:729-732, 1995.

70. Smith RC, Osborn G, Hoppe RB, et al: Efficacy of a one-month training block in psychosocial medicine for residents: a controlled study, *J Gen Intern Med* 6:535-553, 1991.

71. Smyth FS: The place of the humanities and social sciences in the education of physicians, *J Med Educ* 37:495-499, 1962.

72. Stewart M, Brown JB, Donner A, et al: The impact of patient-centered care on outcomes, *J Fam Pract* 49:796-804, 2000.

73. Stewart MA: Effective physician-patient communication and health outcomes: a review, *Can Med Assoc J* 152:1423-1433, 1995.

74. Suchman AL, Markakis K, Beckman HB, et al: A model of empathic communication in the medical interview, *JAMA* 277:678-682, 1997.

75. Swartz F: The rehabilitation process: a view from inside, *Rehabil Lit* 3: 203-204, 1970.

76. Thornquist E: Body communication is a continuous process: the first encounter between patient and physiotherapist, *Scand J Prim Health Care* 9:191-96, 1991.

77. Waddell G: *The back pain revolution*, London, 1998, Churchill Livingstone, p 1.

78. Wagstaff GF: A small dose of commonsense—communication, persuasion and physiotherapy, *Physiother Canada* 68:327-329, 1982.

79. Welk F: Managing the hostile patient, *PT Magazine* 8:68-70, 2000.

80. White J, Levinson W, Roter D: "Oh by the way. . .": the closing moments of the medical visit, *J Gen Intern Med* 9:24-28, 1994.

81. Whooley MA, Simon GE: Managing depression in medical outpatients, *N Engl J Med* 3443:1942-1950, 2000.

82. Worthington JJ, Rauch SL: Approach to the patient with depression. In Goroll AH, Mulley AG, editors: *Primary care medicine*, Philadelphia, 2000, Lippincott Williams & Wilkins, pp 1157-1162.

83. Wright V, Hopkins R: What the patient means: a study from rheumatology, *Physiotherapy* 64:146-147, 1978.

84. Zeeger LJ: The effects of sensory changes in older persons, *J Neuroscience Nurs* 18:325-332, 1986.

Examination/Evaluation: The Patient Interview

Prologue

William G. Boissonnault, PT, DHSc, FAAOMPT

Chapters 5 through 11 of Sections II and III present a recommended patient examination scheme; as such the author encourages the learner to read these chapters in order the first time through the text. The seven chapters, each representing an important patient data category, are sequenced in accordance with an actual initial patient visit. The chapters also contain suggested tools, such as patient self-report questionnaires, that promote efficient data collection, and also allow for a smooth examination flow from one patient category to the next.

Figure 1 presents a flow chart illustrating all of the categories of patient data to be collected in a recommended sequence during an initial visit. Sequencing the examination in such a manner allows for a more efficient collection of patient data and for a more effective clinical decision-making process concerning:

- Deciding what questions to include or exclude during the patient history
- Deciding what physical examination/tests and measures to include or exclude
- Choosing interventions to be initiated during the initial visit
- Determining whether a patient referral/consultation is needed

As the patient interview begins, therapists typically begin with more open-ended and general questions that prompt patient responses that set the tone for the remainder of the interview and the physical examination. Several patient data categories should be addressed during the initial visit, but the depth for each of the categories of investigation should differ for each patient. For example, if the history reveals red flags associated with the patient's health status, the focus of the physical examination will differ compared with patients in whom no red flags are noted early in the examination.

Access to patient demographic and social and health history information (Chapter 5) before the start of the patient/family interview is very helpful to promote efficiency and effectiveness during the patient interview. In an inpatient setting, this includes reading the patient medical record, whereas in an outpatient setting, reading physician notes, a completed patient health history self-report form, or both would be options. This information will initiate thought related to potential safety precautions for the examination and intervention procedures, the detail and depth of the medical screening component, diagnosis, and prognosis. For example, the more co-morbid conditions that are present and the greater number of medications a patient is taking, the longer the course of rehabilitation.

Once the interview begins, the initial focus should be on what has precipitated the physical therapy intervention. The emphasis again differs depending on the nature of the visit; is it pain, neurologic complaints, or both that are interfering with function (Chapter 6), or is it an interest in health and wellness issues? Once this part of the interview is completed, screening for symptoms unrelated to the chief presenting complaint (review of systems) takes place (Chapter 7). Finally, in terms of the patient interview process, the concept that the physical examination begins during the history portion of the examination is an important one. In fact, in terms of general observation, the physical examination begins as soon as the therapist makes visual contact with the patient/client and then continues throughout the patient interview (Chapter 8). This element of the physical examination includes a general assessment of posture, skin, and neurologic status.

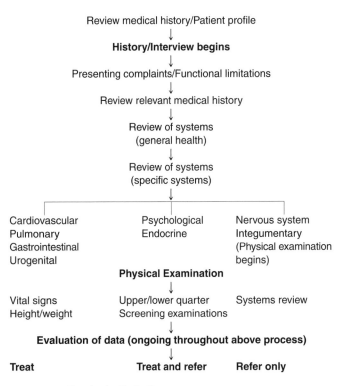

FIGURE 1 Examination/Evaluation.

Chapters 9, 10, and 11 cover the physical examination proper, including elements appropriate for all patients and other elements to be included based on patient history information and initial physical examination findings. Chapter 9 covers topics appropriate for all patients, including vital signs, and patient height and weight. Chapters 10 and 11 describe an upper and lower quarter screening examination scheme from which the clinician will select different components from, depending on the patient's initial presentation. Patient scenarios and cases are presented to summarize important principles in each of these seven chapters, and a formal patient case report is presented in the Epilogue following Chapter 11.

Patient Health History Including Identification of Health Risk Factors

5

William G. Boissonnault, PT, DHSc, FAAOMPT

Objectives

After reading this chapter, the reader will be able to:

1. Identify important patient/client health history information.
2. Explain the relevance of patient/client health history information to physical therapists' (PTs) clinical decision-making in the areas of examination, evaluation, diagnosis, prognosis, and provision of effective and safe interventions.
3. Effectively and efficiently collect patient health history information during an initial patient visit.
4. Explain how patient health history information combined with patient symptoms/signs and systems review can effectively screen patients for depression, domestic violence, chemical dependency, and cancer.

As part of a comprehensive examination, PTs routinely collect patient health history information in both inpatient and outpatient settings.[2] This information, combined with other data collected during the history, including symptom investigation (Chapter 6) and review of systems (Chapter 7), and from the physical examination (Chapters 8, 9, 10, and 11), give the therapist the information necessary to make the essential decision of whether to treat the patient, treat and refer, or refer the patient only. The health history information will give important guidance in the choice of examination and intervention techniques the health status measures to monitor during the treatment, and the establishment of an accurate prognosis.

For example, if a patient with mid-thoracic pain is seen with a co-morbidity associated with loss of bone density (e.g., chronic renal failure), the therapist may choose to assess joint play of the thoracic spine by a method other than that of applying posterior-to-anterior pressure over the thoracic spinous processes with the patient in a prone-lie position. This type of technique with the patient prone could cause "bowing" of the ribs, with the potential for fracture. The joint play information must be collected, but choosing a technique that places less mechanical load on the bony thorax would be in the patient's best interest.

As a second example, if the patient is taking beta-blockers for hypertension and the therapist wants to monitor the patient's general well-being during a conditioning activity, something other than the patient's heart rate should be assessed, considering the physiological effect beta-blockers

have on the cardiovascular system. Finally, the presence of specific co-morbid conditions (e.g., diabetes), or the general presence of additional conditions reported by the patient as a part of the health history, can lead to a prolonged or unsatisfactory response to rehabilitation efforts.

If the decision is made to refer the patient to another health care practitioner, the health history information may provide important data that supports the decision and becomes a part of the information communicated as the referral is made. For example, a patient with a recent history of an infection presents with complaints of chills, fatigue, and a low-grade fever. The chills, fatigue, and low-grade fever could be related to a "benign" virus that is self-limited and not a serious concern, but with the history of a recent infection, this patient should be seen by a physician to ensure that the "recent infection" has not returned or spread to another body region.

The purpose of this chapter is to:

- Describe the types of examination data relevant to a patient's health history investigation and their relevance to the PT's referring a patient to another health care practitioner.
- Describe methods to efficiently collect patient health history information, including where in the examination process one can collect this information.
- Using cancer, depression, domestic violence, and chemical dependency as examples, illustrate how patient health history information, integrated with other examination data, can identify patients who are at high risk for these conditions, facilitating a timely patient referral.

Patient Health History Data

Categories of health history information important to the PT's clinical decision-making needs include:

- Patient demographics (age, sex, race, marital status, level of education)
- Social history (cultural/religious customs/beliefs, occupation and work status, living environment, and family/social support)
- Current and past personal medical history (illnesses, allergies, surgeries, injuries, medication use)
- Social habits (exercise; yes/no, frequency, intensity) including substance use (tobacco use, alcohol and caffeine intake)
- Family medical history

Patient Demographics

Patient demographics and identifying data are important to the medical screening component of the examination. Certain diseases are associated more often with specific age ranges and specific genders. For example, 99% of breast cancer occurs in women, with those aged 60 years or older being the highest-risk group.[22] Prostate cancer accounts for more than one-third of all male cancers, again with those aged 60 years or older being the highest-risk group.[22] Besides these two cancers, other disorders also are more common in one gender than the other, and at younger ages. Thyroid disease, rheumatoid arthritis, and depression all are more common in women, and the age of initial onset is approximately 20 to 40 years. Race also may predispose certain groups to a higher incidence of certain disorders. For example, prostate cancer and sickle cell disease are found more often in the African American population, while skin cancer is more common in the Caucasian population. These examples show that not all patients carry the same risk for diseases, so the degree of medical screening and the goals of our screening will vary in part based on the client's age, race, and other demographics.

Patient Social History

The patient's occupation, leisure activities, customs, and beliefs all expose the patient to various health risks. In addition, this information may reveal potential obstacles to a successful rehabilitation outcome. An occupation that includes repetitive activity or prolonged static body postures or positions, or a leisure activity that places similar demands on the body, carries the risk of development of repetitive, overuse conditions, such as stress fractures or tendonitis. If the work demands cannot be altered or the patient is unwilling to modify the leisure activity, recovery from the condition may be hampered.

Customs, beliefs, and value systems can vary considerably from person to person and can dictate how a person responds to the therapist's requests or instructions. Chapter 3 offers several examples that should raise one's awareness of how such issues may be the key to rehabilitation outcome. Finally, investigating the client's living environment and family/social support network may identify challenges to the delivery of care. The living environment may present obstacles to patient mobility, and many clients depend on others for a number of needs at various points during the recovery from an illness or surgical intervention. Issues such as these may prompt the therapist to initiate a consultation or referral for a variety of services.

Personal Medical History

Although personal health history findings (illnesses, surgeries, or injuries) from the distant past may be relevant for some patients, and should be documented, current health history reports are always relevant and warrant detailed investigation during the initial patient visit. Follow-up questions to the positive health history are keys to determining the clinical relevance of these findings. For example, if a patient acknowledges a history of illness, (e.g., heart problems), follow-up questions should include:

- Can you describe the condition to me—what type of heart problem is it?
- Are you currently receiving care for the illness/condition, or is it something from the past that has fully resolved?
- If the condition is current, what symptoms or warning signs do you typically have?
- Have the symptoms recently changed (e.g., intensity, frequency) in any way?
- How is the condition currently being managed (e.g., diet, exercise, medication?), and by whom?

If a patient acknowledges a heart problem, the therapist should ask, "What type of heart problem, and is it something for which you are currently being treated?" The condition may be a heart arrhythmia, mitral valve prolapse, or ischemic heart disease, all of which carry different precautions or clinical guidelines. A description of the usual symptoms associated with the heart condition gives the therapist baseline information that can be used for comparison with new and possibly related complaints. For example, a worsening of a chronic condition such as ischemic heart disease may result in the onset of new symptoms, and instead of the usual left chest pain, the patient would complain of epigastric pain, or instead of the symptoms being associated with physical exertion, they now occur at rest. The patient may associate this new pain with indigestion, not the heart problem, but an astute therapist will be vigilant for all possible symptoms (see Chapters 6 and 7) associated with ischemic heart disease, including upper abdominal pain.

A patient report of recent surgery or major trauma should alert the therapist to the potential risk of infection or venous thrombosis. Researchers have noted long latency periods between a surgical intervention and the onset of symptoms associated with the resultant infection,[29] and about 50% of patients with a deep venous thrombosis are pain-free.[15] Knowing the possible symptoms (see Chapters 6 and 7) associated with these conditions is paramount to early suspicion and report of concerns to the physician. In addition to knowing the potential for serious complications associated with the trauma/surgery, one should ask the important follow-up question, "Are you currently limited or restricted in any way as a result of the surgery or injury?"

Finally, current medical treatment (e.g., medications) for a condition may be as relevant as, or more relevant than, the underlying disorder itself. Patients seeking services from PTs take a variety of medications,[5,6] some of which may require the therapist to alter or modify his or her usual examination or intervention schemes. For example, therapists should monitor items other than heart rate during physical activity for patients taking beta-blockers because this drug dampens heart rate response to exertion. Many of these drugs also carry significant risk for adverse drug events; therapists can screen for these risks by using the *review of systems* checklists described in Chapter 7.[7] Appendix A presents a summary of drugs and their potential for adverse events for each of the body systems, and Chapter 16 describes additional strategies for screening drug side effects. Understanding the physiological events associated with the various medications and their common side effects will help the therapist identify the body functions to monitor or the symptoms and signs for which to watch. An important principle to guide this screening process is that about 80% of adverse drug events are an extension of the therapeutic effects of the drug (see Chapter 16). For example, the primary adverse drug event associated with antihypertensive medications is hypotension.

Finally, the therapist identifies the patients who need counseling from their physician or pharmacist about proper use of their medications. Important follow-up questions about the use of medications include:

- What is the reason that you are taking the medication?
- Do you feel the medication is helping you?
- What is the dose and schedule for taking the medication? Are you following the dose schedule?
- Who prescribed the medication?
- Have you noticed any side effects from taking the medication?

For patients taking over-the-counter (OTC) medications, (those *not* prescribed by a physician), important additional questions include:

- Is your physician aware that you are taking this medication?
- Have you recently needed to take more of the medication than usual?

An example of how OTC drug use can raise suspicion of potential serious drug complications was described by Boissonnault and Meek.[7] Of the 1817 surveyed patients taking nonsteroidal antiinflammatory drugs (NSAIDs), 28% also were taking OTC antacids, and another 10% were taking histamine-H_2 antagonists (e.g., cimetidine [Tagamet], ranitidine [Zantac]). These drugs are taken for symptoms such as indigestion and heartburn that could be related to NSAID-induced gastrointestinal (GI) ulcers. If the patient reports needing to increase his or her dosage of these OTC drugs (that are not curative of GI ulcers) in order to get the same degree of relief as in the past, this may be a signal that a potentially serious GI condition is worsening.

Social Habits

The investigation of social habits includes, but is not limited to, questions about caffeine and alcohol intake, and tobacco use. This baseline patient information not only identifies risk factors for developing disease but also may affect the patient prognosis and alert the therapist to symptom etiology. Caffeine intoxication can occur with ingestion of as little as 100 mg of caffeine per day and may be marked by several manifestations. The *Diagnostic and Statistical Manual of Mental Disorders*, fourth edition (DSM IV) describes diagnostic criteria for caffeine intoxication[3] (that can be used by the therapist as a screening tool) including:

- Recent consumption of caffeine, usually more than 250 mg (the equivalent of two to three cups of coffee or more)
- Five or more of the following developing during or shortly after caffeine consumption:
  Restlessness
  Nervousness
  Excitement
  Insomnia
  Flushed face
  Diuresis
  GI disturbance
  Muscle twitching
  Rambling flow of thought/speech
  Tachycardia or cardiac arrhythmia
  Periods of inexhaustibility
  Psychomotor agitation
- The effects listed above cause clinically significant distress or impairment in social, occupational, rehabilitation, school, or other settings.
- The aforementioned manifestations are *not* due to a general medical condition

Therapists also should know the possible manifestations of caffeine withdrawal, including headache, lethargy, fatigue, muscle pain and stiffness, and dysphoric mood changes. Research has suggested that these symptoms can occur in people who drink as little as 2.5 cups (or the equivalent of 235 mg of caffeine) of coffee per day,[32] and studies have demonstrated that a patient's postoperative headaches could be related to caffeine withdrawal.[14]

Alcohol intake also is important to document, although quantity alone is not the key issue in determining whether one is alcohol dependent. Another key item to consider when investigating this aspect of patient health history is to avoid using one's own level of use (or non-use) as a reference point to "judge" a patient's level of intake. For example, if the therapist drinks no alcohol, he or she may think that drinking one or two drinks per day most days is at-risk drinking, when in fact evidence suggests that one to two alcoholic drinks per day may reduce the risk of adverse cardiovascular events in certain populations. On the other hand, a therapist who drinks four to five drinks 5 days per week might think that drinking any less than that is not a problem, when in fact long-term consumption of more than seven drinks per week (for women) is considered at-risk drinking.

Therapists can use the guidelines (based on health risks) published by the National Institute on Alcohol Abuse and Alcoholism (NIAAA)[26] to identify at-risk drinking:

- Men: more than 14 drinks/week or more than 4 drinks/occasion
- Female: more than 7 drinks/week or more than 3 drinks/occasion

The at-risk drinking criteria from the NIAAA correspond to the World Health Organization's category of "hazardous use."[31] Potential health risks associated with the described levels of alcohol intake include[19]:

- Hypertension
- Hepatitis
- Cirrhosis
- Gastritis
- Pancreatitis
- Impotence/loss of libido
- Cardiomyopathy

Beyond the at-risk drinking guidelines, *alcohol abuse* is defined by the American Psychiatric Association[3] as:

- A maladaptive pattern of alcohol use leading to clinically significant impairment or distress manifested within a 12-month period by one or more of the following;
  - Failure to fulfill role obligations at work, school, or home (at rehabilitation?)
  - Recurrent use in hazardous situations
  - Legal problems related to alcohol
  - Continued use despite alcohol-related social or interpersonal problems

Generally speaking, alcohol abuse is marked by repetitive consequences associated with the use. If the therapist notes a potential issue associated with alcohol use, he or she can use a screening tool, the CAGE instrument, to help determine the need for a consult. The CAGE instrument consists of four questions:

Have you ever felt you should **C**ut down on your drinking?

Have people **A**nnoyed you by criticizing your drinking?

Have you ever felt bad or **G**uilty about your drinking?

Have you ever had a drink first thing in the morning to steady your nerves or get rid of a hangover (**E**ye-opener)?

The sensitivity of the CAGE questionnaire for identifying lifetime alcohol problems in patients ranges from 60% to 95%, and the specificity ranges from 40% to 95% when the cut-off is set at two or more positive responses.[11,16,25] Finally, additional screening evidence that therapists may note is a pattern of being late or missing appointments, inappropriate behaviors directed toward staff or inappropriate interactions with staff, outbursts of anger or mood swings, and undue defensiveness when asked about alcohol (or drug) use.[4] Initiating a consult when at-risk drinking or alcohol abuse is suspected is extremely important because brief intervention strategies have been shown to be effective in individuals who have not yet progressed to the stage of alcohol dependence.[27]

Tobacco use is associated with increased risk for a number of disorders, including a variety of cardiovascular and pulmonary conditions as well as kidney and bladder cancers. Tobacco use also can impede patients' recovery from injury or surgery, as delayed bone and soft tissue healing has been reported in tobacco users.[10,24] Physical therapists see many patients after injury or surgery and use many factors to establish the initial prognosis for recovery. Tobacco use in these populations does not preclude a recovery from the trauma, but the patient might not progress at the expected speed; this tendency might prompt the therapist to modify goals when developing the plan of care.

Family History

Collecting family history at the initial visit, especially of first-degree relatives (parents and siblings), is important in identifying potential health risks to the patient. Many disorders tend to be passed on through the generations, and if a disorder appears in the family history, it may prompt a modified screening approach for the individual. Identifying patients with significant family histories, such as patients whose parents had heart problems diagnosed in their 40s, could prompt

the therapist to help the patient establish a relationship with a family practice physician. The therapist must make a point of asking detailed family history follow-up questions during the initial visit when the therapist has significant concerns about the patient's current health status. At this point, the decision to contact a physician about the health concerns essentially has been made, so gathering information relevant to the referral is warranted. If the patient reveals a family history of heart disease, the following questions become relevant:

- Who in your family has the heart disease?
- What type of heart disease do/did they have?
- At what age were they diagnosed?
- What is their current health status? If they have passed away, was it from the heart problem, and at what age?

The age of diagnosis is an important factor in the risk for the patient. For example, the risk of someone developing heart disease increases with a younger age of onset for the parents (e.g., diagnosed at age 40 versus 75 years). Knowing the health status of the family member reveals information about the patient's support system, or may reveal demands that the patient faces in providing care for the family member.

Methods Used to Collect Patient Health History Information

A challenge to all clinicians is to collect all of the necessary information in an effective and timely fashion. Patient health history data can be gathered from many different sources and through a variety of methods. In the inpatient setting, the patient medical record should contain a current health history record, while in the outpatient settings, access to the computerized health records, including physician reports, can produce the information. The therapist must consider, however, whether the information found in these sources is in fact accurate and up-to-date.

In the outpatient setting, having the patient complete a health history questionnaire before starting the interview can save time. The patient can fill out the form before the actual starting time of the scheduled patient appointment, and the therapist then can scan the questionnaire before beginning the interview. This allows for the identification of health issues that may fall outside the primary reason for the therapy visit, Knowledge of such issues before investigating the chief complaint (Chapter 6) allows the clinician to adjust his or her usual interview format to ensure that time is available to adequately address the potential health issues.

Appendices are included at the end of this chapter that offer examples of patient self-report questionnaires designed to collect patient health history information. Appendix B illustrates a questionnaire used by the author for more than 15 years in adult outpatient orthopedic clinics. Experience has shown that patients take about 6 to 8 minutes to complete the form. This form not only enables the therapist to collect health history information, but also allows the therapist to begin the review-of-systems (Chapter 7) investigation for issues such as general health, depression, and domestic violence. Appendix C is the same adult questionnaire translated into Spanish. Appendix D offers an example of a form designed for the pediatric population; the parents or other caregivers would complete this questionnaire. Finally, the *Guide to Physical Therapist Practice*[2] contains templates for data collection in both inpatient and outpatient settings.

Patient self-reports have long been advocated for use in ambulatory medical settings,[9,18,20,30] demonstrating reliability and validity in most cases, and if appropriate for the therapist's patient population, may save time by improving data-collection efficiency.[1,17,21,23,28] Care must be taken in developing the questionnaire, however, because open-ended and medication-related questions can lead to less-than-optimal accuracy of patient answers. For example, Boissonnault and Badke[8] reported that of 98 health history questionnaire items (illnesses, surgeries, medication use, and demographics) completed by outpatients with orthopedic conditions, 11 demonstrated poor-to-fair accuracy (per kappa statistics). Of these 11 questionnaire items, 5 were open-ended questions (list "other illnesses"), and 5 were inquiries about specific medications (e.g., Tylenol, "yes or no"). To avoid such open-ended questionnaire items, however, the clinician would need to add an all-inclusive list of items, such as illnesses, producing a form that is unrealistically long. Survey research describes a medical history profile of adult outpatients (primarily with orthopedic conditions) seeking physical therapy services[5,6] that can serve as a basis for items to include on a health history questionnaire. Discussing the content of the form with staff and with physician and pharmacist colleagues is highly recommended.

As described earlier, the questionnaire illustrated in Appendix B allows for the collection of information beyond the patient health history, as it includes screening elements for issues such as depression and domestic violence. Midway down the second column of Appendix B are four questions that fall within the category of *review of systems* for depression, domestic violence, and pregnancy. Why should all patients be asked questions about these particular issues? Our screening tools should address conditions and situations that therapists are likely to see most frequently and that have significance for patients' general well-being, morbidity, and mortality. In the author's clinic, many of the female patients are in their childbearing years, warranting the question, "Are you currently pregnant?" as a part of the form. The two questions for depression ("depressed mood or apathy") have been shown to be a useful instrument in screening for depression.[33] These questions have been found to have a sensitivity of 96% and a specificity of 57% for the diagnosis of depression; thus a negative response to both questions makes the presence of depression very unlikely, but a yes answer to one or both of the items would warrant further screening (see Chapter 7). Major clinical depression carries a lifetime prevalence of 10% to 25% for women and 5% to 12% for men, and also carries a risk that up to 15% of those with major clinical depression commit suicide.[3] Therefore screening for this condition warrants priority on any questionnaire. In Appendix B the screening questions for this issue include:

- Are you currently under the care of a psychiatrist/psychologist?
- Have you ever been diagnosed with depression?
- The two-question case-finding instrument ("depressed mood or apathy")
- Family history of mental illness?
- Have you recently noted fatigue or weight change (from the General Health Checklist, Chapter 7)?

The remaining two-part question ("Do you ever feel unsafe at home," and "Has anyone at home hit you or tried to injure you in any way?") screens for domestic violence, an extremely common health issue (more than 90% of cases involve women being abused by men):

- One in four women seeking care in an emergency department is a victim
- One in six women who are pregnant is abused during the pregnancy
- One in four women seen in primary-care settings has been abused at some point in her life

The two-part screening question for domestic violence has a sensitivity of 71% and a specificity of 85% in detecting domestic violence.[12,13] In most cases a victim probably will not volunteer a "yes" reply to this question to someone (the therapist) during the initial meeting, but at least the subject has been broached and a window of opportunity is available to the victim. Even with a "no" response, the therapist can affirm the patient's response, state that if she (or he) is ever in a threatening situation, there are resources available, and then briefly describe the resources. If the patient answers "yes" to either of these questions, the therapist should follow up by investigating:

- The nature of the abuse
- The dates/times of the abusive events
- The circumstances of the events
- Any previous assaults and resultant injuries
- Detailed documentation of any bruises, lacerations, or other signs

All facilities should have a specific procedure in place for handling such situations. The American Physical Therapy Association website (www.apta.org) is a good resource for more information on this topic.

Finally, in the author's clinic, many female patients are in their child-bearing years, warranting the question "Are you currently pregnant or think you might be?" as part of the form. If your clinical setting provides primarily women's health services, the questionnaire would contain many other items unique to this population (see Chapter 13).

When During the Patient Interview Should the Health History Be Reviewed?

As noted previously, ideally the therapist can review the patient's health history before beginning the interview, but the interview itself should begin with a discussion of what has precipitated the physical therapy examination (see Section Two Prologue). Discussing the patient's chief presenting complaint and primary goals will give the therapist important guidance for the remainder of the examination. After this discussion, the pertinent elements of the patient's health history can be discussed.

Summary

Integrating the patient demographic and health history information with the additional data collected during the history will give the therapist tools that will guide all aspects of clinical decision-making in the encounter with the patient. For example, this information may raise or lower the suspicion of an underlying serious disorder such as occult cancer of the skeletal system. The age groups at highest risk for this disease are those under the age of 20 years and over the age of 50 years, with the latter group involved most often. For those over the age of 50, the skeletal cancer is typically metastatic, with breast, lung, prostate, kidney, and thyroid cancers being the primary cancers that most often metastasize to the bony skeleton. Therefore patients with a recent history of any of these five primary cancers should be scrutinized for any warning signs of a return or spread of the cancer. This vigilance will carry over to the investigation of symptoms (Chapter 6) and the review of systems (Chapter 7). Skeletal metastasis occurs most often in the axial skeleton, including the shoulder girdle, rib cage, and proximal portions of the femur and humerus; thus any onset of new pain in this body area must be investigated closely. Because metastasis represents a systemic illness, the General Health Checklist described in Chapter 7 may reveal other important findings.

Developing an effective and efficient method for collecting patient health history information should be a priority of all practitioners. Being able to access patients' medical records or physicians' notes certainly produces valuable information, but do these sources contain all of the available reports, and has the patient's health status changed since the patient last saw the physician? These questions emphasize the fact that therapists working in most settings should be collecting patient health history information at the initial visit. One result of this detailed information gathering is that the therapist will often be able to add new, important information to the patient's permanent medical record.

REFERENCES

1. Abrahamson JH: The Cornell medical index—as an epidemiological tool, *Am J Public Health* 56:287-298, 1966
2. American Physical Therapy Association: *Guide to physical therapy practice*, ed 2, *Phys Ther* 81:9-744, 2001.
3. American Psychiatric Association: *Diagnostic and statistical manual of mental disorders*, ed 4, text revision, Washington, DC, 2000, American Psychiatric Association.
4. Bilkey WJ, Koopmeiners MB: Screening for psychological disorders. In Boissonnault W: *Examination in physical therapy practice, screening for medical disease*, New York, 1995, Churchill Livingstone, pp 277-302.
5. Boissonnault W, Koopmeiners MB: Medical history profile: orthopaedic physical therapy outpatients, *J Orthop Sports Phys Ther* 20:2-10, 1994.
6. Boissonnault W: Prevalence of comorbid conditions, surgeries, and medication use in a physical therapy outpatient population: a multicentered study, *J Orthop Sports Phys Ther* 29:506-525, 1999.
7. Boissonnault WG, Meek PD: Risk factors for anti-inflammatory-drug or aspirin-induced gastrointestinal complications in individuals receiving outpatient physical therapy services, *J Orthop Sports Phys Ther* 32:510-517, 2002.
8. Boissonnault W, Badke MB: Collecting patient health history information: the accuracy of a self-administered questionnaire in an orthopedic outpatient population (submitted for publication).
9. Brodman K, Erdmann AJ. The Cornell medical index, an adjustment to medical interview, *JAMA* 140:530-534, 1949.
10. Brown CS, Orune TJ, Richardson HD: The rate of pseudoarthrosis (surgical nonunion) in patients who are smokers and patients who are non-smokers: a comparison study, *Spine* 11:942-943, 1988.
11. Buschbaum DG, Welsh J, Buchanan RG, et al: Screening for alcohol abuse using CAGE scores and likelihood ratios, *Ann Intern Med* 115:774-777, 1991.
12. Eisenstat SA, Bancroft L: Domestic violence, *N Engl J Med* 341:886-892, 1999.
13. Feldhaus KM, Kozial-McLain J, Amsbury HL, et al: Accuracy of 3 brief screening questions for detecting partner violence in the emergency room, *JAMA* 277:1357-1361, 1997.
14. Fennelly M, Galletly DC, Purdie GI: Is caffeine withdrawal the mechanism of postoperative headache? *Anesth Analg* 72:449-453, 1991.
15. Ferree BA, Stern PJ, Jolson RS, et al: Deep venous thrombosis after spinal surgery, *Spine* 18:315-319, 1993.
16. Fleming MF, Barry KL: The effectiveness of alcoholism screening in an ambulatory care setting, *J Stud Alcohol* 52:33-36, 1991.
17. Gilkison CR, Fenton MV, and Lester JW: Getting the story straight: evaluating the test-retest reliability of a university health history questionnaire, *JCAH* 40:247-252, 1992.
18. Hall GH: Experiences with outpatient medical questionnaires, *Br Med J* 1:42-45, 1972.
19. Hanna EZ: Approach to the patient with alcohol abuse. In Goroll AH, Mulley AG, eds: *Primary care medicine*, ed 4, 2000, Baltimore, Lippincott Williams & Wilkins, pp 1169-1177.
20. Hershberg PI: Medical diagnosis: the role of a brief, open-ended medical history questionnaire, *J Med Educ* 44:293-297, 1969.
21. Inui TS, Jared RA, Carter WB, et al: Effects of a self-administered health history questionnaire on new-patient visits in a general medical clinic, *Medical Care* 17:1221-1228, 1979.
22. Jemal A, Tiwari RC, Murray T, et al: Cancer statistics, 2004, *CA Cancer J Clin* 54:8-29, 2004.
23. Katz JN, Chang LC, Sangha O, et al: Can comorbidity be measured by questionnaire rather than medical interview? *Medical Care* 34:73-83, 1996.
24. Lind J, Kramhoft M, Bodtker S: The influence of smoking on complications after primary amputations of the lower extremity, *Clin Orthop* 267:211-217, 1991.
25. Liskow B, Campbell J, Nickel EJ, et al: Validity of the CAGE questionnaire in screening for alcohol dependence in a walk-in (triage) clinic, *J Stud Alcohol* 56:277-281, 1995.
26. National Institute on Alcohol Abuse and Alcoholism: *The physicians' guide to helping patients with alcohol problems* (NIH publication no 95-3769), Washington, DC, 1995, Government Printing Office.
27. O'Connor PG, Schottenfeld RS: Patients with alcohol problems, *N Engl J Med* 338:592-602, 1998.
28. Pecoraro RE, Inui TS, Chen MS, et al: Validity and reliability of a self-administered health history questionnaire, *Public Health Records* 94:231-238, 1979.
29. Rasul AT, Tsukayama O, Gustilo RB: Effect of time of onset and depth of infection on the outcome of total knee arthroplasty infections, *Clin Orthop* 273:98-104, 1991.
30. Rockart JF, McLean ER, Hershberg PI, et al: An automated medical history system, *Arch Intern Med* 132:348-358, 1973.
31. Saunders JB, Aasland OG, Babor TF, et al: Development of the alcohol use disorders identification test (AUDIT): WHO collaborative project on early detection of persons with harmful alcohol consumption—II, *Addiction* 88:791-804, 1993.
32. Silverman K, Evans SM, Strain EC, et al: Withdrawal syndrome after the double-blind cessation of caffeine consumption, *N Engl J Med* 327:1109-1114, 1992.
33. Whooley MA, Avins AL, Miranda J, et al: Case-finding instruments for depression; two questions are as good as many, *JGIM* 12:439-445, 1997.

Appendix **A** **Review of Systems: Drug Side Effects/Subjective Complaints***

1. Gastrointestinal distress (dyspepsia, heartburn, nausea, vomiting, abdominal pain, constipation, diarrhea, bleeding)
   Salicylates
   NSAIDs
   Opioids
   Corticosteroids
   β-Blockers
   Calcium channel blockers
   Skeletal muscle relaxants
   Diuretics
   ACE inhibitors
   Digoxin
   Nitrates
   Cholesterol-lowering agents
   Antiarrhythmic agents
   Antidepressants (TCAs and MAO inhibitors, lithium)
   Neuroleptics
   Antiepileptic agents
   OCAs
   Estrogens and progestins
   Theophylline
2. Pulmonary (bronchospasm, shortness of breath, respiratory depression)
   Salicylates
   NSAIDs
   Opioids
   β-Blockers
   ACE inhibitors
3. Central nervous system (dizziness, drowsiness, insomnia, headaches, hallucinations, confusion, anxiety, depression, muscle weakness)
   NSAIDs
   Skeletal muscle relaxants
   Opioids
   Corticosteroids
   β-Blockers
   Calcium channel blockers
   Nitrates
   ACE inhibitors
   Digoxin
   Antianxiety agents
   Antidepressants (TCAs and MAO inhibitors)
   Neuroleptics
   Antiepileptic agents
   OCAs
   Estrogens and progestins
4. Dermatologic (skin rash, itching, flushing of face)
   NSAIDs
   Corticosteroids
   β-Blockers
   Opioids
   Calcium channel blockers
   ACE inhibitors

   Nitrates
   Cholesterol-lowering agents
   Antiarrhythmic agents
   MAO inhibitors and lithium
   OCAs
   Estrogens and progestins
   Antiepileptics
5. Musculoskeletal (weakness, fatigue, cramps, arthritis, decreased exercise tolerance, osteoporosis)
   Corticosteroids
   β-Blockers
   Calcium channel blockers
   ACE inhibitors
   Diuretics
   Digoxin
   Antianxiety agents
   Antiepileptic agents
   Antidepressants
   Neuroleptic agents
6. Cardiac (bradycardia, ventricular irritability, AV block, PVCs, ventricular tachycardia)
   Opioids
   Diuretics
   β-Blockers
   Calcium channel blockers
   Digoxin
   Antiarrhythmic agents
   TCAs
   Neuroleptics
   Oral antiasthmatic agents
7. Vascular (claudication, hypotension, peripheral edema, cold extremities)
   NSAIDs
   Corticosteroids
   Diuretics
   β-Blockers
   Calcium channel blockers
   ACE inhibitors
   Nitrates
   Antidepressants (TCAs and MAO inhibitors)
   Neuroleptics
   OCAs
   Estrogens and progestins
8. Genitourinary (sexual dysfunction, urinary retention, urinary incontinence)
   Opioids
   Diuretics
   β-Blockers
   Antiarrhythmic agents
   Antidepressants (TCAs and MAO inhibitors)
   Neuroleptics
   OCAs
   Estrogens and progestins

9. HEENT (tinnitus, loss of taste, headache, lightheadedness, dizziness)
Salicylates
NSAIDs
Opioids
Skeletal muscle relaxants
β-Blockers
Nitrates
Calcium channel blockers
ACE inhibitors
Digoxin

Antiarrhythmic agents
Antianxiety agents
Antidepressants (TCAs and MAO inhibitors)
Antiepileptic agents

From Boissonnault W: *Examination in physical therapy practice, screening for medical disease*, ed 2, New York, 1995, Churchill Livingstone. *TCAs*, Tricyclic antidepressants; *MAO* inhibitors, monoamine oxidase; *ACE*, angiotensin-converting enzyme; *OCAs*, oral contraceptive agents; *AV*, atrioventricular; *PVCs*, premature ventricular contractions; *HEENT*, head, eyes, ears, nose, throat; *NSAIDs*, nonsteroidal antiinflammatory drugs.
*In order of most common occurrence.

Appendix B

To ensure you receive a complete and thorough evaluation, please provide us with the important background information requested on the following form. If you do not understand a question leave it blank and your therapist will assist you. Thank you!

NAME:_____ LEISURE ACTIVITIES:_____
OCCUPATION:_____

ALLERGIES: List any medication(s) you are allergic to:
_____
Are you latex sensitive? YES NO
List any allergies we should know about:
_____

Please check (√) any of the following whose care you're under:
__Medical doctor (MD)   __Psychiatrist/ Psychologist   Other_____
__Osteopath   __Physical Therapist
__Dentist   __Chiropractor

If you have seen any of the above during the past 3 months, please describe the reason (e.g., illness, medical condition, physical):
_____
_____

Have you EVER been diagnosed as having any of the following conditions?

YES NO Cancer. If YES, describe what kind:_____
YES NO Heart problems
YES NO High blood pressure
YES NO Circulation problems
YES NO Asthma
YES NO Emphysema/Bronchitis
YES NO Chemical dependency (e.g., alcoholism)
YES NO Thyroid problems

YES NO Diabetes
YES NO Multiple sclerosis
YES NO Rheumatoid arthritis
YES NO Other arthritic conditions
YES NO Depression
YES NO Hepatitis
YES NO Tuberculosis
YES NO Stroke
YES NO Kidney disease
YES NO Anemia
YES NO Epilepsy
YES NO Other

For Office Use

During the past month have you been feeling down, depressed, or hopeless? YES NO
During the past month have you been bothered by having little interest or pleasure in doing things? YES NO
Do you ever feel unsafe at home or has anyone hit you or tried to injure you in any way? YES NO
FOR WOMEN: Are you currently pregnant or do you think you might be pregnant? YES NO

Please list any surgeries or other conditions for which you have been hospitalized, including the approximate date and reason for the surgery or hospitalization:

DATE   REASON FOR SURGERY/HOSPITALIZATION

1. _____
2. _____
3. _____
4. _____
5. _____
6. _____

Please describe any significant injuries for which you have been treated (including fractures, dislocations, sprains) and the approximate date of injury:

DATE   INJURY   DATE   INJURY
____ ____ ____ ____
____ ____ ____ ____

Has anyone in your immediate family (parents, brothers, sisters) ever been treated for any of the following?

YES NO Diabetes
YES NO Tuberculosis
YES NO Heart disease
YES NO High blood pressure
YES NO Stroke
YES NO Kidney disease
YES NO Alcoholism (chemical dependency)

YES NO Cancer
YES NO Arthritis
YES NO Anemia
YES NO Headaches
YES NO Epilepsy
YES NO Mental illness

Which of the following OVER-THE-COUNTER medications have you taken in the last week?

YES NO Aspirin
YES NO Tylenol
YES NO Advil/Motrin/Ibuprofen
YES NO Laxatives
YES NO Decongestants
YES NO Antihistamines
YES NO Antacid
YES NO Vitamins/mineral supplements
YES NO Other_____

For Office Use

Please list any PRESCRIPTION medication you are currently taking (INCLUDING pills, injections, and/or skin patches):

1. _____ 2. _____ 3. _____
4. _____ 5. _____ 6. _____

How many caffeinated coffee or caffeine-containing beverages do you drink per day?_____
How many packs of cigarettes do you smoke a day?_____
How many days per week do you drink alcohol?_____
If one drink equals one beer or glass of wine, how much do you drink at an average sitting?_____

Have you recently noted:
YES NO Weight loss/gain
YES NO Nausea/vomiting
YES NO Dizziness/Lightheadedness
YES NO Fatigue
YES NO Weakness
YES NO Fever/chills/sweats
YES NO Numbness or tingling

For Office Use

Therapist signature   Date   Patient signature   Date

Apéndice C

Para asegurarnos de que usted recibe una evaluación completa, sea tan amable de proveernos con la información más importante de su historial médico. Si usted no entiende alguna de las siguientes preguntas, déjelas sin contestar, y su terapista físico le ayudará. Gracias por su cooperación.

NOMBRE:_____ PASATIEMPOS:_____
TRABAJO:_____

ALERGIAS: Indique aquellos medicamentos a los que usted es alérgico:
_____
¿Es usted sensible o alérgico al látex? SÍ NO:_____
Mencione aquellas alergias que usted entiende debemos conocer: _____

¿Ha declarado usted el "Directiva Avanzada Médica" de no resucitar? SÍ:___ NO:___

Favor de marcar (√) a aquellos de los siguientes especialistas que manejan el cuidado de su salud:
___Doctor en Medicina (MD) ___Siquiatra/Sicólogo Otro____
___Osteópata   ___Terapista Físico   ____
___Dentista   ___Quiropráctico

Si usted ha visitado alguno de los especialistas arriba mencionados en los últimos 3 meses, por favor indique cuál fue la razón de la visita (e.j., enfermedad, condición médica, examen físico):
_____
_____

¿Ha sido usted diagnosticado ALGUNA VEZ con cualquiera de las siguientes condiciones?

SÍ NO Cáncer. Si es SÍ, indique cuál tipo:_____
SÍ NO Problemas cardíacos
SÍ NO Alta presión sanguínea
SÍ NO Problemas circulatorios
SÍ NO Asma
SÍ NO Emfisema/Bronquitis
SÍ NO Dependencia química (e.j., alcoholismo)
SÍ NO Problemas de la tiroide
SÍ NO Diabetes
SÍ NO Esclerosis múltiple
SÍ NO Artritis reumatoide
SÍ NO Otras condiciones artríticas
SÍ NO Depresión
SÍ NO Hepatitis
SÍ NO Tuberculosis
SÍ NO Infarto cerebral
SÍ NO Enfermedad renal (riñón)
SÍ NO Anemia
SÍ NO Epilepsia
SÍ NO Otro

Para el uso de la oficina

¿Se ha sentido triste, deprimido(a), o desesperado(a) en el pasado mes? SÍ NO

En el pasado mes, ¿se ha preocupado porque siente que tiene poco interés o placer haciendo actividades que normalmente goce? SÍ NO

¿Se has sentido alguna vez inseguro(a) en su propia casa, o alguna vez alguien le ha golpeado o tratado de lastimar de alguna manera? SÍ NO

SOLO MUJERES: ¿Está embarazada o piensa que podría estarlo? SÍ NO

Favor indicar cualquier tipo de cirujía u otro tipo de condición por la cual usted haya sido hospitalizado(a), incluyendo la fecha aproximada y la razón para la cirujía/ hospitalización:

FECHA   RAZON PARA CIRUJÍA/HOSPITALIZACIÓN
1. _____ _____
2. _____ _____
3. _____ _____
4. _____ _____

Por favor, indique si usted ha recibido alguna lesión grave por la cual haya sido tratado (incluya fracturas, dislocaciones, desgarre/estiramiento de ligamentos/tendones) y la fecha aproximada de la lesión:

FECHA   LESIÓN   FECHA   LESIÓN
_____ _____ _____ _____

_____ _____ _____ _____

¿Ha sido un miembro de su familia inmediata (padres, hermanos[as]) tratado alguna vez por alguna de las siguientes condiciones?

SÍ NO Diabetes   SÍ NO Cáncer
SÍ NO Tuberculosis   SÍ NO Artritis
SÍÍ NO Enfermedad cardíaca SÍ NO Anemia
SÍ NO Alta presión sanguínea SÍ NO Dolor de cabeza
SÍ NO Infarto cerebral   SÍ NO Epilepsia

SÍ NO Enfermedad renal (riñón) SÍ NO Enfermedad mental
SÍ NO Alcoholismo (dependencia química)

¿Cúal de los siguientes medicamentos SIN PRESCRIPCION usted ha tomado en la última semana?

SÍ NO Aspirina   SÍ NO Antihistamínicos
SÍ NO Tylenol   SÍ NO Laxantes
SÍ NO Advil/Motrin/Ibuprofen SÍ NO Antiácido
SÍ NO Descongestionantes SÍ NO Suplementos vitamínicos/ minerales

SÍ NO Otros _____

Favor de indicar los medicamentos bajo PRESCRIPCION que usted está actualmente tomando (INCLUYA pastillas, inyecciones, cremas medicadas, y/o parchos de piel)

1. _____ 2. _____ 3. _____
4. _____ 5. _____ 6. _____

¿Cuánto café cafeinado o bebidas carbonatadas con cafeína usted consume por día? _____

¿Cuántos paquetes/cajetillas de cigarrillos usted fuma al día? _____

¿Cuántos días a la semana usted toma bebidas alcohólicas? _____

Si una bebida es equivalente a una cerveza o copa de vino, ¿cuánto usted toma al día? _____

¿Ha notado recientemente:

SÍ NO Aumento/pérdida de peso? SÍ NO Debilidad?
SÍ NO Nauseas/vómitos? SÍ NO Fiebre/sudores/ escalofrios?
SÍ NO Fatiga?   SÍ NO Adormecimiento u hormiguilleo?

_____ _____
Therapist Signature (Firma del Terapista) _____ Date (Fecha)

_____ _____
Patient signature   Date

Appendix D Gibson-Pike-Warrick Special Education Cooperative-General Health Form

To ensure your child receives a complete and thorough evaluation, please provide us with the important background information on the following form. If you do not understand a question, your therapist will assist you. Thank you.

Child's Name_____
   Birthdate_____
School_____
   Teacher_____
Parent/Guardian_____
   Home Phone_____
Address_____

Work Phone_____

Has the child seen any of the following in the past 3 months? If Yes, who?

Yes No Medical Doctor_____
Yes No Psychiatrist/Psychologist_____
Yes No Orthopedic_____
Yes No Eye Doctor_____
Yes No Osteopath_____
Yes No Physical Therapist_____
Yes No Dentist_____
Yes No Chiropractor_____

Please describe the reason the child visited the above person (illness, medical, surgery):

_____
_____
_____
_____
_____
_____
_____

For what problem is the child being evaluated by the therapist?

_____
_____
_____

Has the child EVER been diagnosed as having any of the following?

Yes	No	Cancer
Yes	No	Heart problems
Yes	No	High blood pressure
Yes	No	Asthma/Breathing problems
Yes	No	Thyroid problems
Yes	No	Diabetes
Yes	No	Arthritis
Yes	No	Depression
Yes	No	Hepatitis
Yes	No	Tuberculosis
Yes	No	Stroke
Yes	No	Kidney disease
Yes	No	Anemia
Yes	No	Epilepsy
Yes	No	Seizures
Yes	No	Cerebral palsy
Yes	No	Muscular dystrophy
Yes	No	Spina bifida/myelomeningocele
Yes	No	ADD/ADHD
Yes	No	Other

Please list any surgeries or other conditions for which the child has been in the hospital:

_____
_____
_____
_____
_____
_____
_____
_____
_____
_____

Has anyone in the child's immediate family (parents, brothers, sisters) ever been treated for any of the following?

Yes	No	Diabetes
Yes	No	Tuberculosis
Yes	No	Heart disease
Yes	No	High blood pressure
Yes	No	Stroke
Yes	No	Kidney disease

Yes	No	Cancer
Yes	No	Arthritis
Yes	No	Anemia
Yes	No	Headaches
Yes	No	Epilepsy
Yes	No	Mental illness
Yes	No	Alcoholism or chemical dependency

Please list all of the prescription medications and the dosage that the child is currently taking:

_____
_____
_____
_____
_____
_____
_____
_____

List any over-the-counter medications the child frequently takes:

_____
_____

Has the child recently experienced any of the following?

Yes	No	Weight loss or gain
Yes	No	Nausea/vomiting
Yes	No	Fatigue
Yes	No	Unusual weakness
Yes	No	Fever/chills/sweats

How many caffeine-containing beverages does the child drink daily? _____

Does the child have allergies? _____

Does the child have special equipment? What? _____
_____
_____

What functional problems is the child having at home? _____
_____
_____
_____

Person completing form? _____
   Date _____
Form reviewed by therapist with parent/guardian? Yes No
   Date _____

_____
 (Therapist)
Date _____

Symptom Investigation 6

Joseph J. Godges, DPT, MA, OCS
William G. Boissonnault, PT, DHSc, FAAOMPT

Objectives

After reading this chapter, the reader will be able to:

1. Describe the types of patient data that fall under the category of symptom investigation, including the information that constitutes a red flag requiring physician contact.
2. Summarize symptoms/signs associated with medical disorders that may result in patient pain syndromes common to the practice of physical therapy.
3. Describe medical-screening questionnaires and incorporate them into an examination scheme for patients with common pain syndromes.

Investigating a patient's presenting disorder usually reveals the reason the patient has consulted the physical therapist (PT). Symptoms such as lower back, shoulder, or knee pain that interferes with daily activities motivates many people to seek physical therapy services.[4,14,23] Many of these patients assume that the symptoms are related to a sprain, strain, poor posture, or arthritic condition. For a percentage of these patients, however, the symptoms are related to a more serious medical condition. For example, low back pain, an extremely common reason that patients seek care in ambulatory clinics, can be mechanical in nature or related to cancer, infection, visceral disease, or fractures. Jarvik and Deyo[20] estimate that of the patients with low back pain presenting to ambulatory primary-care clinics, 4% will have symptoms associated with an osteoporosis-related fracture, 2% with a spondylolisthesis/spondylolysis, 2% with visceral disease, 0.7% with cancer, and 0.5% with infection. The clinician must promptly recognize the patient at risk for such conditions and make the appropriate referral.

A primary objective of the examination process is deciding whether: (1) PT intervention is appropriate, (2) consultation with another health care provider is required along with PT intervention, or (3) PT intervention is not indicated and the patient needs to be managed by another provider.[10] The patient's description of symptoms, being the initial focus of the patient-interview process, often is the point in the examination process at which the PT's suspicion of a potentially serious etiology of symptoms is first raised. This suspicion is based on an atypical description of symptoms provided by the patient, a description that does not make sense based on the PT's understanding of basic and clinical sciences, and the PT's clinical experiences.

The symptom investigation includes subcategories of symptom location, onset (history) of symptoms, and behavior of symptoms. The patient's description of the symptoms will lead to the PT's questions about when and how the symptoms began and how the symptoms fluctuate over a defined period of time (e.g., 24 hours). Just as important, the location of symptoms should alert the PT to other possible "pain generators" (disease entities) that would warrant a referral if present. The PT must know what diseases could produce local pain or referred pain in a region so he or she can screen for other symptoms or signs associated with these conditions.

This chapter discusses the medical screening principles used in the investigation of patients' chief presenting symptoms. The follow-up questions associated with red flags also will be discussed. For example, night pain (pain that wakes a patient from sleep) is considered a red flag and is possibly associated with serious pathology. Yet some authors have associated night pain with degenerative joint disease, especially of the lumbar spine, hip, and knee joints, and others have noted that night pain occurs in a large proportion of patients who apparently do not have a serious disease. So, when is night pain a red flag, suggestive of a potentially life-threatening disorder? Can the clinician determine the seriousness of this symptom with further questioning after the patient reveals the night pain?

In addition, the chapter lists and describes the diseases that are possible "pain generators" in the low back, pelvis/hip/thigh, knee/leg/ankle/foot, thorax, cervical spine/shoulder, head/face, and elbow/wrist/hand regions. Many of these diseases, if suspected, would prompt communication with a physician. Initiating a plan of care for an apparent musculoskeletal disorder that is actually produced by a more serious underlying medical condition can cause grave consequences to the patient.

For example, delaying referral of a patient who complains of lower leg pain and swelling resulting from an acute anterior compartment syndrome while a trial of physical agents is undertaken to relieve the leg pain and inflammation could result in unnecessary serious disability (e.g., paresis or paralysis) for the patient. In another example, a patient might seek physical therapy services for management of a calf pain. Implementing a treatment of soft tissue mobilization/manipulation, ultrasound, and therapeutic exercise could result in medical complications for the patient if the actual cause of the symptoms is a deep vein thrombosis. This chapter describes other potential symptoms and signs besides pain associated with each of the disorders. Finally, a summary table and a self-report medical screening questionnaire for each of the seven body regions are offered as "quick clinical reference guides."

Symptom Investigation

Location of Symptoms

To help document symptoms, the authors recommend the use of a body diagram for noting the exact location of symptoms, including pain, paresthesia, numbness, and weakness. The questioning should start with the patient's chief symptom, that is, the symptom(s) that are most interfering with function, assuming this is the reason physical therapy services have been initiated.

After the PT has determined the description of the chief symptom (e.g., ache, stiffness, pressure), the PT asks, "Do you have symptoms anywhere else?" For example, Figure 6-1 shows that this patient presented with low lumbar and right buttock pain (dull ache). After reporting these symptoms, the patient stated, "That is all of the symptoms I have."

The next follow-up question is: "So you don't experience any pain, pins and needles, weakness, or numbness down the backs of your legs, on the bottoms of your feet, up the front of your body, including the pelvis, stomach, chest, neck, or face, or between your shoulder blades, and you don't experience any headaches?" Noting where the patient *does not* have symptoms is just as important as documenting where the patient does have symptoms. Patients may not volunteer that they have belly pain or facial pain. Their rationale may be, "Why does the PT need to know if my stomach hurts? I am here for my low back pain," or "My physician takes care of my stomach problem, not my PT."

In addition, one of the ways disease-related symptoms may be missed is that the patient has such severe or intense symptoms in one area that he or she pays little attention to a mild ache that was present before the injury. This aching may not be limiting function at all, and if the patient has seen a physician, the patient might not have mentioned the ache. Asymptomatic areas should be noted on the body diagram with a check mark or some other notation, as shown in Figure 6-1.

The investigation of symptoms also includes the patient's description of the symptoms. Sometimes the patient may use more than one descriptor for a symptom. For example, the patient may state that he or she has pain and stiffness, aching, and sharp soreness over the right iliac crest region. The PT must assess each descriptor independently of the others, including the onset and pattern of symptoms. Hearing a similar pattern (aggravating and alleviating factors) for each of the descriptors would lead the PT to believe all three symptoms are related to the same lesion, but hearing different patterns for the symptoms should lead the PT to consider that iliac crest symptoms might have more than one source.

Pain from visceral structures typically would be thought to be located in the anterior chest wall or abdominal regions, but a number of viscera are located in the retroperitoneal region of the trunk. These structures include portions of the duodenum, ascending and descending colon, abdominal aorta, pancreas, and kidneys, and if diseased, may be manifested as back pain rather than belly pain. This leads to considerable "overlap" between pain location patterns associated with visceral disorders and common musculoskeletal disorders (Figure 6-2 and Table 6-1). In addition, many pain-generating diseases simply present as a dull ache, stiffness, or mild to moderate soreness in their early or middle stages; these also are very common conditions for many patient populations. The location of the symptoms by itself rarely is significant in deciding whether a referral is in order. Exceptions to this rule are the patient with symptoms of chest pain or pressure with pain extending into the left upper extremity. PTs (and many patients) rightly would suspect possible involvement of the heart in that scenario. Descriptors such as throbbing, pulsating, and pounding also suggest involvement of the vascular system rather than pain of musculoskeletal origin.

Although the symptom location only occasionally helps to differentiate diseases from impairments, these patient data do play an important role in the medical screening process. Knowledge of potential pain patterns associated with viscera can guide the PT in selecting the organ systems to screen with review-of-systems questioning (see Chapter 7). Finally, knowing the pain patterns associated with various diseases will help PTs know which disorders should be suspected as he or she carries out the examination.

Symptom History

For many patients, the current episode of symptoms is not the first episode, but the most relevant information in the initial visit is a description of the most recent injury or flare-up. If the patient is asked, "When did your symptoms begin?" the reply may be "20 years ago," and after a 5-minute discussion of the incident of 20 years ago, the PT might conclude that he or she has learned nothing that influences today's clinical decision-making.

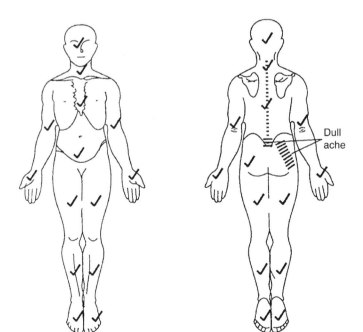

Dull ache

FIGURE 6-1 Example of a body diagram used to illustrate symptomatic and asymptomatic body regions. (From Boissonnault WG: *Examination in physical therapy practice: screening for medical disease*, ed 2, New York, 1995, Churchill Livingstone, p 5.)

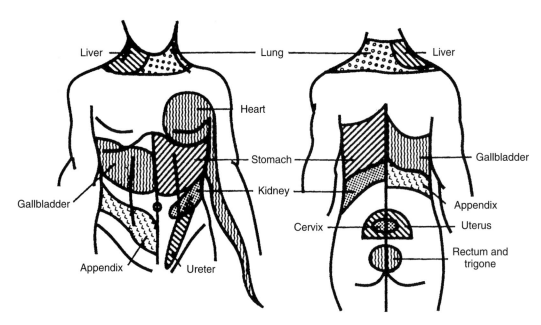

FIGURE 6-2 Possible local and referred pain patterns of visceral structures. (From Boissonnault WG: *Examination in physical therapy practice: screening for medical disease*, ed 2, New York, 1995, Churchill Livingstone, p 6.)

To promote practice efficiency, start with the current or most recent episode, and then work backward chronologically to the initial event.

Impairment-related symptoms typically are associated with a traumatic incident, an accident, repetitive overuse, or sustained postural strains. These events may include lifting an object, falling, or taking an extended car ride or plane trip, or the patient may report shoulder or back pain after a day of heavy yard work. However, many patients cannot relate the onset of their symptoms to any particular incident or accident. Careful questioning by the PT will reveal a likely cause, such as the patient beginning to run after not running for 3 months, being promoted to an administrative position that requires sitting for 8 hours per day, or beginning gardening or yard work after a winter of inactivity. If the onset of symptoms is truly insidious, if new symptoms occur insidiously during the course of treatment, or if resolved symptoms return for no apparent mechanical reason, the PT should be concerned about the underlying nature of the condition.[50]

Investigation of previous episodes of the chief presenting complaint also may produce relevant examination information. One way pain-generating diseases may "slip through" the health care system occurs when a patient with chronic neck pain has a new episode. In the patient's mind, this is their "usual" neck pain, and if a PT already has seen this patient a few times for these symptoms, the PT also may make the same assumption. These assumptions may lead the patient to fail to report a unique finding about his or her current episode and may cause the PT to skip steps in the examination process. In the past, the flare-ups might have always been associated with prolonged travel or time at a computer, but neither might be the case for this episode. The current episode could in fact be related to the previous condition, but any change in the symptom descriptors, onset of symptoms, or 24-hour report of symptoms compared with previous episodes should alert the PT that this condition may have a different etiology.

Behavior of Symptoms

The patient report of symptom site and intensity changes over a defined period of time produces information vital to the medical screening process. The PT should ask questions about:

- The relationship symptoms have to rest, activities, time of day (morning, midday, evening, or night) and positions/postures
- The constancy, frequency, and duration of symptoms, including fluctuations in intensity[30]

For many patients with neuromusculoskeletal disorders, a description of how symptoms do or do not change over a 24-hour period is adequate. For patients with disorders such as multiple sclerosis, stroke, or head injury, the timeframe may be 3 to 6 months.

Besides insidious onset of symptoms, a report of an unexpected or atypical *behavior of symptoms* may be the initial clue that raises the suspicion of a serious underlying condition. Symptoms associated with impairments or movement disorders typically fluctuate accordingly as the mechanical loads on the body increase or decrease with time of day, onset or cessation of specific activities, and the assumption or avoidance of certain postures. This expected *behavior of symptom* pattern fits many patients seeking physical therapy services, with or without a pathoanatomical etiology of symptoms. Boissonnault and DiFabio[5] found in a study of pain profiles for patients with low back pain that there was no difference in the time of day pain was most intense, movements and postures that altered symptoms, or frequency of night pain in patients with disk pathology (degeneration, internal disruption, herniation, or bulging) versus those with no pathoanatomical findings on magnetic resonance imaging (MRI) or computed tomography

TABLE 6-1
Visceral Local and Referred Pain Patterns

Structure	Segmental Innervation	Possible Areas of Pain Location
PELVIC ORGANS		
Uterus including uterine ligaments	T1-L1, S2-S4	Lumbosacral junction Sacral Thoracolumbar
Ovaries	T10-T11	Lower abdominal Sacral
Testes	T10-T11	Lower abdominal Sacral
RETROPERITONEAL REGION		
Kidney	T10-L1	Lumbar spine ((ipsilateral) Lower abdominal Upper abdominal
Ureter	T11-L2, S2-S4	Groin Upper abdominal Suprapubic Medial, proximal thigh Thoracolumbar
Urinary bladder	T11-L2, S2-S4	Sacral apex Suprapubic Thoracolumbar
Prostate gland	T11-L1, S2-S4	Sacral Testes Thoracolumbar
DIGESTIVE SYSTEM ORGANS		
Esophagus	T4-T6	Substernal and upper abdominal
Stomach	T6-T10	Upper abdominal Middle and lower thoracic spine
Small intestine	T7-T10	Middle thoracic spine
Pancreas	T10	Upper abdominal Lower thoracic spine Upper lumbar spine
Gallbladder	T7-T9	Right upper abdominal Right middle and lower thoracic spine, aspect scapula
Liver	T7-T9	Right middle and lower thoracic spine Right cervical spine
Common bile duct	T8-T10	Upper abdominal Middle thoracic spine
Large intestine	T11-L1	Lower abdominal Middle lumbar spine
Sigmoid colon	T11-T12	Upper sacral Suprapubic Left lower quadrant of abdomen
CARDIOPULMONARY SYSTEM		
Heart	T1-T5	Cervical anterior Upper thorax Left upper extremity
Lungs and bronchi	T5-T6	Ipsilateral thoracic spine Cervical (diaphragm involved)
Diaphragm (central portion)	C3-C5	Cervical spine

From Boissonnault W, Bass C: Pathological origins of trunk and neck pain: parts I, II, III, *J Orthop Sports Phys Ther* 12(5):191-221, 1990.

(CT) scans. If the symptom pattern reveals no pattern, the PT should begin questioning whether physical therapy intervention is warranted. This inconsistent symptom pattern should alert the PT to screen specific body systems later in the examination (see Chapter 7).

Symptoms associated with visceral disease will vary in their behavior depending on the severity of the disorder and the function of the structure. Therefore a patient report of intermittent pain does not rule out the possibility of disease. If the patient's thoracic-spine pain is the result of a duodenal ulcer, gastrointestinal system activity may alter the symptoms. For example, the pain associated with the ulcer probably will be reduced shortly after the patient eats, because the food acts as a buffer, and a few hours after eating the pain will return or intensify. The patient probably will not make the connection between eating and pain level; in fact the patient may attribute the symptoms to certain activities or to working at a computer for a number of hours. Careful questioning about the change of symptoms over a 24-hour period may reveal inconsistencies that catch the clinician's attention.

Another example of visceral pain that may mimic mechanical pain patterns is colicky pain. Spasm of the smooth muscle wall of a hollow visceral structure will result in a deep cramping, gnawing, achy sensation that is intermittent. The pain intensity will vary depending on the intensity of the spasm of the smooth muscle wall; the spasms often are mild initially but build to a crescendo over a period of minutes. Although the spasms may come at a variety of times (while the patient is sitting, standing, lying down, or walking) the patient may be pain free much of the time. Gastroenteritis, constipation, menstruation, gallbladder disease, and ureteral obstruction all have been implicated in causing colicky pain experienced in the belly or back areas.[33]

Finally, an inconsistent pattern of change in symptom intensity is not the only warning sign that may be discovered during behavior-of-symptom questioning. Symptoms that move from one body location to another for no apparent mechanical reason are also an atypical report for many patients seeking physical therapy services. For example, a patient may note right shoulder and wrist pain during the initial visit and at the second visit report right and left shoulder and left elbow and wrist pain. This patient cannot describe any reason why the apparently new pains have started. Primary neurologic, endocrine, or rheumatic disorders, or adverse drug reactions may account for a symptom pattern such as this (see Chapter 7).

The investigation of symptom behavior over a defined period of time (often 24 hours) includes questions about night pain. Night pain (pain that wakes someone from sleep) has been associated with serious diseases such as cancer and infection.[3,35,43,46] Many studies also describe night pain as being associated with degenerative joint disease, especially of the lumbar, hip, and knee regions.* In addition, a significant percentage of patients with low back pain reported night pain with no evidence of serious disease. So, when is night pain a red flag? When night pain is reported, follow-up questions should be:

• How many nights per week?
• Is there a consistent time when you wake up?
• How does the intensity of the night pain compare with the pain experienced at other times of the day?
• What do you have to do to fall back asleep?

Boissonnault and DiFabio[5] noted that 53% of patients with a complaint of back pain reported night pain. Only one of this group stated that the night pain was more intense than the pain in the morning, midday, or evening, and almost 80%

stated that they simply had to change position in bed to fall back to sleep. This pattern would be expected for the patient with non-acute low back pain. The practitioner would assume that the low back area would be mechanically loaded to a greater degree, and therefore more painful, when the patient was physically active. In addition, many patients with low back pain start the night sleeping supine with a pillow under the knees or side-lying with a pillow between the legs to support the lumbar region, but wake up with the pillows on the floor and lying halfway onto their stomach. Low back discomfort wakes them up, but they fall back to sleep with minimal effort after the pillows are back in place. More concern would be warranted if the night pain was the patient's most intense pain and if it took more than minimal effort to fall back to sleep (nonacute conditions).

Finally, another patient report that would cause concern is a report that the night pain episodes were becoming more frequent and severe without any "mechanical" explanation for the worsening. Based on the current evidence, one must conclude that the presence of night pain as the sole red flag has little diagnostic value but must be considered in context of the other examination findings.

In summary, the symptom investigation often is the step that first alerts the PT to the possible need for a patient referral. Careful questioning will reveal a pattern of symptoms that is unusual for patients with impairment-driven conditions. Using a body diagram to document the location of symptoms and a description of the symptoms can save documentation time for the PT. A well-organized sequence of questions will allow a patient to give an accurate history of his or her reasons for seeking medical care:

• In which area are symptoms most interfering with functions or daily activities?
• Describe the symptom(s) to me (e.g., ache, pins and needles)
• Do these symptoms spread to any other body regions or parts?
• Was there a recent injury or flare-up? If so, when?
• If not, can you explain why these symptoms may have begun?
• Are the symptoms constant or do they come and go?
• What makes the symptoms worse or better?
• Can you rate the intensity of the symptoms on a 0-10 scale?
• Do the symptoms wake you up at night?
• Have you had any previous episodes like this?
• Do you have symptoms anywhere else? (If so, repeat the above line of questioning.)

Regional Pain Patterns and Associated Diseases and Disorders

Low Back Pain

Consider a 55-year-old patient with a recent history of low back pain who is being examined by a PT. Four serious conditions that may present as low back pain are tumors, spinal infections, vertebral fracture, and cauda equina syndrome.[3] As this patient is describing the pain and activity limitations, he reports that his pain has not resolved with rest or antiinflammatory medications over the past 6 weeks. The PT recalls that

---

*References 1, 16, 17, 21, 24, 36.

lack of improvement for a patient over the age of 50 years with acute low back pain is a red flag, increasing the index of suspicion that the patient's low back pain is caused by a tumor, rather than by a relatively less serious musculoskeletal disorder such as a lumbar or sacroiliac ligament sprain.[13]

This patient's reported lack of improvement leads the PT to verify the patient's age and ask whether the patient has a history of cancer or has experienced recent, unexplained weight loss. Evidence supporting the value of these inquiries is found in a study by Deyo and Diehl on patients with low back pain who had cancer. Deyo and Diehl[12] reported that, of the 13 patients whose low back pain was caused by cancer (out of a total subject pool of 1975 patients with low back pain), all 13 were over 50 years of age, had a history of cancer, had experienced unexplained weight loss, or had failed to improve with conservative therapy.

The PT thus asks our 55-year-old patient the following questions to increase or decrease the index of suspicion that this patient's low back pain is caused by cancer:

- Do you have a history of cancer? If so, what type of cancer (e.g., lung, breast, prostate)?
- Have you recently lost weight, even though you have *not* been attempting to eat less or exercise more? If so, how much?

In our example, the patient responds "no" to each question. Next, the PT considers three other serious pathologies that may cause low back pain. One of these conditions is a back-related infection, such as spinal osteomyelitis.[45] The red flags that raise suspicion of osteomyelitis as a cause of the low back pain all are factors that put the patient at risk for spinal infection. These factors are current recent bacterial infection (e.g., urinary tract or skin infections), intravenous drug use and or abuse, and concurrent suppression of the patient's immune system. The PT thus asks the following questions to increase or decrease the index of suspicion that this patient's low back pain is caused by a back-related infection:

- Have you recently had a fever?
- Have you recently taken antibiotics or other medicines for an infection?
- Have you been diagnosed with an immunosuppressive disorder?
- Does your pain ease when you rest in a comfortable position?

Again, the patient responds "no" to the all of the above questions. Negative responses to the first three questions reduce the suspicion that this patient has a back-related infection. A negative response to the fourth question, however, suggests that the patient's low back pain is *not* due to a musculoskeletal disorder, because pain related to musculoskeletal disorders typically is eased when the patient rests in a comfortable position.

To rule out the likelihood of spinal fracture as a cause of this patient's low back pain, the patient is asked whether any trauma to the spine triggered the onset of pain. In addition, the PT asks whether the patient has any history of osteoporosis, because minor strains or falls may produce an unsuspected spinal fracture in an individual with osteoporosis. The PT also asks whether the patient has a history of other disorders that increase the risk of decreased bone density, including hyperparathyroidism, renal failure, chronic gastrointestinal disorders, and long-term use of corticosteroids:

- Have you recently had a major trauma, such as a vehicle accident or a fall from a height?
- Have you ever had a medical practitioner tell you that you have osteoporosis or other disorders that could cause "weak bones?"

The PT asks our 55-year-old patient these questions and receives negative responses, which greatly reduces the suspicion of fracture as a cause of this patient's low back pain.

Finally, to rule out cauda equina syndrome associated with this patient's low back pain, the PT relies on both historical and physical examination data. The PT asks the following questions:

- Have you noticed a recent onset of difficulty with retaining your urine?
- Have you noticed a recent need to urinate more frequently?
- Have you noticed a recent onset of numbness in the area of your bottom where you would sit on a bicycle seat?
- Have you recently noticed your legs becoming weak while walking or climbing stairs?

A positive response to any of these questions increases the suspicion that the patient has a cauda equina syndrome. The PT follows these inquiries with a physical examination, assessing the sensory integrity of the perianal and perineal areas, as well as the L4, L5, and S1 dermatomes. The PT also assesses the motor integrity of the L4 (quadriceps and tibialis anterior), L5 (extensor hallucis longus and foot everters), and S1 (ankle plantar flexors) musculature (see Chapter 11). In our example, all of the history and physical-examination findings suggesting a cauda equina lesion were negative. Table 6-2 summarizes the red flags for the low back region, and a low back medical screening questionnaire is given in Table 6-3.

TABLE 6-2
Red Flags for the Low Back Region

Condition	Red Flags
Back-related tumor[12]	Age >50 years
	History of cancer
	Unexplained weight loss
	Failure of conservative therapy
Back-related infection (spinal osteomyelitis)[43]	Recent infection (e.g., urinary tract or skin infection)
	Intravenous drug user/abuser
	Concurrent immunosuppressive disorder
Cauda equina syndrome[3]	Urine retention or incontinence
	Fecal incontinence
	Saddle anesthesia
	Global or progressive weakness in the lower extremities
	Sensory deficits in the feet (i.e., L4, L5, S1 areas)
	Ankle dorsiflexion, toe extension, and ankle plantarflexion weakness
Spinal fracture[3,13]	History of trauma (including minor falls or heavy lifts for osteoporotic or elderly individuals)
	Prolonged use of steroids
	Age >70 years

TABLE 6-3		
Medical Screening Questionnaire for the Low Back Region		
Question	**Yes**	**No**
1. Have you recently had a major trauma, such as a vehicle accident or a fall from a height?		
2. Have you ever had a medical practitioner tell you that you have osteoporosis?		
3. Do you have a history of cancer?		
4. Does your pain ease when you rest in a comfortable position?		
5. Have you recently had a fever?		
6. Have you recently lost weight even though you have not been attempting to eat less or exercise more?		
7. Have you recently taken antibiotics or other medicines for an infection?		
8. Have you been diagnosed as having an immunosuppressive disorder?		
9. Have you noticed a recent onset of difficulty with retaining your urine?		
10. Have you noticed a recent need to urinate more frequently?		
11. Have you noticed a recent onset of numbness in the area of your bottom where you would sit on a bicycle seat?		
12. Have you recently noticed your legs becoming weak while walking or climbing stairs?		

Adapted from Bigos S, Bowyer O, Braen G, et al: *Acute lower back problems in adults. Clinical practice guideline no 14*. AHCPR publication no 95-0642, Rockville, MD, December 1994, Agency for Health Care Policy and Research, Public Health Service, US Department of Health and Human Services.

In summary, our patient's response that his pain does not ease when he rests in a comfortable position suggests a non-spinal pathology mimicking a back problem. This justifies an examination for a possible serious condition in an adjacent region (see the discussion below on colon cancer). However, the PT found no other red flags suggesting a back-related tumor or infection, spinal fracture, or cauda equina syndrome. Reviewing the function of the gastrointestinal, urogenital, and vascular systems may be especially helpful in patients with low back pain whose presentation and symptomatology suggest a nonmusculoskeletal disorder.

Pelvis, Hip, and Thigh Disorders

The serious medical conditions that may mimic common musculoskeletal disorders of the pelvis, hip, and thigh include colon cancer, pathologic fractures of the femoral neck, osteonecrosis of the femoral head, Legg-Calvé-Perthes disease, and slipped capital femoral epiphysis. Colon cancer, the third-most-common cancer for both women and men,[22] is a result of malignant neoplasms that develop in the large intestine, from the cecum to the rectum. Colon cancer is most common in people 50 years and older and who have a family history of colon cancer. The initial symptoms usually are a change in bowel habits, such as blood in the stools (if the lesion is near the rectum) or black stools (if the lesion producing the bleeding is located in the more proximal portion of the colon).

Colon cancer is an especially deadly disease because malignant neoplasms can develop undetected for many years before the onset of bowel symptoms. Thus PTs, along with other health care professionals, must stress to patients the importance of routine screening examinations for colon cancer (e.g., sigmoidoscopy and colonoscopy) for individuals with a family history of this disorder. Polyps, which are the precursor to cancerous lesions in the colon, often can be excised if they are discovered during a colonoscopy examination. In the later stages of colon cancer, a palpable mass may be felt in the abdominal cavity.

Because PTs often see patients with midback and thoracic-cage pain, they should remember that the most common metastatic presentation of colon cancer includes the thoracic spine and ribcage. The following information, collected by a PT during a history or physical examination, could be red flags for colon cancer:[40]

- Age greater than 50 years
- History of colon cancer in an immediate family member (first-degree relative; see Chapter 5)
- Bowel disturbances (e.g., rectal bleeding or black stools; see Chapter 7)
- Unexplained weight loss (see Chapter 7)
- Back or pelvic pain that is unchanged by positions or movement

Disorders of the proximal femur are another type of serious condition that the PT may encounter. As the elderly population increases, PTs will be more likely to detect and manage patients with pathologic fractures of the femoral neck. Pathologic fractures of the femoral neck occur secondary to disease and often in the absence of trauma. These fractures are most common in people older than 50 years (women more often than men) who have a history of metabolic bone disease, such as osteoporosis or Paget's disease. A history of a fall from a standing position is often reported, along with a feeling of a sudden, painful snap in the hip region and a giving way. Acute groin pain usually is reported, but pain also may be felt in the anteromedial thigh or in the trochanteric region. The physical examination usually reveals that the involved extremity appears shortened when compared with the contralateral side and typically is held in an externally rotated position.[41]

Another serious disorder of the proximal femur is osteonecrosis (also known as avascular necrosis) of the femoral head. Osteonecrosis of the femoral head is a result of insufficient arterial supply to this region. This ischemic process eventually results in death of the bony tissue of the femoral head and can be associated with hip trauma, such as fractures or dislocations. It also can be associated with nontraumatic conditions, such as sickle cell disease, and with long-term corticosteroid administration, as in patients receiving corticosteroid therapy for management of rheumatoid arthritis, systemic lupus erythematosus, or asthma.

Nontraumatic osteonecrosis of the femoral head may be bilateral in up to 60% of cases.[39]

A similar condition that occurs in children (most common in 5-to-8-year-old boys) is Legg-Calvé-Perthes disease. This condition results from an idiopathic loss of blood supply from the lateral ascending cervical artery to the femoral head. Patients with osteonecrosis and Legg-Calvé-Perthes disease often report pain in the groin, thigh, and knee that worsens with weight-bearing activities; resulting in an antalgic gait. Common clinical findings in children with Legg-Calvé-Perthes disease also include shortening of the involved extremity and limited internal rotation and abduction of the involved hip.[48] Internal rotation typically is tested in these cases with the patient prone, with both extremities simultaneously internally rotated, and with the angles of the tibial shaft relative to the table compared. Abduction is tested with the patient supine in the hook lying position (with the knees flexed to approximately 90 degrees and both feet positioned on the table adjacent to the midline). The patient then is instructed to relax his or her adductor muscles and to allow the knees to fall out to the "frog-leg" position (i.e., horizontally abducted toward the table). This test allows easy comparison of the involved and uninvolved hips; abduction is measured by using the angles of the tibial shaft relative to the table, with the femurs in approximately 45 degrees of hip flexion.[11]

A hip disorder that occurs in adolescence is slipped capital femoral epiphysis, which involves progressive displacement of the femoral head relative to the neck through the open growth plate. It is more common in males (male-to-female ratio, 2.5:1) who are typically, but not always, overweight. Patients with slipped capital femoral epiphysis usually experience groin, thigh, or knee pain that is described as diffuse and vague (i.e., difficult to pinpoint). Common findings of the physical examination are antalgic gait, involved extremity positioned in external rotation, and hip internal rotation range-of-motion limitations.[8] The red flags for slipped capital femoral epiphysis as well as the other serious conditions of the pelvis, hip, and thigh region are listed in Table 6-4. Table 6-5 offers a self-report questionnaire that can help in screening for these conditions.

Knee, Lower Leg, and Ankle/Foot Pain

The remaining regions of the lower quarter to consider are the knee, leg, ankle, and foot regions. Two of the important conditions, compartment syndrome and deep vein thrombosis (DVT), will be described in detail, as will three other potentially serious conditions of the knee, leg, ankle, and foot that a PT is likely to encounter: peripheral arterial occlusive disease, septic arthritis, and cellulitis.

Peripheral arterial occlusive disease, also known as peripheral vascular disease, is the manifestation of atherosclerosis below the bifurcation of the abdominal aorta. This disease is common, which is not surprising when we consider that the risk factors for heart disease that are so widespread in our society (i.e., history of type II diabetes, smoking, sedentary lifestyle) are also the risk factors for peripheral arterial occlusive disease. In fact, people who have a history of ischemic heart disease should be assumed to have peripheral arterial occlusive

TABLE 6-4	
Red Flags for the Pelvis, Hip, and Thigh Region	
Condition	**Red Flags**
Colon cancer[40]	Age >50 years
	Bowel disturbances (e.g., rectal bleeding, black stools)
	Unexplained weight loss
	History of colon cancer in immediate family
	Pain unchanged by positions or movement
Pathologic fractures of the femoral neck[41]	Older females (>70 years) with hip, groin, or thigh pain
	History of a fall from a standing position
	Severe, constant pain, worse with movement
	A shortened and externally rotated lower extremity
Osteonecrosis of the femoral head[39] (also known as avascular necrosis)	History of long-term corticosteroid use (e.g., in patients with RA, SLE, asthma)
	History of AVN of the contralateral hip
	Trauma
Legg-Calvé-Perthes disease[46]	5- to 8-year-old boys with groin/thigh pain
	Antalgic gait
	Pain symptoms aggravated with hip movement, especially hip abduction and internal rotation
Slipped capital femoral epiphysis[8]	Overweight adolescent
	History of a recent growth spurt or trauma
	Groin aching exacerbated with weight-bearing
	Involved leg held in external rotation
	ROM limitations of hip IR and abduction

RA, Rheumatoid arthritis; *SLE*, systemic lupus erythematosus; *AVN*, avascular necrosis; *ROM*, range of motion; *IR*, internal rotation.

disease until proven otherwise. A primary clinical feature of this disease is intermittent claudication. A patient with intermittent claudication often complains of aching in the buttock and of thigh and calf pain that is precipitated by walking, intensifies with walking, and disappears with rest. In addition, the patient may complain of the distal extremities feeling cold. The physical-examination findings that suggest peripheral occlusive arterial disease include decreased pedal pulses (i.e., posterior tibialis and dorsalis pedis arteries; see Chapter 11), a unilateral cool extremity, and wounds and sores on the toes or feet.

Two special tests that the PT can perform that aid in confirming the presence of peripheral vascular disease are the reactive hyperemia test and the ankle-to-arm systolic pressure (ankle/brachial index; ABI) index. The reactive hyperemia test assesses the integrity of the vascular system in redistributing blood with postural changes. One performs this test by elevating the leg of a patient who is lying supine to 45 degrees of hip flexion (i.e., a unilateral straight leg test to 45 degrees). The lower extremity is maintained in this position for 1 to 3 minutes, or until the color of the foot, ankle, and lower leg is blanched. The examiner then lowers the limb and measures the number of seconds required for the limb to turn pink. The normal time is 1 or 2 seconds. A venous filling time of greater than 20 seconds indicates peripheral occlusive arterial disease.

The PT obtains the ankle-to-arm systolic pressure index by measuring the highest systolic blood pressure at the ankle

TABLE 6-5

Medical Screening Questionnaire for the Pelvis, Hip, and Thigh Region

Question	Yes	No
1. Have you recently had a trauma, such as a fall?		
2. Have you ever had a medical practitioner tell you that you have osteoporosis?		
3. Have you ever had a medical practitioner tell you that you have a problem with the blood circulation in your hips?		
4. Are you currently taking steroids or have you been on prolonged steroid therapy?		
5. Does your pain ease when you rest in a comfortable position?		
6. Do you have a history of cancer?		
7. Has a member of your immediate family (i.e., parents or siblings) been diagnosed with cancer?		
8. Have you recently lost weight even though you have *not* been attempting to eat less or exercise more?		
9. Have you had a recent change in your bowel functioning, such as black stools or blood in your rectum?		
10. Have you had diarrhea or constipation that has lasted for more than a few days?		
11. Do you have groin, hip, or thigh aching or pain that increases with physical activity, such as walking or running?		

(using the dorsalis pedis and posterior tibial arteries) with a hand-held Doppler flowmeter and dividing it by the blood pressure in the brachial artery. An ankle-to-arm systolic pressure index that is less than 0.97 indicates the presence of peripheral occlusive arterial disease.[6,31] See Chapter 9 for a detailed description of the ABI.

One of the major therapies for patients with peripheral vascular disease is aerobic exercise, such as progressive walking. Thus PTs often may help design and monitor exercise programs for patients with this disorder. However, the PT must remember that when a screening examination of a lower-extremity musculoskeletal disorder suggests peripheral occlusive vascular disease, the PT must also assume the presence of ischemic heart disease until proven otherwise. Therefore a physician evaluation (often including an exercise tolerance test) and medical management (often including medications; see Chapter 16) of the underlying cardiovascular disorder are essential so the PT can proceed with the plan of care confident in the patient's safety.

Another serious condition of the lower extremity that may initially appear as a musculoskeletal strain is DVT. A DVT is a spontaneous obstruction of the popliteal vein of the calf and may present as a gradual or sudden onset of calf pain, typically intensified with standing or walking and reduced with rest and elevation. Up to 50% of patients with DVT will not experience the calf pain. The risk factors that predispose an individual to DVT are recent surgery, malignancy, trauma, prolonged immobilization of the extremities (including placement of the limb in a cast or immobilizer and a long car ride or plane trip, especially for those already at risk for DVT), and pregnancy. Physical-examination findings that increase the suspicion of a DVT are localized calf tenderness, calf swelling and edema, and skin warmth. The diagnosis of DVT is confirmed with contrast venography or other imaging procedures. The potential that the blood clot may travel proximally toward or into the pulmonary vessels is the risk that makes a DVT a serious condition that requires referral to a physician for a medical examination and possible intervention, including anticoagulant medication. The red flags that suggest the presence of a DVT are listed in Table 6-6.

PTs often help in the management of patients who have experienced trauma or overuse (i.e., repetitive trauma) strains

to the legs. The inflammatory phase of healing that accompanies these traumas can lead to an abnormal rise in pressure in one of the fascial compartments of the leg. This abnormal rise in pressure resulting from acute swelling inside a fascial connective tissue compartment is called a compartment syndrome.

TABLE 6-6

Red Flags for the Knee, Leg, Ankle, or Foot Region

Condition	Red Flags
Peripheral arterial occlusive disease[6,31]	Age >60 years old History of type II diabetes History of ischemic heart disease Smoking history Sedentary lifestyle Concurrent intermittent claudication Unilaterally cool extremity Decreased pedal pulses: posterior tibial artery, dorsalis pedis artery Prolonged venous filling time Abnormal ankle-to-arm systolic pressure
Deep vein thrombosis[47]	Calf pain, edema, tenderness, warmth Calf pain that is intensified with standing or walking and relieved by rest and elevation Recent surgery, malignancy, pregnancy, trauma, or leg immobilization
Compartment syndrome	History of blunt trauma, crush injury, or unaccustomed exercise Severe, persistent leg pain that is intensified with stretch applied to involved muscles Swelling, exquisite tenderness, and palpable tension (hardness) of involved compartment Paresthesia, paresis, and pulselessness
Septic arthritis[47]	Constant aching and/or throbbing pain, joint swelling, tenderness, warmth History of recent infection, surgery, or injection Coexisting immunosuppressive disorder
Cellulitis[47]	Pain, skin swelling, warmth, and an advancing, irregular margin of erythema/reddish streaks Fever, chills, malaise, and weakness History of recent skin ulceration or abrasion, venous insufficiency, CHF, or cirrhosis

CHF, Congestive heart failure.

The vascular occlusion and nerve entrapments that are possible sequelae of a compartment syndrome make this condition a medical emergency. Thus the PT must know the red flags that signify the presence of a compartment syndrome when examining musculoskeletal disorders of the lower extremity.

Patients with compartment syndromes have a history of a blunt trauma or crush injury, or of participating in an unaccustomed physical activity involving the lower extremities, such as rapidly increasing the amount of running distance (e.g., while training for a marathon) or walking distance (e.g., while participating in a long hike). The patient often reports severe, persistent leg pain that is intensified when stretch is applied to the involved muscles. The physical examination reveals swelling, exquisite tenderness, and palpable tension (i.e., hardness) of the involved compartment. The nerve entrapment or compression found in this condition results in paresthesias and potentially in paresis or paralysis. The vascular compromise accompanying this condition results in diminished peripheral pulses (i.e., dorsalis pedis or posterior tibial). A mnemonic that clinicians use to remember the signs of a compartment syndrome are the *five "P's": pain, palpable tenderness, paresthesias, paresis, and pulselessness.*

The two remaining potentially serious conditions that may mimic lower extremity musculoskeletal disorders are related to infections. One is septic arthritis, which is an inflammation in a joint caused by a bacterial infection, and the other is cellulitis, which is an infection in the skin and underlying tissues following bacterial contamination of a wound. Patients who have septic arthritis complain of a constant aching and or throbbing pain and swelling in a joint. The involved joint is usually tender and warm when palpated. Patients who develop septic arthritis often are immunosuppressed or have preexisting joint disease. This immunosuppression may be a result of corticosteroid administration, alcohol abuse, renal failure, malignancy, diabetes mellitus, intravenous drug abuse, collagen vascular disease, organ transplantation, or acquired immunodeficiency syndrome.

Examples of preexisting joint diseases that predispose individuals to septic arthritis are rheumatoid arthritis, osteoarthritis, and psoriatic arthritis. The cause of the septic arthritis also is usually associated with a local or distant site of infection, or a history of a recent joint surgery or intraarticular injection. An example of a distant infection site in a patient is a gonococcal infection. Thus individuals who are sexually active and exposed to gonorrhea may develop gonococcal septic monoarthritis or gonococcal septic polyarthritis.[49]

Infection in the tissues—cellulitis—exhibits the classic signs of pain, skin swelling, warmth, and an advancing, irregular margin of erythema or reddish streaks. Upon further inquiry, patients with these findings also may report other classic signs of infection: fever, chills, malaise, and weakness (see Chapter 7). Individuals predisposed to developing cellulitis are those with congestive heart failure, lower extremity venous insufficiency, diabetes mellitus, renal failure, liver cirrhosis, and advancing age. The precipitating factor to developing cellulitis is typically a recent skin ulceration or abrasion.[49]

The management of septic arthritis and cellulitis includes (of course) monitored administration of antibiotic therapy,

---

TABLE 6-7

Medical Screening Questionnaire for the Knee, Leg, Ankle, or Foot Region

Question	Yes	No
1. Have you recently had a fever?		
2. Have you recently taken antibiotics or other medicines for an infection?		
3. Have you recently had surgery?		
4. Have you recently had an injection to one or more of your joints?		
5. Have you recently had a cut, scrape, or open wound?		
6. Have you been diagnosed as having an immunosuppressive disorder?		
7. Do you have a history of heart trouble?		
8. Do you have a history of cancer?		
9. Have you recently taken a long car ride, bus trip, or plane flight?		
10. Have you recently been bedridden for any reason?		
11. Have you recently begun a vigorous physical training program?		
12. Do you have groin, hip, thigh, or calf aching or pain that increases with physical activity, such as walking or running?		
13. Have you recently sustained a blow to your shin or any other trauma to either of your legs?		

---

and thus referral of the patient to a physician should be expedited. The red flags and medical-screening questionnaires for peripheral arterial occlusive disease, DVT, compartment syndrome, septic arthritis, and cellulitis are found in Tables 6-6 and 6-7.

Thoracic Pain

CARDIAC/PULMONARY DISORDERS. The thoracic spine and rib cage lie close to many organ systems that, when diseased, usually result in local or referred pain to the thoracic cage. In addition, both metastatic disease and bone diseases usually manifest as pathologic fractures of the thoracic vertebrae and ribs.[46] Thus the PT should remember that the patient who reports "back pain" may have an underlying serious medical condition when the reported back pain is in the thoracic region. This section will briefly discuss the clinical presentation and red flags of cardiac (myocardial infarction, unstable and stable angina), pulmonary (lung cancer, pneumothorax, pneumonia, pleurisy, and pulmonary embolus), gastrointestinal (peptic ulcers and cholecystitis), and urogenital (pyelonephritis) conditions.

Myocardial infarction (MI; an acute blockage of a coronary artery resulting in death to a portion of the myocardium) has the highest mortality rate of any of the disorders discussed in this chapter. A cardinal clinical feature of MI is angina, chest symptoms described as discomfort, pressure, tightness, or squeezing with potential referral into the arms, neck, or jaw regions. The classic presentation of pain in the left chest and left upper extremity is not necessarily the norm for women or the elderly. Pain experienced in the epigastric, midthoracic spinal, or right shoulder/neck regions may be the presentation for these patients. PTs should realize that one of every three patients diagnosed with MI did not have chest pain on initial presentation to a hospital emergency room.[9] Instead of pain as the primary manifestation, myocardial infarction may appear with the clinical features of dyspnea, nausea or vomiting, palpitations, syncope, or cardiac arrest. The risk factors for this atypical presentation of MI are a history of diabetes, older age, female sex, nonwhite racial or ethnic group, and a history of congestive heart failure and stroke.[9]

Two related terms that PTs should understand are stable and unstable angina pectoris. Stable angina, as the name implies, is substernal chest pain or pressure with possible pain referral to the left upper extremity that occurs with predictable exertion or known precipitating events, such as exercise or exertion at an intensity level higher than usual. The chest pain that occurs with stable angina also is predictably alleviated with change in the precipitating event (e.g., rest) or with self-administration of sublingual nitroglycerin. Chest pain that occurs with stable angina is relatively benign, especially if relief is gained with rest and administration of nitroglycerin.

Unstable angina, also as the name implies, is chest pain that occurs outside of a predictable pattern and that does not respond to nitroglycerin. Individuals experiencing unstable angina must be closely monitored (see Chapter 9). Signs suggesting MI, such as substernal squeezing or crushing pressure, pain radiation to both arms, shortness of breath, pallor, diaphoresis, or angina lasting more than 30 minutes, should alert the PT that this is an emergency condition, and that immediate transportation to an appropriate emergency room or coronary-care facility is indicated. The survival rate of those experiencing an MI is greatly improved if therapy known to improve survival is available and used appropriately. These therapies include thrombolysis of primary angioplasty, aspirin, beta-blocker therapy, and heparin.[18]

Chest pain that extends to the left shoulder and possibly down the left arm also may be pericarditis. This chest pain usually is accompanied by fever and increases with lying down, inhalation, or coughing, and is alleviated with forward lean while sitting. Pericarditis is an inflammation of the pericardium, a sac that surrounds the heart to keep it in place, to prevent overfilling with blood, and to protect the heart from chest infections. The pericardium becomes inflamed by bacterial, viral, or systemic diseases, such as kidney failure, systemic lupus, rheumatoid disease, heart failure, or increased fluid around the heart when there is leakage from an aortic aneurysm. This inflammation around the heart prevents complete expansion, because the additional pressure from the resulting inflammation results in less blood leaving the heart. To make up for the reduced stroke volume and to get enough oxygen to the tissues, the heart beats faster. If increased heart rate cannot compensate enough, the person may start to breathe heavily, the veins in the neck may distend, and blood pressure may drop drastically during inhalation. This condition is termed cardiac tamponade and is often a medical emergency. Emergency medical care is needed to remove the pressure on the heart and restore proper cardiac output.

Pulmonary embolus is a pulmonary condition that may produce angina-like pain. An acute massive pulmonary embolism can even produce crushing chest pain that mimics MT, especially if the blood clot, usually traveling from the calf, thigh, or pelvic veins, reaches a major pulmonary artery. The location of the chest pain usually is substernal, but it can be located anywhere in the thorax depending on the location of the embolus. This may include shoulder pain or upper-abdominal pain. In addition to chest pain, patients with a pulmonary embolus may develop dyspnea, wheezing, and a marked drop in blood pressure. Factors that increase the risk of blood clots in the lower extremities or pelvis and subsequent embolus include immobilization or recent surgery; these are two patient types that PTs frequently treat. Pulmonary embolism also has a high mortality rate, so if the PT suspects this condition, he or she should immediately refer the patient to emergency care so that a definitive diagnosis can be made and appropriate anticoagulant therapy (e.g., intravenous streptokinase, heparin) can be administered.

Two other pulmonary conditions that can cause chest pain are pleurisy and pneumothorax. Pleurisy is an irritation of the pleural membranes that make up the lining between the lungs and the inner surface of the ribcage. The pain that pleurisy produces is characteristically described as sharp and stabbing and is worsened by deep inspiration and other ribcage movements, such as a cough. Passive-movement testing of the ribcage and thoracic spine also may produce pleuritic pain. Pleurisy may have multiple causes, such as viral infections or tumors, and also is associated with disorders such as rheumatoid arthritis. Each of these conditions requires a definitive diagnosis and intervention by a physician. Suspicion of this disorder should lead the PT to auscultate over the thorax, listening for a "pleural rub" sound. See Chapter 9 for an overview of auscultation of heart and breath sounds.

A pneumothorax, air in the thoracic cage—also produces chest pain that is intensified with deep inspiration. A pneumothorax can be a spontaneous, usually pathologic event associated with rupture of the wall of the lung lining. Such a rupture prevents the lung from maintaining negative pressure during diaphragmatic and ribcage motions. A simple pneumothorax may begin without any precipitating event, or it may follow a bout of extreme coughing or strenuous physical activity. The physical-examination findings that are associated with a pneumothorax include limited ability of the affected side of the chest to expand, hyperresonance of the affected area upon percussion, and markedly reduced breath sounds. A small pneumothorax may resolve within a few days without therapy. A large pneumothorax, however, will require aspiration of the air from the lung. Factors predisposing individuals to pneumothorax are menstruation (in young women), asthma, chronic obstructive lung disease, cystic fibrosis, and lung cancer. A tension pneumothorax usually is a consequence of a trauma, such as a penetrating wound to the ribcage or a severe blow to the ribcage that may occur in contact sports or during an automobile injury (with the patient hitting the steering wheel). The signs of a tension pneumothorax include severe pleuritic-type chest-wall pain, extreme shortness of breath, tracheal deviation, distended neck veins, tachycardia, hypotension, and hyperresonance to percussion of the involved (painful) side of the chest. Tension pneumothorax can be an extreme emergency requiring insertion of a chest tube with a seal or Heimlich valve.[49]

Finally, another cause of pleuritic-type chest pain is pneumonia, which is a bacterial or viral infection of the lungs. The signs of systemic infection, such as chills, fever, malaise, nausea, and vomiting, typically accompany the pleuritic pain. The fever may be absent in the elderly, with onset or worsening of confusion being the primary manifestation (see Chapter 7). A distinguishing characteristic of pneumonia is a cough that produces sputum of varying coloration, from light green to dark brown.

GASTROINTESTINAL DISORDERS. Gastrointestinal disorders are common in the general population and may present as co-morbidities during the examination process. The PT should routinely ask patients about bowel movement characteristics, vomiting, unexplained weight loss, or extended use of nonsteroidal antiinflammatory drugs (see Chapter 7). Common gastrointestinal disorders include gastric or peptic ulcer disease and cholecystitis. Ulcers occur when the lining of the digestive tract is exposed to digestive acids and are named according to their anatomical location. An ulcer in the duodenum is called a duodenal ulcer and is associated with the presence of *Helicobacter pylori* bacteria in the stomach. Duodenal ulcers present as dull, gnawing, or burning pain in the epigastric region, in the midthoracic (T6-T10) region, or in the supraclavicular region. These symptoms occur when the stomach is empty and are relieved with eating or taking of antacids. Relief is temporary, however, and the symptoms return within 2 to 3 hours. If the ulcer is located in the stomach (a gastric ulcer), eating may increase, rather than relieve, the symptoms. These ulcers are more common in the elderly secondary to increased use of NSAIDs (see Chapter 5).

Unlike duodenal ulcers, gastric ulcers can be malignant and need the attention of a doctor even if symptoms spontaneously resolve when the drugs are stopped. With esophageal ulcers, the person experiences pain with swallowing or when lying down. Symptoms of these ulcers include black, tarry-colored stools; bright red or reddish-brown clumps (coffee-ground emesis) in the vomit, relief or intensification of pain with eating; and pain in the chest, back, or supraclavicular area.

The other common gastrointestinal disorder is cholecystitis, an inflammation of the gallbladder. The initial symptom often is pain in the right upper abdominal quadrant or in the interscapular or right scapular regions,[15] which can be constant and intense. Pain usually is severe enough to cause nausea and vomiting. Murphy's sign is positive (inspiration inhibited by pain on local palpation in the right upper abdominal quadrant) in more than 50% of patients with cholecystitis.[27] Patients initially may seek pain control from a PT but should be referred to their physician or local emergency room. Inflammation of the gallbladder usually is caused by a gallstone lodged in the cystic duct, and medical help is needed to remove the gallstone.

KIDNEY DISORDERS. Disorders of the kidney such as pyelonephritis and renal stones result in pain in the posterior lateral aspect of the thoracic cage and upper lumbar area. PTs may see the terms *costovertebral angle (CVA)* or *flank* in physician notes referring to this region. Both conditions present with chills, fever, nausea, vomiting, and renal colic. Renal colic is excruciating intermittent pain from the CVA or flank that spreads across the lower abdomen into the labia in women and into the testicles and penis in men. The pain is associated with spasms in a ureter and may extend as far down as the inner thighs.

Pyelonephritis is an infection in the kidney, usually caused by an infection of the ascending urinary tract. Thus those at risk for pyelonephritis are individuals with recent or coexisting urinary tract infections. Blood-borne pathogens or conditions causing obstruction of urine flow (benign prostatic hyperplasia or kidney stones) also may cause renal infections.

Kidney stones (nephrolithiasis if in the kidney, urolithiasis if anywhere else in the urinary tract) are hard masses of salts that precipitate from the urine when it becomes supersaturated with a particular substance. Most stones are composed of calcium, and less common are stones composed of uric acid, cystine, or struvite (a combination of magnesium, ammonium, and phosphate). Risk factors for developing kidney stones are warm, humid atmospheric temperatures and diseases (such as leukemia) that involve high cell turnover. The incidence of kidney stones in men is four times greater than in women.[47] Caucasian men have three times as many stone episodes as black men. About 5% to 15% of the population is expected to have kidney stones during their lifetime.[47] Still, the best predictor for kidney stones is a past episode, as about 50% of patients experience at least one recurrence.[34] A PT who suspects these conditions should refer the patient for medical attention. Tables 6-8 and 6-9 offer a summary of the red flags for thoracic symptoms and a questionnaire for screening.

Shoulder and Cervical Pain

Patients with shoulder and cervical symptoms make up a large portion of an orthopedic PT's caseload.[4,14,23] There are fewer serious disorders involving the shoulder and neck regions compared with the thorax. For example, metastasis does not occur in the cervical region nearly as often as in other regions of the axial skeleton.[46] PTs should be familiar with a few conditions, however, including central cord syndromes, ligamentous instability, brachial plexus neuropathies, and Pancoast's tumor.

The PT should rule out a ligamentous injury after trauma such as a motor vehicle accident or a fall, but trauma is not the only condition that should alert the PT to the possibility of ligamentous instability. People with rheumatoid arthritis, Down syndrome, or ankylosing spondylitis, and even people who merely use oral contraceptives, should be screened for ligamentous instability of the neck. The alar and transverse ligaments maintain the proper relationship of C1 on C2, while the ligamentum flavum, anterior and posterior longitudinal ligaments, and interspinous and intertransverse ligaments help maintain the proper alignment through the entire cervical region. Resultant instability can lead to significant neurologic and cardiovascular consequences, and PTs should routinely screen for such symptoms.

Neurologic symptoms associated with ligamentous instability can include the typical presentation of tingling, numbness, weakness, or burning pain. The PT should be concerned about possible compromise of the spinal cord if the patient has these

TABLE 6-8

Red Flags for the Thoracic Spine and Rib Cage Region

Condition	Red Flags
Myocardial infarction	Chest pain
	Pallor, sweating, dyspnea, nausea, palpitations
	Presence of risk factors: previous history of coronary artery disease, hypertension, smoking, diabetes, elevated blood serum cholesterol (>240 mg/dL)
	Men over age 40, women over age 50
	Symptoms lasting longer than 30 minutes and not relieved with sublingual nitroglycerin
Unstable angina pectoris	Chest pain that occurs outside of a predictable pattern
	Not responsive to nitroglycerin
Stable angina pectoris	Chest pain/pressure that occurs with predictable levels of exertion
	Symptoms are predictably alleviated with rest or sublingual nitroglycerin
Pericarditis	Sharp/stabbing chest pain that may be referred to the lateral neck or either shoulder
	Increased pain with left-side lying
	Relieved with forward lean while sitting (supporting arms on knees or a table)
Pulmonary embolus	Chest, shoulder, or upper abdominal pain
	Dyspnea
	History of, or risk factors for developing, a deep vein thrombosis
Pleurisy	Severe, sharp, "knife-like" pain with inspiration
	Dyspnea, decreased chest wall excursion
	History of a recent or concurrent respiratory disorder (e.g., infection, pneumonia, tumor, tuberculosis)
Pneumothorax	Chest pain, intensified with inspiration
	Difficulty ventilating or expanding rib cage
	Recent bout of coughing or strenuous exercise or trauma
	Hyperresonance on percussion
	Decreased breath sounds
Pneumonia	Pleuritic pain, may be referred to shoulder
	Fever, chills, headaches, malaise, nausea
	Productive cough
Cholecystitis	Colicky pain in right upper abdominal quadrant with accompanying right scapular pain
	Symptoms may worsen with ingestion of fatty foods
	Symptoms not increased by activity nor relieved by rest
Peptic ulcer	Dull or gnawing pain or "burning" sensation in the epigastrium, midback, or supraclavicular regions
	Symptoms relieved with food
	Localized tenderness at the right epigastrium
	Constipation, bleeding, vomiting, tarry-colored stools, coffee ground emesis
Pyelonephritis	Recent or coexisting urinary tract infection
	Enlarged prostate
	Kidney stone or past episode of kidney stone
Nephrolithiasis (kidney stones)	Sudden, severe back or flank pain
	Chills, fever, nausea, or vomiting
	Renal colic
	Symptoms of urinary tract infection
	Residence in hot and humid environment
	Past episodes of kidney stone; 50% of patients experience a recurrence

symptoms in more than one extremity. In addition, dizziness, vertigo, or nystagmus associated with head or neck movements should alert the PT. Symptoms such as these in a patient who has been involved in a traumatic event or has a positive history of the disorders mentioned above that can lead to instability should prompt the PT to conduct special stability tests such as the Sharp-Purser test and the alar and transverse ligament stress tests. Other potential signs to note during the physical examination are clonus and a positive Babinski sign.[32]

Brachial plexus neuropathies can occur secondary to repetitive overuse, postural syndromes, and trauma. Nerves affected by such neuropathies can be of three categories: sensory, motor, or mixed. The emphasis will be on motor nerves, but the therapist should remember that there is no such thing as a pure motor nerve. A motor nerve carries efferent commands to the muscles but also returns with information from the muscles, joints, and associated ligamentous structures. A nerve that innervates a muscle also augments the sensation from the joint upon which that muscle acts. Pain produced by a motor-nerve-entrapment neuropathy is not well localized, is present at rest, and has a retrograde distribution. The muscles innervated can be tender to palpate, and if the neuropathy has been present for an extended time, there will be muscle atrophy, although the patient may not be aware of the weakness. The greatest challenge with entrapment neuropathies is not treatment but diagnosis. These neuropathies are more often the cumulative result of many small traumata or longstanding compression, or are of mechanical origin.

TABLE 6-9

Medical Screening Questionnaire for the Thoracic Spine and Rib Cage Region

Question	Yes	No
1. Do you have a history of heart problems?		
2. Have you recently taken a nitroglycerin tablet?		
3. Do you have diabetes?		
4. Do you take medication for hypertension?		
5. Have you been or are you now a smoker?		
6. Does your pain ease when you rest in a comfortable position?		
7. Have you had recent surgery?		
8. Have you recently been bedridden?		
9. Have you recently noticed that it is difficult for you to breathe, laugh, sneeze, or cough?		
10. Have you recently had a fever, infection, or other illness?		
11. Have you recently received a blow to the chest, such as during a fall or motor-vehicle accident?		
12. In the past few weeks, have you noticed that when you cough, you easily cough up sputum?		
13. Are your symptoms relieved after eating?		
14. Does eating fatty foods increase your symptoms?		
15. Do you currently have a urinary tract infection, or have you had one in the past 2 months?		
16. Do you currently have a kidney stone, or have you had one in the past?		
17. Do you experience severe back or flank pain that comes on suddenly?		

With the evaluation of any new patient, the PT should conduct a thorough examination of motor and sensory function and reflexes in the area of interest (see Chapters 10 and 11). The PT should carefully observe the area, preferably with the area disrobed to allow for bilateral comparison of muscle bulk and to note possible atrophy. If the PT suspects a specific nerve, he or she should consider the muscles and sensory distribution that would be affected. The PT should palpate bilaterally along the path of the suspected nerve, looking for bone, joint, or soft-tissue abnormalities. Local tenderness or a positive Tinel sign will help identify the site of nerve entrapment. Suspicion can be confirmed by use of electromyography (EMG) and/or nerve conduction studies (NCS).[26]

If a patient presents with weakness of shoulder abduction and cannot shrug a shoulder, the PT should suspect a nerve entrapment of the spinal accessory nerve. The patient typically will have dull pain, weakness, and drooping of the shoulder. The patient will have paralysis of the trapezius muscle, and winging of the scapula usually is present. The spinal accessory nerve can be injured by blunt trauma to the posterior triangle of the neck or a traction injury, or can be a result of cervical surgery, such as for head or neck cancers.[28] The spinal accessory nerve is susceptible to trauma at the posterior triangle because of its superficial location, but the SCM would be spared because the injury would be distal to its innervation. A traction force that depresses the shoulder while laterally flexing the head in the opposite direction stretches the nerve and can damage the nerve. The patient will notice damage to the spinal accessory nerve when he or she notices a reduced ability to use his or her shoulder secondary to lack of scapular stabilization or a reduced ability to shrug the shoulder.

Weakness of shoulder abduction and flexion should raise the suspicion of a possible axillary nerve entrapment or injury. The axillary nerve arises from the posterior cord of the brachial plexus and has fibers from C5 and C6 nerve roots. After branching from the brachial plexus, the nerve travels laterally and downward, passing just below the shoulder joint and into the quadrilateral space.[28] The nerve then curves around the posterior and lateral portion of the proximal humerus to innervate the deltoid and teres minor muscles, while supplying the sensation of the lateral aspect of the upper arm.[28] A typical axillary nerve injury is caused by trauma, either a direct blow to the shoulder or a dislocation that stretches the nerve where it curves around the humerus. Patients will be aware of weakness with shoulder flexion and abduction, but numbness will not necessarily be present. The PT should refer such a patient to his or her doctor for surgical intervention.

Scapular winging may be due to trapezius involvement or related to serratus anterior paralysis. The serratus anterior is innervated by the long thoracic nerve after it branches from cervical roots 5, 6, and 7. The nerve passes down the posterolateral aspect of the chest wall, and its superficial course makes it susceptible to injury. The nerve can be damaged by excessive use of the shoulder, prolonged traction to the nerve, or trauma to the lateral chest wall. A patient with entrapment or injury of the long thoracic nerve will experience pain in the shoulder girdle, a reduction in active shoulder motions caused by a loss of scapulohumeral rhythm, and scapular winging that becomes especially evident when doing a wall push-up.

Poorly localized shoulder pain also may be related to a rotator cuff tear or to suprascapular nerve entrapment. Suprascapular nerve entrapment often is confused with rotator cuff tear, because both have wasting of the supraspinatus or infraspinatus with loss of strength in abduction and external rotation of the shoulder. The suprascapular nerve, like the long thoracic nerve, is a motor nerve, and pain resulting from its irritation is deep and poorly localized. The suprascapular nerve derives from the upper trunk of the brachial plexus, formed from the roots of C5 and C6. The nerve runs in the posterior triangle of the neck, sometimes passing through the body of the middle scalene, and past the anterior border of the trapezius on its way to the upper border of the scapula. After arriving at the scapula, the suprascapular nerve passes through the suprascapular notch. The notch is roofed by the transverse scapular ligament, making the U-shaped notch into a foramen. Here the nerve gives off innervation for the supraspinatus muscle, then it continues around the lateral border of the spine of the scapula. The nerve passes through the spinoglenoid notch to reach its destination in the infraspinatus muscle.[28]

Entrapment of the suprascapular nerve most often occurs at the suprascapular foramen, resulting in weakness and atrophy of both the supraspinatus and infraspinatus muscles. Entrapment also has occurred, however, at the spinoglenoid notch, resulting in the isolated involvement of the infraspinatus muscle. Trauma, whether in the form of repetitive microtrauma or distal trauma, causes a traction injury to the suprascapular nerve. A person with poor scapular stability will have additional motion at the suprascapular foramen against the suprascapular nerve, causing pain and inflammation through repetitive microtrauma.

A distal trauma can result from a fall onto an outstretched arm that is fully supinated, extended, and somewhat adducted. With this type of fall, the scapula remains fixed at the end of the upper extremity, while the inertia of the trunk keeps the body moving down, and the nerve is directly injured before protective crumpling or a Colles' fracture occurs. Conservative treatment of rest, nonsteroidal antiinflammatory drugs, and physical therapy is often unsuccessful, and surgical decompression may be necessary.[28]

As stated earlier, shoulder and cervical pathologies make up a large portion of an orthopedic PT's caseload. Thoracic outlet syndrome, cervical disk disease, and intrinsic shoulder disorders (e.g., bursitis, tendonitis, or frozen shoulder) all are very common disorders. Most PTs think that they fully understand these diagnoses and can confidently guide a patient through rehabilitation, but do they understand the relationship of these diagnoses with Pancoast's tumor? All of these diagnoses are common misdiagnoses of Pancoast's tumor.

Pancoast's tumor is a malignant tumor in the upper apices of a lung, and also may be called a superior pulmonary sulcus tumor. Pancoast's tumor has the highest occurrence in men over 50 with a history of cigarette smoking. In more than 90%

of patients, shoulder pain, rather than pulmonary symptoms, appears first.[38] Pulmonary symptoms are rare, and shoulder or disk problems are suspected because the tumor grows into the thoracic inlet, affecting the eighth cervical and first thoracic nerve roots, the subclavian artery and vein, and the sympathetic chain ganglions.

The patient with Pancoast's tumor initially suffers only "nagging" pain in the shoulder and along the vertebral border of the scapula as the tumor irritates the parietal pleura. As the tumor continues to invade the thoracic inlet, the pain becomes more burning, extending down the arm and into the ulnar nerve distribution. Over time, the intrinsic hand muscles atrophy, and the tumor occludes the subclavian vein. Occlusion causes venous distention of the ipsilateral arm. It is during this progressive decline that the patient seeks medical attention, and the disorder is misdiagnosed for an average of 6.8 months (ranging from 1 to 24 months).[38] The misdiagnosis by doctors and mistreatment by PTs and chiropractors reduce the odds of survival, as with any malignant cancer.

The goal is to prevent metastasis to the mediastinal lymph nodes or other peripheral sites. If a PT is treating a patient (especially one with the above profile: male older than 50 years and a smoker) for neck or shoulder diagnoses mentioned above and does not notice any change in pain after three to four treatments, a referral back to the doctor may be warranted. Table 6-10 summarizes the red flags for patients with

---

TABLE 6-10

Red Flags for the Cervical Spine and Shoulder Region

Condition	Red Flags
Myocardial infarction	Chest pain
	Pallor, sweating, dyspnea, nausea, palpitations
	Presence of risk factors: previous history of coronary artery disease, hypertension, smoking, diabetes, elevated blood serum cholesterol (>240 mg/dL)
	Men over age 40, women over age 50
	Symptoms lasting longer than 30 minutes and not relieved with sublingual nitroglycerin
Cervical ligamentous instabilities with possible cord compromise	Major trauma such as a motor-vehicle accident or a fall from a height
	Rheumatoid arthritis or ankylosing spondylitis
	Oral contraceptive use
	Long track neurologic signs, especially present in more than one extremity, dizziness, nystagmus, vertigo with head/neck movements/positions, clonus, positive Babinski sign
Cervical and shoulder girdle peripheral entrapment neuropathies	Paresthesias
	Pain present at rest and possibly with a retrograde distribution
	Muscles innervated can be tender to palpate
	Muscles and sensory distribution follow specific nerve pattern
Spinal accessory nerve	Weakness of shoulder abduction
	Inability to shrug the shoulders
	Dull pain, weakness, and drooping of the shoulder
	Lack of scapular stabilization
Axillary nerve	Weakness of shoulder abduction and flexion
	Lack of sensation of the lateral aspect of the upper arm
Long thoracic nerve	Serratus anterior weakness with scapular winging
	Loss of scapulohumeral rhythm
Suprascapular nerve	Presentation similar to rotator cuff tear because of wasting of the supraspinatus and/or infraspinatus muscles
	Loss of strength in abduction and external rotation of the shoulder
	Pain is deep and poorly localized
Pancoas's tumor[38] (superior sulcus lung tumor)	Men older than 50 years with a history of cigarette smoking
	"Nagging"-type pain in the shoulder and along the vertebral border of the scapula
	Pain that has progressed from nagging to burning in nature, often extending down the arm and into the ulnar nerve distribution

TABLE 6-11

Medical Screening Questionnaire for the Cervical Spine and Shoulder Regions

Question	Yes	No
1. Have you had a direct blow to your shoulder or a shoulder dislocation?		
2. Have you recently used your shoulder excessively?		
3. Have you had a traction injury to your arm?		
4. Have you had a direct blow to the lateral chest wall?		
5. Have you recently fallen onto an outstretched arm?		
6. Have you noticed difficulty lifting your arm or any other muscle weakness?		
7. Have you been experiencing pins and needles anywhere in your body?		
8. Do you experience pain that does not improve with rest?		
9. If you do have pain, where is your pain?		
10. Does your pain move into the arm?		
11. Do you currently smoke?		
12. Do you have a history of smoking?		

cervical and shoulder pain, and Table 6-11 offers a medical screening questionnaire for these patients.

Craniofacial Pain

PTs have become increasingly involved in the treatment of conditions of the head, face, and temporomandibular joint (TMJ). When seeing a patient for TMJ dysfunction, Bell's palsy, stroke, or even conditions of the back or neck, PTs should consider the possibility of meningitis, a primary brain tumor, or a subarachnoid hemorrhage. Quick detection of all of the aforementioned conditions by an alert PT can greatly increase the chance of survival and possibly minimize morbidity.

Meningitis is a relatively rare infection that affects the meninges, causing brain swelling, bleeding, and death in 10% of cases.[7] The most common and most serious type of meningitis is bacterial meningitis. Bacteria that are responsible for bacterial meningitis are present in the external environment and even in our own respiratory systems. The bacteria somehow cross the blood-brain barrier after a head injury, because of a depressed immune system, or for some unidentifiable reason. Bacterial meningitis can cause death within hours, and a child less than 2 years old with an unexplained fever should immediately be seen by a doctor.

Viral meningitis, caused by a viral intestinal infection, mumps, or a herpes infection, is generally the least serious, clearing on its own within 1 to 2 weeks. Antiviral medications may be used in more serious cases of infection, depending on the type of viral infection. Acyclovir is effective against herpes simplex, which can cause herpes encephalitis and severe brain damage if not treated. Acyclovir, although effective against the herpes virus, does little to most other viruses and must be given before the person lapses into a coma.

Fungal meningitis affects 10% of patients with AIDS and should be considered when seeing these patients.[7] Fungal meningitis is spread from pigeon droppings and is treated with antifungal medications after it is detected.

Meningitis is more common in people with compromised immune systems, such as patients with AIDS and those who have suffered a facial trauma leading to infection that spreads to the cerebrospinal fluid (CSF). In addition, meningitis is most common in children less than 2 years old and people living in close quarters, such as college dormitories or military training camps.

If meningitis is suspected, a slump test is performed. In this test, the neck and trunk are fully flexed, causing pain that is relieved when the neck flexion ceases. Different variants are used with the trunk flexed and the leg straightened, but all forms stress the meninges.[30] If a meningeal inflammation is present, a positive test should result, as pain in the back, neck, or head that is relieved when the meninges are no longer stressed. Other signs are headaches, high fever, stiff neck, nausea and vomiting, photophobia, confusion, sleepiness, and seizures. A patient with this type of presentation should be referred immediately to an emergency room or back to his or her primary-care physician for proper testing. A physician must perform a lumbar puncture to get a sample of CSF for analysis, to make the diagnosis, and to determine appropriate treatment.

Another possible intracranial disorder that requires vigilance is *brain cancer*. A primary brain tumor occurs relatively infrequently, in six to nine people per 100,000,[37] but the CNS also is a common site for metastasis. Lung cancer accounts for about one-half of all metastatic brain lesions, and breast cancer and melanomas often metastasize to the brain. Therefore PTs treating patients with a history of these primary cancers should be vigilant for symptoms suggesting CNS metastases. Although headache is a symptom associated with a brain tumor, neurologic deficits are a more common symptom in the early and mid stages of this disorder.[19] Change in mentation, vomiting with or without nausea, visual changes, seizures, ataxia, and speech impairment all are possible presentations, with or without the headache. Symptoms of this type would warrant a detailed neurologic screening (see Chapter 10).

The third condition affecting the head, face, and TMJ region is *subarachnoid hemorrhage*. Hemorrhage is most often caused by a rupture of a saccular intracranial aneurysm or rupture of an arteriovenous malformation. The signs and symptoms can be very similar to those of a brain tumor and of meningitis. A patient will describe a headache of sudden onset that is the worst headache of his or her life, and the patient may even experience a brief loss of consciousness. Meningeal irritation symptoms and signs (nuchal rigidity, fever, photophobia, nausea, and vomiting) and brain tumor symptoms and signs (neurologic dysfunction, nausea, and vomiting) also are possible. If a PT suspects a subarachnoid hemorrhage, emergency medical care should be instituted. Early diagnosis is critical and can prevent devastating neurologic effects. See Table 6-12 for a summary of the red flags for patients with

TABLE 6-12

Red Flags for the Head, Face, and Temporomandibular Joint Regions

Condition	Red Flags
Meningitis	Positive slump sign
	Headache
	Fever
	Gastrointestinal signs of vomiting and symptoms of nausea
	Photophobia
	Confusion
	Seizures
	Sleepiness
Primary brain tumor	Ataxia
	Speech deficits
	Sensory abnormalities
	Headache
	Gastrointestinal signs of vomiting and symptoms of nausea
	Visual changes
	Altered mental status
	Seizures
Subarachnoid hemorrhage	Headache of sudden onset (the worst headache of his or her life)
	A brief loss of consciousness
	Brain tumor signs (neurologic dysfunction, nausea and vomiting)
	Meningeal irritation signs (nuchal rigidity, fever, photophobia, nausea and vomiting)

TABLE 6-13

Medical Screening Questionnaire for the Head, Face, and Temporomandibular Joint Regions

Question	Yes	No
1. Do you have a depressed immune system?		
2. Have you recently had an intestinal infection, mumps, or herpes?		
3. Have you had recent contact with pigeons or pigeon droppings?		
4. Have you recently been living in close quarters, such as in a dormitory or military training camp?		
5. Have you recently had a head trauma?		
6. Do you currently have a high fever, or have you had a fever recently?		
7. Have you been experiencing nausea or vomiting?		
8. Have you had difficulty with light sensitivity?		
9. Have you noticed a recent inability to concentrate?		
10. Have you recently had a seizure?		
11. Do you experience abnormal sensations in the skin?		
12. Have you recently had difficulty with speaking?		
13. Have you noticed an increased clumsiness or lack of coordination?		
14. Have you recently experienced a loss of consciousness?		

craniofacial pain and Table 6-13 for a medical-screening questionnaire for these patients.

Elbow, Wrist, and Hand Pain

Injuries involving the elbow, wrist, and hand are common, and pain in specific locations should alert the PT to the possibility of a more serious disorder. For example, a patient with osteoporosis or other conditions that can compromise bone density who suffers a fall is more likely to sustain a fracture. A patient who takes corticosteroids for chronic respiratory problems will be more likely to suffer a tendon rupture or ligamentous injury secondary to the same fall. Finally, a patient who is immunosuppressed for any number of reasons is more susceptible to a space infection in the hand. This section will cover the red flags associated with specific fractures, tendon ruptures, space infections of the hand, Raynaud's disease, and complex regional pain syndrome (reflex sympathetic dystrophy).

Fractures

A fracture at the elbow will likely have been caused by a fall onto an outstretched arm or by direct trauma to the elbow itself. An *olecranon fracture* will cause posterior pain, swelling, and tenderness. Elbow extension will be the function most impaired, and there may be a palpable gap between the olecranon and the trochlear notch of the humerus. A fall also may cause anterolateral pain and tenderness, cause an inability to supinate and pronate the forearm, or cause the arm to be held against the side with the elbow flexed. This would be more typical of a radial head fracture, and having the elbow flexed produces the least pressure within the elbow capsule. This loose packed position of 70 degrees of ulnohumeral flexion and 10 degrees of supination also will compensate for the effusion of the elbow joint that is usually present.[29]

The radius also may be fractured distally during a fall onto an outstretched arm. A fracture of the distal radius, *Colles' fracture*, typically presents with local pain, tenderness, swelling, and ecchymoses, and wrist extension in particular will be painful.[29] The same fall onto an outstretched arm and extended wrist can cause a *scaphoid fracture*. The patient will have similar signs and symptoms, but localized to the anatomical snuffbox. The wrist also will be very stiff secondary to the swelling. Radiographs, if performed with all four views plus a navicular view, have a 100% diagnostic sensitivity.[49] If films are negative, however, the patient is put into a spica cast and radiographs are repeated after 2 weeks. The main concern with scaphoid fractures is the possibility of avascular necrosis secondary to disruption of the blood supply.

The final type of fracture that will be discussed is a lunate fracture or dislocation and capitate fracture. Lunate fractures are rare and often are related to osteonecrosis. Lunate fractures can cause diffuse synovitis with generalized wrist swelling, pain, decreased motion, and even decreased grip strength. The best way to identify a lunate fracture is by radiographic imaging, especially a T1-weighted MR image to detect loss of bone marrow. A capitate fracture is more common and will present with similar symptoms of wrist pain, swelling, and tenderness at the mid-dorsal wrist area. Capitate fractures, however, are the result of trauma involving maximal wrist flexion or extension, rather than of osteonecrosis.

Soft-Tissue Injuries

Falls, traumas, and sports-related injuries cause problems not only with bones but also with local soft tissue structures. The flexor forearm muscle mass, including the pronator teres, flexor carpi radialis, palmaris longus, and flexor carpi ulnaris, can be strained or even ruptured. A grade I muscle strain is a stretching of the muscle fibers without disruption. A grade II tear is a partial tearing of the muscles with maintenance of the overlying fascia. This injury will include local tenderness, swelling, muscle spasms, a hematoma, and pain with motion and with passive elongation of the tissue. Strains of grade I and II can be treated conservatively with the RICE (*rest*, *ice*, *compression*, *elevation*) technique. Grade III tears are a complete tearing of the muscle and its investing fascia. This injury results in a total loss of motion, and surgical repair will be needed. Swelling, tenderness, ecchymoses of the overlying skin, and a palpable defect in the muscle are characteristic of a grade III rupture of the flexor forearm muscle mass and would warrant referral of the patient to a physician as soon as possible.

Infection

The hand often is traumatized secondary to puncture wounds, abrasions, cuts, or other injuries, and a break in the skin brings the increased possibility of an infection. Hands have several spaces (e.g., midpalmar space, web space, and thenar space) that can serve as prime areas for infection to develop and spread. Fingers also have such spaces on the volar surface, such as the pulp space of the proximal, middle, and distal phalanx. Any of these spaces can become infected after a direct puncture, formation of an abscess, or purulent tenosynovitis of tendons that pass through the space. These spaces can become infected as a result of trauma or poor nail care. A patient will present with the typical signs of local inflammation, and the swelling will cause the finger pads to be tense and painful with a resultant loss of motion. Infections must be treated quickly, or the infection will spread to the adjacent web space of the hand and beyond.

If the web space becomes infected, the swelling, pain, tenderness, warmth, and erythema will be present in the palm and over the dorsum of the hand proximal to the involved area of the involved space. The edema can cause the metacarpal bones to become splayed, resulting in loss of the normal hand shape. The causes are similar to those listed above, and, as mentioned, can be caused by progression of a pulp space infection.

Midpalmar-space infections appear very similar to web-space infections in their presentation, with inflammation of the palm and dorsum of the hand and loss of the concavity of the palm secondary to swelling. Even the midpalmar space can be infected by the second, third, and fourth web spaces through the lumbrical canals.[49] Direct puncture also can infect the midpalmar space or produce tenosynovitis of the flexor tendons of the second or fourth finger.

The thenar space is the equivalent of the midpalmar space, but for the thumb. Direct puncture, tenosynovitis of the second flexor tendon or from an adjacent space, such as the midpalmar space, can infect this area. This space is treated the same as the spaces mentioned previously, by drainage with a course of antibiotics specific to the organism causing the infection. If the patient is not seen by a doctor quickly, the infection could drain through a necrotic area of the skin, increasing the possibility of osteomyelitis or septic arthritis. The infection also can spread, causing high fever, chills, weakness, and malaise. Ultimately, the infection could lead to sepsis and amputation of fingers or parts of the hand.[25] As with any infection, people who are immunocompromised are at the greatest risk. Space infections also have been seen in recipients of cardiac transplants, because of the need for long-term immunosuppression to prevent rejection of donor hearts.[25]

Raynaud's Disease

Another disorder that may affect patients seeing PTs is *Raynaud's disease*, or *Raynaud's phenomenon*. This disorder affects one or both hands and the feet. One or more digits may be involved, and progression of the disease involves more digits. When a person is exposed to cold or to emotional upset, the hands blanch, become cyanotic, and then turn red. During the rubor stage the patient has pain and paresthesias as the blood returns to the hands or feet. This entire phase lasts only 15 to 20 minutes, and the patient can alleviate it by running the hands under warm water. As mentioned, exposure to cold or stress usually precipitates episodes, but Raynaud's phenomenon is also more common in patients with rheumatoid arthritis or occlusive vascular disease, those who smoke, and people taking beta-adrenergic blocking drugs to treat migraine, angina, or hypertension.

Reflex sympathetic dystrophy (RSD; also known as complex regional pain syndrome) is a disorder that varies in severity, but often follows trauma to the elbow, wrist, or hand. The trauma may include a fracture, sprain, dislocation, crush injury, or surgery such as a carpal tunnel procedure. There is often a lag period between the injury and the onset of the symptoms of complex regional pain syndrome. Symptoms include severe aching, stinging, cutting, or boring pain that is out of proportion to the injury, corrective surgery, or normal tissue healing.[42,43] The pain does not respond to typical analgesics, and regional nerve blocks usually produce only temporary relief. The hand often becomes swollen, warm, and erythematous.

Hyperhidrosis is also often present. The other hand may support the involved limb, and the patient is often resistant to let a practitioner handle the hand because of hypersensitivity. Nerve blocks are a common treatment, in conjunction with physical therapy to maintain function and assist the patient with strategies for pain management.

See Table 6-14 for a summary of the red flags for patients with distal upper extremity pain and Table 6-15 for a medical screening questionnaire for these patients.

TABLE 6-14

Red Flags for the Elbow, Wrist, and Hand Regions

Condition	Red Flags
Fractures	Recent fall or trauma
	Pain, tenderness, swelling and ecchymosis
	History of osteoporosis
	Extended use of steroids (e.g., respiratory problems)
	Pathologies with improper bone remodeling
Radial head fracture	Fall onto an outstretched arm that is supinated
	Anterolateral pain and tenderness at the elbow
	Inability to supinate and pronate the forearm
	Elbow held against the side with 70 degrees of flexion and slightly supinated
Distal radius (Colles') fracture	Fall onto outstretched arm with forceful wrist extension
	Wrist held in neutral resting position
	Wrist swelling
	Movements into wrist extension are painful
Scaphoid fracture	Fall onto outstretched arm
	Wrist swelling
	Wrist held in neutral position
	Pain in the "anatomical snuff box"
Lunate fracture or dislocation	Diffuse synovitis
	Generalized wrist swelling and pain
	Decreased motion
	Decreased grip strength (Rule out capitate fracture)
Long flexor tendon rupture	Grade I and II muscle tear: local tenderness, swelling, muscle spasms, hematoma, pain with motion and with passive stretch
	Grade III muscle rupture: total loss of motion and palpable defect in the muscle, swelling, tenderness, ecchymosis of the overlying skin
Space infection of the hand	Recent puncture of skin
	Presence of an abscess
	Purulent tenosynovitis of tendons that go through a space
	Typical signs of inflammation: swelling in palm, dorsum of hand, or finger tips
	Pain, tenderness, warmth, and erythema
	Signs of longstanding infection: high fever, chills, weakness, and malaise
Raynaud's phenomenon or Raynaud's disease	Hands or feet that blanch, go cyanotic and then red when exposed to cold or emotional stress
	Pain and tingling in hands or feet when they turn red
	Past medical history significant for rheumatoid arthritis, occlusive vascular disease, smoking, or use of beta-blockers
Complex regional pain syndrome (reflex sympathetic dystrophy)	Trauma including fracture, dislocation, or surgery
	Severe aching, stinging, cutting, or boring pain that is not typical of injury; hypersensitivity
	Area swollen (pitting edema), warm, and erythematous
	Pain does not respond to typical analgesics

TABLE 6-15

Medical Screening Questionnaire for the Elbow, Wrist, and Hand Regions

	Yes	No
1. Have you recently had a trauma, such as a fall?		
2. Has a medical practitioner ever told you that you have osteoporosis?		
3. Are you currently taking steroids or have you been on prolonged steroid therapy?		
4. Do you have a pathology with improper bone remodeling?		
5. Have you noticed an inability to move your elbow normally?		
6. Have you noticed an inability to move your wrist normally?		
7. Do you have difficulty turning you hand upwards or downwards (e.g., turning a doorknob)?		
8. Have you recently had an infection?		
9. Do you have any open wounds, cuts, swelling, or redness on your hands or arms?		
10. Have you noticed weakness of you hands or frequent dropping of objects?		
11. Have you recently experienced a high fever, chills, weakness, or malaise?		
12. Do your hands or feet blanch, go blue, and then turn red when exposed to cold or emotional stress?		
13. Do you have a medical history of rheumatoid arthritis, occlusive vascular disease, or use of beta-blockers?		
14. Do you currently smoke or have a history of smoking?		
15. If you have pain, does it respond to typical pain medications?		

Summary

The investigation of symptoms produces information vital in determining why the patient has sought physical therapy services. While the patient describes the location, onset, and behavior of symptoms, the PT must decide whether the patient's narrative makes sense based upon our understanding of basic and clinical sciences and our experiences. This information helps the PT make a diagnosis and decide whether to refer the patient to a physician. This information, gathered during the initial patient visit, also helps guide the PT in choosing the body systems to screen (Chapter 7) later during the history, helps in determining whether a lower-quarter (Chapter 10) or upper-quarter (Chapter 11) screening examination is warranted, and helps identify the components of these exams that are most relevant.

Finally, the location of symptoms should alert the PT to the possibility of certain disorders that may be responsible for the patient's symptoms. Knowledge of such disorders will enable the PT to recognize the specific symptoms and warning signs for these disorders. Many of these warning signs (e.g., fever), and the specific appearance that makes the finding a red flag, are described in Chapter 7. The clinician also is encouraged to use the accompanying tables and figures to collect this patient information in a more effective and efficient manner.

REFERENCES

1. Acheson RM, Chan YK, Payne M: New Haven survey of joint diseases: The interrelationships between morning stiffness, nocturnal pain and swelling of the joints, *J Chron Dis* 21:533-542, 1969.
2. Bianco AJ: Low back pain and sciatica. Diagnosis and indications for treatment, *J Bone Joint Surg*, 508A:170-181, 1968.
3. Bigos S, Bowyer O, Braen G, et al: *Acute lower back problems in adults. Clinical practice guideline no 14.* AHCPR publication no 95-0642, Agency for Health Care Policy and Research, Public Health Service, US Department of Health and Human Services, Rockville, MD, December, 1994.
4. Boissonnault W: Prevalence of comorbid conditions, surgeries, and medication use in a physical outpatient population: a multicentered study, *J Orthop Sports Phys Ther* 29:506-519, 1999.
5. Boissonnault W, DiFabio R: Pain profile of patients with low back pain referred to physical therapy, *J Orthop Sports Phys Ther* 24:180-191, 1996.
6. Boyko EJ, Ahroni JH, Davignon D, et al: Diagnostic utility of the history and physical examination for peripheral vascular disease among patients with diabetes mellitus, *J Clin Epidemiol* 50:659-668, 1997.
7. Bruce M, Rosenstein N, Capparella J, et al: Risk factors for meningococcal disease in college students, *JAMA* 286:688-693, 2001.
8. Busch MT, Morrissy RT: Slipped capital femoral epiphysis, *Orthop Clin North Am* 18:637-647, 1987.
9. Canto JG, Shlipak MG, Rogers WJ, et al: Prevalence, clinical characteristics, and mortality among patients with myocardial infarction presenting without chest pain, *JAMA* 283:3223-3229, 2000.
10. Delitto A, Erhard RE, Bowling RW: A treatment-based classification approach to lower back syndrome: identifying and staging patients for conservative treatment, *Phys Ther* 75:470-489, 1995.
11. DeRosa GP. The child. In D'Ambrosia RD, ed: *Musculoskeletal disorders: regional examination and differential diagnosis*, ed 2, Philadelphia, 1986, JB Lippincott, pp 595-598.
12. Deyo RA, Diehl AK: Cancer as a cause of back pain: frequency, clinical presentation, and diagnostic strategies, *J Gen Intern Med* 3:230-238, 1988.
13. Deyo RA, Rainville J, Kent DL: What can the history and physical examination tell us about lower back pain? *JAMA* 268:760-765, 1992.
14. DiFabio R, Boissonnault W: Physical therapy and health-related outcomes for patients with common orthopaedic diagnoses, *J Orthop Sports Phys Ther* 27:219-230, 1998.
15. Doran FSA: The sites to which pain is referred from the common bile-duct in man and its implication for the theory of referred pain, *Br J Surg* 54:599-606, 1967.
16. Farrell JP, Twomey LT: Acute low back pain: comparison of two conservative approaches, *Med J Aust* 1:160-164, 1982.
17. Foldes K, Balint P, Gaal M, et al: Nocturnal pain correlates with effusions in diseased hips, *J Rheumatol* 19:1756-1758, 1992.
18. Henderson JM: Ruling out danger: differential diagnosis of thoracic spine, *Phys Sports Med* 20:124-131, 1992.
19. Isaacs ER, Bookhout MR: Screening for pathologic origins of head and facial pain. In Boissonnault WG, ed: *Examination in physical therapy practice: screening for medical disease*, ed 2, New York, 1995, Churchill Livingstone, pp 181-182.
20. Jarvik JG, Deyo RA: Diagnostic evaluation of low back pain with emphasis on imaging, *Ann Intern Med*, 137:586-597, 2002.
21. Jayson MI, Sims-Williams H, Young S, et al: Mobilization and manipulation for low back pain, *Spine* 6:409-416, 1981.
22. Jemal A, Murray T, Samuels A, et al: Cancer statistics, 2003, *CA Cancer J Clin* 53:5-26, 2003.
23. Jette AM, Davis KD: A comparison of hospital-based and private outpatient physical therapy practices, *Phys Ther* 71:366-375, 1991.
24. Jonsson B, Stromquist B: Symptoms and signs in degeneration of the lumbar spine: a prospective, consecutive study of 300 operated patients, *J Bone Joint Surg* 75B:381-385, 1993.
25. Klein M, Chang J: Management of hand and upper-extremity infections in heart transplant recipients, *Plast Reconstr Surg* 106:598-601, 2000.
26. Kopell H, Thompson W: *Peripheral entrapment neuropathies*, FL, 1976, Robert I Krieger Publishing, pp 146-153,156,167.
27. Liu, K, Atten M: Coping with kidney stones, *Am Surg* 63:519-525, 1997.
28. Lorei M, Hershman E: Peripheral nerve injuries in athletes, *Sports Med* 16:130-147, 1993.
29. Magee DJ: *Orthopedic clinical assessment*, New York, 1997, WB Saunders, p 38.
30. Maitland GD, Hengeveld E, Banks K, et al, eds: *Maitland's vertebral manipulation*, ed 6, Oxford, 2001, Butterworth/Heinemann, pp 41-43.
31. McGee SR, Boyko EJ. Physical examination and chronic lower-extremity ischemia: a critical review, *Arch Intern Med* 158:1357-1364, 1998.
32. Meadows JTS: *Orthopedic differential diagnosis in physical therapy*, New York, 1999, McGraw-Hill.
33. Raj PP: Prognostic and therapeutic local anesthetic block. In Cousins MJ, Bridenbaugh PO, eds: *Neural blockade in clinical anesthesia and management of pain*, ed 2, Philadelphia, 1988, JB Lippincott, p 908.
34. Saklayen M: Medical management of nephrolithiasis, *Med Clin North Am* 81:785-799, 1997.
35. Schofferman L, Schoffmerman J, Zucheman J, et al: Occult infection causing persistent low back pain, *Spine* 14:417-419, 1989.
36. Siegmeth W, Noyelle RM: Night pain and morning stiffness in osteoarthritis: a crossover study of flurbiprofen and diclofenac sodium, *J Intern Med Res* 16:182-188, 1988.
37. Snyder H, Robinson K, Shah D, et al: Signs and symptoms of patients with brain tumors presenting in the emergency department, *J Emerg Med* 11:253-258, 1993.
38. Spengler D, Kirsh M, Kaufer H: Orthopaedic aspects and early diagnosis of superior sulcus lung tumor, *J Bone Joint Surg* 55:1645-1650, 1973.
39. Stulberg BN, Bauer TW, Belhobek GH, et al: A diagnostic algorithm for osteonecrosis of the femoral head, *Clin Orthop* 249:176-182, 1989.
40. Suadicani P, Hein HO, Gyntelberg F: Height, weight, and risk of colorectal cancer. An 18-year follow-up in a cohort of 5249 men, *Scand J Gastroenterol* 28:285-288, 1993.
41. Tronzo RG: Femoral neck fractures. In Steinburg ME, ed: *The hip and its disorders*, Philadelphia, 1991, Saunders, pp 247-279.
42. Van de Vusse AC, Stomp-van den Berg SGM, de Vet HWC, et al: Interobserver reliability of diagnosis in patients with complex regional pain syndrom, *Eur J Pain* 7:259-265, 2003.
43. Vanharanta H, Sachs BI, Spivey M, et al: A comparison of CT/discography, pain response and radiographic disc height, *Spine* 13:321-324, 1988.
44. Veldman PH, Reynen HM, Arntz IE, et al: Signs and symptoms of reflex sympathetic dystrophy: prospective study of 829 patients, *Lancet* 342:1012-1016, 1993.

45. Waldvogel FA, Vasey H: Osteomyelitis: the past decade, *N Engl J Med* 14:360-370, 1980.
46. Weinstein JN, McLain RF: Primary tumors of the spine, *Spine* 12:843-851, 1987.
47. Wells K: Nephrolithiasis with unusual initial symptoms, *J Manipulative Physiol Ther* 23: 196-205, 2000.

48. Wenger DR, Ward WT, Herring JA: Current concepts review: Legg-Calve-Perthes disease, *J Bone Joint Surg* 73:778-788, 1991.
49. Wiener SL: *Differential diagnosis of acute pain by body region*, New York, 1993, McGraw-Hill, pp 532, 542, 616, 645, 678, 680.
50. Zohn DA, Mennell JM: *Diagnosis and physical treatment, musculoskeletal pain*, Boston, 1976, Little, Brown, pp 20, 36, 49.

Review of Systems

7

William G. Boissonnault, PT, DHSc, FAAOMPT

Objectives

After reading this chapter, the reader will be able to:

1. Create checklists for general health and for each of the body organ systems.
2. Describe strategies for determining whether a "yes" answer to any checklist item is a "red flag" or a "yellow flag."
3. Discuss the types of patients and the patient visits (initial or follow-up) for which each of the checklists is appropriate.
4. Describe strategies to efficiently integrate the review of systems checklists into a patient examination scheme.

The *review of systems (ROS)* is an important category of data that are collected during the patient interview. These data, in conjunction with a patient's medical history and symptoms and signs, is vital to the physical therapists' (PT) role in medical screening and differential diagnosis as described in the *Guide to Physical Therapist Practice*.[3] The ROS investigation includes the use of checklists of common symptoms relevant to each of the body systems. The purpose of the ROS is to identify symptoms that may have been overlooked during the investigation of the patient's chief presenting symptoms.[8,39]

The systematic review of each of the body systems may reveal symptoms that are in fact related to the reason the patient initiated physical therapy, but, equally important, it may identify symptoms that are not. These "adjunct" symptoms may be associated with one or more existing co-morbid conditions, with occult disease, or with adverse drug reactions. Detecting such symptoms that were not previously reported to the patient's physician, or that represent a worsening of preexisting manifestations of a co-morbidity or medication use, would prompt contact with the appropriate health care provider.

These checklists are *not* intended to rule out specific diseases or enable the therapist to differentiate diseases; these are tasks of the physician. These checklists are based on body-system physiology; so if the system is malfunctioning in some capacity, the patient may report the symptoms identified in these checklists, assuming the therapist has asked the appropriate questions.

The addition of the ROS checklists to the PT's examination scheme may cause some therapists to ask; "Where do I find time to add even more questions to the patient interview?" The checklists, presented later in the chapter, are relatively short. The checklists' being manageable from a time perspective, but adequate from a screening perspective, depends on where in the history these questions are asked. The assumption is made that the therapist already has investigated the patient's symptoms and functional limitations (see Chapter 6) and has reviewed the relevant portions of the patient's demographics and medical history (see Chapter 5).

With regard to the amount of time required, the cardiovascular checklist (Box 7-1) has only seven items. The PT could legitimately say that this checklist by itself is inadequate for screening patients for cardiovascular conditions. One might ask, "Where is the item for chest pain or claudication? Where is the item for history of heart problems? Where is the item for family history of heart problems?" If the therapist has investigated the patient's symptoms using a body diagram, any chest pain will have been documented already. If the therapist has investigated the pattern of symptoms (with the 24-hour report), claudication would have been identified already. If the patient's medical history already has been reviewed, a history of heart problems, hypertension, or peripheral vascular disease would have been revealed, as would a positive family history of cardiovascular disease. The key to keeping the checklists manageable is to perform the detailed investigation of the patient's medical history and presenting symptoms *before* implementing the ROS checklists.

In addition, the PT need not use every checklist in the examination of every patient. The general health checklist should be used in the initial visit of all patients, but the rest of the body-specific checklists should be used only if appropriate for the location and description of the patient's symptoms and medical history. After the PT chooses the appropriate body-specific checklists for the patient, the next decision is whether to use these checklists during the initial visit or at a later visit. This important decision will depend on the patient data already collected: the patient medical history, the investigation of symptoms, and the general health checklist.

Another challenge to the PT is deciding whether a positive response ("yes" response) on a checklist constitutes a *red flag* (requiring communication with another care giver) or a *yellow flag* (something to note in the PT's documentation and to monitor, but not something that warrants immediate communication with a physician). This is especially challenging with general findings such as fatigue or weakness. This chapter discusses the guidelines clinicians can use to make this important decision, including follow-up questions for the various checklist items. In addition to helping the therapist differentiate between a red flag and yellow flag, these follow-up questions

---

BOX 7-1

Cardio/Peripheral Vascular Systems Checklist

- Dyspnea
- Palpitations
- Syncope
- Pain with sweats
- Cough
- Peripheral edema
- Cold hands/feet
- Open wounds
- Skin discoloration

---

elicit information that will be a vital part of what the PT communicates to the physician.

General Health Checklist

Some symptoms can result from many diseases of individual body systems, from multisystem disorders, from systemic illnesses, and from adverse drug reactions (Box 7-2). Using a checklist of these symptoms (general health checklist) can give the PT a valuable first level of medical screening during an initial patient visit. See Appendix 5-B to see how some of this information can be collected on a patient self-report questionnaire. Some symptoms (e.g., fatigue and malaise) are vague but may be the initial manifestation of a very serious illness. After the patient acknowledges such symptoms, follow-up questions are key in determining their significance.

BOX 7-2

General Health Checklist: All Patients at Initial Visit

1. Fatigue
2. Malaise
3. Fever/chills/sweats: significant if 99.5° F or higher for more than 2 weeks
4. Weight loss/gain: 5%-10% of body weight increase/decrease, unexplained
5. Nausea/vomiting
6. Dizziness/lightheadedness
7. Paresthesia/numbness
8. Weakness
9. Change in mentation/cognitive abilities

FOR ANY "YES" ANSWER, DETERMINE:
1. Is there an explanation for it?
2. Has patient mentioned this to a physician?
3. If a physician is aware of it, has it become worse?

Fatigue

Concern about fatigue accounts for about 10 million primary-care office visits per year in the United States.[25] Many serious illnesses can cause fatigue, including some psychological disorders, infections, cancers (typically advanced disease), and endocrine disorders (Box 7-3). In addition, fatigue may be associated with medication use, including antihypertensives, cardiovascular and psychotropic medications, and antihistamines.[28] The challenge to the PT is to differentiate the fatigue associated with everyday

---

BOX 7-3

Conditions Presenting as Chronic Fatigue[9]

PSYCHOLOGICAL
- Depression
- Anxiety
- Somatization disorder

ENDOCRINE/METABOLIC
- Hypothyroidism
- Diabetes mellitus
- Pituitary insufficiency
- Addison's disease
- Chronic renal failure
- Hyperparathyroidism

INFECTIOUS
- Endocarditis
- Tuberculosis
- Mononucleosis
- Hepatitis
- HIV infection

NEOPLASMS
- Occult malignancy

CARDIOPULMONARY
- Congestive heart failure
- Chronic obstructive pulmonary disease

CONNECTIVE TISSUE DISEASE
- Rheumatic disorders

SLEEP DISTURBANCES
- Sleep apnea
- Esophageal reflux

ALLERGIC RHINITIS

---

life from the potentially serious fatigue. After the patient reports fatigue, the PT should ask the following questions:
- "What do you mean by fatigue? Describe your fatigue to me."
- "When did the fatigue begin?"
- "Do you know why you are so tired?"

Many patients say they are simply tired or worn out. PTs must follow up with questions such as, "Does the tiredness interfere with your ability to function?" Fatigue becomes a red flag when the tiredness interferes with the patient's ability to carry out typical daily activities at home, work, social settings, school, or during rehabilitation, and when the fatigue has lasted for 2 to 4 weeks or longer.[4,28] For example, a patient may say that up until 3 weeks ago she typically worked 8 to 9 hours per day, went home and helped take care of dinner, and then was active until she went to bed at 11 PM. Now she struggles to make it through her workday, and in fact she went home early twice this week because of her fatigue. When she comes home from work now, she barely makes it through dinner, and has been going to bed by 9 PM. This report represents a change in the patient's ability to carry out her everyday activities. If the patient describes true fatigue, the PT should ask the following questions:
- "Was the onset quick, or was it a slow, gradual process?"
- "Have you told your physician about the fatigue?"

When communicating concerns about fatigue to the physician's office, the PT must describe the specifics of the condition. Simply reporting that the patient is tired will not alarm anyone, but describing the functional limitations associated with the fatigue will.

Malaise

Malaise is a sense of uneasiness or general discomfort, an "out-of-sorts" feeling. Patients may describe this uneasiness as an intuition that "something isn't right" or that they are "coming down with something." Malaise often is noted with conditions that generate fever (e.g., infectious disorders).[21,35] A patient may describe malaise by saying, "I have felt like I am coming down with the flu for weeks, but haven't yet become ill." Another patient with an existing history of heart problems or cancer might start experiencing new symptoms or a return of previous symptoms. This patient may say, "I am worried that the cancer has come back." On review of Appendix 5-B, *malaise* is not included in the general health checklist. Most patients will not know if they feel malaise or not, so this symptom is generally identified by the therapist, based on patient comments.

Fever/Chills/Sweats

Fever/chills/sweats are symptoms and signs most often associated with systemic illnesses such as infections, cancers, and connective-tissue disorders such as rheumatoid arthritis.[7,29] Fever associated with a pathologic condition is a result of the release of pyrogens into the bloodstream by toxic bacteria or from degenerating body tissues, which cause the "set point" of the hypothalamic thermostat to rise. The sense of feeling "chilled" is often associated with fever.

When the blood temperature is lower than the hypothalamic set point, the body reacts by increasing core body temperature via the normal responses, including cutaneous vasoconstriction (Fig. 7-1). This superficial vasoconstriction produces a drop in skin temperature that can lead to *shaking chills* or *rigor*. If the body temperature reaches 39.5° C (103° F), however, the patient typically no longer feels chilled or hot.[23] The therapist should watch for patients with an occult fever. If the patient answers

"yes" to fever on the questionnaire, follow-up questions are in order. As with any other "yes" answer on these checklists, the therapist should determine whether the patient knows why he or she has the fever (e.g., "I have the flu or a sinus infection"). If the patient complains of persistent chills or sweats but does not know whether he or she has a fever, the therapist should take the patient's temperature.

When assessing fever, the PT should understand that normal body temperature is not defined by a single value, 37° C (98.6° F), at a single point in time. Body temperature (mean rectal temperature) typically follows a circadian rhythm, ranging from about 36.1° C (97° F) in the morning to 37.4° C (99.3° F) in the late afternoon.[35] Fever has been defined as body temperature greater than 37.5° C (99.5° F).[13]

To qualify as a red flag, the fever should have some longevity, as with the symptom of fatigue. If the fever has been present for 2 weeks or longer, and a physician has not seen the patient for this symptom, the patient should be referred to a physician. The 2-week window accounts for the common self-limited viruses that can be accompanied by a fever but of shorter duration. If the patient does not know whether he or she has a fever, the therapist can ask the patient whether he or she feels the same today as he or she has felt for the past 2 weeks or more. If the answer is yes, and the patient has a temperature of 37.5° C (99.5° F) or higher via the clinical reading, the therapist should assume the patient has had this fever for 2 or more weeks until proven otherwise. The referral takes on a more urgent nature if the therapist gets a reading of 39° C (102° F) or higher. Such a fever may require hospitalization.[13]

Normal body temperature also varies among age groups. Studies have shown that the amount of fluctuation in the circadian body temperature was lower in an elderly population, as were the baseline body temperatures.[42] Therefore screening guidelines may vary depending on the population in question. One study[11] of an elderly population found that an oral temperature of 37.2° C (98.9° F) carried a sensitivity of 83% and a specificity of 89% for the detection of infection. Thus the authors recommended that a persistent temperature (taken orally) of greater than 37.2° C, or an increase of 1.3° C above the patient's baseline body temperature in an elderly person, be considered cause for concern. Therapists can use this guideline to help determine whether to contact the physician about a patient's health.

Finally, therapists should remember that a perceived absence of fever does not preclude the possibility that the patient has an infection. The elderly population is especially vulnerable to this phenomenon. Reduced thermoregulatory responses in the aged may be responsible for the differences in fever response to infection between the elderly and younger populations.[29] This finding is in part responsible for the increased morbidity and mortality associated with infectious processes. For example, pneumonia is the most common cause of infectious death in the geriatric population because of the frequent absence of the expected fever, productive cough, and pleuritic pain.[18] The PT must watch for the other warning signs (see the following discussion of confusion/change in mentation) that may manifest and alert the PT that the patient may have a serious condition.

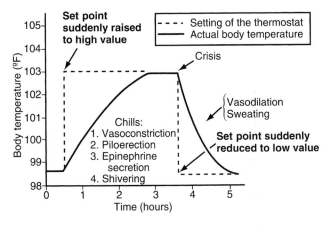

FIGURE 7-1 Effects of changing the set point of the hypothalamic temperature controller. (From Guyton AC, Hall JE. *Textbook of medical physiology*, ed 10, Philadelphia, 2000, WB Saunders, p 831.)

Unexplained Weight Change

Unexplained weight loss or gain also is a red flag. Involuntary weight loss is associated with many potentially serious disorders, but much like fatigue, it is a sensitive but nonspecific finding. The potential causes of weight loss can be summarized by physiological categories (Table 7-1). Not all of these disorders occur with equal frequency.

Thompson and Morris[40] investigated unexplained weight loss in an elderly population (aged 63 years and older; 67% female), identifying those who had lost 7.5% or more of their baseline body weight over a 6-month period. The patients then were followed for up to 24 months, or until the definitive cause of the weight loss had been determined. The disorders most frequently associated with the weight loss were depression (18%), cancer (16%), and gastrointestinal disease other than cancer (11%).

Marton et al[27] investigated involuntary weight loss in a patient population (mean age 59 years ± 17.5 years; 99% males) at a Veterans Medical Center, identifying those who had lost at least 5% of the usual body weight during the previous 6 months. The causes most often noted included cancer (19%), gastrointestinal disorders (14%), and psychiatric and cardiovascular disorders (9%). The definition of a significant weight loss varies. Goroll and Mulley[21] use a loss of about 5 to 10 lb as a general range, and Swartz[39] suggests a loss of 5% to 10% of body weight over 6 months to 12 months as a warning sign of underlying disease. The author's personal communication with physicians over the years has prompted the author to use a loss of 5% to 10% of body weight as a guideline. The exception to this general rule is women who are pregnant; a loss of more than 5 lb during the first trimester should be reported.[8]

People lose weight for reasons other than disease, so what makes weight loss a red flag? If a patient reports weight loss during the examination, appropriate follow-up questions include:

- How much weight have you lost?
- Over what period of time?
- Do you know why you have lost weight?

The third question is the most important in determining the importance of the weight loss. If the patient has purposely changed his or her diet or increased his or her physical activity during the time of the weight loss, the therapist's concern can drop considerably. If the patient reports a loss of 5% to 10% of body weight with no purposeful change in diet or activity level, the weight loss becomes a red flag and should be reported to the patient's physician. The patient may say he or she is eating less because, "I'm just not as hungry as I used to be." If this is the only explanation the patient offers, the therapist must be concerned, especially if the patient has risk factors for serious disease (see Chapter 5).

Although weight gain is not noted as a red flag as often as weight loss, excessive weight gain also can be a manifestation of serious disease. Rapid weight gain often is associated with fluid retention (edema or ascites) that can be a manifestation of conditions such as congestive heart failure, liver or renal disease, and preeclampsia.[39,43] In these conditions, the PT may detect the initial warning sign of a relatively rapid onset of edema and check the patient's weight. Of course, this assumes that the PT knows the patient's usual weight and can compare it to the new weight (see Chapter 9).

The extremities are the area most often affected by dependency-related edema, but the face and neck regions also can be involved in patients with preeclampsia.[33] Other conditions that can manifest as unexplained weight gain are depression,

---

TABLE 7-1

Physiological Categories Associated with Weight Loss

Physiological Categories	Symptoms	Diseases
Decreased caloric intake	Anorexia or satiety	Depression/dementia/anxiety disorders
	Loss of sense of taste	Poor dentition
	Dry/sore mouth	Upper gastrointestinal tract disease
	Difficulty with chewing/ swallowing	Malignancies
	Nausea/vomiting	Infections
		Alcoholism
		Chronic congestive heart failure
		Medications: NSAIDs/amphetamines/antitumor drugs/digitalis excess
Maldigestion/malabsorption	Diarrhea	Gallbladder/pancreatic disorders
	Fatty malodorous stools	Infection (giardiasis)
	Food particles in stools	Small bowel disease
		Crohn's disease
Excessive demand/requirements	Fever	Infection
	Change in appetite	Hyperthyroidism
		Malignancies
		Manic disorders
Increased loss/excretion	Diarrhea	Uncontrolled diabetes
	Increased urination	Burns
	Excessive vomiting	Occult gastrointestinal bleeding

Adapted from Goroll AH, Mulley AG. Evaluation of weight loss. In Goroll AH, Mulley AG, eds: *Primary care medicine*, ed 4, Philadelphia, 2000, Lippincott Williams & Wilkins, p 49; and from Swartz MH: *Textbook of physical diagnosis*, ed 4, Philadelphia, 2002, WB Saunders, p 81.

hypothyroidism, and Cushing's syndrome. The same general guideline used to qualify weight loss as a red flag (i.e., 5% to 10% unexplained loss of body weight) can be used for weight gain. An exception to this rule for weight gain would be that a weight gain of 5 lb or greater in a 1-week period during pregnancy is a warning sign and is potentially associated with preeclampsia[12] (see Chapter 13).

Nausea and Vomiting

Intuitively, the PT may intuitively would link nausea with the gastrointestinal checklist rather than the general health checklist, but nausea can be a manifestation of primary disease of other organ systems, of systemic illnesses (metastatic disease), and of adverse drug reactions (Box 7-4). In most cases of persistent vomiting, the physician already has been contacted, but low-level nausea may go unreported for several months. The PT must ask follow-up questions when a patient reports nausea:

- Describe your nausea to me (constant or intermittent, how frequent?).
- How long have you been experiencing the nausea?
- Do you know why you are nauseated?
- Is your physician aware of the nausea? (If the answer is yes, has it gotten any worse since your last physician contact?)
- Is the nausea associated with vomiting or any other symptoms?
- Do you have vomiting without nausea?
- How are you treating the nausea?

As with other findings, if the patient's physician is not aware of the nausea or vomiting, or if the symptoms have worsened since the last physician contact, and the PT has not found an explanation for these symptoms that satisfies the therapist, then this finding becomes a red flag. Over-the-counter treatments for nausea and indigestion could be masking a serious underlying gastrointestinal disorder. For example, patients coming for physical therapy widely use antacids and histamine H_2 antagonists (e.g., cimetidine, ranitidine).[10] If the patient reports such use, the therapist must ask why the patient is taking these medications, for how long, and whether the patient's physician knows of this drug use. The PT also should ask, "Do you need more of the medication to feel comfortable compared with a few weeks or months ago?" An affirmative answer may reveal a serious condition that is worsening.

Paresthesia, Numbness, or Weakness

Besides primary neurologic disorders, several other conditions can be manifested as paresthesia, number, and weakness, including certain renal and endocrine diseases as well as adverse drug reactions. As described in Chapters 5 and 6, the therapist should ask all patients questions about changes in sensation and strength during the first visit because of the possible urgency of a progressive neurologic loss. For example, Jarvik and Deyo[24] state that an important goal of the diagnostic process in patients with low-back pain being seen in primary care settings is to determine whether the patient has a neurologic impairment that requires surgical evaluation. The primary red flags for this patient population include progressive sensory or strength deficits (based on patient report and detection of a deficit during the physical examination (see Chapters 10 and 11), as well as any symptoms of "saddle" anesthesia, urinary retention, increased urinary frequency, and overflow incontinence.[9]

In addition to the progressive neurologic symptoms that seem to suggest a deficit of a spinal nerve root or a peripheral nerve entrapment, the PT should watch for descriptions unusual for the orthopedic outpatient population. These include the following:

- Glove-and-stocking distribution of altered sensation
- Bilateral extremity deficits (sensory/motor)
- Combination of upper extremity and lower extremity deficit patterns (sensory/motor)

Chronic renal failure, multiple sclerosis, and hypothyroidism are examples of disorders that could present with these findings.

Many patients may report weakness, but much like the symptom of fatigue, this finding often does not become a red flag. These scenarios often include general symptoms of weakness, rather than frank weakness such as reports of foot drop. The PT must ask whether the weakness has caused a change in normal daily activities. If the patient reports an inability to carry out usual activities because of the weakness, this finding would warrant a detailed neurologic screening of the upper and lower quarters (see Chapters 10 and 11) once the physical examination begins. If the patient has no other neurologic symptoms such as sensation changes, balance problems, visual symptoms, or taste, smell, or hearing deficits and if the results of the neurologic screening are negative, then the symptom of weakness becomes a yellow flag and not a red flag.

Dizziness/Lightheadedness

Dizziness can be associated with disorders of most body systems as well as multisystem disease and adverse drug reactions. See Box 7-5 for examples of causes of dizziness. Use the

---

BOX 7-4

Some Common Causes of Nausea and Vomiting (Other than Primary Gastrointestinal Disorders)

AS ACUTE PREDOMINANT OR INITIAL SYMPTOM
- Ketoacidosis
- Inferior myocardial infarction
- Hepatitis
- Drug withdrawal
- Early pregnancy
- Medication use: opiates, digitalis, cancer chemotherapeutic agents

RECURRENT OR CHRONIC
- Psychogenic disorders (bulimia)
- Metabolic disorders (adrenal insufficiency, uremia)
- Bile reflux after gastric surgery
- Pregnancy

IN ASSOCIATION WITH NEUROLOGIC SYMPTOMS
- Increased intracranial pressure
- Vestibular disturbances
- Migraine headaches
- Midline cerebellar hemorrhage

Adapted from Swartz MH: *Textbook of physical diagnosis*, ed 4, Philadelphia, 2002, WB Saunders, p 386.

BOX 7-5

Potential Causes of Dizziness

NEUROLOGIC DISORDERS
- Multiple sclerosis
- Benign positional vertigo
- Ménière's disease
- Acoustic neuromas
- Ototoxic drugs
  - Aminoglycoside antibiotics (streptomycin, gentamicin)
  - Antineoplastics (cisplatin, vincristine)
  - Diuretics (furosemide, bumetanide, mannitol)
  - Environmental toxins (mercury, tin, lead, carbon dioxide)
- Basilar insufficiency

CARDIAC AND VASCULAR DISORDERS
- Critical aortic stenosis
- Carotid sinus hypersensitivity
- Volume depletion
- Severe anemia
- Diminished vascular reflexes (the elderly)

OTHER
- Diabetes mellitus
- Cervical spondylosis
- Anxiety
- Psychosis
- Hypoxia

Adapted from Allison L, Fuller K: Balance and vestibular disorders. In Umphred DA, ed: *Neurological rehabilitation*, ed 4, St Louis, 2001, Mosby, pp 617-619; and from Pruitt AA: Evaluation of dizziness. In Goroll AH, Mulley AG, eds: *Primary care medicine*, ed 4, Philadelphia, 2000, Lippincott Williams & Wilkins.

---

following questions to elicit a precise description of what the patient means by *dizzy:*
- Do you feel lightheaded or faint?
- Is there a spinning sensation in your head?
- Is the room spinning around you?
- Is it associated with specific postures or movements?
- Is it associated with nausea, vomiting, diaphoresis, hearing loss, tinnitus, visual disturbance, or hemiparesis?
- Have you fallen because of the dizziness?

Lightheadedness or the feeling of faintness often is associated with cardiac and vascular insufficiency. Such symptoms typically worsen on standing and improve with recumbence. Vestibular disease often manifests with sensations of the head spinning or the room spinning around the patient. Symptoms also may be described as headache, weaving, seasickness, rocking, sensation of things moving, or a feeling that the ground is rising and falling. Nausea and vomiting can be associated with severe vestibular disorders and migraine headaches. The associated hearing loss and tinnitus could be manifestations of Ménière's disease and labyrinthitis. Finally, symptoms of visual disturbance or hemiparesis along with the dizziness could be signs of vertebral basilar insufficiency.[2,30,39]

For patients with the symptom of dizziness, the PT should include the Romberg test, Hautart's test, vertebral artery test, and Dix-Hallpike maneuver in the physical examination (see Chapters 10 and 11).

Change in Mentation

The onset of confusion or disorientation, or a change in these symptoms, can be a manifestation of multiple disorders including delirium, dementia, head injury, adverse drug reactions, and infection. If the mentation issues are discovered during the history-taking process, the PT should point out the observation to the patient, caregiver, and family member and ask whether they noted the difficulties. The observations may include the following[8]:
- Level of consciousness: alertness or state of awareness
- Attention: ability to focus on a task or activity
- Memory: short-term versus long-term
- Orientation: personal identity, place, and time
- Thought processes: logical and coherent thoughts leading to selected goal
- Judgment: ability to evaluate alternatives and follow appropriate values while choosing a course of action

If the patient reports that these issues have been present since the head injury or stroke and that they have not worsened since the last visit to the physician, the observation becomes a yellow flag. If the difficulties represent a new onset or a worsening of the symptoms, then follow-up questions are in order:
- When did you first note the changes?
- Do you know the cause (e.g., a fall, blow to the head, a new medication)?
- Did the problem come on quickly, or slowly and gradually?
- Have you noted the onset of any other problems along with the onset of these symptoms?

The onset of confusion can be a particularly challenging and important finding in the elderly. For example, pneumonia is the most common cause of death from infection in the elderly population because of its atypical clinical presentation. The expected productive cough, pleuritic pain, and fever often do not appear in this group, and confusion and mental deterioration are the primary manifestations.[18,25] Because altered mentation and confusion are such general terms, the onus is on the PT to be as specific as possible when collecting these data and communicating these concerns to a physician. The more detail the therapist can provide about the situation, the more likely the physician wil take the concerns seriously.

Because altered mentation and confusion are such general terms, the onus is on the PT to be as specific as possible when collecting these data. The PT next communicates these concerns to a physician, and the more detail the therapist can give about the concerns, the more likely the physician will take the concerns seriously.

General Health Checklist Summary

Because the general health checklist covers symptoms associated with multiple body systems, disease states, and adverse drug reactions, the PT can use this tool to screen the entire body. Therefore the PT is strongly encouraged to use this checklist during every *initial visit* regardless of the patient's age or diagnosis. Using the general health checklist before the remaining body-system-specific checklists will help the PT determine the priority of the remaining checklists. For example, if the patient's medical history reveals nothing urgent (see Chapter 5), if there are no red flags in the patient's presenting symptoms, and if the patient reports no symptoms on the general health checklist, the PT has much less to worry about regarding the patient's health status. Thus the PT could consider postponing other checklists for this patient until the second or third visit.

Checklist for Cardiac and Vascular Systems

Box 7-1 presents the checklist for the cardiac and vascular systems. This checklist overlaps (in dyspnea and cough) with the checklist for the pulmonary system. *Dyspnea* is the subjective sensation of difficult or uncomfortable breathing and is most often associated with chronic heart and lung disease. This entity must be distinguished from tachypnea, or rapid breathing. Dyspnea can be related to activity, exertion, or body position. Examples include *orthopnea*, difficulty breathing when recumbent (lying flat); and *platypnea*, difficulty breathing when sitting upright and ease of breathing when recumbent. Finally, *trepopnea* is ease of breathing that is improved by assuming a sidelying position. Important follow-up questions for this patient include[39]:

- When did the shortness of breath (SOB) begin?
- Did the SOB begin suddenly or slowly over time?
- Do you wake up suddenly at night with severe SOB (paroxysmal nocturnal dyspnea)?
- Do you know why the SOB started?
- Is the SOB constant?
- Does SOB occur with exertion only? At rest? When in certain positions; lying flat (orthopnea) or when sitting up (platypnea)?

See Table 7-2 for causes of shortness of breath.

Palpitations are described as uncomfortable sensations in the chest and are associated with a variety of arrhythmias. Patients may use terms such as fluttering, jumping, pounding, irregularity, stopping, or skipping beats to describe this sensation. The PT should ask follow-up questions about frequency, duration, and associated symptoms such as chest pain, syncope, lightheadedness, and dyspnea when investigating this report.[19] *Syncope* is a sudden loss of consciousness accompanied by an inability to maintain postural tone, followed by spontaneous recovery; that patients often describe as fainting.[37]

These "blackouts" usually are due to a reduction in blood flow to the brain, but other potential causes of syncope include metabolic and psychogenic origins.[8] The incidence of syncope increases with age, marked by a sharp increase in patients older than 70 years.[37] Most patients or their caregivers will be sufficiently alarmed to report to the physician any episodes of fainting or blackouts, but the incident may simply be described as a fall.

During the history portion of the examination, one patient may report that he has fallen four times in the past 6 months and it is unclear whether the physician knows of the number of recent falls. The therapist must consider the multitude of possible reasons for the repeated falls, including the presence of syncope, especially in patients with risk factors for reduced cerebral blood flow.

Investigation of pain was discussed in Chapter 6, and the topic of sweats was covered in the General Health Checklist section for fever/chills/sweats in this chapter. The onset of *pain with sweats* is relevant when the PT screens the cardiovascular system. Diaphoresis is a common finding associated with an acute myocardial infarction. If the patient has chest pain or tightness extending into the left upper extremity, along with the onset of diaphoresis, both the patient and the PT probably will grasp the seriousness of these symptoms. Besides this classic presentation, though, the location of pain associated with ischemic heart disease can vary considerably (see Chapter 6), and can include the jaw, neck, tooth, right shoulder, epigastric, and midthoracic regions. Women and the elderly are the two groups most likely to present with pain patterns such as these. A patient with pain in these locations accompanied by reports of sweats should raise the PT's suspicion, especially in a patient who has risk factors for cardiac disease.

Like dyspnea, the presentation of a *cough* should trigger concern about the pulmonary system, but this finding is associated with disorders of the cardiovascular system as well. Cough, especially at night (nocturnal cough), can be associated with heart failure[19] and is also a side effect of some of the calcium channel–blocking agents.[16] A cough can be considered chronic if the duration is 3 weeks or longer.[21] The most common causes of cough are cigarette smoking (as a result of the direct bronchial irritation), allergies, and postnasal drip. The finding also may be associated with very serious disorders such as asthma, pneumonia, and heart failure. So how does the PT determine the seriousness of a cough? Follow-up questions are the key, including the following:

- What is the duration?
- What is the cause (from the patient's perspective)?
- Is it constant/persistent or intermittent?
- Is the cough related to position or posture?
- Is it a productive cough (including color and odor of sputum)?
- Are there associated symptoms (dyspnea and items from the General Health Checklist)?

A productive cough that has lasted 3 weeks or longer and that is associated with any other relevant symptoms should raise the PT's concern. Sputum should be odorless and clear to whitish gray in color. Sputum that is yellow, red or bloody (hemoptysis),

TABLE 7-2
Possible Causes of Positional Dyspnea

Type	Possible Causes
Orthopnea	Congestive heart failure
	Mitral valve disease
	Severe asthma (rarely)
	Emphysema (rarely)
	Chronic bronchitis (rarely)
	Neurologic diseases (rarely)
Trepopnea	Congestive heart failure
Platypnea	Status postpneumonectomy
	Neurologic diseases
	Cirrhosis (intrapulmonary shunts)
	Hypovolemia

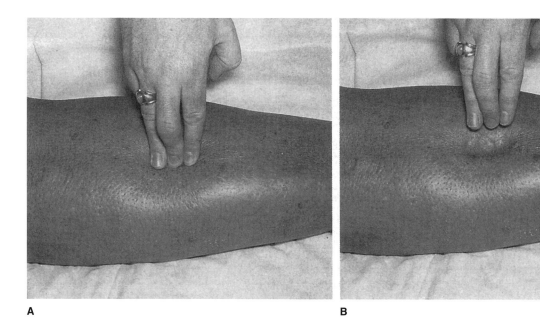

FIGURE 7-2 A, Palpating for pitting edema; the examiner pressing into the lower leg. **B,** The indentation that remains after the pressure is removed from the limb, demonstrating the pitting edema. (From Swartz MH: *Textbook of physical diagnosis,* ed 4, Philadelphia, 2002, WB Saunders, p 381.)

pink, rust, green, or a combination of these colors suggests the presence of pathology. A cough associated with heart failure typically will be noted with a recumbent position.[19,39] A PT concerned with a cough should auscultate the chest (see Chapter 9).

Finally, *peripheral edema* may be observed at any point during the history-taking process (see Chapter 8). This finding can be associated with many serious disorders, including venous insufficiency, congestive heart failure, deep venous thrombosis (DVT), and pulmonary hypertension. The PT must note whether the edema is unilateral or bilateral. Unilateral edema may be associated with DVT, while a bilateral presentation is associated more often with the other disorders listed above. Important follow-up questions to ask include:
- What was the onset of the edema (slow versus fast)?
- Is it related to dependent limb position?
- Is it related to time of day or not?
- Are there any other associated symptoms or signs (e.g., pain, cyanosis, jaundice, redness of the limb[s], clubbing of the nails)?

After the PT has investigated the edema, he or she should palpate the limb(s) at some point during this patient visit. Does the patient have pitting edema (Fig. 7-2), local tenderness, altered skin temperature (cold or warmth), or a palpable cord along a vein? Is there any discoloration of the limb? The PT should take circumferential measurements of the limb. Unilateral edema is marked by a difference of 1 cm or more just above the ankle or 2 cm or more at the midcalf regions.[8]

Pulmonary System Checklist

Box 7-6 is the checklist of screening items for the pulmonary system. See the discussion on dyspnea and cough in the above section Checklist for Cardiac and Peripheral Vascular Systems,

---

> **BOX 7-6**
> ### Pulmonary System Checklist
>
> - Dyspnea
> - Cough
> - Clubbing of the nails
> - Wheezing/stridor

and see Chapter 8 for a discussion of clubbing of the nails. *Stridor* and *wheezing* are abnormal respiratory sounds audible to the ear. Wheezing is a high-pitched noise caused by a partial obstruction of the airway; stridor is a high-pitched sould also associated with obstruction of the larynx or trachea. Relevant follow-up questions to this finding include the following:
- Have you noticed this noise?
- How long has it been present?
- How often does it occur?
- What are the precipitating factors (e.g., odors, food, animals, emotions)?
- Are there any associated symptoms?[39]

The wheezing may be resolved by the opening of the airway or a further narrowing of the airway. The PT should watch for additional signs of well-being or of distress and pulmonary distress, and perform auscultation to identify the reason for the decrease in the wheezing.

Gastrointestinal System Checklist

See Box 7-7 for the gastrointestinal system checklist. Two items obviously missing from this checklist are nausea and vomiting, but the reader is reminded that they are part of the general health checklist and would have been covered before the PT adds this checklist to a patient visit. *Swallowing difficulties*

Gastrointestinal System Checklist

- Swallowing difficulties
- Indigestion/heartburn
- Food intolerance
- Bowel dysfunction
    Color of stool
    Shape/caliber of stool
    Constipation
    Diarrhea
    Difficulty initiating
    Incontinence

(dysphagia) typically are a result of a loss of coordinated local muscle activity or a mechanical obstructive disorder. Myasthenia gravis, multiple sclerosis, amyotrophic lateral sclerosis, and Parkinson's disease are examples of disorders that could result in the local muscle uncoordination. Tumors, thyroid goiter, osteophytes of the cervical spine, and aortic aneurysm could be causes of the mechanical obstruction.[39] Table 7-3 provides a comparison of manifestations of motor versus obstructive causes of dysphagia. Follow-up questions about the swallowing difficulties should determine the presence or absence of each manifestation. Other questions include the location where the patient senses the difficulty (e.g., back of the throat, behind the sternum); whether it is associated with swallowing solids, liquids, or both; and whether pain accompanies the difficulty (odynophagia).

Indigestion and heartburn are common symptoms that fall under the category of dyspepsia, which can have an organic cause (peptic ulcer, gastroesophageal reflux disease) or a functional source (no ascertainable cause). Use of nonsteroidal antiinflammatory drugs also has been associated with these upper gastrointestinal tract symptoms.[38] The patient usually feels these symptoms retrosternally or in the epigastric region. Important follow-up questions for these symptoms include the following:

- How long have you had these symptoms?
- Do you know what is causing them?

A Comparison of Symptoms—Motor Versus Mechanical Etiology of Dysphagia

Manifestation	Dysphagia, Motor	Dysphagia, Mechanical
Onset	Gradual onset	Faster onset
Progression	Slow	Faster
Swallowing solid food versus liquids	Equal difficulty	More difficulty swallowing solids
Swallowing cold substances	Worsening of swallowing difficulties	Swallowing difficulties not affected by temperature
Bolus passage	Facilitated by repeated swallowing, Valsalva, or throwing back the head and shoulders	Can be accompanied by regurgitation

- Are they constant or intermittent?
- How are you treating the symptoms?
- Are there any associated symptoms?

These questions may reveal important information, such as the fact that the symptoms have become more persistent or more intense and that the need for self-treatment has increased. Many over-the-counter medications, such as antacids (e.g., Milk of Magnesia Alu-Tab, Tums, Maalox) and histamine H_2 antagonists (e.g., Tagamet, Zantac, Pepcid AC), are designed to relieve heartburn and indigestion.[16] Even though these drugs may bring symptomatic relief, they do not cure the underlying organic causes. Therefore if the patient reports the need to take increasing amounts of the drug to attain relief, then the PT should communicate with the patient's physician.

Food intolerance associated with the provocation or alleviation of symptoms can be a warning sign of underlying pathology. A patient who realizes that symptoms appear only after ingesting certain foods probably will report this fact to a physician, but if the symptoms appear only in the back (not in the anterior chest wall or abdominal area), the patient might not associate the symptoms with the food. A classic example is pain referred from gallbladder disorders, often noted in the midthoracic or right scapular regions.[15,41] The patient may relate the onset of these symptoms to his or her posture or excessive time spent at the computer rather than the ingestion of fatty foods, which stimulates gallbladder activity. Another example in which the ingestion of foods may trigger symptoms is the tendency of cheese, chocolate, citrus fruits, nuts, and red wine to trigger migraine headaches in some people.[30]

The screening of the lower gastrointestinal tract is based on questions about bowel function, including color of stools, shape and caliber of stools, constipation, diarrhea, difficulty initiating a bowel movement, and incontinence. The PT may initiate this line of questioning with a general question, such as, "Have you recently noted any problems or difficulties with bowel function?" Regardless of the patient response, however, the PT must complete the entire checklist in Box 7-7. Many patients initially answer the general question by reporting "no problems," but later answer "yes" when the PT asks specific questions from the list. Many of these patients assume that if no pain is associated with defecation there are no problems.

The color of stools is an important indicator of serious health issues. Melena, or the passage of black tarry stools (sticky and shiny), represents gastrointestinal bleeding (most likely from upper gastrointestinal structures including the esophagus, stomach, or duodenum), with a blood loss of 150 to 200 mL or greater being necessary to produce a consistent or regular presentation.[34] If the patient reports melena, the PT should ask these important follow-up questions:

- How long have you been having black, tarry stools?
- Have you felt lightheaded?
- Have you had any nausea, vomiting, diarrhea, fatigue, abdominal or back pain, or sweats associated with these stools?

In addition, the PT should check the patient's heart rate and blood pressure (see Chapter 9).

These questions produce important information for the physician about the acuteness of the situation.[39] Black, nonsticky stools can be associated with the ingestion of iron and bismuth salts (e.g., Pepto-Bismol), black licorice, and some commercial chocolate cookies.[8]

Hematochezia, or the passage of bright, blood-red stools, usually originates in the left side of the colon or the anorectal area.[32] With this symptom, the PT should ask the following questions:

- How long have you noticed bright red blood in your stools?
- Is the red blood mixed within the stools (red streaks) or not?
- Are there any associated symptoms, such as difficulty in initiating bowel movements or a feeling of lightheadedness or fatigue?

In addition, the PT should check the patient's heart rate and blood pressure (see Chapter 9).

Reddish but nonbloody stools can be a result of ingestion of beets.[8] Finally, light gray or pale stools (acholic; without bile) can be associated with obstructive jaundice.[8] If this is reported, the PT should ask these follow-up questions:

- How long have you noticed the light, pale-colored stools?
- Have you noticed an atypical color (dark) of your urine? (See the genitourinary system checklist on page 97.)
- Have you noticed any associated symptoms, such as fatigue, fever, chills, unexplained weight change, or nausea?

The PT can broach the subject of atypical stool color by asking, "Have you noticed any unusual color of your stools recently, such as black, tarry, bloody red, or light pale-colored stools?"

A change in shape or caliber of stools also is a potentially significant finding. Stools that are pencil-thin in diameter or flat and ribbonlike are suggestive of an anal or distal-colon carcinoma. There may not be any pain associated with these types of lesions. Thus, if the patient experiences no problems with going to the bathroom, he or she may answer the general question about bowel problems with, "I have no problems."

Constipation and *diarrhea* are conditions most everyone experiences for relatively brief periods at various times in their lives, but for some patients these symptoms can represent serious underlying pathology. Table 7-4 lists potential causes of constipation and diarrhea. When a patient reports constipation, the PT should ask what the patient means by being constipated. A report of "hard stools that are difficult or painful to push out" warrants follow-up questions by the PT, including the following:

- How long have you been constipated?
- When was the last time you had a bowel movement?
- Do you ever have periods of constipation alternating with periods of diarrhea (a pattern noted in some patients with colon cancer or diverticulitis)?
- Do you have any associated symptoms, such as malaise, a sensation of abdominal fullness or bloating, fever, agitation, or altered mental status?

The associated symptoms described in the last question are potential manifestations of fecal impaction and should prompt immediate communication with the patient's physician.[1] If the patient reports that the constipation is due to a current medication he or she has been taking, such as an opiate, the PT

TABLE 7-4
Potential Causes of Constipation and Diarrhea

Mechanism	Etiology
CONSTIPATION	
Impaired motility	Inadequate dietary fiber
	Inactivity
	Diverticulitis
	Hypothyroidism
	Hypercalcemia
	Scleroderma
Neurologic dysfunction	Multiple sclerosis
	Spinal cord injury
Psychosocial dysfunction	Depression
	Situational stress
	Anxiety
DIARRHEA	Infectious agents
	Laxative abuse
	Colon cancer
	Irritable bowel syndrome
	Crohn's disease
	Ulcerative colitis
	Diabetic enteropathy

must ask whether the constipation has gotten worse since the last physician visit. If the patient is having bowel movements and the constipation is not getting worse, the PT should document the information provided by the patient and every subsequent week or two ask the patient whether the constipation has changed. The PT may learn a few weeks after the initial visit that the condition has worsened and now warrants physician contact.

Diarrhea is described as excessively frequent passage of watery and unformed stools.[8] Episodes that are brief and self-limited do not require reporting, but diarrhea that becomes severe raises concern about the underlying cause and may carry the risk of dehydration. With a patient report of diarrhea, the PT should ask these follow-up questions[39]:

- How many episodes do you have each day?
- How long have you had diarrhea?
- Do you ever have periods of diarrhea alternating with periods of constipation?
- Is the diarrhea worse at certain times of the day?
- Do family members or companions have similar symptoms?
- Do you have any associated symptoms, such as fever, chills, nausea, vomiting, abdominal pain, or distention?

The last two items on the checklist are difficulty initiating bowel movements and incontinence. The difficulty with initiating bowel movements may be a part of the patient's description of the constipation. This symptom also may be associated with a condition called *tenesmus* in which the patient has an intense urge to defecate but with little or no result. This painful and ineffective straining can be associated with inflammation or cancer at the anorectal region.[39] Fecal incontinence may bring the patient to physical therapy, depending on the nature of the therapist's practice, but in most settings, reports of this nature should raise considerable concern. The therapist should approach this symptom like all others: If the patient does not provide a good explanation for the finding, if the physician is unaware of the symptoms, or if the condition has worsened since the last communication with the physician, then this finding becomes a red flag.

Genitourinary System Checklist

The checklist illustrated in Box 7-8 represents two physiological functions, urination and reproduction. As with the screening of bowel function, the PT may want to start with the general question of, "Do you have any trouble with urination?" Regardless of the patient's response, the PT must ask the patient to complete the checklist. Reddish or dark (brownish-colored) urine can be associated with several disorders. *Hematuria*, or blood in the urine, can be a manifestation of virtually every disease of the genitourinary (GU) tract.[17] Reddish-colored urine also may occur for reasons other than the presence of blood, including ingestion of vegetable dyes, heavy ingestion of beets, and use of medications such as Pyridium. Important follow-up questions to better identify the symptoms include:

- How long have you noticed the red urine?
- Do you have a history of bleeding problems (see Chapter 5)?
- What medications are you currently taking (see Chapter 5)?
- Do you currently have, or have you recently recovered from, an upper-respiratory infection or sore throat?
- Have you noticed whether the urine "starts red" and then clears; starts clear and then turns red; or is red throughout?

BOX 7-8
Genitourinary System Checklist

URINATION
- Color
- Flow
    - Frequency
    - Urgency
    - Output
    - Retention
    - Dysuria
- Reduced caliber or force of urine stream
- Difficulty initiating urine stream
- Incontinence

REPRODUCTION
Male
- Urethral discharge
- Sexual dysfunction
- Pain during intercourse/ejaculation

Female
- Vaginal discharge
- Pain with intercourse
- Menstruation
    - Frequency of periods and length of cycle
    - Dysmenorrhea
    - Blood flow
- Number of pregnancies and deliveries
- Menopause
    - Perimenopausal
    - Postmenopausal vaginal bleeding or spotting

- Do you have any associated symptoms, such as items on the general health checklist, including fever, weight loss, fatigue, or flank or abdominal pain (see Chapter 6)?

Red urine noted 1 to 2 weeks after an upper-respiratory-tract infection may be associated with acute glomerulonephritis.[39] Dark urine can be associated with hepatic or biliary obstructive disease and with acute exertional rhabdomyolysis. A case report by Baxter and Moore[6] described a patient presenting to physical therapy with shoulder pain and weakness, and a report of dark urine. The resultant laboratory tests led to the diagnosis of acute exertional rhabdomyolysis.

Urinary frequency, urgency, output, and dysuria also are important indicators of GU system disorders, with urinary frequency being the symptom reported most often.[39] Increased frequency may be most noticeable with *nocturia* (urination at night) because most patients recognize when a pattern of not waking to urinate changes to waking two to three times a night to urinate. Urinary urgency, the intense and immediate sensation of the need to urinate, can be associated with infection or irritation. *Dysuria*, pain on urination, can occur with inflammation, infection, and sudden distention of a structure.[8,39] *Polyuria*, increased amounts of urine, can be associated with diabetic conditions. The PT should ask these follow-up questions after reports of a change in urinary flow:

- Have these changes occurred quickly or over a long period of time?
- Have you been drinking more fluids (with an excessive thirst) than usual lately?
- What medications are you taking (diuretics)?
- Have you noticed that despite the urge to urinate you cannot start urination?
- After urine flow has stopped, do you experience the sensation of still needing to urinate?
- Do you have any associated symptoms, such as headaches or visual problems (possibly diabetes related), or items on the general health checklist, such as fever, nausea, and weight loss?

Symptoms of a reduced force or caliber of urine flow and difficulty in starting the urine stream are common symptoms associated with obstructive disorders, including benign prostatic hyperplasia (BPH). For patients with BPH, the physician will know of the urinary difficulties, but the PT should forward any reports that the urinary-flow problems may be worsening. The term *benign* can be misleading, because BPH can result in complications of hydroureter and renal failure.[5] True urinary retention is associated with serious conditions such as cauda equina syndrome. A recent onset of urinary dysfunction (problems of retention, frequency, or overflow incontinence) and "saddle" anesthesia is a red flag in patients with low back pain.[9]

The final urinary disorder to consider is *incontinence*, a very common disorder in the adult population for which many patients receive physical therapy services. When incontinence is not the reason for the physical therapy, the same screening principles apply to this symptom. Important follow-up questions to ask patients who report incontinence include the circumstances, causes, timing, frequency, and volume of urine loss; the presence of any warning signs: and the intactness of perineal and bladder sensation.[20] See Chapter 13 for a related discussion of incontinence in the obstetric population.

Reproductive function is the other important GU aspect to screen. Areas of overlap among men and women are discharge and sexual dysfunction. Discharge from the penis or the vagina suggests the possibility of infection. The PT should follow such reports by asking the following questions:

- What is the frequency?
- Is it a continuous flow, spotting, or sporadic episodes?
- What is the color of the discharge?
- Is the discharge accompanied by an odor?
- Are there associated symptoms, such as pruritus (itching), local pain or inflammation, fever, nausea, or dyspareunia?

Early treatment of urinary tract infections and sexually transmitted infections is important, as untreated infections may increase the risk of developing an ectopic pregnancy and also may lead to infertility.[21,26,31]

Some patients presenting with mechanical low back, sacroiliac, and hip joint conditions report *dyspareunia*, pain during or after sexual intercourse. One way to help differentiate pain of mechanical dysfunction from pain of internal pelvic disease or disorders is to investigate the pain pattern (see Chapter 6). Pain of mechanical origin (nonacute) will be associated with specific intercourse positions, while pain associated with pelvic organ disease likely will occur regardless of the intercourse position. If the patient reports that a physician has examined her and ruled out disease, then the PT should refer the patient to a PT who specializes in women's health.

Besides pain during intercourse, sexual dysfunction may include *erectile dysfunction* (inability to achieve or maintain an erection), which can be associated with neurologic conditions resulting from spinal cord injury, herniated disk, postsurgical complications (radical prostate, bladder, or colon procedures), diabetes mellitus, medication side effects, and psychogenic disorders.[21]

The PT should ask these important follow-up questions:

- How long has the condition been present?
- How constant or intermittent is the problem?

The PT also should ask questions about the patient's history of conditions such as diabetes mellitus and medication use (see Chapter 5).

Questions about menstruation have the same goal as the investigation of cough and bowel and bladder function: They look for a change from the usual pattern. The items to assess include frequency and length of periods, dysmenorrhea, and blood flow. Abnormal vaginal bleeding is described as bleeding at an inappropriate time or in excessive amounts. The general time frame for inappropriate bleeding is less than 21 days and more than 36 days since the last period. Secondary amenorrhea (the absence of periods after they have been established) has been associated with female long-distance runners, anorexia, and diseases of the endocrine system.[8,21]

As a general rule, blood flow lasting more than 7 days should be considered excessive. The menstrual cycle tends to shorten as menopause approaches. Menopause can be associated with hot flashes, flushing, sweats, and sleep disturbances. Postmenopausal

bleeding, that is, vaginal bleeding for 6 to 8 months or longer after the cessation of periods, warrants a consultation with the physician.[8,21] Dysmenorrhea (pain with menstruation) is common, but a screening that reveals pain that is atypical in its location, where in the cycle it occurs, intensity, quality, and duration may raise the PT's suspicion about the causes of the symptoms. Another challenge in the screening of menstruation is that fact that some women do not generally experience a regular pattern. In such a case, a primary care physician should regularly monitor the woman's health. The PT should ask the following questions about menstruation:

- When was your last period?
- Was it a normal period for you (timing of the period compared with her normal cycle, pain pattern, and blood flow)?
- Have you experienced any vaginal bleeding between periods?

The PT also should investigate the woman's obstetric history. Depending on the nature of the PT's practice, the PT should at minimum learn the number of pregnancies and any residual complications or limitations associated with the pregnancies and deliveries. In a women's health practice, the questioning is much more extensive (see Chapter 13).

Other Body Systems

The screening of the remaining body systems—nervous, endocrine, integumentary, psychological, and musculoskeletal—is different from that of the aforementioned systems. The screening moves away from the use of a short checklist and relies more heavily on the physical examination. Despite the different methods of screening these body systems, the PT must remember that the general health checklist also helps screen these particular body systems.

Nervous System

The PT usually screens the nervous system during the investigation of symptoms (see Chapter 6), which takes place before the specific review-of-systems questioning. Using the entire body diagram and noting the locations of any symptoms (including pain, numbness, pins and needles, and weakness) are key elements of the examination process. To help ensure that the report reveals any neurologic symptoms, the general health checklist asks about numbness, tingling, and weakness. In addition, the PT performs a nervous system screening during the patient observation that begins with the interview process (see Chapter 8) and continues with the upper or lower quarter examination (see Chapters 10 and 11).

Endocrine System

Considering the physiology of the endocrine system, one can understand that malfunction in this system could lead to symptoms involving multiple body systems. For example, people who have hypothyroidism may experience any or all of the following:

- Joint or muscle pain
- Paresthesias
- Dry, scaly skin or brittle hair and nails
- Cold intolerance
- Reduced sweating

- Weight gain
- Constipation
- Fatigue
- Dyspnea
- Periorbital edema
- Bradycardia
- Hoarseness of voice
- Slow reflex relaxation

Many of the items on this list would be noted in other parts of the data collection process (other than review of systems). The paresthesia and joint and muscle pain would be noted on the body diagram during symptom investigation (see Chapter 6). An atypical symptom pattern (e.g., insidious onset, symptoms that come and go for no apparent mechanical reason, no consistent time of day when symptoms are better or worse) may raise the suspicion that the endocrine system is involved. Following is a summary checklist for the endocrine system:

- General health (fatigue, unexplained weight change, weakness)
- Psychological/cognitive (personality changes, memory loss, confusion, irritability)
- Gastrointestinal (nausea, vomiting, anorexia, dysphagia, diarrhea, constipation)
- Urogenital (impotence, intermittent urine stream, dribbling, straining to void, impotence)
- Musculoskeletal (muscle weakness and cramps, arthralgias, myalgias, stiffness, bone pain)
- Sensory (paresthesia, numbness)
- Dermatologic (foot ulcerations, edema, dry/coarse skin, impaired wound healing)
- Miscellaneous (temperature intolerances, visual changes, orthostatic hypotension, increased bruising)

Integumentary System

A significant portion of the integumentary system screening takes place through observation during the physical examination. As with the screen of the general nervous system, screening of the integumentary system begins when the patient interview begins (see Chapter 8), and it continues throughout the physical examination as more skin becomes visible (in the postural assessment and regional examinations). The PT can note wounds, abrasions, and bruises on the body diagram used during the symptom investigation and then can examine these findings in more detail during the physical examination.

Psychological System

The range of mental disorders is so extensive that providing screening protocols for this entire category of illness is beyond the scope of this textbook. The *Diagnostic and Statistical Manual of Mental Disorders*, fourth edition, is an excellent resource for the clinician in screening this system.[4]

The general health checklist and the investigation of symptoms (see Chapter 6) will act as general screens for many of these disorders. Fatigue, unexplained weight change, a change in mentation, or an onset of confusion are symptoms associated with many psychological disorders, and an atypical symptom report also may indicate any of a variety of mental disorders (see Chapter 6).

Three specific mental disorders—major clinical depression, chemical dependency, and abuse—are discussed in this text because of their incidence and their potential for serious complications (morbidity and mortality). (See Chapter 5 for a detailed discussion of screening for these disorders.)

Musculoskeletal System

The checklist for the musculoskeletal system consists primarily of items discussed in Chapters 5 and 6, including the patient's medical history, the symptom investigation, the general health checklist, and the physical examination. Items such as onset of symptoms; how and when symptoms change with the time of day, posture, and activity; night pain; the ease or lack of decreasing the symptom intensity; and correlation of symptoms with the findings of the physical examination are key elements to the screening of this system.

Determining whether a symptom "story" from the patient makes sense according to our understanding of basic and clinical sciences is the basis for the decision to communicate with the physician or not. See Box 7-9 for a list of findings that suggest pathologic origins of musculoskeletal pain. The four categories of serious musculoskeletal disorders are cancers, infections, fractures, and inflammatory arthritis conditions.

Chapter 5 contains information about screening for cancers and infections of the musculoskeletal system. The most common cancers (especially for those aged 50 and older) of the musculoskeletal system are metastatic, having spread to the skeletal system from other primary cancers. The general health checklist helps screen for many of these malignancies and infections that have become systemic disorders.

FRACTURES. Fractures can be classified into three general categories: (1) sudden impact (most common), (2) stress, and (3) pathologic.[22,94] The most common manifestations of fractures include the following:

- Pain and local tenderness
- Deformity
- Edema
- Ecchymosis
- Loss of general function and mobility

A mechanism of injury or an onset of symptoms that includes sudden impact should raise the PT's concern about a possible fracture. The PT also should remember that a patient with compromised bone density may sustain a fracture as a

---

BOX 7-9

Musculoskeletal System Checklist

- Insidious onset of symptoms (Chapter 6)
- Atypical pain pattern (Chapter 6)
- Night pain (Chapter 6)
- Inadequate relief with rest or rehabilitation (Chapter 6)
- General Health Checklist items
- Inability to alter symptoms during the physical examination (Chapters 10 and 11)
- Lack of impairments that match the patient's functional limitations (Chapters 10 and 11)
- Atypical findings of physical examination

result of relatively minor trauma, such as sneezing, lifting a gallon of milk out of a car, or opening a window that is stuck. These patients often do not come into therapy with a diagnosis of osteoporosis, but other items in their medical history may catch the PT's attention. Box 7-10 lists a wide variety of disorders, medications, and substances that may compromise bone density. The PT should assume that patients with these items in their medical history have reduced bone density, and thus the PT should adjust the choice of physical examination and intervention techniques to minimize external load on the patient's skeletal system. See the "Diagnostic Imaging Rules" section in Chapter 17 to identify cases in which the PT should recommend plain films because of the suspicion of fracture in specific patient populations.

Stress fractures typically are associated with an onset of symptoms that sounds like a repetitive or overuse syndrome, and symptoms will worsen with weight-bearing activities. The diagnosis of stress fractures, including diagnostic imaging issues, is described in Chapter 17. Finally, pathologic fractures can be associated with local cancerous or infectious lesions and are described in Chapter 5.

INFLAMMATORY ARTHRITIS. Inflammatory arthritic conditions usually manifest as syndromes of joint or muscle pain, but unlike degenerative arthritis, require a timely diagnosis to prevent irreversible tissue damage. An important consideration is that disorders such as rheumatoid arthritis (RA) are systemic illnesses, not local joint disorders like osteoarthritis. Therefore the general health checklist is an important tool in screening for conditions such as RA. See Figure 7-3 for a summary of systemic features associated with RA. Figure 7-4 compares joint involvement associated with RA and that associated with osteoarthritis. In addition, joint pain or stiffness associated with RA often includes an insidious onset of symptoms and bilateral joint symptoms. In addition, RA symptoms can wax and wane without the expected associated changes in postures, physical activity, and time of day described in Chapter 6. Another feature that distinguishes RA from osteoarthritis is "post-rest gel." Patients with either condition may complain of joint stiffness after prolonged static postures (e.g., sitting, sleeping), but patients with osteoarthritis generally loosen up more quickly. General findings with this clinical disorder are that morning joint stiffness secondary to osteoarthritis typically resolves or starts to resolve within 30 minutes, while morning post-rest gel secondary to RA may last for long periods and may not resolve completely even after activity is initiated.[36] If the PT suspects that a rheumatic disorder may have developed, all of the previously described checklists may be important to cover.

Adverse Drug Reactions

We screen for adverse drug reactions by using the same tools (checklists) described above for the screening of potential occult disease; all of these tools are relevant in the screening for side effects of medication. Ultimately, physicians will determine whether the symptoms or signs we bring to their attention are related to disease or to medications. The challenge to PTs is to decide which checklists are relevant for each group of medications, remembering that the general health checklist screens to some degree for all medications. Box 7-11 lists groups of medications that may adversely affect the health of the various body systems. Even though some medications, such as nonsteroidal antiinflammatory drugs (NSAIDs), are found under many of the listed body systems, certain body systems are involved more often than others. For example, the two body systems most often associated with NSAID use are the upper GI and renal systems. Chapter 16 includes a detailed description of potential adverse drug reactions associated with commonly used drugs.

Checklist Use: Based on Symptom Location/Pattern

Not all checklists must be used with every patient. The location and pattern of symptoms can help guide these choices because part of the rationale for the use of the checklists is that individual organs making up each particular body system are potential symptom generators. Because of this, the PT will use more checklists in the examination of a patient with symptoms located in the trunk (including pelvis) than with patients who have symptoms located only from mid-humerus to fingers and mid-femur to toes, because more non-neuromusculoskeletal structures are located in the trunk than at the periphery of the body.

Chapter 6 presents a detailed description of symptoms (both local and referred-pain patterns) associated with non-neuromusculoskeletal diseases. Certain body systems may not present with a predictable pain location (local or referred) but rather present with an atypical pattern of symptoms that move from one body region to another. The symptoms may be inconsistent in their intensity, increasing and decreasing regardless of time of day, posture, and physical activity (see Chapter 6).

BOX 7-10
Disorders, Medications, and Substances Associated with Compromised Bone Density

DISORDERS
- Chronic renal failure
- GI malabsorption syndrome
- Rheumatoid arthritis
- Ankylosing spondylitis
- Hyperparathyroidism
- Hypogonadism
- Multiple sclerosis
- Chronic alcohol dependency
- Cushing's syndrome

MEDICATION OR SUBSTANCE USED
- Aluminum
- Anticonvulsants
- Corticosteroids
- Cytotoxic drugs
- Excessive thyroxine
- Heparin
- Caffeine
- Tobacco
- Soft drinks

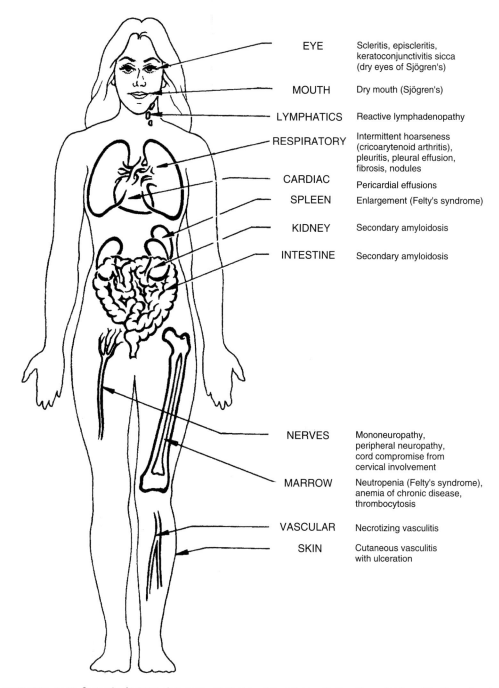

EYE	Scleritis, episcleritis, keratoconjunctivitis sicca (dry eyes of Sjögren's)
MOUTH	Dry mouth (Sjögren's)
LYMPHATICS	Reactive lymphadenopathy
RESPIRATORY	Intermittent hoarseness (cricoarytenoid arthritis), pleuritis, pleural effusion, fibrosis, nodules
CARDIAC	Pericardial effusions
SPLEEN	Enlargement (Felty's syndrome)
KIDNEY	Secondary amyloidosis
INTESTINE	Secondary amyloidosis
NERVES	Mononeuropathy, peripheral neuropathy, cord compromise from cervical involvement
MARROW	Neutropenia (Felty's syndrome), anemia of chronic disease, thrombocytosis
VASCULAR	Necrotizing vasculitis
SKIN	Cutaneous vasculitis with ulceration

FIGURE 7-3 Systemic features that may accompany rheumatoid arthritis. (From Caldron PH: Screening for rheumatic disease. In Boissonnault W, ed: *Examination in physical therapy practice; screening for medical disease*, ed 2, New York, 1995, Churchill Livingstone, p 262. Courtesy Healthwest Regional Medical Center, Phoenix, AZ.)

Box 7-12 matches the specific ROS checklists with locations and patterns of symptoms.

Checklist Use: Based on Patient Medical History

The patient's report of current illnesses also will guide the PT in selecting the body systems to screen. For example, if the patient reports heart problems, one of the follow-up questions to ask is, "What symptoms do you have with your heart problem?" If the patient replies, "Chest pain and shortness of breath," the PT

then should ask whether the patient has ever experienced any of the other items on the cardiovascular checklist to make sure the patient has not left out any important information. The same approach applies if the patient reports a GI or GU disorder.

Checklist Use: At Which Patient Visit?

The general health checklist applies to all patients and should be used during the initial visit. The PT selects the remaining checklists based on the patient data collected

Rheumatoid arthritis   **Osteoarthritis**

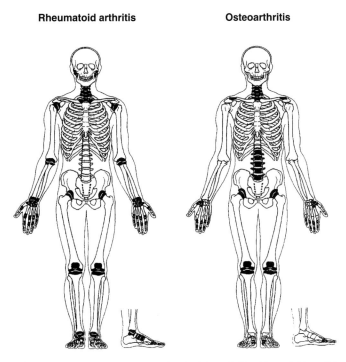

FIGURE 7-4 Joints commonly involved in arthritis. (From Caldron PH: Screening for rheumatic disease. In Boissonnault W, ed: *Examination in physical therapy practice; screening for medical disease*, ed 2, New York, 1995, Churchill Livingstone, p 262. Courtesy Healthwest Regional Medical Center, Phoenix, AZ.)

before reaching the ROS portion of the history. If the patient's medical history reveals nothing that concerns the PT (see Chapter 5), the patient's symptom description makes sense to the PT based on his or her understanding of basic and clinical sciences (see Chapter 6), and the general health checklist is negative for all of the items it lists, the PT has much less concern about the patient's health status. In such cases, the PT could considering leaving them for a subsequent visit (ideally the second visit).

If the patient's medical history contains an item of concern (e.g., recent infection, a diagnosis of cancer within the previous 5 years), the symptom report includes an insidious onset of symptoms or night pain, or the general health checklist reveals two "yes" answers that are unexplained or have worsened since the last physician contact, then the remaining appropriate checklists assume a higher priority within the initial visit.

In such cases, one method the PT can use to make time for the remaining checklists is to ask these questions when the patient is resting or when the PT is performing some physical task with the patient. For example, suppose the PT plans to perform soft tissue mobilization on a patient's shoulder or stretch a patient's hip flexor. The PT explains to the patient what he or she plans to do and the feedback the patient should give during the intervention. Then, the PT also can ask the patient a few questions during the procedure.

BOX 7-11

Review of Systems: Medication Side Effects and Subjective Symptoms (in Order of Most Common Occurrence)

A. GASTROINTESTINAL DISTRESS (DYSPEPSIA, HEARTBURN, NAUSEA, VOMITING, ABDOMINAL PAIN, CONSTIPATION, DIARRHEA, BLEEDING)
Salicylates
Nonsteroidal antiinflammatory drugs (NSAIDs)
Opioids
Corticosteroids
Beta-blockers
Calcium channel blockers
Skeletal muscle relaxants
Diuretics
Angiotensin-converting enzyme (ACE) inhibitors
Digoxin
Nitrates
Cholesterol-lowering agents
Antiarrhythmic agents
Antidepressants (tricyclic antidepressants [TCAs], monoamine oxidase inhibitors [MAOIs], lithium)
Neuroleptics
Antiepileptic agents
Oral contraceptives
Estrogens and progestins
Theophylline

B. PULMONARY (BRONCHOSPASM, SHORTNESS OF BREATH, RESPIRATORY DEPRESSION)
Salicylates
NSAIDs
Opioids
Beta-blockers
ACE inhibitors

C. CENTRAL NERVOUS SYSTEM (DIZZINESS, DROWSINESS, INSOMNIA, HEADACHES, HALLUCINATIONS, CONFUSION, ANXIETY, DEPRESSION, MUSCLE WEAKNESS)
NSAIDs
Skeletal muscle relaxants
Opioids
Corticosteroids
Beta-blockers
Calcium channel blockers
Nitrates
ACE inhibitors
Digoxin
Antianxiety agents
Antidepressants (TCAs and MAOIs)
Neuroleptics
Antiepileptic agents
Oral contraceptives
Estrogens and progestins

D. DERMATOLOGIC (SKIN RASH, ITCHING, FLUSHING OF FACE)
NSAIDs
Corticosteroids
Beta-blockers
Opioids
Calcium channel blockers
ACE inhibitors
Nitrates
Cholesterol-lowering agents
Antiarrhythmic agents
MAOIs and lithium

BOX 7-11

Review of Systems: Medication Side Effects and Subjective Symptoms (in Order of Most Common Occurrence)—cont'd

Oral contraceptives
Estrogens and progestins
Antiepileptics

E. MUSCULOSKELETAL (WEAKNESS, FATIGUE, CRAMPS, ARTHRITIS, REDUCED EXERCISE TOLERANCE, OSTEOPOROSIS)
Corticosteroids
Beta-blockers
Calcium channel blockers
ACE inhibitors
Diuretics
Digoxin
Antianxiety agents
Antiepileptic agents
Antidepressants
Neuroleptic agents

F. CARDIAC (BRADYCARDIA, VENTRICULAR IRRITABILITY, AV BLOCK, CHE, PVCS, VENTRICULAR TACHYCARDIA)
Opioids
Diuretics
Beta-blockers
Calcium channel blockers
Digoxin
Antiarrhythmic agents
TCAs
Neuroleptics
Oral antiasthmatic agents

G. VASCULAR (CLAUDICATION, HYPOTENSION, PERIPHERAL EDEMA, COLD EXTREMITIES)
NSAIDs
Corticosteroids
Diuretics
Beta-blockers

Calcium channel blockers
ACE inhibitors
Nitrates
Antidepressants (TCAs and MAOIs)
Neuroleptics
Oral contraceptives
Estrogens and progestins

H. GENITOURINARY (SEXUAL DYSFUNCTION, URINARY RETENTION, URINARY INCONTINENCE)
Opioids
Diuretics
Beta-blockers
Antiarrhythmic agents
Antidepressants (TCAs and MAOIs)
Neuroleptics
Oral contraceptives
Estrogens and progestins

I. HEENT (TINNITUS, LOSS OF TASTE, HEADACHE, LIGHTHEADEDNESS, DIZZINESS)
Salicylates
NSAIDs
Opioids
Skeletal muscle relaxants
Beta-blockers
Nitrates
Calcium channel blockers
ACE inhibitors
Digoxin
Antiarrhythmic agents
Antianxiety agents
Antidepressants (TCAs and MAOIs)
Antiepileptic agents

ACE, Angiotensin-converting enzyme; *MAOIs*, monoamine oxidase inhibitors; *NSAIDs*, nonsteroidal antiinflammatory drugs; *OCAs*, oral contraceptive agents; *TCAs*, tricyclic antidepressants; *HEENT*, head, eyes, ears, nose, and throat.
From Cain SD, Janos SC: Clinical pharmacology for the physical therapist. In Boissonnault W, ed: *Examination in physical therapy practice; screening for medical disease*, ed 2, New York, 1995, Churchill Livingstone, pp 350-351.

BOX 7-12

Selection of Body Systems to Screen Based on Symptom Location

- All patients—First visit
  General Health Checklist
- Cervical and left/right shoulder pain (including shoulder girdle region)
  Cardiovascular
  Pulmonary
  Gastrointestinal (potential referral to scapular and shoulder strap regions)
- Thoracic spine pain
  Cardiovascular
  Pulmonary
  Gastrointestinal
  Genitourinary (thoracic-lumbar junction)

- Lumbopelvic pain
  Gastrointestinal
  Urogenital
  Peripheral vascular
- Midhumerus/femur to digits pain
  Peripheral vascular
- Inconsistent symptom pattern
  Psychological
  Endocrine
  Neurologic
  Rheumatic disorders
  Adverse drug reaction

Summary

Considering the amount of data that PTs collect during symptom investigation, the review of the patient's medical history, and the ROS, the PT's medical screening examination is very extensive. At this point, the physical examination proper, including the systems review, has not yet even begun. The ROS is a very important component of the examination because it enables the PT to recognize clinical manifestations, other than the patient's presenting complaints, that require a referral to another health care provider. At the same time, the PT should avoid "crying wolf" about a patient's health status whenever possible. Asking the follow-up questions about the patient's symptoms, learning whether the patient's physician is aware of the symptoms, learning whether the symptoms have worsened, and, finally, judging the patient's ability to give an accurate history, all contribute to the PT's ability to distinguish between a red flag and a yellow flag. Erring on the side of patient safety, however, always should be the PT's priority.

REFERENCES

1. Ahronheim JC: Special problems in the geriatric patient. In Goldman L, Bennett JC, eds: *Cecil textbook of medicine*, ed 21, Philadelphia, 2000, WB Saunders, pp 22-25.
2. Allison L, Fuller K: Balance and vestibular disorders. In Umphred DA, ed: *Neurological rehabilitation*, ed 4, St. Louis, 2001, Mosby, pp 617-619.
3. American Physical Therapy Association: *Guide to physical therapy practice*, ed 2, *Phys Ther* 81:9-744, 2001.
4. American Psychiatric Association: *Diagnostic and statistical manual of mental disorders*, ed 4, Washington, DC, 2000, American Psychiatric Association, pp 317-328.
5. Barry MJ, Goodson JD: Approach to benign prostatic hyperplasia. In Goroll AH, Mulley AG, eds. *Primary care medicine*, ed 4, Philadelphia, Lippincott Williams & Wilkins, 2000, pp 794-798.
6. Baxter RE, Moore JH: Diagnosis and treatment of acute exertional rhabdomyolysis, *J Orthop Sports Phys Ther* 33:104-108, 2003.
7. Berland B, Gleckman RA: Fever of unknown origin in the elderly, *Postgrad Med* 92:197-210, 1992.
8. Bickley LS: *Bates' guide to physical examination and history taking*, ed 7, Philadelphia, 1999, JB Lippincott, pp 3-4, 456.
9. Bigos S, Bowyer O, Braen G, et al: *Acute low back problems in adults. Clinical practice guideline*, quick reference guide number 14 [AHCPR pub no 95-0643], Rockville, MD, December, 1994, US Department of Health and Human Services, Public Health Service, Agency for Health Care Policy and Research.
10. Boissonnault WG, Meek PD: Risk factors for anti-inflammatory drug or aspirin-induced gastrointestinal complications in individuals receiving outpatient physical therapy services, *J Orthop Sports Phys Ther* 32:510-517, 2002.
11. Castle SC, Yeh M, Toledo S, et al: Lowering the temperature criterion improves detection of infections in nursing home residents, *Aging Immunol Infect Dis* 4:67-76, 1993.
12. Chesley LC: *Hypertensive disorders in pregnancy*, New York, 1978, Appleton-Century-Crofts.
13. Dale DC. The febrile patient. In Goldman L, Bennett JC, eds: *Cecil textbook of medicine*, ed 21, Philadelphia, 2000, WB Saunders, pp 1564-1565.
14. Dirckx JH: *Stedman's concise medical dictionary for the health professions*, ed 4, Philadelphia 2001, Lippincott Williams & Wilkins, p 586.
15. Doran FSA: The sites to which pain is referred from the common bile duct in man and its implication for the theory of referred pain, *Br J Surg* 54:599-606, 1967.
16. *Drug facts and comparisons 2003*, St Louis, 2002, Facts and Comparisons, pocket version, p 252.
17. Fang LS: Evaluation of the patient with hematuria. In Goroll AH, Mulley AG, eds: *Primary care medicine*, ed 4, Philadelphia, 2000, Lippincott Williams & Wilkins, pp 751-754.
18. Gladman JRF, Barer D, Venkatesan P, et al: The outcome of pneumonia in the elderly: a hospital survey, *Clin Rehabil* 5:201-204, 1991.
19. Goldman L: Cardiovascular diseases. In Goldman L, Bennett JC, eds: *Cecil textbook of medicine*, ed 21, Philadelphia, 2000, WB Saunders, pp 160-162, 212-213.
20. Goodson JD: Approach to incontinence and other forms of lower urinary tract dysfunction. In Goroll AH, Mulley AG, eds: *Primary care medicine*, ed 4, Philadelphia, Lippincott Williams & Wilkins, 2000, pp 776-782.
21. Goroll AH, Mulley AG: *Primary care medicine*, ed 4, Philadelphia, 2000, Lippincott Williams & Wilkins, p 43.
22. Gunta K: Alterations in skeletal function: trauma and infection. In Mattson-Porth C, ed: *Pathophysiology: concepts of altered health states*, ed 4, Philadelphia, 1994, JB Lippincott, pp 1203-1209.
23. Guyton AC, Hall JE: *Textbook of medical physiology*, ed 10, Philadelphia, 2000, WB Saunders, pp 830-832.
24. Jarvik JG, Deyo RA: Diagnostic evaluation of low back pain with emphasis in imaging, *Ann Intern Med* 137:586-597, 2002.
25. Johanson WG: Overview of pneumonia. In Goldman L, Bennett JC, eds: *Cecil textbook of medicine*, ed 21, Philadelphia, 2000, WB Saunders, pp 436-438.
26. Kumar V, Cotran RS, Robbins SL, et al: *Robbins basic pathology*, ed 7, Philadelphia, 2003, WB Saunders, pp 701-702.
27. Marton KI, Sox HC, Krupp JR: Involuntary weight loss: diagnostic and prognostic significance, *Ann Intern Med* 95:568-574, 1981.
28. Morrison RE, Keating HJ: Fatigue in primary care, *Prim Prev Care Obstet Gynecol* 28:225-240, 2001.
29. Norman DC: Fever in the elderly, *Clin Infect Dis* 31:148-151, 2000.
30. Pruitt AA: Evaluation of dizziness. In Goroll AH, Mulley AG, eds: *Primary care medicine*, ed 4, Philadelphia, 2000, Lippincott Williams & Wilkins.
31. Rebar RW, Erickson GF: Menstrual cycle and fertility. In Goldman L, Bennett JC, eds: *Cecil textbook of medicine*, ed 21, Philadelphia, 2000, WB Saunders, pp 1338-1339.
32. Richter JM: Evaluation of gastrointestinal bleeding. In Goroll AH, Mulley AG, eds: *Primary care medicine*, ed 4, Philadelphia, 2000, Lippincott Williams & Wilkins, pp 404-408.
33. Roberts JM: Pregnancy-related hypertension. In Creasy RK, Resnick R, eds: *Maternal-fetal medicine*, ed 4, Philadelphia, 1999, WB Saunders, p 837.
34. Rockey DC: Occult gastrointestinal bleeding, *N Engl J Med* 341:38-46, 1999.
35. Simon HB: *Evaluation of fever in primary care medicine*, ed 4, Philadelphia, 2000, Lippincott Williams & Wilkins, pp 57-63.
36. Smith-Pigg J, Bancroft DA: Alterations in skeletal function: rheumatic disorders. In Mattson-Porth C, ed: *Pathophysiology: concepts in altered health status*, ed 4, Philadelphia, 1994, JB Lippincott, pp 1246-1249.
37. Soteriades ES, Evans JC, Larson MG, et al: Incidence and prognosis of syncope, *N Engl J Med* 347:878-885, 2002.
38. Straus WL, Ofman JJ, Maclean C, et al: Do NSAIDs cause dyspepsia? A meta-analysis evaluating alternative dyspepsia definitions, *Am J Gastroenterol* 97:1951-1958, 2002.
39. Swartz MH: *Textbook of physical diagnosis*, ed 4, Philadelphia, 2002, WB Saunders, pp 28-30, 320-322, 434.
40. Thompson MP, Morris LK: Unexplained weight loss in the ambulatory elderly, *J Am Geriatr Soc* 39:497-500, 1991.
41. Tucker LE: Back pain due to visceral disease, *Hosp Med* July, 125-145, 1985.
42. Weitzman ED, Moline ML, Czeisler CA, et al: Chronobiology of aging: temperature, sleep-wake rhythms, and entrainment, *Neurobiol Aging* 3:299-309, 1982.

The Patient Interview: The Physical Examination Begins

William G. Boissonnault, PT, DHSc, FAAOMPT

Objectives

After reading this chapter, the reader will be able to:

1. Describe patient observation findings that suggest the presence of underlying disease.
2. Provide follow-up questions to ask once the concerning observations are noted.
3. Provide follow-up physical examination screening tools to implement once the concerning observations are noted.

The goals of the initial patient visit include establishing rapport with the patient (and care-giver), collecting sufficient examination data, establishing a diagnosis, initiating an intervention program, establishing a prognosis, and formulating a plan of action with the patient. Having to do all this in a 30- to 45-minute visit can be overwhelming to any clinician. One characteristic that master clinicians tend to demonstrate[10] that can enhance efficiency is the ability to multitask during the visit. An example of multitasking is starting the physical examination (patient observation) when first meeting the patient and continuing to do so throughout the history-taking process.

Patient data collected by observation, although general in nature, can affect the remainder of the history taking and the physical examination. For example, during the interview of a patient with low back pain, the physical therapist (PT) observes asymmetric pupil size. This observation warrants follow-up questioning regarding the patient's vision and a cranial nerve screening, items that are not routinely incorporated into the examination of patients with low back pain. This chapter discusses potential observational findings relevant to making the decision of whether to initiate a referral to, or consultation with, another health care practitioner. The observational findings include an integumentary systems screen, atypical surface anatomy, and a general nervous system screen. The description includes the examination data to be collected and the evaluation of these data relating to clinical decision-making.

General Observation: Integumentary System

The elements of the integumentary system most relevant to observation during the interview include skin, hair, and nails and then continue during the remainder of the physical examination. Findings noted by the PT may represent changes associated with aging, exposure to the environment, local skin disease or trauma, or a manifestation of organ disease and systemic illness.

Skin Color/Condition

Skin color varies considerably from individual to individual and is generally determined by the presence of melanocytes, carotene, oxygenated hemoglobin, and local blood flow. Melanocytes, found in the deep basal layer of the epidermis, contain brown granules called melanin. Besides contributing to skin color, melanin provides protection during episodes of sun exposure. Carotene found in subcutaneous fat tissue contributes to the yellowish color of the skin. This substance is especially concentrated in the palms of the hands and soles of the feet. Lastly, the normal reddish color of skin is attributed to the presence of oxygenated blood being transported through the arteries and capillaries.

Certain skin colors may represent serious disease, including pallor (pale), cyanosis (blue), jaundice or icterus (yellow), gray, and hyperpigmentation (brown). Table 8-1 summarizes these abnormal states, including the underlying physiological features and associated causes of the color. The physiological events may result in observable changes other than those noted in the skin. For example, there are two forms of cyanosis, central and peripheral. Central cyanosis results from low arterial oxygen levels and is best identified by color changes in the lips, tongue, and oral mucosa. Peripheral cyanosis results from a decrease or slowing of cutaneous blood flow, which allows for tissues to extract increased levels of oxygen from the circulating blood. The bluish hue noted in the hands, feet, or nails can be of central or peripheral origin.[2] Another example is excessive bilirubin, associated with the yellowish hue of the skin, which can result in the sclera of the eyes or mucous membranes assuming a similar hue. Lastly, severely jaundiced individuals may have a greenish hue to the skin resulting from the oxidation of bilirubin to biliverdin.[19,22]

In addition to general skin color changes, local alterations can also indicate a condition that should be reported to a physician. Local redness accompanied by local heat, edema, and tenderness that develops within a few days may be a manifestation of cellulitis, a bacterial infection. This infection may be accompanied by red streaks extending proximally, which are associated with secondary lymphangitis.[24] Local skin changes could also be a result of chronic arterial insufficiency. Ischemic ulcers, thin and shiny skin, hair loss, paleness of an elevated extremity, and intense rubor when the limb assumes a dependent position are all possible manifestations of this condition. Although cuts and bruises are fairly common, their presence on the head, face, and neck may be an indication of physical

TABLE 8-1

Abnormal Color Changes of the Skin

Color Change	Physiological Change	Common Causes
White, pale (pallor)	Absence of pigment or pigment change; blood abnormality; temporary interruption or diversion of blood flow; internal disease	Albinism (albinos); lack of sunlight; anemia; lead poisoning; vasospasm; syncope; stress; internal bleeding; chronic gastrointestinal disease; cancer; parasitic disease; tuberculosis
Blue (cyanosis)	Decreased oxygen in blood (deoxyhemoglobin)	Methemoglobinemia (oxidation of hemoglobin); high blood iron level; cold exposure; vasomotor instability; cerebrospinal disease
Yellow	Jaundice, excess bilirubin in blood (2-2.5 mg/100 mL), excess bile pigment; high levels of carotene in blood (carotenemia); high level of metals in body	Liver disease; gallstone blockage of bile duct; hepatitis (conjunctiva also yellow); ingestion of food high in carotene and vitamin A
Gray	Disturbances of adrenocortical hormones	Increased iron, bronze/gray; increased silver, blue/gray
Brown (hyperpigmentation)	Disturbances of adrenocortical hormones	Adrenal or pituitary glands, Addison's disease

Shapiro C, Skopit S: Screening for skin disorders. In Boissonnault W: *Examination in physical therapy practice: screening for medical disease,* ed 2, New York, 1995, Churchill Livingstone.

abuse. Also, similar findings on the forearms may be indicative of defensive injuries sustained while trying protect oneself.[6,16] Additional information regarding screening for domestic abuse can be found in Chapter 5.

Nails

As with skin color, changes in the nails may also indicate the presence of occult disease. The changes may occur in the nail itself or in the surrounding tissues. See Figure 8-1 for an illustration of normal nail anatomy and Figure 8-2 for a comparison between normal and abnormal nail appearances. The PT may also observe "clubbing" of the digits, an abnormality associated with chronic hypoxia and lung cancer (Figure 8-3).[2] *Clubbing* is manifested by three abnormal appearances: the distal phalanx appears rounded and bulbous, the nail plate is convex shaped, and the proximal nail fold and plate angle (Lovibond's angle) increases to 180 degrees or more.

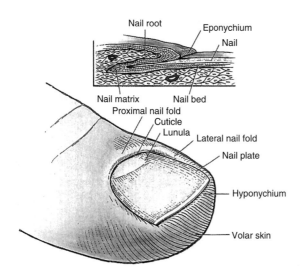

FIGURE 8-1 Nail anatomy.[21] (From Sams WM Jr: Structure and function of the skin. In Sams WM, Lynch PJ, editors: *Principles and practice of dermatology,* ed 2, New York, 1996, Churchill Livingstone.)

Hair

Hair is normally found over the entire body except for the soles of the feet, palms of the hands, and portions of the genitalia. A vascular network located in the dermal layer of the skin provides the necessary nourishment to hair follicles (Figure 8-4). If the local circulation is compromised, as in arterial insufficiency, hair loss will occur along with the other manifestations previously mentioned. If the disorder has progressed so that these skin changes have occurred, the patient will likely state that the extremity is cold. Hair loss (alopecia) of the scalp, although most often associated with male- and female-pattern baldness, can be a result of a variety of diseases or a side effect of medication use (Box 8-1).[17,24] As a general rule, hair loss that occurs quickly or that does not begin in the frontoparietal scalp should cause concern.[25] Lastly, brittle hair leading to hair breakage can also indicate illnesses such as hypothyroidism.[18] The broken hair may be noted later in the examination after the patient sits up after lying on a sheet or pillow case.

Skin Lesions

The term *skin lesion* implies the loss or change of local tissue continuity, structure, or function. Although skin lesions are benign, many characteristics are associated with disorders such as skin cancer. The American Cancer Society projects more than 1 million new cases of basal and squamous cell carcinomas in the United States during 2004. This estimation is much higher than the projections for any other cancer. In addition, more than 37,000 new cases of melanoma are projected over the same period.[9] Of the skin cancers, melanoma is the most aggressive type in terms of metastasis, and metastasis to the spine appears to be on the rise.[26] Early detection of the disease is important for a good patient prognosis, and who initially detects the lesion seems to be linked with the severity of disease at the time of diagnosis. Cutaneous melanomas first detected by physicians were found to be thinner at the time of diagnosis compared with lesions first detected by the patient, the spouse, or others.[7] The concerning finding of a study by Epstein et al,[7] however, was that only 24% of the melanomas

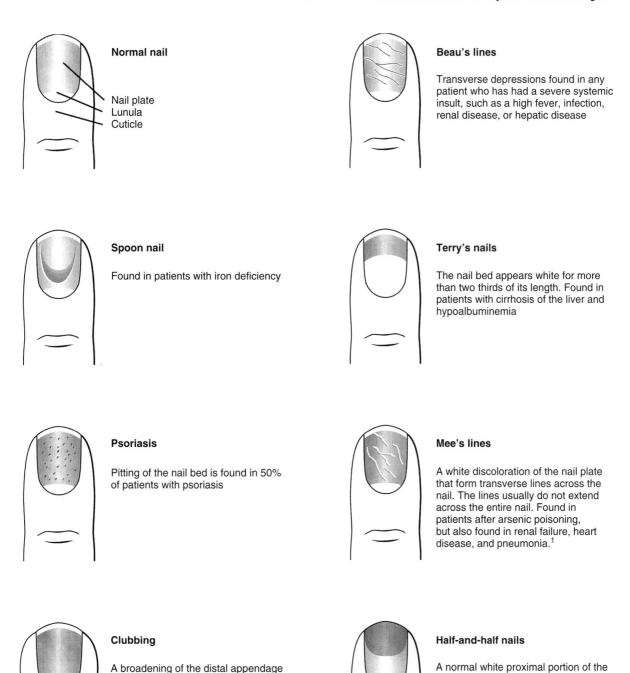

Normal nail

Nail plate
Lunula
Cuticle

Beau's lines

Transverse depressions found in any patient who has had a severe systemic insult, such as a high fever, infection, renal disease, or hepatic disease

Spoon nail

Found in patients with iron deficiency

Terry's nails

The nail bed appears white for more than two thirds of its length. Found in patients with cirrhosis of the liver and hypoalbuminemia

Psoriasis

Pitting of the nail bed is found in 50% of patients with psoriasis

Mee's lines

A white discoloration of the nail plate that form transverse lines across the nail. The lines usually do not extend across the entire nail. Found in patients after arsenic poisoning, but also found in renal failure, heart disease, and pneumonia.[1]

Clubbing

A broadening of the distal appendage with an increased Lovibond's angles as viewed from the lateral side

Half-and-half nails

A normal white proximal portion of the nail with a distinct brownish distal portion, the latter is more than one third of the nail plate. Indicates chronic renal failure

FIGURE 8-2 Normal nail appearance and common systemic diseases manifested in changes in the nail.[23] (From Shapiro C, Skopit S: Screening for skin disorders. In Boissonnault W: *Examination in physical therapy practice: screening for medical disease,* ed 2, New York, 1995, Churchill Livingstone.)

were initially detected by a physician, with the majority of the lesions being discovered by the patient or his or her spouse. Early detection is extremely important for a positive prognosis; the long-term survival rate for a localized lesion is 92% but only 5% for metastatic melanoma.[15] The PT's role does not include differentiating a melanoma from squamous cell cancer, but does include recognizing atypical skin lesion characteristics that require a physician consultation. This consultation may lead to a lesion being biopsied and diagnosed earlier in the course of the disease. PTs are rarely included in discussions of secondary prevention and skin cancer,[11] but considering how much skin PTs tend to "see" during a patient visit and the

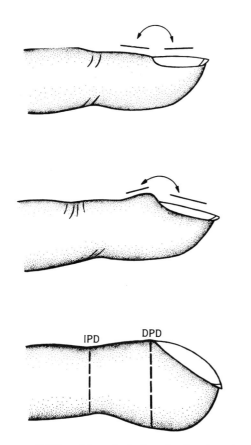

FIGURE 8-3 Clubbing of the nails. **A,** Normal nail configuration. **B,** Mild digital clubbing with increased hyponychial angle. **C,** Severe digital clubbing.[28] (From Wilkins RL, Sheldon RL, Krider SJ: *Clinical assessment in respiratory care,* ed 4, St Louis, 2000, Mosby.) *IPD,* Interphalangeal diameter; *DPD,* distal phalangeal diameter.

high incidence of skin cancer, PTs could be valuable members of the team screening for such lesions. See Plates 8-1 through 8-16 for examples of skin lesions including skin cancer and Table 8-2 for characteristics typical of a benign versus a pathologic skin lesion. The first four criteria represent the "ABCD rule," an acronym related to warning signs of melanoma: *a*symmetry, *b*order irregularity, *c*olor variation or black color, and *d*iameter greater than 6 mm.[12] Each criterion is not weighted equally. For example, a lesion 3 mm in diameter, but black and having indistinct borders, needs to be examined by a physician. Friability and ulceration imply weakened or damaged tissue and may be represented by an area that is scabbed over or by a lesion that is bleeding. The PT may note a spot of blood showing through the patient's clothing. These are findings more commonly associated with basal and squamous cell carcinomas. Basal cell carcinomas also frequently have a depressed center surrounded by raised, firm border, and squamous cell cancers often present with scaling, crusty nodules or plaques. If any atypical characteristics are observed by the PT, follow-up questions should be asked:

• Have you noticed this skin lesion?
• Has it recently changed in terms of size, color, shape, or surface appearance?
• Has a physician looked at the lesion? If so, what did the physician say about it?

If the patient states that a physician has not looked at the lesion, or the patient questions whether the lesion has changed since the physician has checked it, the PT should refer the patient to his or her primary care physician. If the patient states the lesion has been there as long as he or she can remember and no change in the lesion has occurred, then

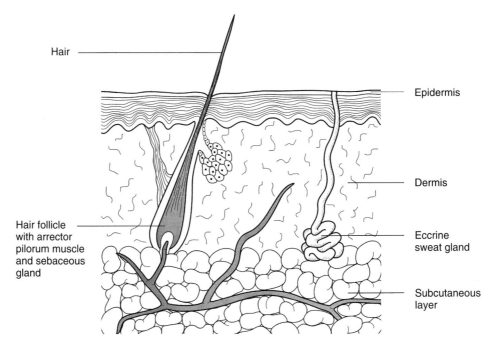

FIGURE 8-4 Normal human skin, including hair and associated vascular supply.[23] (From Shapiro C, Skopit S: Screening for skin disorders. In Boissonnault W: *Examination in physical therapy practice: screening for medical disease,* ed 2, New York, 1995, Churchill Livingstone.)

Diseases and Medications Associated with Hair Loss Diseases/Conditions/Therapy

INFECTIONS
Hypothyroidism
Iron deficiency
Systemic lupus erythematosus
Neoplasms
Pregnancy
Radiation therapy to the scalp
Crash diets

MEDICATIONS
Allopurinol
Amphetamines
Anticonvulsants
Antidepressants
Beta-blockers
Coumadin
Heparin
Oral contraceptives
Chemotherapy

a referral is not necessary as long as the PT has confidence in the patient's ability to be an accurate historian. If the skin lesion is on a body part that is not readily visible to the patient, then the therapist should assume that a physician should examine the lesion.

Two common benign vascular skin lesions that therapists may observe include spider and cherry angiomas. Both lesions tend to be small, with the cherry angioma ranging up to 3 mm in diameter, and the spider angioma ranging up to 2 cm. These lesions are marked by a bright or fiery red color, but whereas the cherry angioma is round with smooth borders, the spider angioma presents with a central body surrounded by radiating red "legs." Pressure applied to the central body of the spider angioma will cause blanching of the "legs." The spider angioma can occur in women who are pregnant and may be a manifestation of liver disease or vitamin B deficiency. Cherry angiomas, although they may increase in size and

TABLE 8-2

Skin Characteristics: Benign Versus Cancerous Lesions

Characteristics	Benign	Malignant
Size	<6 mm	>6 mm
Color	Uniform	Varied/black
Borders	Distinct/smooth	Irregular/indistinct
Shape	Symmetric	Asymmetric
Consistency	Soft to firm	Firm to hard
Friability	None	Often
Ulceration	Seldom	Often
Mobility	Mobile	Mobile/nonmobile
Rate of change (color, shape, size, surface)	Slow	Slow or rapid

number as one ages, are not typically associated with a pathologic condition.[2,27]

Observation: Surface Anatomy and Body Contour

During the interview the face, neck, anterior shoulder girdle, hands, and feet are typically visible. Besides the elements of the skin, the PT should also be vigilant for abnormal body contours that may be manifestations of masses or abnormal fluid accumulation (edema). Masses may not necessarily be manifested by a lump or bump on the body surface, but instead by the absence of a notch or body concavity. Enlarged tissues located within a fossa or notch may simply "fill in" the notch. Examples include the sternal notch completely or partially filled in by an enlarged thyroid gland, or the supraclavicular fossa filled in by an enlarged supraclavicular lymph node. Cervical masses may also be manifested by a tracheal deviation. When observing the patient from the front, the trachea should be vertically oriented. If a mass is present the trachea may appear to be "pushed" to one side. The observation of any abnormality will direct the PT to palpate the area once the physical examination begins and then ask follow-up questions including:

- Are you aware of this bump/lump?
- Is the lump painful? (If so, could be an inflammatory process/infection)
- Has the lump changed within the past few months? (Size, shape, consistency)
- Is your physician aware of the lump? If so, what did he or she say about it?

As with skin lesions, if the physician is not aware of the finding or the mass has changed since the last physician visit, the PT should initiate a referral.

Neck Masses (Palpation)

The structures most likely to present as a neck mass include the thyroid, parotid, and submandibular glands and the local lymph nodes (Figures 8-5 and 8-6). Glandular surfaces tend to be lobulated and irregular compared with the smaller lymph nodes, which tend to be round or ovoid in shape, and smooth. Glands normally tend to be nontender, soft to firm to touch, and hard nodules should not be present within the structure. Table 8-3 summarizes characteristics of normal versus abnormal lymph nodes. Abnormal lymph nodes may be exquisitely tender in the presence of acute inflammation but may also be nontender in the presence of a slow- to moderate-growing mass. This nontender lymph node will be firm to hard. A nontender mass is often the initial manifestation of head and neck cancers.[4] Pain generated from an inflamed lymph node often presents as a dull, diffuse, nonlocalized ache instead of the pinpoint pain expected from a structure that is up to a few centimeters in diameter. Palpation within the area of the ache will reveal a local lump that is exquisitely painful and firm to hard in consistency.

During a patient examination questions may arise as to whether the palpable mass is a band within a muscle belly or is an adjacent involved lymph node. To clarify the involved structure, the PT can elicit a light contraction of the local

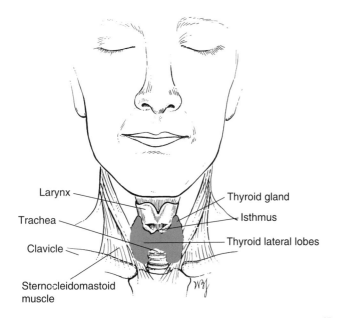

FIGURE 8-5 The thyroid gland located in the sternal notch.[27] (From Swartz MH: *Textbook of physical diagnosis*, ed 4, Philadelphia, 2002, WB Saunders.)

muscle while palpating the lump. If the lump does not change from a palpation perspective, the mass is probably superficial to the muscle belly. If the lump changes or disappears under the fingers palpating the area, the lump may be within the muscle belly or deep to the muscle. In this scenario, pal-

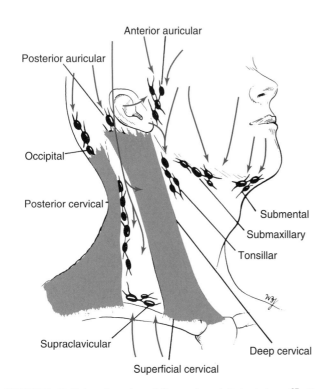

FIGURE 8-6 Lymph nodes of the neck and their drainage.[27] (From Swartz MH: *Textbook of physical diagnosis*, ed 4, Philadelphia, 2002, WB Saunders.)

TABLE 8-3

Characteristics of Normal and Abnormal Lymph Nodes

Characteristics	Normal	Abnormal
Size	<1 cm	Can be >1 cm
Consistency	Soft, squishy	Firm to hard
Mobility	Mobile	Mobile to nonmobile
Pain/tenderness	Nontender	Tender or nontender

pating posterior to the muscle belly (if possible) would be warranted to discern if the mass is within the muscle belly. Palpable bands within a muscle belly may be associated with a trigger point as described by Travell and Simons.[29] If this is the PT's conclusion, the patient's response to treatment is key in terms of deciding whether a physician needs to be contacted.

Anterior Shoulder Girdle Masses (Palpation)

If the patient is not wearing a shirt or has a tank top or sports bra on, the therapist may be able to observe the infraclavicular and the anterior glenohumeral joint regions. Figure 8-7 illustrates the infraclavicular fossa within which lymph nodes are located. Enlarged local lymph nodes or a breast mass may "fill in" this fossa. Breast tissue extends up toward the anterior glenohumeral joint region (upper and outer quadrant of the breast), and in some women the tissue can extend into the axilla (Figure 8-8). The upper and outer breast quadrant is often the site of neoplasms.[5] As described earlier, the PT who palpates a lump in this region should attempt to determine if the mass is within the local musculature (e.g., pectoralis major muscle) or within tissue superficial to the muscle (e.g., breast tissue). If the mass is superficial to the muscle, the PT will probably not note a change in the lump while eliciting a gentle contraction of the local musculature. If the therapist has any concerns about

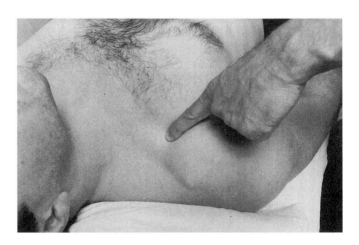

FIGURE 8-7 Palpation of the infraclavicular fossa.[3] (From Boissonnault W: *Examination in physical therapy practice: screening for medical disease*, ed 2, New York, 1995, Churchill Livingstone.)

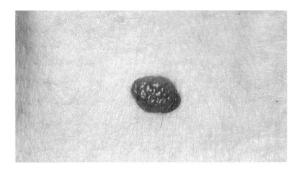

PLATE 8-1 Benign lesion.

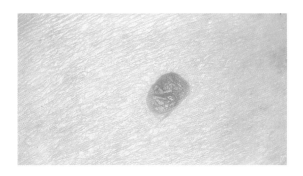

PLATE 8-2 Benign lesion.

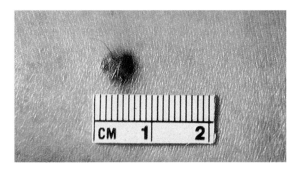

PLATE 8-3 Melanoma.

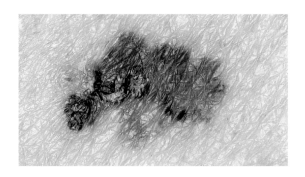

PLATE 8-4 Melanoma.

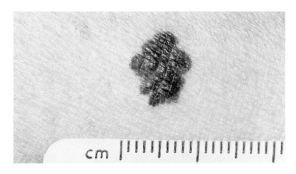

PLATE 8-5 Melanoma.

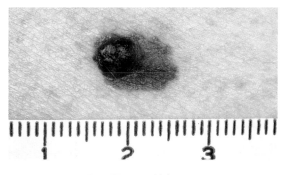

PLATE 8-6 Melanoma.

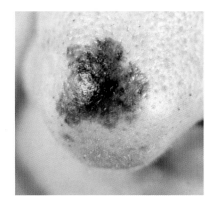

PLATE 8-7 Melanoma.

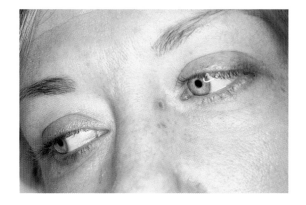

PLATE 8-8 Basal cell carcinoma.

PLATES 8-1 THROUGH 8-16. Skin lesions, including cancer. (Plates 8-1 through 8-16 from the American Skin Cancer Foundation.)

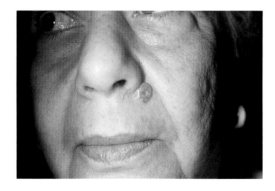

PLATE 8-9 Basal cell carcinoma.

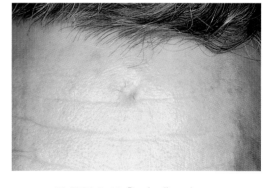

PLATE 8-10 Basal cell carcinoma.

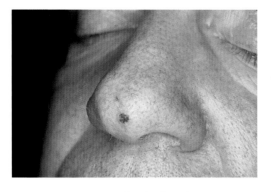

PLATE 8-11 Basal cell carcinoma.

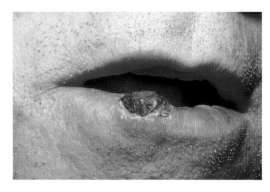

PLATE 8-12 Squamous cell carcinoma.

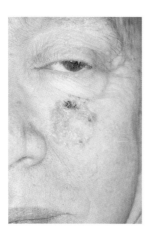

PLATE 8-13 Squamous cell carcinoma.

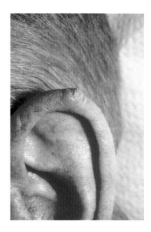

PLATE 8-14 Squamous cell carcinoma.

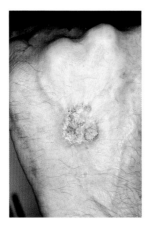

PLATE 8-15 Squamous cell carcinoma.

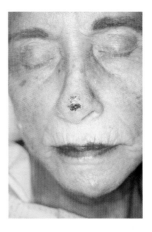

PLATE 8-16 Squamous cell carcinoma.

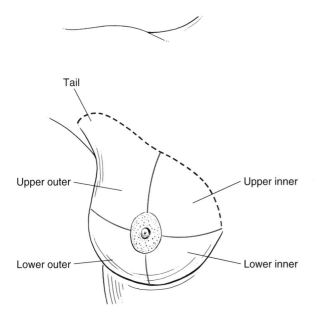

FIGURE 8-8 The four breast quadrants.[27] (From Swartz MH: *Textbook of physical diagnosis*, ed 4, Philadelphia, 2002, WB Saunders.)

the nature of the noted mass, follow-up questions should be asked, including:

- Have you noticed this lump?
- Has a physician examined this area?

If the answer to the second question is no or the patient states the lump has changed since the physician examined it, then the following questions are warranted:

- Has the lump changed (shape, size, consistency, numbers of)?
- Is the lump tender?
- Have you noticed any changes of the skin overlying the breast (color, puckering, scaliness, dimpling, peau d'orange)?
- Have you noticed any nipple discharge or retraction?

Approximately 1% of breast cancers occur in men, so the same principles apply to finding a mass in this region in a male patient.[9]

Observation: Nervous System Screen

A general nervous system screen can also begin as soon as the PT sees the patient, including:

- Gross movement patterns
- Gait
- Balance
- Tremors
- Asymmetric facial features
  - Pupils
  - Ptosis
  - Strabismus
  - Facial contour
- Hearing

If the PT meets the patient in the waiting area, watching the patient rise from the chair and walk back to the treatment area provides information about gross muscle strength, coordination, and balance. Once the patient interview begins, the

therapist can be vigilant for tremors and areas of muscle atrophy.

Facial Inspection

Careful inspection of the face, including the pupils, eyelids, gaze, and movement of the eyes, during the interview can reveal important findings associated with nervous system function. See Figure 8-9 for the identification of normal external landmarks of the eye. Although a small percentage of the population has a normal anatomic variant of up to 1 mm in diameter, pupils are normally equal in size and round, with smooth margins.[20,27] An abnormal pupil may be enlarged (mydriasis) or constricted (miosis). Mydriasis may be associated with medication use (sympathomimetics and dilating drops; see Chapter 15) or conditions such as acute glaucoma. Miosis may be associated with parasympathomimetic medications (see Chapter 16) or conditions such as Horner's syndrome and inflammation of the iris. See Table 8-4 for a summary of the more common pupillary abnormalities. Although not associated with a nervous system disorder, a specific pattern of eye redness should alert the PT to ask follow-up questions listed below. An intense circle of redness (vasodilated vessels) around the iris, called ciliary flush, is associated with inflammation of the iris or cornea or acute glaucoma.[1] Observation of *ciliary flush* would warrant an immediate consultation with the patient's physician.

Drooping of the upper eyelid (ptosis) may also be a manifestation of a normal anatomic variant or of a pathologic condition, including myasthenia gravis, lesion of the oculomotor nerve, and involvement of the cervical sympathetic chain. Normally the upper eyelid covers the upper margin of the iris and the sclera above, while a thin strip of the sclera is usually visible between the lower lid and the bottom margin of the iris. The space between the upper and lower eyelids is called the palpebral fissure. Because of connective tissue changes in the skin associated with aging, the elderly may have bilateral drooping of the upper eyelids (senile ptosis).[13] Unilateral ptosis is a classic component of Horner's syndrome. To maintain the visual field the patient may compensate by contracting the frontalis (resulting in wrinkling the forehead) to raise the upper eyelid.[20] In summary, bilateral ptosis in the non-elderly population and unilateral ptosis in any population should raise concern on the part of the PT.

The final component of the static assessment of the eyes is gaze. Normally, both of the patient's eyes should meet the

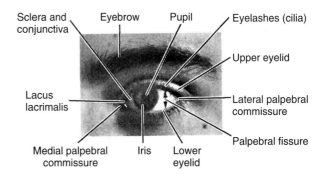

FIGURE 8-9 External features of the eye.[14] (From Magee DJ: *Orthopedic physical assessment*, ed 4, Philadelphia, 2002, WB Saunders.)

TABLE 8-4

Pupillary Abnormalities

	Adie's Tonic Pupil	Argyll Robertson Pupil	Horner's Syndrome
Etiology	Unknown	Diabetes, tertiary syphilis	Lesions of the brain stem, cervical root, carotid artery dissection, apex of the lung, orbit
Laterality	Often unilateral	Bilateral	Unilateral
Reaction to light	Minimally reactive	Nonreactive	Reactive
Accommodation	Sluggishly reactive	Reactive	Reactive
Pupillary size	Mydriatic	Miotic	Miotic
Other signs	Absent or diminished tendon reflexes	Absent knee-jerk reflexes	Slight ptosis and anhidrosis

Adapted from Swartz MH: *Textbook of physical diagnosis, history and physical examination,* ed 4, Philadelphia, 2002, WB Saunders.

PT's during the interview process. Misalignment of the two eyes is called strabismus. In this case, one eye is focused on the PT, but the other is not. Observation of any of the earlier described abnormalities would warrant follow-up questions, including:

- Have you noticed the abnormality (ptosis, pupil asymmetry, strabismus)? If so, how long has the abnormality been present, and what brought it on?
- Have there been any recent changes in your vision, including acuity or sharpness of vision, flashes, photophobia, loss of visual field(s), diplopia or double vision, colored halos around lights, difficulty in seeing in dim light, or altered colored vision? (See Table 8-5 for a summary of visual abnormalities and potential disease states.)
- Is there any pain in or around your eye(s)?
- Is your physician aware of the condition?

Additional follow-up questions regarding nervous system status should also be asked, including:

- Have you noticed any recent changes in your ability to smell, taste, swallow, talk, or hear?
- Have you noticed any recent changes in your balance, memory, ability to concentrate, or attention span?

If the patient states he or she is unaware of the abnormality of the eyes or gives equivocal answers to the above questions, the PT should include some tests in the physical examination to gather more information about the status of the relevant cranial nerves. For example, the pupillary reaction test can be used to test elements of the second and third cranial nerves (Figure 8-10). The pupils of both eyes should constrict briskly and to the same degree in response to the light stimulus. Also, ocular movements can be used to assess function of the third, fourth, and sixth cranial nerves and associated muscles (Figure 8-11). The PT

TABLE 8-5

Common Visual Symptoms and Possible Disease States

Symptom	Disease States
Loss of vision	Optic neuritis, detached retina, retinal hemorrhage, central retinal vascular occlusion, central nervous system disease
Spots	Impending retinal detachment, fertility drugs
Flashes	Migraine headaches, retinal detachment, posterior vitreous detachment
Loss of visual field, presence of shadows	Retinal detachment, retinal hemorrhage
Glare, photophobia	Iritis, meningitis
Distorted vision	Retinal detachment, macular edema
Impaired vision in dim light	Myopia, vitamin A deficiency, retinal degeneration
Colored halos around lights	Acute narrow angle glaucoma, opacities in the lens or cornea
Colored vision changes	Cataracts, medication such as digitalis (increases yellow vision)
Double vision (diplopia)	Extraocular muscle paresis or paralysis

Adapted from Swartz MH: *Textbook of physical diagnosis; history and examination,* ed 4, Philadelphia, 2002, WB Saunders.

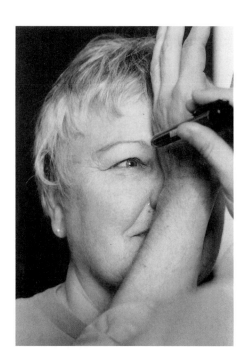

FIGURE 8-10 Pupillary light reaction test should be performed in a dimly lit room with the patient told to look at a distant object. The PT's hand divides the patient's visual field and shines the light into one eye, watching that pupil for the response (direct response). The PT then shines the light in the *same* eye, watching the *opposite* pupil for the response (consensual response). This process is repeated while shining the light in the other eye.

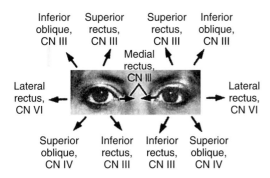

Inferior oblique, CN III   Superior rectus, CN III   Superior rectus, CN III   Inferior oblique, CN III

Medial rectus, CN III

Lateral rectus, CN VI   Lateral rectus, CN VI

Superior oblique, CN IV   Inferior rectus, CN III   Inferior rectus, CN III   Superior oblique, CN IV

FIGURE 8-11 Six cardinal fields of gaze with the associated eye muscles and cranial nerves responsible for the movements.[14] (From Magee DJ: *Orthopedic physical assessment,* ed 4, Philadelphia, 2002, WB Saunders.)

holds a finger approximately 10 to 15 inches from the patient's nose[14,27] and slowly traces a large "H" in front of the patient's face (Figure 8-12). The patient is asked to follow the finger with his or her eyes, and the eyes should track together. The PT then asks the patient to follow the finger as it moves toward the tip of the patient's nose; again, the eyes should converge together. If the eyes do not track together, or, in the presence of strabismus, the degree of misalignment varies depending on which direction the eyes are moving (paralytic strabismus), especially when accompanied by diplopia, the patient's physician should be contacted. Once again, abnormalities that the patient or physician is unaware of or abnormalities that have worsened since that last physician visit warrant communication with the patient's physician.

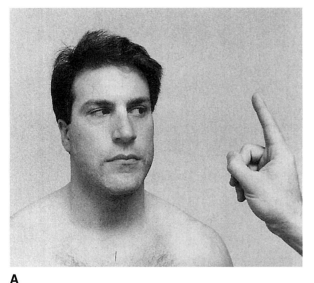

A

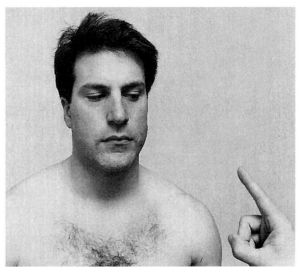

B

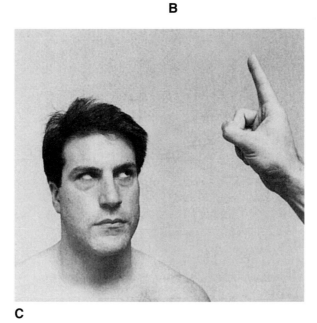

C

FIGURE 8-12 A, The PT's finger moving laterally to the patient's left. **B,** The PT's finger moving down and away from the patient's nose. **C,** The PT's finger moving up and away from the patient's nose. All three movements would be repeated to the patient's right side.[3] (From Boissonnault W: *Examination in physical therapy practice: screening for medical disease,* ed 2, New York, 1995, Churchill Livingstone.)

Hearing

During the interview a hearing deficit may be suspected by the PT or reported by a concerned patient. Impaired hearing has many potential causes, including neurologic conditions. There are three types of hearing loss: conductive (involvement of the middle ear, outer ear, or both), sensorineural (involvement of the inner ear), or a combination of both. Ultimately the patient's physician will determine the type of lesion once the PT refers the patient with a suspected occult hearing impairment. If the patient reports the suspected hearing loss is of new onset or has recently worsened, tests should be included in the physical examination. The first auditory acuity test used should be the *whisper test* because the outer, middle, and inner ear are all assessed simultaneously. The PT whispers familiar bisyllabic words (e.g., weather, thirteen, hot dog) and asks the patient to repeat the words that were whispered. To test one ear at a time and to ensure the patient cannot lip-read, the PT should stand behind and off to one side of the patient while whispering. To ensure unilateral assessment the patient should cover the ear not being tested. If a unilateral or bilateral deficit is noted or if the findings are equivocal, follow-up testing with a 512-Hz tuning fork should occur.[2,8]

The *Weber test* allows for bilateral hearing assessment. After striking the tuning fork in the palm of the hand, the PT places the fork firmly on the vertex of the cranium or mid-forehead (Figure 8-13). The patient is then asked, "Do you hear the sound? If so, equally in both ears?" A normal response should be "Yes, I hear it equally in both ears." If the sound lateralizes to one ear (heard more loudly in one ear), this finding and the subjective complaints and the whisper tests results, should be reported to the patient's physician.

Summary

Although one of the goals of this chapter is to foster efficient clinical practice, it might appear that the recommended observations, follow-up questions, and physical examination techniques could actually disrupt the natural flow of the initial visit. Depending on the make-up of the therapist's patient population, the abnormal observations noted in this chapter will often have nothing to do with the health issues that have precipitated the physical therapy visit. In that case, following the normal examination scheme and organization is important for the sake of efficiency, but at some point during the visit (often toward the end) the observation warranting concern needs to be addressed. For example, a patient comes to physical therapy for upper body pain, and a suspicious looking skin lesion is noted on the lower leg. The PT can complete the usual examination for the upper body pain and associated functional limitation, but as the visit is concluding the PT could state "Before we finish for the day, I would like to talk to you about a spot I noticed on the outside of your right leg." This statement then could be followed up by the questions and the physical examination techniques described throughout this chapter. The observations described are not just germane to the initial patient visit. The PT should make an effort to remain vigilant during any subsequent visits for the surface anatomy, skin, and nervous system findings that were described. Clinical manifestations can be easily overlooked during a hectic initial visit, especially when they are not directly related to the reason for the physical therapy visit, and new manifestations can develop after the initial visit.

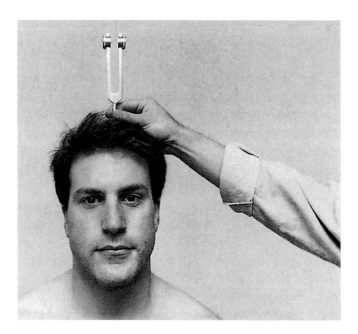

FIGURE 8-13 Weber test. The 512-Hz tuning fork, once struck, is placed firmly at the vertex of the cranium.[3] (From Boissonnault W: *Examination in physical therapy practice: screening for medical disease,* ed 2, New York, 1995, Churchill Livingstone.)

REFERENCES

1. Berson FG: *Basic ophthalmology for medical students and primary care residents,* San Francisco, Calif, 1993, American Academy of Ophthalmology, p 64.
2. Bickley LS: *Bates' guide to physical examination and history taking,* ed 7, Philadelphia, 1999, JB Lippincott, pp 145-149.
3. Boissonnault W: *Examination in physical therapy practice: screening for medical disease,* ed 2, New York, 1995, Churchill Livingstone, pp 93, 216, 217, 404.
4. Concus AP, Singer MI: Head and neck cancer. In Goldman L, Bennett JC, editors: *Cecil textbook of medicine,* ed 21, Philadelphia, 2000, WB Saunders, pp 2257-2261.
5. Damjanov I: *Pathology for the health-related professions,* ed 2, Philadelphia, 2000, WB Saunders, p 397.
6. Eisenstat SA, Bancroft L: Domestic violence, *N Engl J Med* 341:886-892, 1999.
7. Epstein DS, Lange JR, Gruber SB, et al: Is physician detection associated with thinner melanomas? *JAMA* 281:640-643, 1999.
8. Guyla AJ: Evaluation of hearing loss. In Goroll AH, Mulley AG, editors: *Primary care medicine,* ed 4, Philadelphia, 2000, Lippincott Williams & Wilkins, pp 1108-1112.
9. Jemal A, Tiwari RC, Murray T, et al: Cancer statistics, 2004, *CA Cancer J Clin* 54:8-29, 2004.
10. Jensen GM, Shepard KF, Gwyer J, et al: Attribute dimensions that distinguish master and novice physical therapy clinicians in orthopedic settings, *Phys Ther* 72:711-722, 1992.
11. Koh HK, Geller AC, Miller DR, et al: Prevention and early detection strategies for melanoma and skin cancer, *Arch Dermatol* 132:436-443, 1996.
12. Koh HK: Cutaneous melanoma, *N Engl J Med* 325:171-182, 1991.
13. Lewis CB, Bottomley JM: *Geriatric physical therapy; a clinical approach,* Norwalk, Conn, 1994, Appleton & Lange.

14. Magee DJ: *Orthopedic physical assessment,* ed 4, Philadelphia, 2002, WB Saunders, pp 70, 100.

15. Miller BA, Ries LAG, Hnakey BF, et al, editors: *Cancer statistics review: 1973-1990.* Bethesda, Md, 1993, National Cancer Institute, National Institutes of Health publication 93-2789.

16. Muelleman RL, Lenaghan PA, Pakieser RA: Battered women: injury locations and types, *Ann Emerg Med* 28:486-492, 1996.

17. Parker F: Skin diseases of general importance. In Goldman L, Bennett JC, editors: *Cecil textbook of medicine,* ed 21, Philadelphia, 2000, WB Saunders, pp 2293-2294.

18. Porth CM, Jurwitz LS: Alterations of endocrine controls of growth and metabolism. In Porth CM, editor: *Pathophysiology: concepts of altered health states,* ed 4, Philadelphia, 1994, JB Lippincott, pp 915-917.

19. Richter JM: Evaluation of jaundice. In Goroll AH, Mulley AG, editor: *Primary care medicine,* ed 4, Philadelphia, 2000, Lippincott Williams & Wilkins, pp 399-404.

20. Ross RT: *How to examine the nervous system,* ed 3, Stamford, Conn, 1999, Appleton & Lange, pp 56-57, 61-66.

21. Sams WM Jr: Structure and function of the skin. In Sams WM, Lynch PJ, editors: *Principles and practice of dermatology,* ed 2, New York, 1996, Churchill Livingstone, p 6.

22. Scharschmidt BF: Bilirubin metabolism, hyperbilirubinemia, and the approach to the jaundiced patient. In Goldman L, Bennett JC, editors: *Cecil textbook of medicine,* ed 21, Philadelphia, 2000, WB Saunders, pp 770-775.

23. Shapiro C, Skopit S: Screening for skin disorders. In Boissonnault W: *Examination in physical therapy practice: screening for medical disease,* ed 2, New York, 1995, Churchill Livingstone, pp 304, 305, 313.

24. Shellow WVR: Approach to bacterial skin infections. In Goroll AH, Mulley AG, editors: *Primary care medicine,* ed 4, Philadelphia, 2000, Lippincott Williams & Wilkins, pp 1040-1042.

25. Shellow WVR: Approach to the patient with hair loss. In Goroll AH, Mulley AG, editors: *Primary care medicine,* ed 4, Philadelphia, 2000, Lippincott Williams & Wilkins, pp 1015-1019.

26. Spiegel DA, Simpson JH, Richardson WJ, et al: Metastatic melanoma to the spine. Demographics, risk factors, and prognosis in 114 patients, *Spine* 20:2141-2146, 1995.

27. Swartz MH: *Textbook of physical diagnosis,* ed 4, Philadelphia, 2002, WB Saunders, pp 182, 204, 415.

28. Wilkins RL, Sheldon RL, Krider SJ: *Clinical assessment in respiratory care,* ed 4, St Louis, 2000, Mosby.

29. Travell J, Simons DG: *Myofascial pain and dysfunction,* vol 2, Baltimore, Md, 1992, Williams & Wilkins.

SECTION THREE

Examination/Evaluation: The Physical Examination

Review of Cardiovascular and Pulmonary Systems and Vital Signs

9

Steven H. Tepper, PT, PhD

Michael McKeough, PT, EdD

Objectives

After reading this chapter, the reader will be able to:

1. Provide a rationale for the need to measure, monitor, and record vital signs at rest, during activity, and during recovery from activity.
2. Provide a rationale for the need to measure, monitor, and record body mass index.
3. Define blood pressure, heart rate, ventilatory rate, and heart and breath sounds. Describe accurate, reliable, and valid clinical tests for each of these measurements.
4. Describe the expected normal and potential abnormal changes in blood pressure, heart rate, ventilatory rate, and heart and breath sounds at rest and in response to short- or long-term exercise.
5. Describe how abnormal measures of vital signs and body composition are potential risk factors for the development of pathologic conditions, impairment, functional limitation, and disability.
6. Describe how measures of vital signs and body composition can be used to establish treatment goals, assist with the development of a treatment plan, and assess response to intervention (verify treatment effectiveness).

Physiological measures of the cardiovascular and respiratory systems and body composition are important because they may accurately reflect the patient's general health and wellness. Simply, health can be defined as the absence of disease, and wellness can be defined as the ability to respond adaptively to stress. Blood pressure (BP), ventilatory rate, and heart rate (HR) are basic physiological measures of the cardiovascular and pulmonary systems. Heart and lung sounds also help delineate normal function or potential disease. The location of these and other physiological measures is shown in Figure 9-1. Body mass index (BMI) is a measure of body composition and has been shown to be related to the risk of developing many of the diseases commonly seen in the physical therapy clinic. Normal values and ranges have been established for these physiological measures at rest and during activity in various age groups. Significant deviations from these norms may indicate an abnormal condition and are valuable in assessing the risk of developing a disease or disorder. The ability to provide quality health care depends in part on the practitioner's ability to assess and interpret accurately measures of these important physiological parameters (vital signs) at rest and during activity and recovery. In spite of the demonstrated value of these measures in assessing a patient's general health and risk of developing disease and the recommendation by the *Guide to Physical Therapy Practice*,[1] recent evidence indicates that they have not yet become a routine part of physical therapists' assessment.[2]

For most patients, a baseline measurement of vital signs and body composition should be established so changes in these values from exercise, diet, medications, or other factors can be determined. If abnormal values are found at rest, the cause of these abnormal values should be determined before initiating any activity that involves significant stress, physical or psychological. Individuals with abnormal resting values are frequently less able to tolerate physical activity or other stress-producing events. Depending on the extent of these abnormalities, significant life-threatening sequelae may occur.

Measurements of these physiological parameters can be used to determine the need to refer the patient to a physician, establish intervention goals, assist in developing an intervention plan, and assess the individual's response to intervention (establish treatment effectiveness). For example, patients being seen for complications associated with diabetes mellitus (elevated blood glucose levels) are often found to have hypertension (elevated BP), hypercholesterolemia (elevated total cholesterol), lack of endurance, and obesity (elevated BMI). These changes may be caused by a sedentary lifestyle and will usually lead to a more sedentary lifestyle. An intervention plan should be developed that may include drug therapy to help control blood glucose level, hypertension, and cholesterol; an exercise program to help control blood glucose level, hypertension, cholesterol, lack of endurance, and obesity; and dietary modifications to help control blood glucose level, hypertension, cholesterol, and obesity. At 4 weeks into the intervention (a walking program), the short-term goals should include better control of blood glucose level, a lowered total cholesterol, resting and submaximal HR and BP, and a reduction in BMI.[3] By discharge, the patient should have accepted responsibility for controlling his or her comorbidities. Controlling their comorbidities involves a permanent change in lifestyle, including medications (which over time may be reduced or eliminated), regular exercise, and eating a healthy diet. The intervention plan is deemed effective if, by discharge, the measures of physiological parameters are closer to or within normal limits.[4-6]

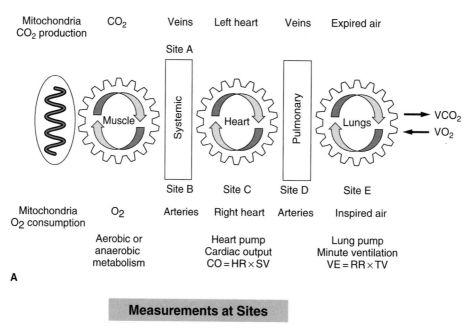

Measurements at Sites

- **Site A**
  - Jugular venous distention
  - Venous pulse
  - Central line*
    - Central venous pressure
    - PvO$_2$

- **Site B**
  - Pulse palpation for:
    - Heart rate
    - Heart rhythm
    - Patency of blood vessel
  - Blood pressure
  - Pulse oxygen or O$_2$ saturation
  - Arterial line*
    - BP
    - PaO$_2$
    - Cardiac output or index

- **Site C**
  - ECG
  - Heart rate
  - Heart rhythm
  - Heart sounds

- **Site D**
  - Swan-Ganz catheter*
    - Pulmonary artery BP
    - Pulmonary capillary wedge pressure

- **Site E**
  - Breath frequency
  - Tidal volume
  - Lung sounds

FIGURE 9-1 Anatomic sites for physiologic measurements. **A,** Oxygen transport system. **B,** Measurements obtained at sites A through E. BP, Blood pressure; CO$_2$, carbon dioxide; CO, cardiac output; PaO$_2$, partial arterial oxygen pressure, PvO$_2$, partial oxygen pressure in mixed venous blood; RR, respiratory rate; VCO$_2$, carbon dioxide output; VE, ventricular ejection; VO$_2$, volume of oxygen utilization. (Adapted from Wasserman K, Hansen JE, Sue DY, et al: *Principles of exercise testing and interpretation*, Philadelphia, 1987, Lea & Febiger.)

Body Mass Index

It is estimated that 64% of the American population is overweight or obese, a condition that leads to increased risks for cardiopulmonary, musculoskeletal, neurologic, and integumentary disorders (Figure 9-2).[8] Many of the disorders lead to disability and functional limitations that motivate these patients to seek the assistance of health care professionals, including physical therapists.[7] Comprehensive health care for these individuals cannot be achieved without addressing the issue of weight as an underlying cause of their functional limitations. The National Institutes of Health, National Heart, Lung and Blood Institute has developed clinical guidelines for adults who are overweight or obese (http://www.nhlbi.nih.gov/guidelines/obesity/ob_home.htm). A free, downloadable copy

Being overweight or obese increases the risk of the following:

- Hypertension*
- Dyslipidemia (abnormalities of the blood lipids)*
- Type 2 diabetes*
- Coronary heart disease*
- Stroke
- Gallbladder disease
- Osteoarthritis
- Sleep apnea and respiratory problems
- Endometrial, breast, prostate, and colon cancer

FIGURE 9-2 Comorbid risks associated with being overweight or obese. (From Clinical guidelines on the identification, evaluation, and treatment of overweight and obesity in adults. *Primary risk factor. Available at: http://www.nhlbi.nih.gov/guidelines/obesity/ob_home.htm.)

Calculation of BMI

- BMI gives comparative weight for height information that is "significantly correlated with total body fat"
  - Non-metric formula = weight (pounds)/height [inches]$^2 \times 704.2$
  - Metric formula = weight (kilograms)/height (meters)^2
- Subject is female
  - Weighs 183 lbs, height 5'4", waist 32"
- BMI = $[183/64^2] \times 7.4.5 = 31.5$
- Using table—subject is at high risk for disease

FIGURE 9-3 Formula to determine body mass index.

of "Clinical Guidelines for the Identification, Evaluation, and Treatment of Overweight and Obesity in Adults" is available on this website.

How to Measure Body Mass Index

BMI (body weight in kilograms divided by the square of the height in meters; Figure 9-3) is the recommended measurement for assessing a patient's level of obesity and risk for disease. Although the validity of the BMI varies and is not useful in individuals who have enlarged muscle mass, this simple clinical measure is endorsed for use by health care professionals. BMI has been correlated with percent body fat and the risk of disease. By coupling the BMI with waist measurement, an even more valid measure of the risk of disease can be achieved (Figure 9-4). Individuals who carry a greater percentage of their weight in the abdominal region have a higher risk of developing disease.[34a]

When to Measure

As part of a shift from a disease-oriented approach to health care to a wellness approach, and because of its value in predicting the risk of developing debilitating disorders, BMI should be assessed as part of the initial examination of all patients, regardless of the reason for the visit. Once established, BMI can then serve as part of the health profile monitored at follow-up visits. Increased physical activity is one approach that has been shown to be effective in reducing BMI. Behavior modification, dietary modification, and pharmacologic and surgical approaches have also been shown to be effective.[9] Reduction in BMI has been associated with a reduction in the development of disease.

Role of the Physical Therapist

By focusing exclusively on the impairments causing a patient's chief symptom, PTs risk overlooking the role of excess body weight in the patient's condition. Excess body weight can cause various musculoskeletal disorders such as low back, hip, knee, and ankle impairments and may lead to various pathologic conditions such as hypertension, stroke, or coronary heart disease. For example, joint degeneration may be the direct cause of a patient's hip replacement. Obesity may have been the original cause of the joint degeneration. Failure to address the excess body weight may shorten the life expectancy of the prosthesis or cause additional joint degeneration, leading to the need for additional hip or knee joint replacements. The epidemic of obesity in the United States today requires that the role of BMI be considered in all cases.[7] It is our professional duty to inform patients that if they want to do something about their body size, we can recommend an activity program and help them seek nutritional counseling. A study of overweight and obese persons who were at high risk of developing diabetes reported that mild changes in diet and physical activity reduced the occurrence of type 2 diabetes by 58% compared with a control group.[10]

Heart disease is the leading cause of death in the United States today. Because the risk of heart failure increases with an increasing BMI, strategies to promote optimal body weight may reduce the incidence of heart failure.[11] During a 14-year follow-up of the 5881 participants in the Framingham Heart Study, 496 subjects (258 women and 238 men) had heart failure develop. After adjusting for established risk factors, there was an increase in the risk of heart failure of 7% for women and 5% for men for each increment of 1 in BMI. Obese subjects had double the risk of heart failure of subjects with normal BMI.

Disease risk relative to normal weight and waist circumference

	BMI (kg/m^2)	Obesity class	Men ≤102 cm (≤40 in) Women ≤88 cm (≤35 in)	>102 cm (>40 in) >88 cm (>35 in)
Underweight	<18.5		–	–
Normal	18.5-24.9		–	–
Overweight	25.0-29.9		Increased	High
Obesity	30.0-34.9	I	High	Very high
	35.0-39.9	II	Very high	Very high
Extreme obesity	≥40	III	Extremely high	Extremely high

FIGURE 9-4 Classification by body mass index, waist circumference, and associated disease risks. (From Clinical guidelines on the identification, evaluation, and treatment of overweight and obesity in adults. Available at: http://www.nhlbi.nih.gov/guidelines/obesity/ob_home.htm.)

Blood Pressure

BP is the force driving the blood through the vascular tree (see Figure 9-1). This pressure is usually measured in the systemic arteries. BP is usually divided into systolic BP (SBP) and diastolic BP (DBP). SBP is the peak lateral force primarily caused by the contraction of the heart ejecting blood, or stroke volume (milliliters of blood ejected from the left ventricle), into the systemic vascular tree. DBP is the minimal lateral force found in the arteries and is primarily related to resistance (total peripheral resistance [TPR]) to blood flowing from systemic arterioles into the capillaries. Capillaries are the functional unit of the vascular tree that enables the exchange of materials, whereas pressure maintains the flow.

BP is usually expressed as SBP/DBP in millimeters of mercury. Mean arterial BP (MABP) is related to cardiac output (HR × stroke volume, which is the amount of blood being ejected from the heart per beat; see Figure 9-1) × TPR. Factors affecting MABP are shown in Figure 9-5. MABP can be estimated by DBP + ⅓ SBP − DBP (or pulse pressure), which shifts the pressure closer to DBP because more time is spent in diastole (Figure 9-6). A minimal MABP of approximately 70 mm Hg is needed to ensure adequate flow of blood to tissues and organs. Pressures lower than this level may lead to complications related to inadequate blood flow. Inadequate blood flow to the brain may result in lightheadedness or reduced mentation, and inadequate blood flow to other organs may result in shock. BP is controlled by multiple mechanisms (e.g., baroreceptors, chemoreceptors, hormones that control fluid balance) under a negative feedback control system. In adults, excessive BP, or hypertension, is defined as a resting SBP of more than 140 mm Hg or a resting DBP of more than 90 mm Hg. Hypertension will lead to damage to tissues (blood vessels) and organs (e.g., renal failure, stroke, myocardial infarction, blindness).

How to Measure Blood Pressure

BP can be *directly* measured through a catheter placed into an artery. This technique is used in more severely ill patients in the acute care setting. The majority of time BP is *indirectly* measured with a sphygmomanometer (BP cuff) and a stethoscope. The reason BP can be indirectly assessed is that the turbulent flow of fluid moving under pressure through a vessel produces an audible sound (bruit). Listening with a stethoscope (auscultation) over a normal artery will usually produce no sound because of laminar (smooth) flow. When cuff pressure exceeds SBP (Figure 9-7), all blood flow ceases in the artery distal to the occlusion and no sound is heard. As cuff pressure gradually decreases, there comes a point where SBP exceeds cuff pressure and blood flow is restored. When the pressure in the artery exceeds the pressure in the cuff, blood squirts through the artery, creating a bruit. The bruit continues until smooth laminar flow is returned.

The technique for measuring brachial artery BP is as follows:
- Explain the procedure if the patient is unaware of this measurement
- Obtain a resting BP after a 5-minute rest period
- Place the cuff on the patient's arm 2 to 4 cm above the antecubital area
- Palpate the brachial artery (medial to the biceps tendon)

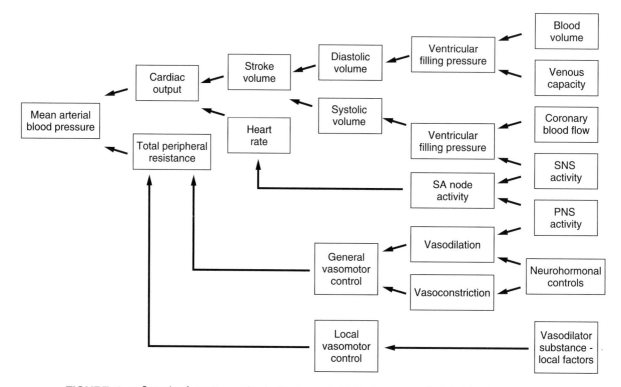

FIGURE 9-5 Cascade of events associated with mean arterial blood pressure. *PNS*, Peripheral nervous sytem; *SA*, sinoatrial; *SNS*, sympathetic nervous system.

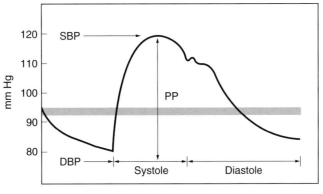

Systolic blood pressure (SBP) = 120 mm Hg
Diastolic blood pressure (DBP) = 80 mm Hg
Pulse pressure (PP) = SBP − DBP = 120 mm Hg − 80 mm Hg = 40 mm Hg
Systole = time during heart contraction
Diastole = time during heart relaxation
Estimate mean arterial blood pressure (MAPB) = DBP + 1/3 PP
MABP = 80 mm Hg + 1/3 × 40 mm Hg = 93 mm Hg

FIGURE 9-6 Example of estimation of mean arterial blood pressure.

- Place the diaphragm of the stethoscope over the brachial artery
- Inflate the cuff by squeezing the pressure bulb to greater than the patient SBP (which can be assessed by palpating the radial artery until the pulse disappears)
- Reduce the cuff pressure at a rate of 2 to 3 mm Hg/heartbeat[25]
- Listen for the first sound you hear (the bruit called Korotkoff 1, considered SBP)
- Listen for the sound to continue (Korotkoff 2 to 4)
- Listen for the last sound (DBP, or Korotkoff 5)
- Express BP in even numbers (e.g., 136/92 mm Hg)
- If this is the first time assessing BP in a patient, the BP should be assessed in both upper extremities, and the higher of the two pressures should be used in subsequent pressure measurements.

Common Errors in Measuring Blood Pressure

Common errors in BP determination are listed in Table 9-1. The most common errors include use of an inappropriate cuff size, inability to hear the bruits (listening through clothing, stethoscope is placed in the ears incorrectly, stethoscope is not correctly set for diaphragm etc.), and an uncalibrated sphygmomanometer.[12]

When Should Blood Pressure Be Assessed?

RESTING. Resting BP should be assessed during the systems review portion of the patient management. Because a large percentage of the population has hypertension that usually occurs without symptoms (the "silent killer"), resting BP should be assessed with all new patients. BP should also be assessed if a patient has any of the symptoms of hypertension or hypotension. Signs of hypertension include the following[15a]:

- Headache (usually occipital and present in the morning)
- Vertigo (dizziness)
- Flushed face

- Spontaneous epistaxis (nosebleed)
- Blurred vision
- Nocturnal urinary frequency

Hypertension is often clinically silent in the early and middle stages of the disease. Signs of hypotension include the following[15a]:

- Lightheadedness
- Syncope
- Mental or visual blurring
- Sense of weakness or "rubbery" legs

ACTIVITY. BP can also be used as an objective assessment of physiological changes from activity.[13] BP may be assessed during or immediately after the activity. With every metabolic equivalent increase in activity, SBP should rise by 9 ± 2 mm Hg. DBP should remain the same or decrease with activity. Changes in BP can also serve as an objective outcome measure of the effectiveness of interventions such as aerobic exercise training. Prolonged aerobic training has been associated with a reduction in resting and submaximal exertion BP.

MEDICAL CONSULTATION OR EMERGENCY SITUATIONS. Finally, BP can also be used to distinguish between a medical emergency (calling a code or dialing 911) and a suggested medical consult. With a high BP (e.g., 180/98 mm Hg), PTs can ask the patient if they could contact the patient's physician to set up an appointment or make sure that the patient contacts his or her physician. If the patient agrees, contact the physician. If he or she doesn't want you to contact the physician, educating the patient of the consequences and proper documentation is essential. A medical emergency would include (1) no BP or an extremely low BP in which a lack of normal mentation or unconsciousness exists and (2) an elevated BP more than 200/110 mm Hg at rest.

RELIABILITY AND VALIDITY OF THE BLOOD PRESSURE MEASUREMENT. BP validity is determined by comparing the values received with the direct BP measurement technique ("gold standard") to the

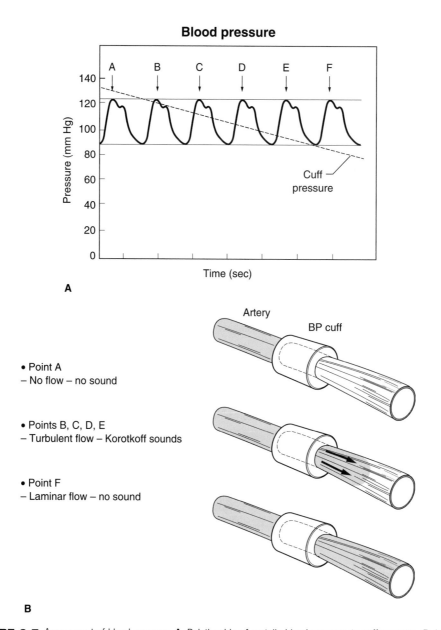

FIGURE 9-7 Assessment of blood pressure. **A,** Relationship of systolic blood pressure to cuff pressure. **B,** Indirect assessment of blood pressure auscultating over a normal artery.

indirect measurement technique. Measurements of resting BP vary from 3 to 24.6 mm Hg.[14-16] Resting BP taken by a trained person is usually within 3 to 5 mm Hg for SBP and 5 mm Hg for DBP. Measurements of BP during exercise or activity are often less valid and reliable. For example, when comparing direct and indirect methods on a cycle ergometer, SBP levels of −2.3 to 12.9 mm Hg and DBP levels of −4.3 to 18.2 mm Hg were found.[17] During peak anaerobic activity, direct and indirect measures of SBP were found to be highly correlated ($r = 0.87$; direct, 197 ± 11 mm Hg; indirect, 191 ± 9 mm Hg). During peak anaerobic activity, measures of DBP were found to be invalid.[18] After exercise, BP drops precipitously (in healthy persons) and therefore may not reflect actual BP during the activity. (Griffen et al.[16] provide a good review of this topic.)

RESTING BLOOD PRESSURE VALUES (NORMAL/ABNORMAL). Normal resting BP ranges, both SBP and DBP, are determined by age.

Table 9-2 lists normal and elevated pressure ranges for children, young adults, and adults. Table 9-3 lists the ranges of resting BP for optimal; normal; high normal; and hypertension stages 1, 2, and 3 in adults.

VALUES THAT MAY CONTRAINDICATE ACTIVITY OR REQUIRE TERMINATION OF ACTIVITY. BP values that contradict initiating activity vary by practice setting. Guidelines from the American College of Sports Medicine (ACSM) suggest activity is contraindicated for persons whose resting SBP is greater than 200 mm Hg or less than 80 mm Hg and DBP greater than 100 mm Hg. In some practice settings, such as the coronary care unit, where PTs are working with patients immediately after myocardial infarction, these critical BP values would be significantly less than those suggested by the ACSM. Termination of exercise is warranted with a rise in SBP greater than 250 mm Hg or DBP greater than 110 mm Hg. Because SBP

TABLE 9-1
Common Problems in Measuring Blood Pressure

Problem	Result	Recommendation
EQUIPMENT		
Stethoscope		
Ear pieces plugged	Poor sound transmission	Clean ear pieces
Ear pieces poorly fitting	Distorted sounds	Angle ear pieces forward
Bell or diaphragm cracked	Distorted sounds	Replace equipment
Tubing too long	Distorted sounds	Length from ear pieces to bell should be 30-38 cm (12-15 in)
Mercury manometer		
Meniscus not at 0 at rest	Inaccurate reading	Replace or remove mercury
Column not vertical	Inaccurate reading	Place manometer on level surface
Bouncing of mercury with inflation/deflation	Inaccurate reading	Clean tubing and air vent, replace mercury
Aneroid manometer		
Needle not at 0 at rest	Inaccurate reading	Recalibrate
Bladder cuff		
Too narrow for arm	Blood pressure too high	Use cuff length 80% of circumference
Too wide for arm	Unable to fit on arm	Use regular but longer cuff
Inflation system		
Faulty valves	Inaccurate reading Difficulty inflating and deflating bladder	Replace equipment
Leaky tubing or bulb	Inaccurate reading	Replace equipment
Observer		
Digit preference	Inaccurate reading	Be aware of tendency; record BP to nearest 2 mm Hg
Cut-off bias	Inaccurate reading	Record to nearest 2 mm Hg
Direction bias	Inaccurate reading	Record to nearest 2 mm Hg
Fatigue or poor memory	Inaccurate reading	Write down reading immediately
Subject		
Arm below heart level	Reading too high	Place patient with midpoint of upper arm at heart level
Arm above heart level	Reading too low	Place patient with midpoint of upper arm at heart level
Back unsupported	Reading too high	Avoid isometric exercise during measurement
Legs dangling	Reading too high	Avoid isometric exercise during measurement
Dysrhythmia	BP level variable	Make multiple measurements and average
Large or muscular arm	Reading too high	Use appropriate cuff size
Calcified arteries	Reading too high	Note presence of positive Osler sign in record
TECHNIQUE		
Cuff		
Wrapped too loosely	Reading too high	Rewrap more snugly
Applied over clothing	Inaccurate reading	Remove arm from sleeve
Manometer		
Below eye level	Reading too low	Place manometer at eye level
Above eye level	Reading too high	Place manometer at eye level
Stethoscope head		
Not in contact with skin	Extraneous noise	Place head correctly
Applied too firmly	Diastolic reading too low	Place head correctly
Not over artery	Sounds not well heard	Place head over palpated artery
Touching tubing or cuff	Extraneous noise	Place below edge of cuff
Palpatory pressure omitted	Danger of missing auscultatory gap Underestimation of systolic pressure	Routinely check systolic pressure by palpation first
Inflation level too high	Patient discomfort	Inflate to 30 mm Hg above palpatory blood pressure
Inflation level too low	Underestimation of systolic pressure	Inflate to 30 mm Hg above palpatory blood pressure
Inflation rate too slow	Patient discomfort Diastolic pressure too high	Inflate at even rate
Deflation rate too fast	Systolic pressure too low Diastolic pressure too high	Deflate at 2 mm Hg/sec or 2 mm Hg per beat
Deflation rate too slow	Forearm congestion Diastolic pressure too high	Deflate at 2 mm Hg/sec or 2 mm Hg per beat Completely deflate cuff at end of measurement

From Perloff D, Grim C, Flack J, et al: Human blood pressure determination by sphygmomanometry, *Circulation* 88(5 pt 1):2460-2470, 1993.
In patients in whom the Korotkoff sounds are faint and difficult to hear, the following technique may help: have the subject raise the arm over the head and make a fist several times. Inflate the cuff while the arm is still overhead but the hand relaxed to a level 50 mm Hg above expected systolic level. Have the patient lower the arm rapidly and measure the BP in the usual manner. Draining the venous blood in this fashion often amplifies the Korotkoff sounds and makes weak sounds, particularly diastolic sounds, more audible.

TABLE 9-2

Normal Ranges for Blood Pressure by Patient Age

		Systolic		Diastolic	
	Age (years)	Maximum	Minimum	Maximum	Minimum
Children	3 to 6	116	80	76	50
	6 to 9	122	84	78	55
Young adults	10 to 13	126	90	82	55
	14 to 19	142	90	86	60
Adults	20 to 60	150	90	90	60
	60+	160	90	95	60

From Blumenthal S: Report on the Task Force on Blood Pressure Control in Children, *Pediatrics* 59(suppl):797, 1977, and from The 1988 Report of the Joint National Committee on Detection, Evaluation, and Treatment of High Blood Pressure, *Arch Intern Med* 148:1023-1038, 1988.

TABLE 9-3

Classification of Blood Pressure for Adults 18 Years or Older*†

Category	SBP (mm Hg)		DBP (mm Hg)
Optimal‡	<120	and	>80
Normal	120-129	and	80-84
High normal	130-139	or	85-89
HYPERTENSION			
Stage 1	140-159	or	90-99
Stage 2	160-179	or	100-109
Stage 3	≥180	or	≥110

From The sixth report of the Joint National Committee on Prevention, Detection, Evaluation, and Treatment of High Blood Pressure, *Hypertension* 23:275-85, 1994, and the 6th Report of the U.S. Department of Health and Human Services, Public Health Service, National Institutes of Health, National Heart, Lung and Blood Institute, Bethesda, Md, 1997.

*Not taking antihypertensive drugs and not acutely ill. When SBP and DBP fall into different categories, the high category should be selected to classify the individual's BP status. In addition to classifying stages of hypertension on the basis of average BP levels, clinicians should specify presence or absence of target organ disease and additional risk factors. This specificity is important for risk classification and treatment.

†Based on the average of two or more readings taken at each of two or more visits after an initial screening.

‡Optimal BP regarding cardiovascular risk is less than 120/80 mm Hg. However, unusually low readings should be evaluated for clinical significance.

during activity increases above resting values, a drop in SBP by more than 10 to 20 mm Hg with maintenance of activity or increasing the load of activity is another reason to terminate activity. Again, depending on the type of patient and practice setting, ACSM guidelines may need to be modified.

OTHER EXAMPLES OF BLOOD PRESSURE MEASUREMENT. The ankle/brachial index (ABI) is a useful means of assessing the likelihood of peripheral arterial vascular disease. Peripheral arterial vascular disease is caused primarily by atherosclerosis (deposition of fibrous fatty plaque in the lining layer [intima] of the artery). Arteries of the lower extremities that are commonly affected include the iliac, femoral, and popliteal. ABI is calculated by dividing the SBP from the upper extremity by the SBP from the lower extremity. With the patient in the supine position, the SBP is measured in all four extremities. In the upper extremities the SBP is measured at the level of the heart (brachial pressure). In the lower extremities the SBP is measured in either the posterior tibial artery or the dorsalis pedis

artery. The ABI is then calculated by dividing each ankle pressure by the highest brachial pressure (Figure 9-8). ABI measurements less than 0.96 are considered abnormal, with lower values representing worsening of the disease (Figure 9-9). If ABI is less than 0.8 or the mean of three readings is less than 0.9, the predictive validity of the patient having significantly altered vessel lumen (e.g., peripheral vascular disease [PVD]) as determined by angiography is 95%.[19] Conversely, if ABI is greater than 1.1 or the mean of three measurements is greater than 1.0, PVD can be ruled out 99% of the time.[19] Usually a pocket Doppler is used to measure the lower extremity SBP, but sometimes the dorsalis pedis can be assessed with a stethoscope.[20] The determination of an abnormal ABI should be followed by a systematic search to locate the vessel lesion (abnormality in tissue structure). The BP cuff is moved progressively up the lower extremity for subsequent segmental SBP measurements (Figure 9-10). Measurements taken below and above the knee help locate the lesion site, which is revealed by a significant change in SBP from one location to another.

Finally, measurements of segmental BP can be used to examine local blood flow. Adequate blood flow is a critical variable in wound healing. Healing of an arterial ulcer requires an SBP more than 60 mm Hg for a patient without diabetes and greater than 80 mm Hg for a person with diabetes.

Common Conditions Related to Blood Pressure and the Physical Therapist's Role

Orthostatic Hypotension

Often in clinical situations, patients report a symptom of lightheadedness on rising from supine to sitting or standing. This rapid change in body position causes blood to pool in the abdomen and lower extremities because of gravity. The resulting reduction in venous return leads to a reduced stroke volume/cardiac output and a lowering of the BP. This drop in BP leads to a lack of activation of the baroreceptors. Reduced baroreceptor firing causes activation of the cardiorespiratory area of the medulla, which leads to a sympathetic discharge. This may help to increase BP by increasing TPR, venous return/cardiac output, and HR. Sometimes the sympathetic compensation is not enough and BP still falls. Reduction in BP by 10 to 20 mm Hg in either SBP or DBP or a rise in HR by 10 to 20 beats/min reveals orthostatic signs. Symptoms of

Abnormal ABI

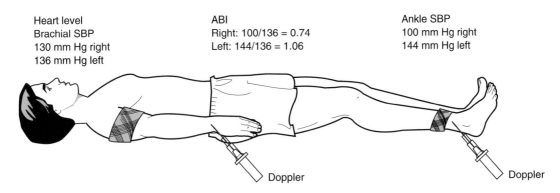

Heart level
Brachial SBP
130 mm Hg right
136 mm Hg left

ABI
Right: 100/136 = 0.74
Left: 144/136 = 1.06

Ankle SBP
100 mm Hg right
144 mm Hg left

Doppler   Doppler

FIGURE 9-8 Calculation of ankle/brachial index. *ABI*, Ankle/brachial index; *SBP*, systolic blood pressure.

orthostasis include lightheadedness, "rubbery legs," and feelings of syncope. Both HR and BP should be monitored in this patient population when going from supine to sitting or standing. When a patient reports orthostatic symptoms or orthostatic signs are revealed, the PT should have him or her sit or lie down. Performing "ankle pumps" while supine may help to equilibrate pressures and facilitate successful standing on the next attempt. If orthostatic signs or symptoms persist, notifying other medical personnel is warranted and standing activities should be discontinued.

Hypertension and Prehypertension

Hypertension can produce serious consequences, including the following:
- Stroke
- Myocardial infarction
- Congestive heart failure (see Figure 9-3)
- Peripheral vascular disease
- Renal failure
- Blindness

In the adult population, hypertension is defined as either SBP greater than 140 mm Hg or DBP greater than 90 mm Hg. Increasing grades of hypertension are shown in Table 9-3. If the pressures are high enough (e.g., more than 200/100 mm Hg), a single measure of BP is enough to diagnose hypertension. If the pressures are only slightly elevated (e.g., 146/92 mm Hg), three consecutive measures are needed to diagnose this borderline hypertension. After a diagnosis of hypertension, it is sometimes difficult to convince patients to comply with drug therapy.

ABI Interpretation

- \>0.96   Normal
- <0.95   Abnormal; stress testing is appropriate
- <0.8   Probable claudication
- <0.5   Multilevel disease or long segment occlusion
- <0.3   Ischemic rest pain; possible tissue necrosis

FIGURE 9-9 Interpretation of ankle/brachial index calculations. *SBP*, Systolic blood pressure. (From *Integrated ultrasound reference guide*, Plano, TX, 1996, Society of Diagnostic Medical Sonographers Education Foundation.)

Hypertension usually occurs without symptoms, and medications often produce side effects. Although hypertension is usually clinically silent, some associated symptoms may include morning headache, dizziness, and blurred vision. The benefits of routine physical activity (a walking program) should be discussed with patients and their physicians. Although treatment including dietary modifications, routine aerobic activities, weight loss, and medications has been shown to reduce hypertension, this regimen has not yet become the standard of care. New guidelines established by the American Heart Association have defined "prehypertension."[21] This new category establishes persons who have a strong potential of becoming hypertensive. This category helps to begin medical management with dietary alterations and increased activity level. Persons whose BP is more than 120/80 mm Hg fall into the prehypertensive range and should be counseled to increase their physical activity, reduce their weight (if increased), and reduce their salt intake.

Congestive Heart Failure: Jugular Venous Pressure, Palpation, and Engorgement

Right-sided congestive heart failure leads to elevated right atrial and systemic venous pressure (see Figure 9-1). If severe, the elevated pressure results in engorgement and distension of the jugular veins. Estimating jugular venous pressure has been shown to be a nonsensitive and nonspecific test for disease. When right atrial pressure increases above 15 mm Hg, the jugular vein will distend, a reliable measure of heart failure if the person is known to have impaired heart function. Other signs and symptoms associated with this rise in systemic venous pressure include increased fluid retention as evidenced by weight gain, dependent and pitting edema, and increased fatigue with activity.

Pulse Palpation for Heart Rate, Rhythm, and Patency of Blood Vessels

The heart pumps blood to the lungs for the exchange of gases and to the body for distribution of oxygen, nutrients, and other vital components in blood. The amount of blood pumped by the heart per minute is referred to as cardiac output and is calculated by multiplying HR by stroke volume (see Figure 9-1).

Segmental BP

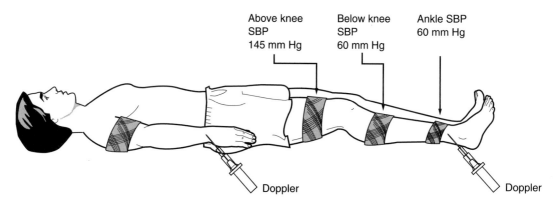

Above knee
SBP
145 mm Hg

Below knee
SBP
60 mm Hg

Ankle SBP
60 mm Hg

Doppler   Doppler

FIGURE 9-10 Segmental blood pressure assessment.

The rate and rhythm of blood pumped during myocardial contraction can be sensed by lightly placing the fingertips over the skin covering peripheral arteries (see Figure 9-1). As the myocardium contracts, a volume of blood is ejected from the left ventricle. The forward-rushing blood produces a pressure wave that extends from the aorta through the arterial system. This traveling pressure wave can be felt by the fingertips as a change in tension in the peripheral vessel. The rate and rhythm of the pressure wave are determined by the rate and rhythm of myocardial contractions. The strength of the peripheral pulse is determined by the difference between SBP and DBP (pulse pressure) and the elasticity of the blood vessels. Pulse pressure can vary from stroke volume (amount of blood ejected per beat) and the resistance to blood flow. With increased filling time, blood volume, or strength of contraction, the stroke volume increases and the pulse becomes stronger. With increased vascular resistance, reduced stroke volume, or hypovolemia (reduced blood volume), there is a reduction in pulse strength.

Because of the electrophysiologic properties of the pacemaker cells of the heart (sinoatrial node), the rate and rhythm of myocardial contraction at rest are usually stable. HR will increase or decrease in response to changes in energy demands, but rhythm usually remains regular because of the sinoatrial node. Factors affecting pulse and HR are shown in Figure 9-11.

- Age—infant increased and over 65 years reduced
- Gender—Male < Female
- Environmental/core temperature/hydration
- Physical activity
- Emotional status
- Medications (β-receptor blocker, Ca^{2+} channel blocker or β-receptor stimulators), chemicals (caffeine), hormones (thyroid hormones)
- Pain
- Pathology—anemia, CHF, autonomic dysfunction (e.g., diabetes, SCI, fever)
- Hydration status
- Physical condition

FIGURE 9-11 Factors affecting pulse rate. *CHF,* Congestive heart failure; *SCI,* spinal cord injury. (From Pierson F, Fairchild S: *Principles and techniques of patient care,* ed 3, Philadelphia, 2002, WB Saunders.)

Dysrhythmias (alterations in rate or rhythm) produce variations in the time of the myocardial contraction (interpulse interval). Unequal time in filling the heart will increase the variation in stroke volume and pulse pressure. A delay in filling leads to a stronger pulse because of increased stroke volume and pulse pressure, and a shortened time of filling leads to a reduced stroke volume and pulse pressure, therefore a weaker or missed pulse. Factors leading to dysrhythmias are shown in Figure 9-12.

HOW TO MEASURE THE PULSE. The pulse can be measured wherever the artery is large enough and close enough to the body surface to be felt with the fingertips. Common sites for pulse palpation include the radial, brachial, carotid, femoral, temporal, popliteal, and posterior tibial arteries. The examiner lightly palpates in the appropriate area for a change in tension. It is recommended that the examiner palpate with the second, third, or fourth digit of the dominant hand. The thumb is a less desirable digit for palpation because it has a particularly strong pulse of its own that sometimes interferes with accurately assessing the patient's pulse.[22,23]

Terms commonly used to describe pulse strength include "bounding" or "full" when the pulse is strong and "thready" or "weak" when the pulse volume is reduced. Pulse strength can also be quantified with a pulse scale. Two pulse scales are shown in Figure 9-13. To date, no validity or reliability studies have been performed with these scales. The rhythm of the pulse is often classified into one of three categories:

- Regular—similar rate (equal interpulse intervals) and volume (e.g., normal sinus rhythm or sinus tachycardia)
- Regularly irregular—the periodic nature of the irregularity comes at a specific time (interpulse intervals are unequal but the pattern is periodic and stable), such as bigeminy (one normal, one abnormal heart contraction) or trigeminy (two normal and one abnormal heart contraction)
- Irregularly irregular—no specific pattern, and rate and volume vary widely (interpulse intervals are unequal and the pattern is unstable), such as atrial fibrillation or multiple premature ventricular contractions not in a row or sequence

- Ischemia/hypoxia of the myocardium
- Sympathetic discharge—anxiety, exercise
- Acidosis
- Alterations in electrolytes (primarily ↓ K^+ <3.2 mEq/dL)
- Excessive stretch of the myocardium (e.g., CHF)
- Pharmacological agents
  —Sympathomimetics—caffeine
  —Antiarrhythmic drugs
  —Digitalis

FIGURE 9-12 Causes of dysrhythmias or ectopic pacemakers. *CHF,* Congestive heart failure.

- **Pulse 0-4 Scale***

  0 Absent pulse
  1 Markedly reduced pulse
  2 Slightly reduced pulse
  3 Normal pulse
  4 Bounding pulse

- **Pulse 0-3 Scale†**

  0 Absent
  1 Weak, thready
  2 Normal
  3 Full, bounding

FIGURE 9-13 Pulse assessment scales. (*From Greenberger NJ, Hinthorn DR: *History taking and physical examination*, St Louis, 1993, Mosby; and †Jarvis C: *Examination and health assessment*, Philadelphia, 1992, WB Saunders.)

COMMON ERRORS IN PALPATING THE PULSE. When palpating for HR and rhythm, the most common problem is examiner error. The inability to locate a pulse can be caused by anatomic variation, but more often the examiner's fingers are placed in the wrong area or are pressing too strongly. Figure 9-14 lists some common causes of false-positive or false-negative results when assessing pulse rate and rhythm. When a patient has a dysrhythmia such as atrial fibrillation or a premature beat, a pulse deficit may be found. The pulse deficit is the difference between the number of heart contractions and the HR as determined by pulse palpation. The mechanism is shown in Figures 9-15 and 9-16. If, because of changes in filling time, the heart contracts before the left ventricle has filled completely, the volume of blood ejected (and therefore the pulse pressure) is reduced. The weakened pulse pressure may then be below threshold by the time the pressure wave has traveled down the vascular system to the point where the examiner is palpating, thereby causing the examiner to miss feeling the beat. When a person has an irregularly irregular pulse, HR should be determined by electrocardiography or auscultation (listening to the heart [apical pulse] with a stethoscope). When checking for the patency (opening) of a vessel, hypovolemia, shock, and obesity may cause a false-negative reading. False-

positive measures of patency may be caused by hypervolemia or anorexia.

When Heart Rate Should be Assessed

RESTING HEART RATE. HR assessment should occur during the systems review in all patients on initial visit. HR is an objective, indirect measure of the status or condition of the cardiovascular system. Baseline measurements should be taken only after a 2- to 5-minute rest period (sitting or reclining). The rest period ensures baseline metabolic conditions. Normal resting values of HR by age are listed in Table 9-4. A 15- to 30-second monitoring period should be used to determine resting HR.[24]

HEART RATE DURING ACTIVITY. During activity HR is an objective, indirect measure of work intensity. HR responds to changes in work load in a relatively linear fashion. Exercise HR should be assessed with a 10-second monitoring period because of the rapid decline in HR with cessation of the activity.[25,26] During training, HR should be assessed to ensure training intensity is within the guidelines set forth by the American Heart Association (target HR). One effect of prolonged aerobic training (weeks to months) is a reduction in HR under resting and submaximal working conditions. Therefore HR can serve as an outcome measure indicating the effectiveness of long-term aerobic training.

Target HR as a measure of exercise intensity must be used in reference to some expected maximal value. In the healthy, normal population, maximal HR can be estimated by subtracting the subject's age from 220. Newer calculations are also available and may improve the prediction of maximal HR.[27] Although this estimate varies by 15 to 20 beats/min, it is often commonly used. This estimate should not be used in persons with underlying pathologic conditions or persons taking medications that affect HR (e.g., β-blockers, calcium channel blockers).

EMERGENCY SITUATIONS. HR should also be assessed in an emergency situation. The HR may differentiate "calling a code" or dialing 911 from merely initiating a medical consult. When signs or symptoms of circulatory decompensation arise in a patient (Figure 9-17), palpation of the pulse is useful but is neither sensitive nor specific. Auscultation of the heart may often aid in determining HR in persons with a weak or irregular pulse. Clinical vascular testing with a Doppler device can be useful for assessing patency of the arteries. This procedure may also be coupled with a sphygmomanometer for determining SBP.

VALIDITY OF MEASUREMENT. The gold standard for determining HR is an electrocardiogram. HR should be assessed as an objective measure of resting metabolic activity. At rest, palpation measurement of HR performed by trained personnel can vary by 3 to 5 beats/min compared with the gold standard. During activity, palpation measurement of HR performed by trained personnel can vary by 3 to 10 beats/min compared with the gold standard. The validity of exercise HR requires the measurement be taken quickly and immediately after the cessation of activity because HR drops precipitously after exercise in a healthy person.[25]

- False positives
  —Anorexia
  —Examiner error (e.g., examiner's digital pulse)
- False negatives
  —Obesity
  —Edema
  —Scar tissue
  —Thickened skin
  —Examiner error (e.g., palpation in wrong area)

FIGURE 9-14 Potential errors in pulse assessment.

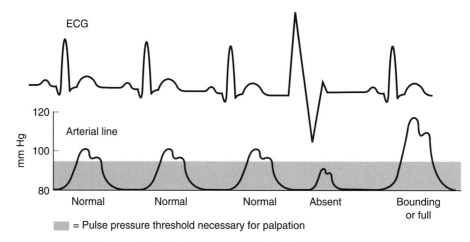

FIGURE 9-15 Palpating pulse with premature contractions (e.g., premature ventricular contraction).

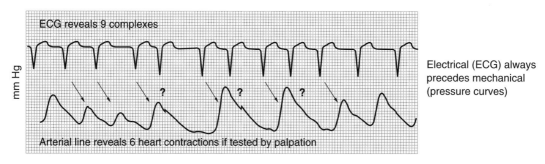

FIGURE 9-16 Pulse "inaccuracy" deficit.

Common Conditions Related to Heart Rate and Rhythm and the Physical Therapist's Role

Dysrhythmias

Physical therapists maybe the first health care practitioner to assess the patient's HR and rhythm at rest and during activity. Dysrhythmias can be an alteration in HR or rhythm. Many dysrhythmias are common and of little concern under certain circumstances. For example, sinus tachycardia (an HR more than 100 beats/min) is usual in a person performing physical activity or in an infant at rest. But sinus tachycardia can be abnormal in a healthy person without any other contributing factors who is resting. Sinus bradycardia, an HR of less than 60 beats/min, is normal in a well-trained aerobic athlete or in a person taking β receptor–blocking medication. Consequently sinus bradycardia of 45 beats/min in an individual who is 65 years old and not in good shape or taking medications that affect HR can also be an ominous sign.

A sudden change in HR (more than 20 to 40 beats/min), either an increase or decrease, at rest or during activity may be a signal of an ectopic pacemaker or conduction abnormality. For example, a patient's resting HR that is 76 beats/min and suddenly rises to 166 beats/min without any physiological or psychological need is abnormal. Likewise a sudden drop with

maintained or increasing level of work is also abnormal. Changes in rhythm can also be either a normal response to workload or a life-threatening malfunction in cardiac regulation. As a basic rule of thumb, if a patient has a normal sinus rhythm and the heart rhythm suddenly becomes irregular, he or she should be asked if a history of cardiac dysrhythmia is present and be monitored for cardiac decompensation. If the person is not showing signs or symptoms of cardiac decompensation, referral to a physician is warranted. Usually more then 6 abnormal beats in a minute, such as with premature ventricular contractions (the most common type of ectopic beat), requires medical attention. Depending on the severity of the symptoms caused by the dysrhythmia, if the patient shows signs of severe cardiac compromise (see Figure 9-17), this may be a medical emergency. If there is no pulse, calling a code or dialing 911 and starting cardiopulmonary resuscitation (CPR) are necessary. If a patient is known to have a dysrhythmia, accurate HR measurement is determined by electrocardiogram or auscultation.[28]

Ventilatory Rate and Rhythm

The ventilatory musculature pumps air into and out of the lungs for the exchange of gases (oxygen and carbon dioxide). The amount of air moved by the lungs per minute is referred to

TABLE 9-4

Resting Pulse Rate

Norms	Average (beats/min)	Limits
Fetal	120-160	—
Newborn	120	70-190
1 year	120	80-160
2 years	110	80-130
4 years	100	80-120
6 years	100	75-115
8-10 years	90	70-110
12 YEARS		
Female	90	70-110
Male	85	65-105
14 YEARS		
Female	85	65-105
Male	80	60-100
16 YEARS		
Female	80	60-100
Male	75	55-95
18 YEARS		
Female	75	55-95
Male	70	50-90
Well-conditioned athlete	50-60	50-100
Adult	—	60-100
Aging	—	60-100

Adapted from Jarvis C: *Physical examination and assessment*, Philadelphia, 1992, WB Saunders, p 202.

as minute ventilation and is calculated by multiplying ventilatory rate by tidal volume (see Figure 9-1). The rate and rhythm of air moved during ventilation can be sensed by observing the chest rise and fall in correlation to time. Normal rate for an adult is 12 to 20 breaths/min. Normal tidal volume in an adult is approximately 500 mL, with expiration being twice as long as inspiration. Tidal volume can be greater or less depending on body size. Observing the rate, volume, and rhythm is necessary during the systems review in the pulmonary screen. Terms to describe ventilatory rate and rhythm or breathing patterns include[29]:

- Apnea: no breathing
- Tachypnea: rate more than 20 breaths/min in an adult
- Bradypnea: rate of less than 12 breaths/min in an adult

- Hyperpnea: normal rate but increased volume
- Hypopnea: normal rate but decreased volume
- Hyperventilation: increased rate and volume
- Hypoventilation: decreased rate and volume
- Cheyne-Stokes: hyperventilation followed by hypoventilation then apnea, with the cycle repeating
- Orthopnea: difficulty breathing while patient is horizontal with easing of breathing with more vertical positioning
- Dyspnea: labored or difficult breathing

How to Measure Ventilation

Ventilation is observed by watching the chest rise and fall in relation to time. Usually this is assessed in a 30-second to 1-minute time interval. Because ventilation is under both involuntary and voluntary control, awareness by the patient of the PT's observation may cause ventilation to be modified from the usual resting pattern. A trick that is often used is to appear as if taking a pulse measurement, but actually observe the rise and fall of the chest.[30] Shallow breathing also makes this assessment more difficult. Ventilatory rate and rhythm should be assessed on the first patient visit during the systems review portion of the examination. If the patient reveals any abnormality in ventilatory rate or rhythm, further examination (auscultation and examination of symptoms) is required.[23a]

VALIDITY OF MEASUREMENT. A study performed on nurses assessing ventilatory rate revealed a 20% error by the nurses one third of the time.[31] Another study on interobserver reliability in physicians, nurses, and respiratory therapists revealed an excellent kappa value when observing children who were being extubated.

Resting Values (Normal/Abnormal)

Normal resting values for breathing rate change with age. See Figure 9-18 for normal values by age.

Activity Values

With activity, ventilatory rate and volume increase to supply the needed oxygen to the active tissues and remove synthesized carbon dioxide. The more strenuous the activity, the greater the oxygen demand. Once a person is performing activity that is above his or her anaerobic threshold (beginning production of lactic acid by the muscles), this metabolic

Symptoms	Signs
• Angina	• Dysrhythmias
• Palpitations	• Syncope
• Dyspnea or shortness of breath	• Dyspnea or shortness of breath (using scale)
• Fatigue	• Dependent edema
	• Hemoptysis (coughing blood)
	• Cyanosis

FIGURE 9-17 Classic cardiac signs and symptoms of decompensation. (Adapted from Swartz MH: *Textbook of physical diagnosis: history and examination*, ed 4, Philadelphia, 2002, WB Saunders, pp 345-390.)

Age	Breaths/min
Neonate	30-40
1 year	20-40
2 year	25-32
4 year	23-30
6 year	21-26
8-10 year	20-26
12-14 year	18-22
16 year	16-20
18 year	12-20
Adult	10-20

FIGURE 9-18 Normal resting respiratory rates. (Adapted from Jarvis C: *Physical examination and assessment*, Philadelphia, 1992, WB Saunders, p 203.)

acidosis is compensated by respiratory alkalosis, which means hyperventilation begins. Clinically this often occurs when the patient has difficulty speaking because of labored breathing. It should be noted that anaerobic threshold decreases with detraining, so with some deconditioned patients anaerobic threshold may occur with even slow ambulation down the hallway.

Values That May Contraindicate Activity or Require Termination of Activity

ACSM[32] recommends not performing an endurance test if the patient's resting respiratory rate is more than 45 breaths/min. If the patient reports dyspnea with activity, the Ranchos Los Amigos Physical Therapy Department recommends the following tool to quantify the level of involvement. The patient is asked to inhale normally and then count to 15 out loud over a 7.5- to 8-second time period:

Level 0: on a single breath
Level 1: requires two breaths
Level 2: requires three breaths

Level 3: requires four breaths
Level 4: unable to count

If the dyspnea is severe enough or a new onset, this may be a reason to decrease or stop activity level. For persons with chest discomfort, see the questions outlined in Figure 9-19.

Other Examples of Measurement

Although not a measure of ventilatory rate or rhythm, oxygen saturation (SaO_2), or pulse oxygen, is a useful measurement to assess the adequacy of ventilation. Pulse oxygen reveals the saturation of oxygen on hemoglobin contained in the erythrocytes (red blood cells). This measurement tells one piece of the oxygen delivery equation: the percentage of oxygen on hemoglobin. To get the full picture of oxygen delivery, the patient's hematocrit and hemoglobin levels must also be known. A person may have normal oxygen saturation, but if he or she is anemic the delivery of oxygen to tissue can be impaired. Normal values for oxygen saturation are between 90% and 100% in systemic arterial blood. If a person has no

If a person reports chest discomfort:

- Stop any activity and place the person in a comfortable position (sitting or lying)
- Monitor vital signs
- Ask if he or she has been diagnosed with heart disease
- If yes, then
  —Ask if this symptom is usual or different
  —Ask if he or she has medication (e.g., nitroglycerin)
  —Allow administration of up to three tablets in a 10-minute period and, if symptoms don't resolve, get the patient to the emergency department or seek medical attention
- If no, then
  —Ask patient to describe the discomfort
  —Ask what precipitated the discomfort
  —Ask whether the discomfort is getting worse or better
  —If signs and symptoms get better and do not appear to be musculoskeletal (movement or revealed by palpation) in origin, have the patient see his or her physician
  —If the signs and symptoms are worsening, get the patient to the emergency department
- Common changes in vital signs with chest discomfort from coronary artery disease
  —Pulse may change from normal sinus rhythm to dysrhythmia (ischemia of heart cells leads to overexcitability and ectopic pacemakers), causing the pulse to change in rhythm
  —Pulse rate may increase (anxiety and pain) or decrease (damage to pacemaker cells)
  —BP may increase (anxiety and pain) or decrease (damage to myocardium)
  —Ventilatory rate usually increases (anxiety and pain) with tidal volume declining (anxiety and pain)
- Auscultate heart for changes in rate, rhythm, or sound (S3)
- Ask if he or she has been diagnosed with lung disease
- If yes, then
  —Ask if this symptom is usual or different
  —Ask if he or she has medication (inhaler)
  —Allow use of the inhaler and see if symptoms resolve. If symptoms don't resolve and are getting worse, get the patient to the emergency department or seek medical attention
- If no, then
  —Ask patient to describe the discomfort
  —Ask what precipitated the discomfort
  —Ask whether the discomfort is getting worse or better
  —If signs and symptoms are getting better and do not appear to be musculoskeletal (movement or revealed by palpation) in origin, have the patient see his or her physician
  —If the signs and symptoms are worsening, get the patient to the emergency department
- Common changes in vital signs with chest discomfort from lung disease
  —Ventilatory rate usually increases with tidal volume increases
  —Pulse rate will usually increase
  —BP may increase (anxiety and pain) or decrease (lack of normal blood flow through lungs or retention of CO_2, which is a potent vasodilator)
  —Auscultate lung for changes in ventilatory sounds (crackles, wheezes, lack of normal ventilation)

FIGURE 9-19 Guidelines for patients with onset of chest pain or discomfort.

known lung pathology and an oxygen saturation of less than 90%, you need to:

- Stop performing any physical activity
- If performing physical activity, then
  - —Stop any activity
  - —Retake the measurement with the patient being still
  - —Check that the device is on properly
  - —If the measurement is valid, notify medical personnel
  - —Continue to monitor the patient

If the person has known lung disease, a resting value of less than 90% is often found. PTs should stop activity if SaO_2 lowers by 5% below resting value or is less than 88% in persons with right-sided heart failure (cor pulmonale). Patients with lung disease should not have a resting SaO_2 of less than 80%. Patients whose lung disease causes their SaO_2 to be less than 88% usually receive supplemental oxygen. Depending on state laws, it is often advisable when performing activity to increase the patient's flow of oxygen to maintain oxygen saturation if needed. The PT must remember to lower the oxygen flow level back to the normal flow once activity has ended.

Auscultation of the Heart and Lungs

Differentiating the various heart and lung sounds that accompany various disorders or pathologic conditions requires skill beyond reading this text. When compared with a gold standard, even physicians who are trained in this skill are often no better than chance at detecting true abnormalities in heart and lung sounds.[33,34] PTs should familiarize themselves with normal heart and lung sounds. The ability to merely differentiate abnormal from normal sounds is an important first step in using auscultation to detect pathologic conditions. Differentiating the type of pathologic feature is beyond the scope of our practice. Some PTs are skilled in auscultation as a diagnostic procedure, particularly those who have received specialized training or are involved in settings that use these techniques.

Using a Stethoscope

The head of a stethoscope usually contains both a bell and a diaphragm (Figure 9-20). The smaller diameter bell is more effective in discriminating low-frequency heart sounds (S_3), whereas the larger diameter diaphragm is more effective in discriminating high-frequency heart sounds (S_1 and S_2), BP, and lung sounds. The bell and diaphragm can be switched by rotating the head of the stethoscope. The price of the stethoscope is determined, in part, by the quality of the head and the sound transmission. Less expensive stethoscopes tend to have poorer quality sound resolution, and more expensive stethoscopes tend to have higher quality sound resolution. A shorter, thicker tube connecting the head of the stethoscope to comfortable, well-fitting earpieces aids in sound quality along with reduced environmental noises.

When using a stethoscope for auscultation of either heart or lung sounds, proper anatomic placement is essential. Firmness of pressure of the stethoscope head onto the body is critical. The pressure should be sufficient to ensure that the entire head of the scope (either diaphragm or bell) is in direct

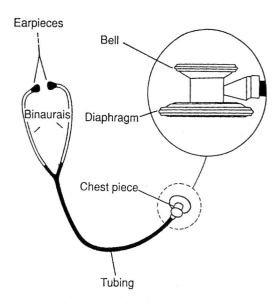

FIGURE 9-20 Components of a stethoscope. (From Boissonnault WG: *Examination in physical therapy practice: screening for medical disease*, ed 2, Philadelphia, 1995, Churchill Livingstone, p 76.)

contact with the underlying skin. Excessive or inadequate pressure leads to extraneous noise and potential inaccuracy of measurement.

When to Measure Heart and Lung Sounds

Measurement of heart and lung sounds should occur in all persons with a history of chronic cardiac or pulmonary conditions or signs or symptoms of cardiopulmonary distress. Differentiation of normal sounds from abnormal should be a goal.

Normal Heart Sounds

The normal heart sound of "lub dub," or S_1 and S_2, is attributed to the vibrations caused by the closure of the heart valves. With the increased pressure caused by contraction of the heart muscle (systole), the right and left atrioventricular (AV) valves (commonly called the tricuspid [T_1] and mitral [M_1] valves) slam shut. This closing of the AV valves causes the S_1 heart sound or the characteristic "lub." This is followed by the opening of the semilunar valves, which are the aortic and pulmonic valves. No heart sound occurs with the opening of normal valves. At the end of systole or the ejection phase of the contraction, the closing of the aortic and pulmonic valves causes the S_2 heart sound, or the characteristic "dub." These sounds can be heard with varying intensity over different areas on the chest (Figure 9-21). Probably the best site for hearing S_1 and S_2 is the apex of the heart. With deep inhalation the S_2 sound can be differentiated into two components, aortic (A_2) and pulmonic (P_2). Deep inhalation creates an interval between A_2 and P_2 because of basic cardiac physiological characteristics. During deep inhalation thoracic pressure is decreased. During the decreased thoracic pressure, venous return to the heart is increased. The increased venous return produces an increased filling of the right side of the heart. The increased venous

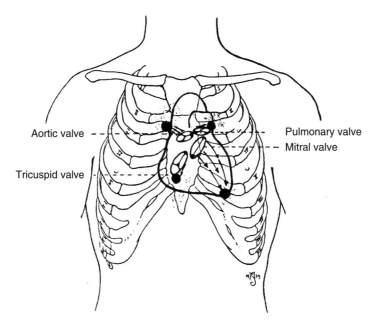

Aortic valve – – –

Pulmonary valve – – –
Mitral valve

Tricuspid valve –

FIGURE 9-21 Anatomic location of heart valves and areas where sounds are best heard. (From Boissonnault WG: *Examination in physical therapy practice: screening for medical disease*, ed 2, Philadelphia, 1995, Churchill Livingstone, p 76; and Delp M, Manning R: *Major physical diagnosis*, ed 8, Philadelphia, 1979, WB Saunders.)

return produces an increased stroke volume and delays the closure of the pulmonic valve, thereby separating the A_2 and P_2 sounds.

Depictions and recordings of these sounds may be found on the Internet at http://blaufuss.org.

Abnormal Heart Sounds

Reliable detection of abnormal heart sounds requires considerable practice. Even with considerable experience, reliability and validity of measurement by physicians are limited.[33] Recognition of murmurs, S_3 or gallop, and pericardial friction are three frequently occurring abnormal heart sounds that PTs should be able to detect.

Murmurs are caused by abnormal vibrations through stenotic valves (narrowed opening), incompetent valves (leaky valves), high flow, or abnormal communication between blood vessels (e.g., patent ductus arteriosus) or heart chambers (ventricular septal defects). Murmurs can be divided into systolic, which produce a "lub-swish-dub" sound; diastolic, which produce a "lub-dub-swish" sound; and continuous, which produce a "lub-swish-dub-swish" sound. For example, a stenotic aortic valve can produce a systolic murmur, whereas an incompetent aortic valve can produce a diastolic murmur. Detection of a murmur is based on a complete understanding of normal anatomy and physiological characteristics of the heart and its valves. Depending on type and severity of murmur, certain types of physical activity might be contraindicated. If a patient is unaware of an existing murmur and the PT detects an abnormal heart sound, a medical consult is in order. Signs and symptoms of moderate to severe murmurs may include cardiopulmonary compromise at rest or with increasing physical activity (see Figure 9-17).

S_3, or gallop, is caused by an excessive amount of high-pressure blood from the atrium hitting a distended ventricular wall during diastole. The S_3 sound is found with either right- or left-sided congestive heart failure (CHF). This sound is normal in children until their 20s but abnormal in persons older than 40 years. The mnemonic "Ken-tuk-ee" is often used to mimic the sound of S_3, which is often compared to a horse galloping. In persons with CHF, this sound may occur at rest or with increasing activity. This can be accompanied by the symptoms of shortness of breath or dyspnea found with left-sided heart failure. Excessive physical activity is contraindicated when the S_3 sound is present.

The pericardial friction rub sound is caused by friction between the outer wall of the heart (epicardium or the visceral layer of the serous pericardium) and the pericardium (parietal layer of the serous pericardium) that occurs with pericarditis. Excessive physical activity is contraindicated with this sign because inflammation would be potentially worsened by increased HR and BP, causing more rubbing of the two surfaces.

Other websites for normal and abnormal heart sounds include the following:
- http://www.medlib.com/spi/coolstuff2.htm
- http://www.wilkes.med.ucla.edu/intro.html
- http://www.bioscience.org/atlases/heart

Normal Lung Sounds

Normal breath sounds occur because of the turbulence of air flow. This turbulence is related to the volume of air moving and the diameter of the lung passageways. The diameter of the lung passageways determines the resistance to the flow, which leads to the turbulence. Depending on the patient's position and anatomic location of assessment, auscultation of normal breath sounds varies. The three major normal breath sounds are as follows[35]:

1. Vesicular sounds are heard over the lung parenchyma, primarily alveoli or smaller air passageways. These sounds, heard primarily on inhalation, are described as "soft," with exhalation occurring without a break (continuous) and lasting only about a third of the inspiratory time. In a normal healthy person, vesicular sounds are heard with auscultation over the peripheral lung fields on the anterior, posterior, and lateral chest walls.

2. Bronchial sounds are heard over the trachea and major bronchi. These sounds are much louder than the vesicular breath sounds because of the large volume of air moving. They have a higher pitch and last for an equal time during inhalation and exhalation. There is a notable pause between inhalation and exhalation (discontinuous). In a normal healthy person, bronchial breath sounds are heard with auscultation over the trachea.

3. Bronchovesicular sounds are heard over the junction of the major bronchi as air moves into the smaller segmental bronchi. These sounds are similar to bronchial sounds but occur without any pause between inhalation and exhalation. In a normal healthy person, bronchovesicular breath sounds are heard with auscultation over the posterior chest wall (lateral to the thoracic spine) at the level of the scapula.

With various pathologic conditions, normal breath sounds may be heard in anatomic areas where they should not occur. For example, listening over the peripheral lung fields in a normal healthy person should reveal vesicular sounds. In the presence of a pathologic condition that causes consolidation within the lung (e.g., pneumonia or significant atelectasis), vesicular sounds are replaced by bronchial sounds in the peripheral lung fields. This is because with consolidation of the lung parenchyma, movement of air in the large airways is transmitted through the nonventilated consolidated areas.

Abnormal "Adventitious" Lung Sounds

The use of auscultation to detect abnormal breath sounds reliably requires considerable practice. PTs, despite practice and experience, have shown limited reliability and validity in using auscultation to detect abnormal breath sounds.[34,36] Abnormal or adventitious (extra) sounds are caused by pathologic alterations in the respiratory process. Because the reliable detection of abnormal breath sounds is difficult, PTs should begin by differentiating abnormal sounds from normal sounds. Three abnormal sounds are of particular importance: crackles, wheezes, and pleural friction rubs.

Crackles are a discontinuous "popping" sound most often heard during inhalation. During inhalation, crackles are caused by the reinflation of closed alveoli. Crackles may also occur during exhalation as air moves over the secretions present in pneumonia and CHF. Crackles are present in pathologic conditions that cause restriction or obstruction of the lung and also during deep breathing in patients with atelectasis. Differentiating whether the crackle occurs during inhalation or exhalation helps with diagnostic categorization.

Wheezes are caused by the faster movement of turbulent air through narrowed passageways that may also contain secretions (mucus). Narrowed passageways with secretions lead to airway obstruction and trapping of air in the distal portions of the lung. Airway obstruction can be classically found with acute conditions such as asthma or chronic obstructive pulmonary disease. Wheezes are considered a continuous adventitious sound that usually occur on exhalation and can be monophonic (single frequency musical note) or polyphonic (multiple musical notes).

Pleural friction rub, as the name implies, occurs when the visceral and parietal layers of the pleural sac become inflamed (pleuritis) or thickened and rub against one another during movement of the chest wall. The friction between inflamed pleural tissues produces a lower pitched sound (compared with crackles) and may be heard during both inhalation and exhalation.

Examination of lung sounds should follow a standardized procedure designed to compare the sounds heard from one lung with those heard from the other. The procedure should include examination of apical, mid, and lower lobes both anteriorly and posteriorly. Examination results should be classified into major categories; their interpretation is shown in Figure 9-22. See Table 9-5 for a description of terms appropriate for documenting sounds and the interpretation of various sounds.

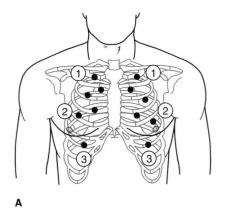
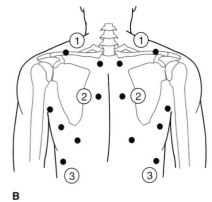

FIGURE 9-22 One method of auscultating the chest. **A,** Anterior chest wall; **B,** posterior chest wall. (From Buckingham EB: *A primer of clinical diagnosis*, ed 2, New York, 1979, Harper & Row.)

TABLE 9-5

Guidelines for the Documentation and Interpretation of Auscultated Sounds

Type of Sound	Nomenclature	Interpretation
Breath sound	Normal	Normal, air-filled lung
	Decreased	Hyperinflation in chronic obstructive pulmonary disease
		Hypoinflation in acute lung disease (e.g., atelectasis, pneumothorax, pleural effusion)
	Absent	Pleural effusion
		Pneumothorax
		Severe hyperinflation
		Obesity
	Bronchial	Consolidation
		Atelectasis with adjacent patent airway
	Crackles	Secretions, if biphasic
		Deflation, if monophasic
	Wheezes	Diffuse airway obstruction if polyphonic; localized stenosis if monophonic
Extrapulmonary adventitious sounds	Pleural rub	Pleural inflammation or reaction
	Pericardial rub	Pericardial inflammation

Adapted from Irwin S, Tecklin JS: *Cardiopulmonary physical therapy*, ed 2, St Louis, 1990, CV Mosby, p 289.

The following websites provide samples of normal and abnormal breath sounds:
- http://www.wilkes.med.ucla.edu/lungintro.htm
- http://www.rale.ca

Common Conditions Related to Heart and Breath Sounds and the Physical Therapist's Role

Approximately 5 million Americans have CHF. The pharmacotherapeutic approach to managing this condition involves administration of iatrogenic agents that improve heart function, vasodilating agents that reduce the resistance to blood flow, and diuretics that reduce blood volume. Proper medical management can lead to a reduction of signs and symptoms of CHF. Physical activity is recommended for persons with mild to moderate CHF. CHF is a commonly seen comorbidity in the physical therapy clinic because it frequently accompanies the primary movement-related disorders for which patients are seen. The competent physical therapy management of patients with CHF requires knowledge of the condition, including signs and symptoms that the condition is becoming worse. If a patient with CHF reports increasing dyspnea, auscultation of the lungs may reveal crackles and auscultation of the heart may reveal an S_3 heart sound. Depending on the practice setting, either of these sounds may warrant a medical referral. If the sounds become worse, this may signal a medical emergency if signs and symptoms of cardiopulmonary compromise occur (see Figure 9-17).

Summary

Physiological measures of the cardiovascular and respiratory systems, as well as measures of body composition, are important because they reflect the patient's general health and wellness. BP, ventilatory rate, and HR provide a basic physiological profile of the cardiovascular and pulmonary systems. Heart and lung sounds can help differentiate persons with normal function from those with disease. BMI has been shown to be related to the risk of developing many of the diseases commonly seen in the physical therapy clinic (osteoarthritis, diabetes, myocardial infarction, stroke, and certain types of cancer). Normal values and ranges have been established for these physiological measures at rest and during activity for various age groups. Significant deviations from these norms may indicate an abnormal condition and are valuable in assessing the risk of developing a disease or disorder. Establishing baseline measurements of vital signs and body composition is a central component of competent health care management. They can be used to help ensure the safety of initiating an exercise program, establish intervention goals, assist in developing an intervention plan, and assess the individual's response to intervention (establish treatment effectiveness). The practitioner's ability to assess and interpret measures of these important physiological parameters (vital signs) accurately at rest and during activity and recovery is an important clinical competency in an environment of increasingly independent physical therapy practice.

REFERENCES

1. *ACSM guidelines for exercise testing and prescription*, ed 6, Philadelphia, 2000, American College of Sports Medicine, Lippincott, Williams & Wilkins.
2. American Physical Therapy Association: Guide to physical therapy practice, ed 2, *Phys Ther* 81:9-744, 2001.
3. Bailey RH, Bauer JH: A review of common errors in the indirect measurement of blood pressure. Sphygmomanometry, *Arch Intern Med* 153: 2741-2748, 1993.
4. Bond Brill J, Perry AC, Parker L, et al: Dose-response effect of walking exercise on weight loss. How much is enough? *Int J Obes Relat Metab Disord* 26:1484-1493, 2002.
5. Brooks D, Wilson L, Kelsey C: Accuracy and reliability of "specialized" physical therapists in auscultating tape-recorded lung sounds, *Physiother Can* 45:21-24, 1993.
6. Brooks D, Thomas J: Interrater reliability of auscultation of breath sounds among physical therapists, *Phys Ther* 75:1082-1088, 1995.
7. Butman SM, Ewy GA, Standen JR, et al: Bedside cardiovascular examination in patients with severe chronic heart failure: importance of rest or inducible jugular venous distension, *J Am Coll Cardiol* 22:968-974, 1993.
8. Campbell NR, Chockalingam A, Fodor JG, et al: Accurate, reproducible measurement of blood pressure, *CMAJ* 143:19-24, 1990.
9. Campbell NR, McKay DW: Accurate blood pressure measurement: why does it matter? *CMAJ* 161:277-278, 1999.
10. Chobanian AV, et al for the National Heart, Lung, and Blood Institute Joint National Committee on Prevention, Detection, Evaluation, and Treatment of High Blood Pressure; National High Blood Pressure Education Program Coordinating Committee: The seventh report of the Joint National Committee on Prevention, Detection, Evaluation, and Treatment of High Blood Pressure: the JNC 7 report, *JAMA* 289: 2560-2572, 2003.
11. Christian K, Roberts C, Nosratola D, et al: Effect of diet and exercise intervention on blood pressure, insulin, oxidative stress and nitric oxide availability, *Circulation* 106:2530, 2002.
12. Clinical guidelines on the identification, evaluation, and treatment of overweight and obesity in adults, http://www.nhlbi.nih.gov/guidelines/obesity/ob_home.htm. Accessed June 2, 2004.

13. Eason JM: Cardiopulmonary assessment, *Cardiopulmonary Phys Ther J* 10:135-142, 1999.
14. Freedman DS, Khan LK, Serdula MK, et al: Trends and correlates of class three obesity in the United States from 1990 through 2000, *JAMA* 288:1758-1761, 2002.
15a. Goodman CC, Snyder TE: *Differential diagnosis in physical therapy*, Philadelphia, 1995, WB Saunders.
15. Frese EM, Richter RR, Burlis TV: Self-reported measurement of heart rate and blood pressure in patients by physical therapy clinical instructors, *Phys Ther* 82:1192-1200, 2002.
16. Griffin SE, Robergs RA, Heyward VH: Blood pressure measurement during exercise: a review. *Med Sci Sports Exerc* 29:149-159, 1997.
17. Hillegass EA, Sadowsky HS: *Essentials of cardiopulmonary physical therapy*, Philadelphia, 1994, WB Saunders.
18. Hollerbach AD, Sneed NV: Accuracy of radial pulse assessment by length of counting interval, *Heart Lung* 19:258-264, 1990.
19. Irwin S, Tecklin JS: *Cardiopulmonary physical therapy*, ed 3, St Louis, 1995, Mosby.
20. Ishmail AA, Wing S, Ferguson J, et al: Interobserver agreement by auscultation in the presence of a third heart sound in patients with congestive heart failure, *Chest* 91:870-873, 1987.
21. Jarvis C: *Physical examination and assessment*, Philadelphia, 1992, WB Saunders.
22. Johnson JH, Prins A: Prediction of maximal heart rate during a submaximal work test, *J Sports Med Phys Fitness* 31:44-47, 1991.
23. Jones A, Jones RD, Kwong K, et al; Effect of positioning on recorded lung sound intensities in subjects without pulmonary dysfunction, *Phys Ther* 79:682-690, 1999.
23a. Kemper KJ, Benson MS, Bishop MJ: Interobserver variability in assessing pediatric postextubation stridor, *Clin Pediatr (Phila)* 31:405-408, 1992.
24. Kenchaiah S, Evans JC, Levy D, et al: Obesity and the risk of heart failure, *N Engl J Med* 347:305-313, 2002.
25. Kispert CP: Clinical measurements to assess cardiopulmonary function, *Phys Ther* 67:1886-1890, 1987.
26. Knowler WC, Barrett-Connor E, Fowler SE, et al: Diabetes Prevention Program Research Group. Reduction in the incidence of type 2 diabetes with lifestyle intervention or metformin, *N Engl J Med* 346:393-403, 2002.
27. Krieger B, Feinerman D, Zaron A, et al: Continuous noninvasive monitoring of respiratory rate in critically ill patients, *Chest* 90:632-634, 1986.
28. Lehmann R, Spinas GA: Role of physical activity in the therapy and prevention of type II diabetes mellitus, *Ther Umsch* 53:925-933, 1996.
29. Lok CE, Morgan CD, Ranganathan N: The accuracy and interobserver agreement in detecting the "gallop sounds" by cardiac auscultation, *Chest* 114:1283-1288, 1998.
30. Mion D, Pierin AMJ: How accurate are sphygmomanometers? *Hum Hypertens* 12:245-248, 1998.
31. O'Flynn I: Three methods of taking the brachial systolic pressure to measure the ankle/brachial index: which one is best? *J Vasc Nurs* 11:71-75, 1993.
32. Oldridge NB, Haskell WL, Single P: Carotid palpation, coronary heart disease and exercise rehabilitation, *Medicine & Science in Sports & Exercise* 13:6-8, 1981.
33. Patel R, Bushnell DL, Sobotka PA: Implications of an audible third heart sound in evaluating cardiac function, *West J Med* 158:606-609, 1993.
34. Perloff D, Grim C, Flack J, et al: Human blood pressure determination by sphygmomanometry, *Circulation* 88:2460-2470, 1993.
34a. Poirier P, Despres JP: Waist circumference, visceral obesity, and cardiovascular risk, *J Cardiopulm Rehabil* 23:161-169, 2003.
35. Pollock ML, Broida J, Kendrick Z: Validity of the palpation technique of heart rate determination and its estimation of training heart rate, *Res Q* 43:77-81, 1972.
36. Racette SB, Deusinger SS, Deusinger RH: Obesity: overview of prevalence, etiology, and treatment, *Phys Ther* 83:276-288, 2003.
37. Roberts CK, Vaziri ND, Barnard RJ: Effect of diet and exercise intervention on blood pressure, insulin, oxidative stress, and nitric oxide availability, *Circulation* 106:2530-2532, 2002.
38. Sagiv M, Hanson PG, Ben-Sira D, et al: Direct vs. indirect blood pressure at rest and during isometric exercise in normal subjects, *Int J Sports Med* 16:514-518, 1995.
39. Sagiv M, Ben-Sira D, Goldhammer E: Direct vs. indirect blood pressure measurement at peak anaerobic exercise. *Int J Sports Med* 20:275-278, 1999.
40. Sneed NV, Hollerbach AD: Accuracy of heart rate assessment in atrial fibrillation, *Heart Lung* 21:427-433, 1992.
41. Stoffers HE, Kester AD, Kaiser V, et al: The diagnostic value of the measurement of the ankle-brachial systolic pressure index in primary health care, *J Clin Epidemiol* 49:1401-1405, 1996.
42. Turjanmaa VM, Kalli ST, Uusitalo AJ: Blood pressure level changes caused by posture change and physical exercise: can they be determined accurately using a standard cuff method? *J Hypertens* 6(suppl):S79-S81, 1988.
43. Yamanouchi K, Shinozaki T, Chikada K, et al: Daily walking combined with diet therapy is a useful means for obese NIDDM patients not only to reduce body weight but also to improve insulin sensitivity, *Diabetes Care* 22:1754-1755, 1999.

Upper Quarter Screening Examination   **10**

Steven C. Janos, PT, MS, OCS
William G. Boissonnault, PT, DHSc, FAAOMPT

Objectives

After reading this chapter, the reader will be able to:

1. Describe the primary objectives of the upper quarter screening examination related to the differential diagnosis process.
2. Describe the specific examination elements making up the upper quarter screening examination.
3. Explain the relevance of each of the specific examination elements as they relate to the differential diagnosis process, including identification of clinical red flags that would result in a patient referral or consultation.

The Screening Examination: Principles

The history, physical examination, and related tests and measures provide much of the examination data physical therapists (PTs) need to face the clinical decision-making challenges associated with patient management. The clinician's goal is to efficiently and quickly develop an effective plan of care designed to meet the individual patient's needs. Chapters 4 through 7 present a detailed description of the history-taking process as it relates to differential diagnosis and clinical decision-making. One of the objectives of the patient history is to help guide the clinician regarding what to prioritize in the physical examination. Both Chapter 8, which presents physical examination information associated with general patient observation, and Chapter 9, which presents information associated with patient vital signs, are relevant for all patients. The focus of most of the initial visit physical examination, though, will be associated with the location of the patient's chief presenting symptom (see Chapter 6) and associated functional limitations. For example, if the chief presenting symptom is knee pain associated with prolonged standing and walking, the clinician will spend a majority of the time examining the knee and related anatomic areas. Little time is spent examining the elbow, wrist, and hand compared with the lumbar spine, pelvis and hip, and foot and ankle regions. Broadening the scope of the examination to the trunk and lower extremity can be prohibitive if these areas are examined in detail, considering the initial visit time constraints many clinicians face. Examining these anatomically related areas, however, is essential, especially when the knee pain is not related to local trauma. The knee pain may be referred from some other body region (e.g., hip or lumbar spine), or treating the foot and ankle region may be the key to resolving a local knee condition that is affecting

standing and walking. Does the clinician have to complete an extensive and detailed examination of the trunk and entire lower extremity to identify the source(s) of the symptoms and the primary impairments associated with the patient's condition? This is not necessary, but the regions need to be adequately screened with a cluster of selected examination tools so by the end of the initial visit the PT has necessary answers. Figure 10-1 illustrates a general decision-making sequence leading to a differential diagnosis and plan of care, including a possible referral of the patient to another provider.

This chapter and the next (Chapter 11) present an upper and a lower quarter screening examination, respectively, designed to:

- Narrow the search for the source(s) of symptoms to a specific body region (and the tissue at fault, if possible).
- Identify red flags that, along with the history findings, suggest that the PT initiate a patient referral/consultation.
- Identify primary contributing impairments related to the patient's symptoms, functional limitations, and disability.
- Determine which body regions or body systems require a more detailed examination during the initial or subsequent patient visits.
- Improve rehabilitation outcomes by avoiding inaccurate diagnoses or by the timely referral of patients to other practitioners.
- Provide guidance, along with the history findings, regarding specific interventions that may help the patient or may be contraindicated.

The first two items are crucial factors to be considered by the PT. Alteration of symptoms during the examination is key to determining the source of symptoms as well as becoming suspicious of a red flag. As described in Chapter 6, symptoms associated with neuromusculoskeletal impairments are typically related to a change in the patient's posture or movement. In most cases symptoms could be reproduced or altered during the palpation, active or passive movement, resisted tests, neurologic tests, or special test segments of the physical examination. If this does not occur, the PT should be suspicious of a functional (psychological) or pathologic condition. However, the fact that symptoms are altered during the examination does not absolutely rule out the presence of a pathologic condition. For example, infection of the intervertebral disc can result in low back pain that may vary in intensity with movement and changes in posture as the spine is mechanically loaded and unloaded. A pathologic fracture caused by a metastatic lesion

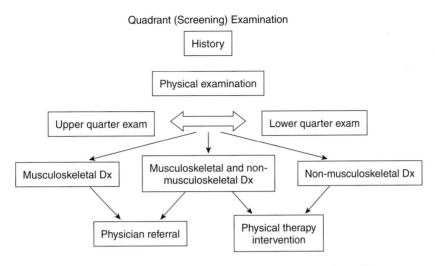

FIGURE 10-1 Flow of patient data collection and clinical decision-making.

may also result in similar findings. In these cases, other information from the history and physical examination should help steer the PT toward the conclusion that the patient's symptoms may not be neuromusculoskeletal in nature. Finally, although therapists should be concerned if they fail to alter a patient's symptomatic presentation, at times symptoms associated with impairments are still the etiology. The patient's condition may not be "irritable" (as defined by Maitland), meaning considerable activity on the patient's part is necessary to provoke the symptoms and the PT cannot clinically stress the tissue sufficiently to bring on or alter the symptoms.

Chapter 4 describes strategies designed to facilitate an effective and efficient patient history. Similar strategies exist to enhance an effective and efficient physical examination as well. First, an adequate-size space is important for efficiency and safety. Next, preparing the examination environment before the patient's arrival in the room is key, making sure the appropriate equipment and supplies are available, such as linen for draping, chairs and stools, and reflex hammers and other examination tools. Having to come and go from the room multiple times can severely disrupt the examination process. Having established positive rapport (see Chapter 4) during the history will enhance the patient's comfort level as the PT begins the "hands-on" portion of the examination. Providing a general description to the patient of what is going to happen next should help alleviate patient anxiety, especially a patient who has never seen a PT before. The better the patient understands what is going to happen and why during the examination, the more information the clinician will be able to efficiently collect. In addition, proper body mechanics are important to prevent injury to the PT and to perform examination techniques effectively.

Also important to the overall success of the visit is protecting patient modesty, which can be influenced by a number of factors such as cultural issues (see Chapter 3). Adequately exposing body areas is especially important for portions of the examination such as observation, palpation, and ROM assessment, but what the PT deems adequate may go beyond the

patient's comfort level. Explaining what the PT plans to do and why is part of the process of receiving consent from the patient to proceed. If the PT is paying attention to patient nonverbal responses to the initial portions of the examination, he or she may pick up signs of discomfort on the patient's part. Important to the patient being comfortable and relaxed is how comfortable and relaxed the clinician is. If the PT is uneasy or nervous about a portion of the examination, the patient will probably be as well. Finally, it is helpful to plan steps to take next during the examination on the basis of data already collected. Avoiding multiple patient or PT position changes can promote practice efficiency and prevent aggravating the patient's acute or subacute condition.

Important general guidelines regarding upper and lower quarter screening examinations described in this chapter and Chapter 11 include the following:

- Include screening as the primary portion of the initial visit physical examination.
- The novice practitioner should use the entire upper quarter screening examination as presented before additional special testing procedures to minimize the chance of misdiagnosis.
- The experienced practitioner, at a minimum, should screen at least one joint/body region above and below the patient's chief symptom. Clinical experience leads to the ability to recognize patterns of patient presentation that will either eliminate diagnostic possibilities that are most probably wrong or very rare and identify the diagnostic possibilities that have the highest probability of being correct.
- If the patient has an acute injury (e.g., sprained knee), or if the visit is after surgery, the emphasis of the initial visit should be on the screening examination components most directly related to the involved joint or body region (e.g., knee). A priority of the physical examination for a patient after trauma is ruling out fracture or ligamentous instability. The remainder of the screening examination is appropriate during follow-up visits once the patient begins to recover from the injury or surgery.

- If the patient has symptoms other than pain associated with a medical condition, such as urinary incontinence, much of the proposed screening examination would probably be irrelevant and should be replaced with an examination that has a different clinical focus.

Upper Quarter Screening Examination

The upper quarter screening examination is organized by patient position: standing, sitting, supine, and prone. This organization minimizes the frequency of changing positions and moving around a patient is asked to do. The specific sequence works well for most patients but will need to be modified in certain circumstances. Data collected during the history regarding symptom description (see Chapter 6) may identify certain positions (e.g., sitting) or movements that significantly increase the symptom intensity to the degree that the PT alters the sequencing of data collection during the physical examination. By ignoring the patient history information and sticking with the examination sequence as listed on paper, the patient's condition may become so aggravated early in the examination that the PT is unable to examine the patient in adequate detail in the other positions and the patient may leave in more pain than before the visit.

The components of both the upper and lower quarter examinations include the standard categories:

- Inspection/observation
- Palpation
- Active range of motion (ROM)
- Passive ROM, including passive overpressures
- Neurologic screening
- Special tests

These categories of patient data will assist in identifying the region or source of symptoms and the primary area of impairment associated with the patient's loss of function. The physical examination and the resultant diagnosis are only as good as the PT performing the examination. Careless or faulty testing techniques produce invalid and inappropriate findings and provide inaccurate diagnosis, treatment plan, and eventual patient outcome.

The upper quarter screening examination process at first glance may appear to be long and cumbersome because it entails performing sample testing of the head, neck, upper thoracic spine (and viscera), and upper extremities, comparing the involved and the uninvolved upper extremity and screening the nervous and peripheral vascular systems. Although this may take somewhat longer to perform than going right to the area of the patient's chief symptom, it typically results in a more cost-efficient and accurate diagnosis and intervention plan. A review of this scope is necessary to meet the objectives expected of an autonomous practitioner and doctor of physical therapy.

The upper quarter screening examination, organized by patient position, is presented in Box 10-1.

BOX 10-1

Upper Quarter Examination Sequence

STANDING
Posture observation
Gait

SITTING
General survey:
  Skin, nails, hair, surface anatomy (see Chapter 8)
  Vital signs (see Chapter 9)
  Weight/height (see Chapter 9)
  Posture assessment (observe during the interview process)
Head, face, neck observation (see Chapter 8)
  Eyes
    Pupils
    Ptosis
    Visual gaze (strabismus)
  Facial contour
    Eyes/mouth (CN VII)
    Cheeks (masseter muscle, CN V)
  Intraoral
    Teeth (dentition and occlusion)
    Gingiva (gums)
    Tongue and other soft tissues
    Anterior neck (trachea and sternal notch)
Head, face, and neck palpation
  Glands (parotid, submandibular salivary, thyroid)
  Lymph nodes (preauricular and postauricular, suboccipital, tonsillar, submental, superficial and posterior cervical, supraclavicular)
  Trachea
  Carotid pulses

Head, face, and neck neurologic screening (see Chapters 7 and 8)
  Follow-up interview questions
    Sense of smell (CN I)
    Visual acuity (CN II)
    Diplopia (double vision) (CN III, IV, VI)
    Sense of taste (CN VII, IX)
    Difficulties with swallowing
    Hearing loss
    Numbness/paresthesia
    Balance/gait difficulties
    Mentation/orientation/behavioral abnormalities
  Physical examination screening (optional)
    Smell (CN I)
    Visual acuity (CN II): Snellen eye chart
    Pupils: light reaction (CN II and III)
    Extraocular eye movements (CN III, IV, and/or VI)
    Sensory (CN V and C2 and 3)
    Motor (CN V and VII, and C1-C3)
    Motor cervical flexion (C1-C3; CN XI: spinal accessory); extension (C1-C8; CN XI: spinal accessory); lateral flexion (C2-C4; CN XI); rotation
    Facial expression: eyes, mouth (CN VII)
    Hearing: air conduction (CN VIII)
    Hearing: bone conduction (CN VIII)
    Gag reflex (CN IX and X)
    Shoulder shrug (CN XI)
    Tongue motor response (CN XII)
Active ROM (with passive overpressure when appropriate)
  Mandibular depression (observe and palpate)
  Cervical spine

BOX 10-1

Upper Quarter Examination Sequence—cont'd

Flexion
Rotation (check vertebral artery signs)
Lateral flexion
Extension
Cervical spine vertical compression/distraction
Shoulder girdle/upper extremity
  Observation
  Palpation
    Lymph nodes (clavicular, axillary, and epitrochlear)
    Pulses (brachial, radial)
    Joint lines and soft tissues
Active ROM (with passive overpressure when appropriate)
  Shoulder girdle
    Elevation, depression, protraction, retraction
  Shoulder
    Hand behind head
    Hand behind back
    Horizontal abduction
  Elbow (may do before shoulder active ROM screening if history of significant elbow injury/pathology)
    Flexion
    Extension
    Pronation
    Supination
  Wrist
    Flexion

Extension
    Radial/ulnar deviation
  Thumb
    Flexion/extension
    Opposition
  Fingers
    Flexion/extension
Upper extremity neurologic screening
  Hoffman's reflex
  Cutaneous sensation (light touch, sharp/dull assessment (C4-T6 dermatomes; see Figure 10-19)
  Myotome testing
    Scapular elevation (CN XI, spinal accessory)
    Shoulder abduction (C4-C6, axillary)
    Elbow flexion (C5, C6; musculocutaneous)
    Elbow extension (C6-C8, radial)
    Wrist extension (C6-C8, radial and ulnar)
    Finger flexors (C7, C8; median)
    Thumb extension (C7, C8; radial)
    Finger abduction/adduction (C8, T1; ulnar)
  Deep tendon reflexes
    Biceps (C5, C6)
    Brachioradialis (C5, C6)
    Triceps (C6, C7)

* All positive neurologic findings in the sitting position should be retested in non-weight-bearing positions.
CN, Cranial nerve.

Description of Examination Elements by Position

Standing

POSTURAL ASSESSMENT. A brief assessment is made of standing posture, primarily focusing on the upper quarter but also screening for significant lumbopelvic or lower extremity findings that may affect upper quarter posture and function. The patient should be viewed from anterior, posterior, and lateral perspectives.

GAIT SCREEN. Although the patient's chief symptoms or functional limitations relate to an upper body region or activity, gathering some information regarding the general gait pattern and its influence on upper quarter posture, movement (or lack of), and symptoms is important. The patient should be instructed to relay information to the examiner regarding at what point during the gait cycle the symptoms are aggravated. As with posture assessment, the gait screening should include viewing the patient from all perspectives (anterior, posterior, and lateral).

Sitting

GENERAL SURVEY. The items listed under "general survey" in Box 10-1 are relevant to all patients. As described in Chapter 8, observing skin, including general color, specific lesions, hair patterns and loss, and nails begins during the patient interview and continues throughout the remainder of the examination. Signs of an inflammatory response (local redness or hyperemia) or ecchymosis indicating bleeding under the skin from injury of underlying tissues may be noted. Scars should also be noted and

examined for their state of healing. In addition, a patient may not inform the PT of a surgical procedure or trauma, so observing the scar can prompt the PT to initiate a line of questioning. The presence of keloid, or excessive scarring, may be an indication of the general response of the patient to trauma and potential complications associated with the healing process. Being vigilant for rashes, such as the malar rash associated with systemic lupus erythematosus, is also important when assessing the head and facial regions. Lastly, calluses and blisters should be noted because they are indicative of excessive friction or irritation of the skin.

Assessing vital signs (see Chapter 9), including blood pressure and heart rate, documenting weight and height, and calculating body mass index may identify important health issues that need to be brought to another health care practitioner's attention or become a focus of the PT's intervention plan. Although sitting posture can also be formally assessed at this point of the examination, a more true picture of how the patient typically sits during their day will probably be more obvious while the patient is being interviewed. Noting head on neck (upper cervical), head and neck on thorax (mid/lower cervical), shoulder girdle on thorax, and overall trunk position will provide direction to the clinician regarding what specific body regions to assess in more detail. Observation of the thorax may reveal structural deformities such as barrel chest, excessive kyphosis, and "pigeon" chest (pectus excavatum). A respiratory screen should also take place at this time, including respiratory pattern (chest vs. abdominal vs. accessory muscles), pursed lip breathing, and so forth.

Head, Face, and Neck Observation

Besides the observation issues noted above, a close look at the eyes and face begins a general nervous system screening (see Chapters 7 and 8). General observation of the eyes includes assessment of the pupils (size and shape), ptosis, gaze, position of the eye relative to the orbit (e.g., exophthalmus), and color (e.g., abnormal patterns of redness). Abnormal findings may include:

- Bulging of the eye(s): exophthalmus from "thyrotoxicosis," hyperthyroidism, Graves' disease; space-occupying mass in the orbit
- Drainage: blockage of nasolacrimal gland/infections
- Ptosis: Horner's syndrome, Pancoast tumor of lung, cranial nerve III dysfunction)
- Color of sclera: yellow for jaundice, hepatitis, liver disease; redness for ciliary flush; inflammation; infection
- Nystagmus: alcohol abuse; upper motor neuron disease; labyrinth irritability
- Abnormal gaze: strabismus (involvement of cranial nerves III, IV, or VI), space-occupying mass in the orbit)

Observing whether the trachea and associated structures are vertically oriented, and whether the sternal notch (bordered by the sternocleidomastoid muscles and the manubrium of the sternum) is present are also important. A space-occupying mass may result in a deviation from the midline of the trachea, and an enlarged thyroid gland or nodules can "fill in" the sternal notch.

Screening intraoral structures includes identifying how many teeth are present, the condition of the teeth, the occlusal pattern, and the condition of associated soft tissue structures. There can be up to eight teeth in each of the four quadrants starting medially and going laterally:

- Central incisor
- Lateral incisor
- Canine
- Bicuspids ("premolars") (two)
- Molars (three)

Absent, chipped, or cracked teeth indicate that an assessment by a dentist is warranted, and shiny, worn spots on teeth may indicate bruxism. The relation of the maxillary to the mandibular incisors when the teeth are in contact may also identify malocclusive or temporomandibular disorders that may suggest the PT should refer the patient to a dentist. The maxillary incisors should vertically overlap the mandibular incisors (overbite) by approximately 30%, with minimal distance noted in the anterior/posterior direction (overjet if excessive). Symptoms and signs of bruxism may indicate an assessment by a PT specializing in craniofacial disorder practice or a dentist. Inflammation or irritation of soft tissues or intraoral bleeding may indicate serious disease or conditions (gingivitis) that require dental intervention. This type of observational screening includes looking at the back of the throat (soft palate, uvula, etc.)

Head, Face, and Neck Palpation

The principles of palpation apply to this body region as in all others. The "layer palpation" approach is recommended, going from superficial to deeper structures as different structures are assessed and identified. General instructions to the patient are also standard, including requesting feedback regarding whether more than just pressure is felt and whether symptoms change, for better or worse, as the area is assessed. General observation of surface anatomy (see Chapter 8) may reveal abnormalities that lead the practitioner to detailed palpation of a region. Do not assume that any lump or bump felt necessarily lies within a muscle belly or fascial layer. A number of glands and lymph nodes are located in the head, face, and neck region (Figures 10-2 and 10-3). Feeling a bump or bump does not automatically indicate a pathologic condition because many of these structures are superficially located. A hard lump or nodule, whether it is tender or not, should lead to questioning the patient about the finding:

- Have you noticed this lump?
- Has a physician checked this spot and told you what the lump is?
- If the physician is aware of the lump, has it changed in size, shape, or consistency since the last visit?

The same abnormal criteria apply to assessment of these nodes as discussed in Chapter 8, including the following:

- More than 1 cm in diameter
- Hard consistency
- Tender, painful node or nontender with hard consistency
- Immobile

A lump that has not been checked by a physician or has changed since the last physician assessment should direct the PT to encourage the patient to make an appointment to get it checked. Finally, palpating along the trachea is important for noting any abnormal anatomy (e.g., deviation from the midline) or abnormal response (e.g., provocation of symptoms) to the pressure applied to the area, and each carotid artery can be palpated near the level of the cricoid cartilage, just medial to

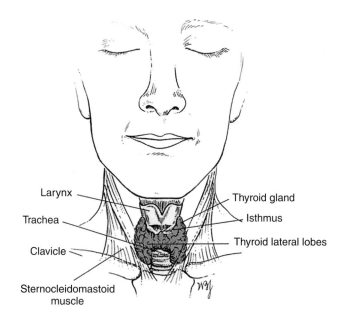

FIGURE 10-2 Anatomic location of thyroid gland. (From Swartz MH: *Textbook of physical diagnosis: history and examination*, Philadelphia, 2002, WB Saunders, p 182.)

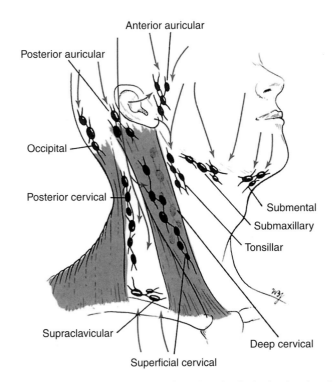

FIGURE 10-3 Anatomic location of lymph nodes in the head and neck regions. (From Swartz MH: *Textbook of physical diagnosis: history and examination*, Philadelphia, 2002, WB Saunders, p 182.)

the sternocleidomastoid muscles. The carotid assessment is primarily for intensity and symmetry of pulsations as well as potentially localized pain provocation.

Head, Face, and Neck Neurologic Screening Physical Examination

Relevant screening questions and tests should be included when the following occur:

- The therapist observes any of the abnormal anatomic findings described above or in Chapters 7 and 8
- The patient describes local head or facial symptoms (Chapter 6) or a pattern of numbness, paresthesia, or weakness that does not fit a peripheral nerve entrapment or a spinal nerve root pattern
- The patient has a history of a primary neurologic condition such as multiple sclerosis or has a history of a stroke or head injury
- The patient describes direct trauma to the head and neck region or a whiplash type of incident

The focus of the screening questions should be to identify findings that are unusual or atypical, representing a change from the norm for the patient. The screening tests can be organized in sequential order of the cranial nerves (I through XII) or by anatomic region (recommended). See Table 10-1 for a summary of cranial nerve screening.

FACE

Sensation (Cranial Nerve V). Light touch, including sharp/dull at a minimum, should be assessed over the forehead (ophthalmic branch), the cheeks (maxillary branch), and the jaw (mandibular branch). It is often helpful to first perform

this over an area of skin that is not within the area of symptoms and is thought to be of normal sensation. The patient should be asked to close the eyes as the face is examined. Ask the patient to report if what is felt is sharp or dull. A loss of sensation in this region suggests either a lesion of the trigeminal nerve or higher sensory pathways.

Motor (Cranial Nerves V and VII). The motor status of the trigeminal nerve is assessed by asking the patient to bite down hard and hold while the therapist palpates the masseter and temporalis muscles bilaterally, noting strength of contraction (degree of tissue resistance during palpation). Subtle asymmetry may be detected in patients with temporomandibular joint or dental occlusion conditions. Next, the status of the facial nerve is assessed by the PT observing for facial symmetry as the patient is asked to perform the following activities:

- Raise both eyebrows
- Frown
- Close both eyes tightly
- Show both the upper and lower teeth
- Smile
- Puff out both cheeks with mouth closed

Cranial nerve VII is also involved in taste sensation of the anterior two thirds of the tongue, so a lesion of this nerve may also have symptoms of altered taste.

EYES

Visual Acuity (Cranial Nerve II). Symptoms of having difficulty seeing should lead to additional screening to determine whether to refer the patient to another practitioner. Visual acuity can be checked with a Snellen eye chart (Figure 10-4). With the patient positioned 20 feet from the chart, using glasses or contact lenses if needed, the patient is asked to cover one eye at a time and read the smallest line of print possible. Visual acuity for each eye is recorded and compared with what the patient knows to be his or her normal vision when checked. If the patient can read at best the 20/200 line, this is interpreted as the ability to read at 20 feet what a person with normal vision can see at 200 feet. If the patient is unable to read any of the lines, the patient is asked to state how many fingers the clinician is holding up in front of the patient's face.

Peripheral Vision (Cranial Nerve II). The patient's temporal or peripheral vision is checked with the patient sitting and the PT in front of and facing the patient. The patient covers one eye while looking straight ahead (as does the therapist). The therapist places his or her hand several feet lateral to the patient on the side of the eye to be tested and slowly brings a finger or object (e.g., pen) toward the midline until the patient states he or she sees it. This is grossly compared to the opposite eye's ability when it is tested. This test can be repeated, moving the finger or object medially in from an upper and lower visual quadrant.

Pupils (Cranial Nerves II and III). After inspecting the pupils for size and symmetry (see Chapter 8), the pupillary reaction test (Figure 10-5) should be performed. In a somewhat darkened room, a penlight is aimed into one eye at a time (either at a 45-degree angle to prevent direct light into the other eye, or

TABLE 10-1

Evaluating the Cranial Nerves

Nerves	Function	Location	Tests	Significant Findings
I—Olfactory	Smell	Olfactory bulb and tract	Odor recognition (unilaterally)	Lack of odor perception on one or both sides
II—Optic	Vision	Optic nerve, chiasm, and tracts	Visual acuity; peripheral vision; pupillary light reflex	Reduced vision
III—Oculomotor	Eye movement; pupil contraction and accommodation; eyelid elevation	Midbrain	Extraocular eye movements; pupillary light reflex	Impairment of one or more eye movements or disconjugate gaze; pupillary dilatation; ptosis
IV—Trochlear	Eye movement	Midbrain	Extraocular eye movements	Impairment of one or more eye movements or disconjugate gaze
V—Trigeminal	Facial sensation; muscles of mastication	Pons	Sensation above eye, between eye and mouth, below mouth to angle of jaw; palpation of contraction of masseter and temporalis muscles	Reduced sensation in one or more divisions of the fifth nerve; impaired jaw reflex; reduced strength in masseter and temporalis muscles
VI—Abducens	Ocular movement	Pons	Extraocular eye movements	Reduced eye abduction
VII—Facial	Facial expression; secretions; taste; visceral and cutaneous sensibility	Pons	Facial expression; taste of anterior two thirds of tongue	Weakness of upper or lower face or eye closure; reduced taste perception (salty, sweet, bitter, sour)
VIII—Acoustic	Hearing; equilibrium	Pons	Auditory and vestibular	Reduced hearing; impaired balance
IX—Glossopharyngeal	Taste; glandular secretions; swallowing; visceral sensibility (pharynx, tongue, tonsils)	Medulla	Gag reflex; speech (phonation); swallowing	Impaired reflex; dysarthria; dysphagia
X—Vagus	Involuntary muscle and gland control (pharynx, larynx, trachea, bronchi, lungs, digestive tract, heart); swallowing and phonation; visceral and cutaneous sensibility; taste	Medulla	Phonation; coughing; gag reflex	Hoarseness; weak cough; impaired reflex
XI—Accessory	Movement of head and shoulders	Cervical	Resisted head; shoulder shrug	Weakness of trapezius and sternocleidomastoid
XII—Hypoglossal	Movement of tongue	Medulla	Tongue protrusion	Deviation, atrophy, or fasciculations of tongue

by the examiner placing a hand at the bridge of the nose to divide the visual field in two). The patient is asked to focus on an object 6 to 10 feet behind the PT and not directly on the light or the PT's hand. Normal response should be twofold: immediate, mild constriction of the ipsilateral pupil (the direct response) and constriction of the pupil of the opposite eye (the consensual response).

Extraocular Movements (Cranial Nerves III, IV, and VI). The patient is asked to focus attention on an object (the PT's finger or a pen) directly in front of him or her at a comfortable distance (approximately 12 inches). Then the patient is asked to follow the object with his or her eyes as it is moved in an H pattern, while holding the head still. The examiner notes the eyes' ability to track the object and symmetry of movement into all quadrants (Figure 10-6), with the expectation that the eyes will move smoothly together and track symmetrically.

EARS

Acuity. The first recommended auditory acuity screening test is the "whisper test" because the outer, middle, and inner ear are all being screened at one time. Standing behind the patient at a 45-degree angle (to ensure the patient cannot read the PT's lips) the PT whispers familiar bisyllabic words (e.g., weather, thirteen, hot dog) and asks the patient to repeat the words that were whispered. To test one ear at a time, the patient should cover the ear not being tested with their hand. If a unilateral or bilateral deficit is noted or if the findings are equivocal, follow-up testing with a 512- or 1024-Hz tuning fork should be performed.

Air/Bone Conduction. Two additional screening tests, the Weber and Rinne tests, can be used if necessary. The Weber test should be performed first because it allows for bilateral hearing assessment, making the test faster to implement than the Rinne test. For the Weber test, after striking the tuning fork in the palm of the hand, the PT places the fork firmly on the vertex of the cranium or mid-forehead (Figure 10-7). (Placing the fork too softly on the cranium can result in a false-positive response.) The patient is then asked, "Do you hear the sound, and, if so, do you hear it equally in both ears?" A normal response would be "Yes, I hear it equally in both ears." If the sound lateralizes to one ear (heard more loudly in one ear), this should be documented and reported to the

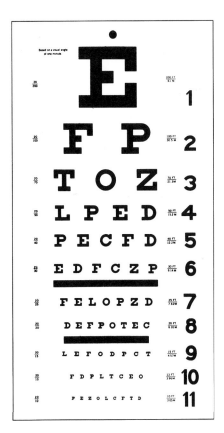

FIGURE 10-4 The Snellen chart, which is used to assess visual acuity. (From American Academy of Ophthalmology, San Francisco, Calif, 1993, p 8.)

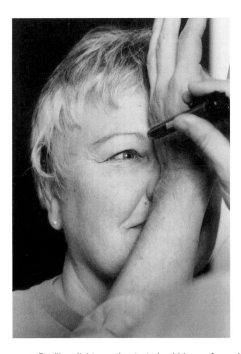

FIGURE 10-5 Pupillary light reaction test should be performed in a dimly lit room with the patient looking at a distant object. The PT's hand divides the patient's visual field and shines the light into one eye, watching that pupil for a direct response. The PT then shines the light in the same eye, watching the opposite pupil for a response (consensual response). This process is repeated by shining the light in the other eye.

patient's physician if the patient does not have a history of current hearing problems.

The Rinne test screens one ear at a time, comparing air conduction with bone conduction. Place the vibrating tuning fork firmly on the mastoid process, behind the ear (the vibrating fork should be pointed back away from the ear), and ask the patient "Do you hear any sound/noise?" A normal response is "Yes, I hear it." The patient is then instructed to report when the sound is no longer heard. At that point the PT moves the still vibrating fork in front of the external auditory meatus and asks the patient whether any sound is heard. The normal response is "Yes, I hear the sound again." The premise for this test is that air conduction should last longer and therefore be greater than bone conduction. The fork vibration slows down enough that the inner ear is no longer being stimulated when it is placed over the mastoid process, but it is still vibrating. So, when the vibrating fork is placed in front of the ear the outer ear picks up the sound waves, carries them to the middle ear, followed by events that result in the inner ear being stimulated again (the sound "comes back").

Balance (Including Vestibular) Testing. If the patient subjectively reports dizziness or balance problems (see Chapter 7), balance testing is in order. The degree of balance problem the patient describes will dictate where the PT will begin with the screening. The lowest level of screening has the patient standing with feet together on a fixed surface (floor) with the eyes open for 20 to 30 seconds. The next level is the same maneuver, but with eyes closed, followed by testing on a soft surface with eyes open. Balance concerns are noted during the history, and the PT should stand close to the patient for safety reasons. Other tests to consider include the Dix-Hallpike maneuver and cervical vertigo tests (body moving on head and the smooth pursuit neck torsion test).

NOSE (CRANIAL NERVE I). If the patient reports difficulty with the sense of smell or if other neurologic deficits are noted during the examination, a follow-up test is in order. To assess the sense of smell, an aromatic stimulus (e.g., orange, coffee, or vanilla) rather than a noxious stimuli is used. The patient's eyes should be closed during the assessment, and he or she is asked to identify the source of the odor. One side (one nostril) should be tested at a time.

MOUTH

Gag Reflex (Cranial Nerves IX and X). PTs should screen for the gag reflex after asking the patient to swallow and noting any difficulties. With the patient's mouth wide open, the PT observes the status of the soft palate and position of the uvula and asks the patient to say "ahh" while observing for symmetric rise of the soft palate and uvula (cranial nerve X). Any deviation of the uvula or asymmetry of the soft palate position indicates possible cranial nerve involvement (Figure 10-8). Lastly, the PT places a tongue blade on the back of the tongue (cranial nerve IX innervates the posterior two thirds of the tongue) and watches for the same motor response seen with the "ahh" action. Again, any deviation of the uvula or asymmetry of the soft palate position indicates possible cranial nerve involvement.

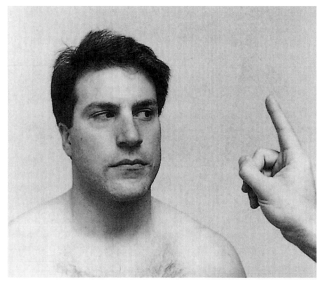

A

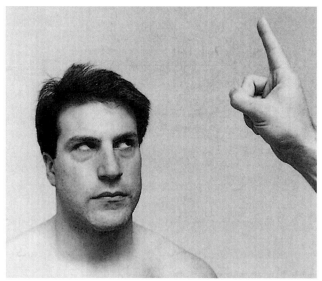

B

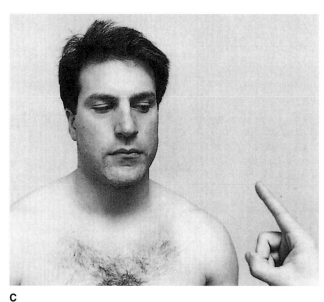

C

FIGURE 10-6 Assessment of gaze into all quadrants. **A,** Eyes following the target to the right (lateral gaze). **B,** Eyes following the target laterally and superiorly. **C,** Eyes following the target laterally and inferiorly. (From Boissonnault W: *Examination in physical therapy practice: screening for medical disease,* ed 2, New York, 1995, Churchill Livingstone, p 216.)

Tongue (Cranial Nerve XII). The patient is asked to protrude the tongue, with the PT observing for symmetry, atrophy, or deviation from the midline. Manual resistance to side-to-side movements of the tongue screens for asymmetry of strength. The PT may ask the patient to push the tongue into the inside of each cheek while providing mild resistance with a few fingers or a tongue blade as the patient holds against the pressure.

Temporomandibular Joint: Active Range of Motion. The joint lines are first palpated (bilaterally) externally over the mandibular condyles, checking for pain provocation, tenderness, and edema. The patient is then asked to open the mouth fully as the PT checks for extent of opening (normal active ROM is approximately 45 to 60 mm), deviation from the sagittal plane, and any alteration of usual condition. Preventing any neck move-

ment during this activity is important because any pain provoked may be referred from the cervical spine.

Cervical Spine

CERVICAL ACTIVE RANGE OF MOTION. The patient should be seated upright with the feet supported to promote a reproducible position as cervical flexion, rotation, lateral flexion, and extension are assessed from anterior, posterior, and lateral views. If symptoms are not altered during active movement assessment, a passive overpressure is applied to exclude the cervical spine as a source of symptoms (Figure 10-9). Besides assessing quantity and quality of motion, the PT must appreciate that during cervical rotation, and to some degree extension, the initial gross assessment for vertebral basilar artery insufficiency has begun. Therefore during the assessment of

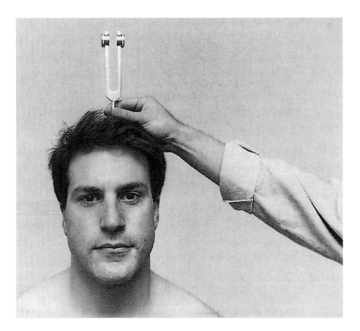

FIGURE 10-7 Weber test. (From Boissonnault W: *Examination in physical therapy practice: screening for medical disease*, ed 2, New York, 1995, Churchill Livingstone, p 217.)

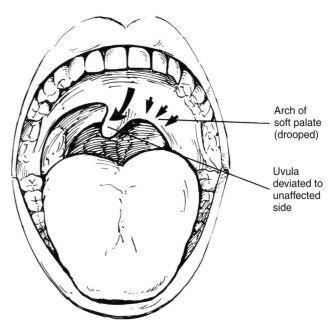

Arch of soft palate (drooped)

Uvula deviated to unaffected side

FIGURE 10-8 Lower motor neuron lesion of the vagus nerve; may be noted during testing of the gag reflex or when the patient says "ahh." (From Wilson-Pauwels, Akesson EJ, Stewart PA: *Cranial nerves: anatomy and clinical comments*, Philadelphia, 1988, BC Decker.)

active cervical left and right rotation, the patient is asked to maintain the head and neck at the end of the movement for an additional 10 to 30 seconds while the PT looks for manifestations that may be related to compromise of the vertebral arteries. The most common manifestations include the following:

- Dizziness
- Dysarthria
- Dysphagia
- Nausea
- Visual disturbances
- Extremity sensory changes

Cervical Vertical Compression and Decompression. With the patient sitting with feet supported, the examiner places his or her hands around the sides and back of the patient's head ("hooking" the mastoid processes on the heel of the hand between the thenar and hypothenar eminences) and gently lifts straight up until the soft tissues of the neck become taut (Figure 10-10). This position is held for approximately 5 seconds. The patient is asked if any change in symptoms is noted. The examiner then places both hands on top of the patient's head and slowly compresses the head and neck, stopping just shy of producing movement of the cervical region (Figure 10-11). This position is also held for approximately 5 seconds, with questioning again regarding any change in symptoms. A pillow is placed between the therapist and the patient to help maintain an upright patient position. This pillow also allows for the maintenance of "personal space" between the therapist and patient.

Upper Extremity Observation

Observe for overall size, contour, symmetry, and posturing of the upper extremities. Look at the hands for clubbing of nails (chronic heart, lung, or liver disease); enlargement of joint

structures, as in Heberden's nodes (distal interphalangeal joints: osteoarthritis) and Bouchard's nodes (interphalangeal and metacarpal phalangeal joints: rheumatoid arthritis) and ulnar drift of the metacarpal phalangeal joints. Observe the skin for sores or ulcerations (e.g., psoriasis), red streaks (local infection, usually distal), swelling (edema and effusion), temperature and color (more diffuse, cold, pallor typically associated with venous or lymphatic conditions; increased warmth and redness more commonly associated with arterial problems), skin texture, and scars. See Chapter 8 for more details regarding interpretation of findings.

Upper Extremity Palpation

The general principles of layer palpation and instructions to the patient also apply to upper extremity palpation. Structures to be aware of include lymph nodes and arteries for pulse assessment (see Chapter 9).

CLAVICULAR LYMPH NODES. There are nodes in the supraclavicular regions, lateral to the distal attachment of the sternocleidomastoid muscles and inferior to the clavicle in the triangle bordered by the anterior deltoid and pectoralis major muscles and the lateral third of the clavicle (Figure 10-12).

AXILLARY LYMPH NODES. There are several sets of lymph nodes in the axillary region, which can be viewed as a pyramid with 4 walls for palpation (Figures 10-13 to 10-16), with lymph nodes present along all 4 walls: medial (thoracic cage), anterior (posterior surface of pectoralis major), posterior (anterior surface of subscapularis, teres major, and latissimus dorsi), and lateral wall (upper shaft and neck of the humerus). The same technique is used to palpate these nodes as in the cervical region, assessing for the same characteristics. As in the cervical spine, it is not uncommon to

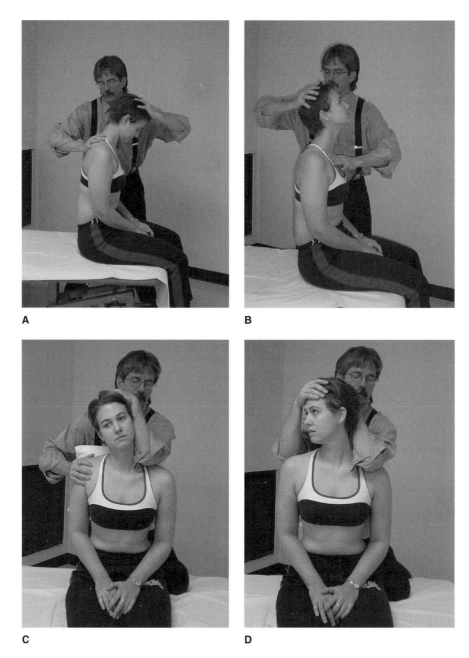

FIGURE 10-9 Passive overpressure of the cervical spine. **A,** Flexion; **B,** extension; **C,** sidebending; and **D,** rotation.

palpate normal nodes in the axillary regions, especially along the medial wall.

EPITROCHLEAR LYMPH NODES. Epitrochlear lymph nodes are located just above the elbow in the proximity of the medial epicondyle of the humerus (Figure 10-17). An awareness of lymph node location is important so PTs don't assume that lumps found during palpation lie within a muscle belly or fascial layer. Specific assessment of lymph node areas is also called for in the presence of diffuse upper extremity swelling, a history of breast cancer (in particular with axillary node involvement), wounds, abrasions, or red streaks noted on the hand, wrist, or forearm regions.

PULSE: BRACHIAL ARTERY. The brachial pulse is assessed at the medial upper arm at the middle/distal third of the humerus, medial to the biceps tendon (Figure 10-18).

PULSE: RADIAL/ULNAR ARTERY. The radial/ulnar pulse is assessed at the volar aspect of the distal forearm, with the radial artery classically used for assessment of heart rate or beats per minute.

Upper Extremity Active Range of Motion with Passive Overpressure

SHOULDER GIRDLE. The movements of elevation (cranial nerve XI when manual resistance is applied), depression, protraction, and retraction should all be assessed while monitoring head and neck posture and movement and glenohumeral motion. Muscle imbalances or joint dysfunction in the shoulder girdle region could lead to multiple compensations throughout this region of the body.

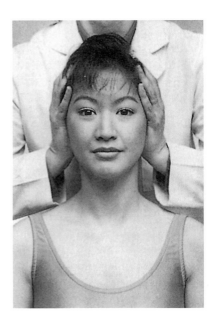

FIGURE 10-10 Vertical cervical distraction. (From Richardson JK, Iglarsh ZA: *Clinical orthopaedic physical therapy*, Philadelphia, 1994, WB Saunders, p 43.)

SHOULDER COMPLEX. In lieu of local trauma to the shoulder or a surgical procedure, the movement screening can begin with combined movements, including having the patient put the hand behind the head, hand behind the back, and horizontal abduction. If movement abnormalities are noted, then a cardinal plane assessment can be performed and measured because a more detailed shoulder examination is warranted. If the active movement findings do not provide definitive guidance, passive overpressure should then be performed to allow the PT to say with confidence whether the shoulder complex is an area that needs to be addressed in the treatment plan.

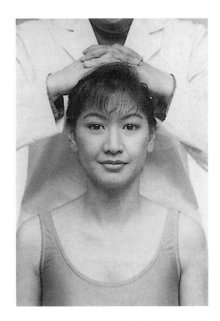

FIGURE 10-11 Vertical cervical compression. (From Richardson JK, Iglarsh ZA: *Clinical orthopaedic physical therapy*, Philadelphia, 1994, WB Saunders, p 43.)

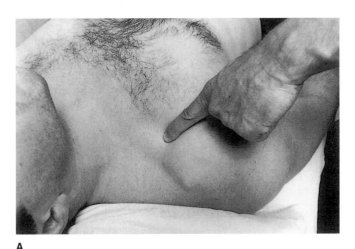

A

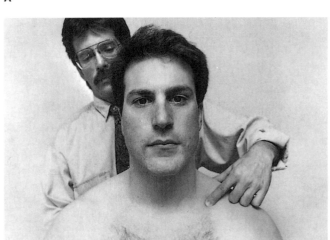

B

FIGURE 10-12 A, Palpating for the infraclavicular lymph nodes between the deltoid and pectoralis major muscles. **B,** Palpating for the supraclavicular lymph nodes lateral to the sternocleidomastoid attachment on the clavicle. (From Boissonnault W: *Examination in physical therapy practice: screening for medical disease*, ed 2, New York, 1995, Churchill Livingstone, p 404.)

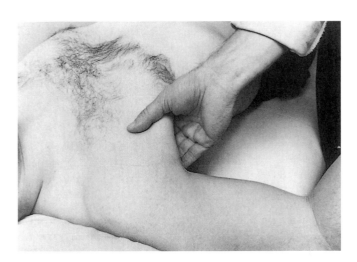

FIGURE 10-13 Palpating for lymph nodes along the anterior axillary wall, posterior surface of pectoralis major. (From Boissonnault W: *Examination in physical therapy practice: screening for medical disease*, ed 2, New York, 1995, Churchill Livingstone, p 404.)

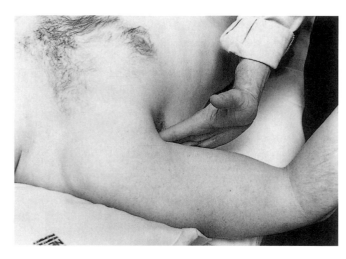

FIGURE 10-14 Palpating for lymph nodes along the lateral axillary wall, along shaft of upper humerus. (From Boissonnault W: *Examination in physical therapy practice: screening for medical disease*, ed 2, New York, 1995, Churchill Livingstone, p 405.)

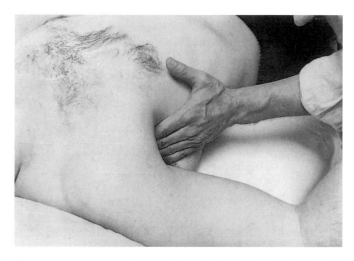

FIGURE 10-16 Palpating for lymph nodes along the medial axillary wall, along thorax. (From Boissonnault W: *Examination in physical therapy practice: screening for medical disease*, ed 2, New York, 1995, Churchill Livingstone, p 406.)

ELBOW. As noted in the screening examination, there may be times when the elbow should be screened before the shoulder is passively examined, such as in patients with a history of significant past or recent trauma to the elbow region. Passive overpressure for many of the shoulder movements will mechanically stress the elbow to the point of potentially exacerbating an underlying condition. To screen the elbow/forearm complex, flexion, extension, pronation, and supination should all be assessed actively as well as passively if indicated. To save time, these active motions can be assessed bilaterally.

WRIST AND HAND. Finally, the wrist/hand complex can be assessed actively and passively, if indicated, including wrist flexion, extension, and radial/ulnar deviation. As with the elbow, these active movements can be assessed bilaterally. For screening the hand, the thumb should be assessed separately

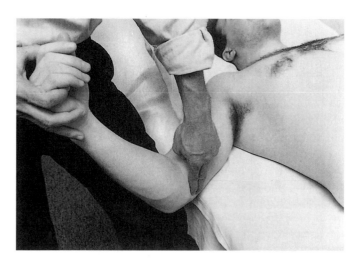

FIGURE 10-17 Palpating for the epitrochlear lymph nodes. (From Boissonnault W: *Examination in physical therapy practice: screening for medical disease*, ed 2, New York, 1995, Churchill Livingstone, p 406.)

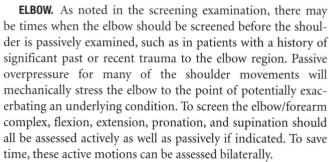

FIGURE 10-15 Palpating for lymph nodes along the posterior axillary wall, anterior surface of teres major and latissimus dorsi. (From Boissonnault W: *Examination in physical therapy practice: screening for medical disease*, ed 2, New York, 1995, Churchill Livingstone, p 406.)

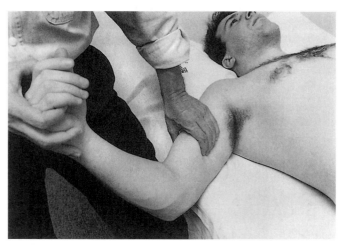

FIGURE 10-18 Assessing pulse at the brachial artery along the medial shaft of the humerus. (From Boissonnault W: *Examination in physical therapy practice: screening for medical disease*, ed 2, New York, 1995, Churchill Livingstone, p 407.)

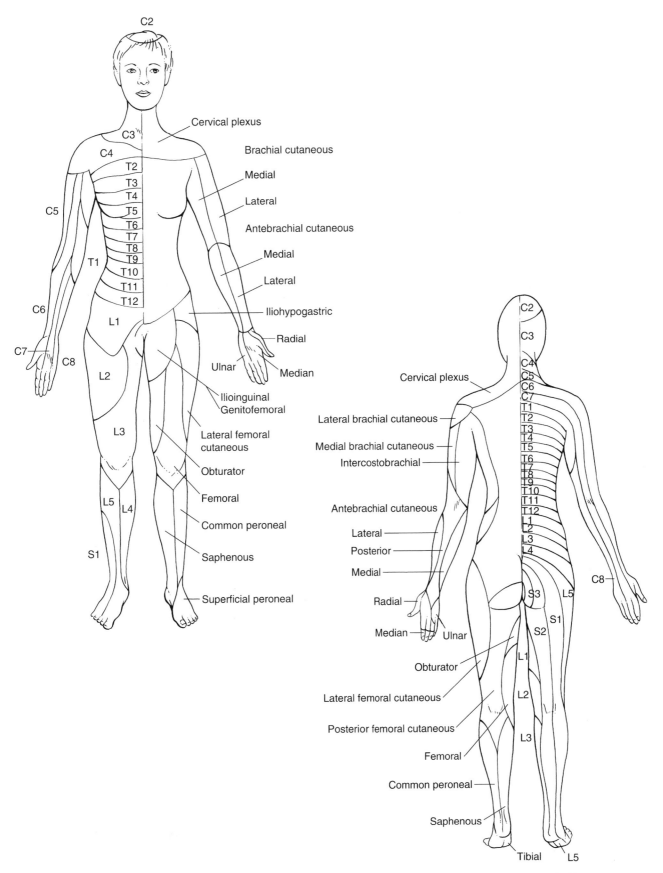

FIGURE 10-19 Segmental distribution of the spinal nerves. (From Swartz MH: *Textbook of physical diagnosis: history and examination*, Philadelphia, 2002, WB Saunders, p 623.)

from the fingers with flexion, extension, and opposition. All the fingers can be actively assessed simultaneously with flexion and extension, followed by passive overpressure if indicated.

Upper Extremity Neurologic Screening Examination

For consistency and reproducibility, the patient should be sitting upright with the feet supported. Controlling head and neck position is essential because certain postures will "open" the cervical foramen and others will "close" them. The patient should be looking straight ahead as the testing is being performed.

MYOTOMES. Selected muscles have been identified to assess the motor status of cervical spinal nerve roots and upper extremity peripheral nerves.

SENSORY. See the description under head, face, and neck sensory assessment, which notes that the patient's eyes should be closed during the assessment. If an alteration in sensation is noted, the examiner will then take the additional time by testing to map the area and make a determination regarding nerve root versus peripheral nerve involvement (Figure 10-19).

DEEP TENDON REFLEXES. For the upper quarter examination, three deep tendon reflexes are assessed: biceps, brachioradialis, and triceps. In each case the tendon in question should be placed slightly stretched from a mid position; it is helpful to support the limb to gain additional feedback by palpation in addition to visual assessment of the reflex. This should be repeated three to five times to ensure a valid response. Grading the reflex response is accomplished by determining the response on a 0 to 4+ scale (Table 10-2). If no response is noted, a Jendrassik maneuver may be used by asking for a contraction of other muscles not involved in the reflex.

Finally, Hoffman's reflex is analogous to the Babinski reflex. The Hoffman reflex assists in the screening for upper motor neuron involvement. While the therapist supports the proxi-

mal phalanges of the second finger, he or she sharply "flicks" the distal phalanx into flexion. A positive finding would be observation of a simultaneous thumb interphalangeal joint flexion.

Summary

The overall examination of the patient is not finished when the testing maneuvers have been completed. At this point (after the history and upper quarter screening examination) the PT should have a strong hypothesis regarding the source of symptoms, primary impairments related to functional limitations, and disability and should have identified potential red flags. In many instances the collected information will provide enough guidance so that treatment can be initiated without further examination. In addition, a determination regarding what joint complexes may require more detailed assessment (which may occur at subsequent visits) will also have been made.

Again, the novice practitioner should complete the screening examination as presented to minimize the chance of a misdiagnosis. Experienced practitioners can recognize patterns of symptoms or signs that will allow them to skip steps in the examination process and initiate effective treatment many times during the examination itself. Finally, when examining a patient after trauma or surgery, the focus of the initial examination should be the involved area. As healing occurs the PT should begin screening other body regions to identify contributing factors related to the injury itself or to help prevent a reinjury.

BIBLIOGRAPHY

1. Bickley LS: *Bates' guide to physical examination and history taking*, ed 8, Philadelphia, 2003, Lippincott Williams & Wilkins.
2. Boissonnault W: *Examination in physical therapy practice: screening for medical disease*, ed 2, New York, 1995, Churchill Livingstone.
3. Cyriax J: *Textbook of orthopaedic medicine: diagnosis of soft tissue lesions*, ed 8, London, 1982, Bailliere-Tindall.
4. Donatelli R, Wooden M: *Orthopaedic physical therapy*, ed 3, New York, 2001, Churchill Livingstone.
5. Goodman C, Snyder T: *Differentiatial diagnosis for physical therapists*, ed 3, Philadelphia, 2000, WB Saunders.
6. Goroll AH, Mulley AG: *Primary care medicine*, ed 4, Philadelphia, 2000, Lippincott, Williams & Wilkins.
7. Magee DJ: *Orthopedic physical assessment*, ed 4, Philadelphia, 2002, WB Saunders.
8. Maitland G, Hengeveld E, Banks K, et al: *Maitland's vertebral manipulation*, ed 6, Oxford, 2001, Butterworth/Heinemann.
9. Meadows J: *Orthopedic differential diagnosis in physical therapy*, New York, 1999, McGraw-Hill.
10. Swartz MH: *Textbook of physical diagnosis: history and examination*, ed 4, Philadelphia, 2002, WB Saunders.

TABLE 10-2

Tendon Reflex Grading Scale

Grade	Description
0	Absent
1+ or +	Hypoactive
2+ or ++	Normal
3+ or +++	Hyperactive without clonus
4+ or ++++	Hyperactive with clonus

Lower Quarter Screening Examination

11

Steven C. Janos, PT, MS, OCS
William G. Boissonnault, PT, DHSc, FAAOMPT

Objectives

After reading this chapter, the reader will be able to:

1. Describe the primary objectives of the lower quarter screening examination as a part of the differential diagnosis process.
2. Describe the specific examination elements making up the lower quarter screening examination.
3. Explain the importance of each specific examination element as part of the differential diagnosis process.

The lower quarter screening examination is performed during the initial patient visit in two scenarios: (1) when the patient's primary symptom(s) are located in the lower half of the body, and (2) when symptom fluctuation is related to movements, postures, or activities that involve primarily the lower portion of the trunk and lower extremities.

The principles associated with the lower quarter screening examination are similar to those of the upper quarter examination. The primary purposes are to identify the regional origin (at times the tissue[s]) of the chief presenting complaint, the associated primary impairments, and medical red flags. This information will direct the physical therapist (PT) to the body regions that he or she should examine in more detail. This information also will help guide the development of the initial intervention plan and will help guide the decision of whether to refer the patient to another health care provider.

Although this procedure is called the lower quarter screening examination, the upper half of the body should not be ignored. The postural assessment is a whole-body assessment, as is the gait screening. In addition, assessment of trunk active range of motion (AROM) includes a close observation of the upper-quarter regions while the patient is moving. Finally, Chapter 8 discusses elements of the physical examination that begin during the history and that are germane to all patients at the initial visit, including the skin assessment and the screen of the general nervous system; and Chapter 9 describes the collection of patient vital signs, again germane to all patients. But as stated previously, the history-taking process has led the PT to believe that the origin of the chief symptom and the primary impairments lie in the lower half of the body.

The lower quarter screening examination is organized by patient position: standing, sitting, supine, and then prone. This organization minimizes the amount of changes in position the patient is asked to make. The recommended sequence works well for most patients but must be modified in certain circumstances. For example, a patient with acute low back pain states that he cannot sit for more than 5 minutes without a significant increase in back and leg symptoms. In such a situation, the PT may choose to perform the sitting portion of the examination last instead of second. If the PT ignores the patient information and strictly adheres to the printed examination procedure, the examination may aggravate the patient's symptoms to the point that the PT cannot examine the patient in sufficient detail in the supine and prone positions, and the patient may leave in more pain than he or she felt before the visit.

The novice PT should perform the entire lower quarter screening examination during the initial patient visit in most cases (see Chapter 10), but there are some exceptions to this rule. If the patient presents with an acute injury to the knee or ankle, the PT should spend most of the initial visit on examining the injured area. The priority in this case is to seek a fracture or serious ligamentous injury (see Chapter 17), and after the PT rules these out, he or she should begin the acute rehabilitation management. When the patient begins to recover from the injury, the remaining portions of the screening examination become appropriate, considering the patient may have impairments elsewhere in the lower quarter that have made the patient susceptible to the original injuries. Other patients who fit this scenario are those seen immediately after surgery. As these patients recover from the surgery, the focus of the examination and interventions should become broader.

Box 11-1 shows the lower quarter screening examination, organized by patient position, followed by a brief description of the various assessment techniques.

Description of Examination Elements by Position
Standing

POSTURE/INSPECTION. Although the PT also assesses standing posture and gait when performing an upper quarter screening examination, these functions typically are examined more precisely in the lower quarter screening examination. The PT can initially provide a simple request, such as "please stand and look straight ahead." This request describes the task at hand, yet the instruction is open ended enough that the patient hopefully will assume a typical posture. The PT usually performs the postural assessment with the patient's shoes

---

BOX 11-1

Lower Quarter Screening Examination

STANDING
- Postural observation
- General palpation
- Gait
- Inspection/palpation, including bony landmarks (ribs, iliac crests, posterior superior iliac spine [PSIS], greater trochanters, popliteal creases/fibular heads, malleoli, calcaneus, medial longitudinal arch, anterior superior iliac spine [ASIS], patella/tibial tuberosity, and forefoot including great toe)
- Standing squat (general clearing of the lumbar, pelvic, hip, knee, foot, and ankle regions)
- Vertical "quick" compression (heel bounce)
- Balance
  - Bilateral stance
  - Unilateral stance
- AROM trunk (with passive overpressures if symptoms *not* produced during the active movements); rotation to be done in sitting position
  - Flexion
  - Right and left lateral flexion
  - Extension
- Neurologic screening; myotome and dermatome testing
- Heel raise (S1, S2) tibial nerve and superficial peroneal nerve
- Toe raise (L4, L5) deep peroneal nerve
- Sensation of posterior lower extremities (LEs) (S1, S2)

SITTING
- Posture (observe during the interview process)
- Active trunk rotation and overpressures
- Thoracic cage: upper and lower respiratory excursion
- Vertical trunk compression and decompression (spine in neutral position)
- Neurologic screening:
  - Sensory
    Trunk: anterior (T7 to T12; abdomen)
    LEs: L1 to S1 (anterior, medial, lateral)
  - Myotome
    Trunk (multisegmental and peripheral nerves) flexion, extension, lateral flexion
    LEs
    Hip flexion: L1, L2, L3 (femoral nerve)
    Adduction: L1, L2, L3 (obturator nerve)
    Abduction: L4, L5, S1 (sup/inf gluteal nerve)
    Knee extension: L2, L3, L4 (femoral nerve)
    Knee flexion: L4, L5, S1, S2 (sciatic-tibial nerve)
    Dorsiflexion: L4, L5 (deep peroneal nerve)
    Extensor hallucis longus: L5 to S1 (deep peroneal nerve)
    Eversion L5 to S1 (superficial peroneal nerve)
    NOTE: already have tested plantarflexors in standing position (S1 and S2, tibial nerve)
  - Deep tendon reflexes (DTR)
    Patellar tendon: (L2, L3, L4)
    Achilles tendon: (S1, S2)

SUPINE
- Posture (compare with Standing findings)
- General palpation (compare with Standing findings)
- Neck flexion dural tension testing
- Thorax/abdomen
  - Layer palpation of abdominal region
  - Abdominal aorta (width and strength of pulse); auscultate if have concerns about the involvement of the aorta (see Chapter 9)
  - Sensory T7 to T12 anterior aspect
  - Superficial abdominal reflex (T7 to L1)
  - Femoral triangle palpation
  - Pulses: femoral artery auscultation for bruit if indicated
  - Lymph nodes: inguinal nodes: vertical and horizontal chains
- Lower extremity palpation
  - Pulses (popliteal artery, posterior tibial artery, dorsalis pedis artery)
- SI gap, compression testing, and ilial shear testing
- Trunk AROM: double knee to chest
- AROM/PROM LEs (add overpressures if symptoms not produced during AROM)
  - Knee flexion and extension
  - Hip flexion
  - Hip internal and external rotation
  - FABER (*f*lexion, *ab*duction, and *e*xternal *r*otation)/FADIR (*f*lexion, *ad*duction, and *i*nternal *r*otation)
  - Ankle dorsiflexion (knee flexed and extended; gastrocnemius versus soleus) and plantarflexion
  - Ankle inversion and eversion
  - Toe flexion and extension
- Straight leg raise
- Neurologic screening
  - Babinski test
  - Repeat or include any or all myotome, sensory, and DTR tests that were positive in sitting or standing, or were not done previously.

PRONE
- Postural observation (compared with other positions and with normal)
- Palpation of posterior lower quarter, as in standing
- AROM/PROM (add overpressures if symptoms not produced during AROM)
  - Prone press-up (if standing trunk extension was symptomatic)
  - Knee flexion
  - Hip extension
- Neurologic screening
  - Sensory testing: S1 to S2 (S2, S3, S4: anal region if patient reports any symptoms suggestive of cauda equina)
  - Myotome testing: hip extension (L5, S1, S2: gluteal and tibial nerves)
  - Femoral nerve tension test

---

and socks off, but considering the effect footwear can have on the lower quarter, the PT should briefly assess the patient's footwear both on and off the patient. The PT should assess the patient's posture from anterior, posterior, and lateral perspectives. The PT should focus on the lower half of the patient's body while briefly scanning the upper body for major deviations. Once this initial assessment is completed, the PT should standardize as much of the remaining postural and inspection examination as possible so that following treatment the PT can reposition the patient and reassess for any resultant changes.

INSPECTION. Inspection includes palpation of specific bony landmarks to help the PT better understand and interpret the patient's postural presentation. Examples of posterior landmarks useful as references include the following:
- Spinous processes (T6 to S2); palpating for a step that suggests possible listhesis deformity
- Inferior angle of the scapula (T7)
- Twelfth ribs
- Iliac crests approximately (L4-L5 level)
- Posterior superior iliac spines (PSIS) (approximately S2 level)

- Superior aspect of the greater trochanters
- Fibular heads (superior aspect)
- Medial malleoli (inferior aspect)
- Calcaneus
- Navicular tuberosities

Inspection of the trunk and lower extremities also includes a general assessment of spinal curves, including the degree of pelvic tilt, as well as general body contour, skin temperature and texture, and muscle tone.

GAIT. As with the postural assessment, the PT should assess *gait* from the anterior, posterior, and lateral perspectives. As mentioned earlier, the PT should assess upper quarter motion (or lack of) during the gait cycle but primarily focus attention from the trunk downward to the foot-ankle complex. The PT notes any gross alterations in the mechanics of gait as well as any change in symptoms and where the symptoms occur during the gait cycle.

STANDING SQUAT. To assess the *squat*, the PT stands in front of the patient and assists the patient in maintaining balance while asking the patient to squat down toward the floor as far as possible. The PT should note any change in symptoms, the overall extent of the movement, and any difficulty or asymmetry while going down and returning to the upright position. The PT also can observe regional ROM contributions (or lack of ROM) of the lumbopelvic, knee, and ankle-feet complexes during the movement. The PT should compare the patient's ability to perform this movement with feet flat versus allowing the heels to rise up in order to screen for length of the gastroc-soleus complex. Finally, the squat maneuver grossly screens for quadriceps (L2 to L4) weakness. If the patient has difficulty performing the squat movement, it should be attempted unilaterally to get a more accurate assessment of strength. If the patient has no change in symptoms and completes the movement fully and easily, it is unlikely that significant impairments exist at the knee, foot, and ankle complexes or the hip. This conclusion would allow the PT to spend more time examining other body regions during the remainder of the visit.

QUICK VERTICAL COMPRESSION. As with the squat testing, this test is a functional method of imparting increased weight-bearing stress on primarily the musculoskeletal structures of the lower trunk and lower extremities. The patient is asked to rise up on the balls of the feet and quickly and vigorously hit down on the heels, using the PT for balance support if needed. The PT notes the patient's willingness to perform the activity and any change in symptoms.

As with the standing-squat screening test, if this test aggravates symptoms, the source may be in any or all of the joint complexes of the lower body. If the patient can complete the movement vigorously and without symptoms, the test does give the PT valuable information about the status of the lower body's weight-bearing structures.

ACTIVE RANGE OF MOTION: TRUNK/HIPS. Active movements of trunk flexion, extension, and lateral flexion continue the evaluation of the functional abilities of the spine and hip joints, and also help in identifying the source of the patient's symptoms. As with postural assessment and bony palpation, the PT should employ a standardized and reproducible position. Once again, the PT can do this by having the patient spread his or her feet apart a specific distance, such as the width of the PT's foot, or the PT can have the patient straddle a tile on the floor.

The PT should observe active movements from multiple angles, and patients should be instructed to go as far as possible before stopping the movement and to report any change in symptoms. Patients are instructed to keep their knees straight. Trunk flexion typically is the first motion tested. A lateral view gives the best picture of the quantity of trunk-flexion motion, while a posterior view gives the best picture of the quality of movement.

The PT's assessment of quantity of motion includes a comparison of the hip and pelvis contribution to the movements versus that of the lumbar and thoracic spine. Overall quantity of trunk range of motion may be excellent (during forward bending of the trunk the patient may able to touch the floor with the fingertips) yet the patient may present with regional limitations (e.g., incomplete reversal of the lumbar lordosis or reduced hip rotation).

In contrast, some patients are hypermobile at the hip or the spine but arbitrarily stop when their fingers touch the floor. This may give the impression that their range of motion is within normal limits, but if they had continued past that point, the PT would have noted their hyperflexibility.

The assessment of quality of motion includes deviation from the desired plane of movement, aberrant speed of motion, experience of an atypical sensation at the end of the motion (e.g., intense stretching sensation noted in the right posterior thigh at end of range-of-trunk flexion).

Finally, symptoms of spinal or hip origin could be altered (increased or decreased) during the motions. These findings will be matched later with the active and passive ROM findings of the hips to identify involvement of the spine or hip joint complex.

If symptoms have not changed during the active motion assessment, the PT can apply a passive overpressure to the spine (Figures 11-1 to 11-3). The passive overpressures are necessary in order to clear the spine as a source of symptoms.

Another method PTs may prefer that places increased mechanical stresses on the spine and hip complex is to have the patient perform repeated active trunk motions, as described by McKenzie.

NEUROLOGIC SCREENING. The final tests in the standing position are classic tests for assessment of several lumbosacral myotomes, heel walking (L4/L5) and toe walking (S1/S2). These particular myotomes, along with quadriceps (L2-L4), are best tested unilaterally to detect subtle weakness. They are a gross assessment that also tests balance mechanisms and proximal stability. The PT performs additional myotome tests later with the patient in the sitting position that also assess the status of these same neurologic levels. The PT also can assess sensory function (S1-S2 dermatomes) of the posterior aspect of the lower extremities with the patient in the standing position.

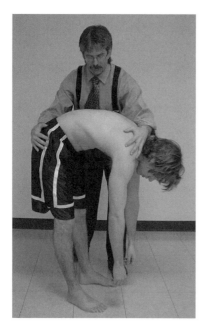

FIGURE 11-1 Passive overpressure with the patient in the position of standing trunk-forward flexion.

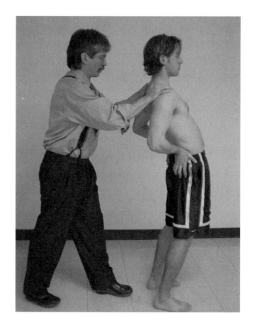

FIGURE 11-3 Passive overpressure with the patient in the position of standing trunk-backward bending.

Sitting

Weight-bearing tests continue with the patient in the sitting position. At this time, the PT should ask the patient whether this change in position has altered the symptoms in any way. The PT briefly assesses trunk posture and compares it with the standing-position findings and with the patient's sitting posture noted during the interview (which may give the most accurate picture of the patient's normal sitting posture).

ROTATION RANGE OF MOTION: TRUNK ROTATION (WITH OR WITHOUT OVERPRESSURES). The patient is asked to cross the arms across the chest and then rotate the trunk to each side. The PT should perform a gross assessment of overall trunk ROM, while specifically observing position changes in the lower thoracic and lumbar spine from a posterior viewpoint. If symptoms are not changed with active movements, the PT then applies passive overpressure in each direction (Figure 11-4). The hips will contribute little movement while the patient is sitting, so a change in symptoms most likely has a spinal origin.

Vertical Trunk Compression/Decompression. These two provocation tests (Figure 11-5) stress primarily the weight-bearing (vertebral bodies, intervertebral disc, facet joints) and ligamentous structures of the spine. The PT first applies a

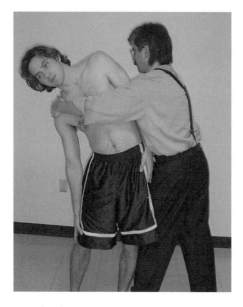

FIGURE 11-2 Passive overpressure with the patient in the position of standing trunk-lateral flexion.

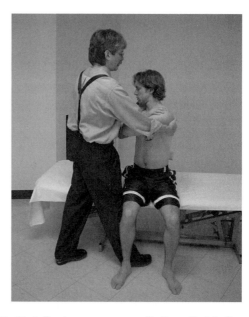

FIGURE 11-4 Passive overpressure with the patient in the position of seated trunk rotation.

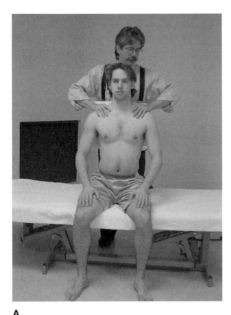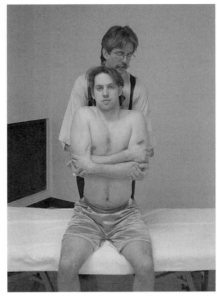

A   **B**

FIGURE 11-5 **A** and **B,** Seated trunk vertical-compression test (stressing weight-bearing structures of the spine).

compression load on the trunk, holding for about 5 seconds and noting any change in symptoms. Next, the PT applies an unloading force, or decompression, to the trunk for the same amount of time and notes its effect (better or worse) on symptoms. The PT must be careful in both of these testing procedures to avoid producing any movement of the trunk except in the vertical plane. A patient response of increased symptoms with vertical compression and relief with unloading should direct the PT to implement traction and other unloading interventions.

Lower Thoracic-Cage Excursion. The PT performs a brief screening of the lower rib cage ROM by observing whether the patient is breathing from the abdomen or the shoulder girdles, and by palpating laterally around the chest wall while having the patient inhale and exhale deeply. The PT should note the amount of rib cage excursion, symmetry, and any change in symptoms. Detecting abnormalities will lead the PT to perform a more extensive examination of this region when the patient is in recumbent positions.

Neurologic Screening: Trunk and Lower Extremities

Myotome testing. The PT can perform this test most easily by starting at the trunk. Again, the PT should ask the patient to "hold" and ask for slow, maximal resistance without any trunk movement. The patient holds this position for 10 seconds, and the PT performs a gross assessment, identifying the patient's performance as weak or strong, and noting any change in symptoms. Because the innervation of these muscles is multisegmental (as in the cervical region, identifying one particular nerve root of the thoracic spine as the reason for any weakness is virtually impossible. The PT continues this screening in the lower extremities, testing the muscle groups listed previously.

Sensory testing. As in the upper-quarter screening examination (see Chapter 10), sharp or dull sensation is assessed for the lower body. Although the PT will need to assess the T6 through S2 dermatomal areas (Figure 11-6), the PT will find

the procedure easiest by beginning with the L1 level and continuing through the S1 level. The PT can best assess the T6 through T12 dermatomes anteriorly with the patient in the supine position, while the posterior of these levels through the S2 level is checked with the patient in the prone position.

Deep tendon reflexes. The two reflexes in the lower extremities most often assessed are the patellar (L2 to L4) and Achilles (S1, S2) reflexes. As in the upper-quarter screening examination (see Chapter 10), the PT must have the patient in a neutral spinal posture (i.e., a reproducible position), sitting comfortably on the examination table.

Supine

The PT questions the patient again about any change in symptoms as the patient assumes the new position, and the PT performs a brief postural observation, comparing findings with the findings of weight-bearing postures. After the general observation is completed, the patient should again assume a standard position, which the PT can produce by asking the patient to perform a bridging activity to reset the position. The general examination sequence is to start at the head and move caudally.

NECK FLEXION (DURAL-TENSION) TESTING. The neck flexion test is a passive neural mobility test, with the PT passively flexing the head and neck on the thorax. If the patient experiences a marked increase in symptoms in the lumbar and posterior thighs accompanied by hip and knee flexion, the PT must be suspicious of meningeal irritation. A patient with an acute lumbar radiculopathy may also experience lumbar and lower extremity pain with the neck flexion.

ABDOMINAL PALPATION AND THORACIC/ABDOMINAL PERCUSSION. The PT next performs palpation of the abdominal area to help rule out nonmusculoskeletal sources of the patient's symptoms and to identify local impairments related to the patient's functional limitations. The palpation is not intended to enable the

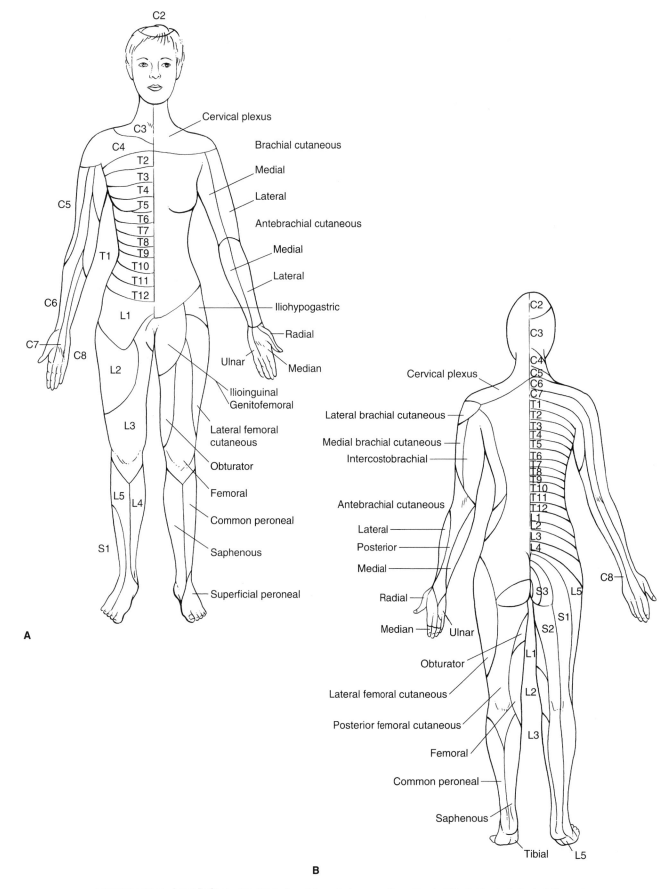

FIGURE 11-6 A and **B,** Segmental distribution of the spinal nerves. (From Swartz MH: *Textbook of physical diagnosis: history and examination*, Philadelphia, 2002, WB Saunders, p 623.)

PT to diagnose a specific visceral problem but to contribute to the overall investigation for potential sources of symptoms. See Chapter 6 for a description of symptom patterns associated with visceral disorders, a number of which could present as back pain.

Many of the visceral structures are difficult to impossible to distinguish via palpation. Therefore the PT can use *manual percussion* to help locate these structures in both the thorax and abdominal cavity. The sound produced from this technique will help determine whether the underlying structure is air filled, fluid filled, or solid. For our purposes, we will be listening for four different sounds or notes produced:

Flatness: Solid, dense tissues like that of the anterior thigh
Dullness: Liver, heart, diaphragm, spleen
Resonance: Lung
Tympany: Gastric (stomach) bubble, bowel

Manual percussion is performed as follows. Hyperextend the middle finger of your nondominant hand. Press its distal interphalangeal (IP) joint firmly on the surface to be percussed. Avoid contact by any other part of the hand, because this could damp the vibrations. Position your other forearm close to the surface, with the hand cocked upward (wrist extended). The middle finger should be partially flexed, relaxed, and poised to strike. With a quick, sharp, but relaxed wrist motion, strike the IP joint of the finger in contact with the skin with your middle finger of the dominant hand. You are simply trying to transmit vibrations through the bones of this joint to the underlying chest wall. Use two strikes, then pause, and then either repeat or move on to another location. The following guidelines can be used for this technique.

• **Liver**: *Percussion*: one starts just above the umbilicus on the right side (along the midclavicular line) and progresses cephalically, noting first tympany of bowel until hearing *dullness* of the liver. When the dullness is noted, continue along the midclavicular line for about 6 to 12 cm (Figure 11-7). If too far cephalad, you will note a new sound, the

resonance of the lung. Palpate on the right side, lateral to the rectus abdominis margin, and below the inferior border of the liver dullness noted during percussion. Place your left hand under the patient's back, around the T10-T11 region on the right, and lift gently. The fingers of the right hand then apply a moderate pressure slightly cephalically and posteriorly. The patient then is asked to hold a deep breath; the PT may note the liver edge as it moves down into the fingers; the PT documents any change or reproduction of symptoms.

• **Spleen**: *Percussion* starts at the lowest rib interspace along the left anterior axillary line. The sound produced should be abdominal tympany. Then move posteriorly to produce splenic dullness, noted in a line from the left ninth to the eleventh ribs (Figure 11-8). *Palpation* of the area of the spleen is similar to that of the liver. The PT positions one hand posteriorly under the patient's left side and lifts upward. The PT places the other hand at the left upper-abdominal region and applies gentle pressure in a cephalic and posterior direction, again having the patient take and hold a deep inspiration, noting any change or reproduction of symptoms.

• **Kidneys**: *Palpation* of the right kidney is difficult (but possible in some patients; the left kidney is seldom palpable) in the absence of significant pathology. To locally stress the area, the technique is similar to that described for palpation in the area of the liver and spleen. The PT places one hand under the patient's back at the area of T12 and L1. The PT lifts upward, and the fingertips of the top hand are just below the liver edge at the midclavicular line. The PT should visualize the kidney lying gently between his or her two hands. Again, the goal is not necessarily to detect anatomical abnormalities, but to mechanically stress this region in order to detect changes or provocation of symptoms. If the PT notes concerns during palpation of this region, he or she can perform *percussion* over the kidneys with the patient sitting. A firm "thumping" with the PT's fist over the left and then right sides of the costovertebral angle (region of the thoracolumbar junction)

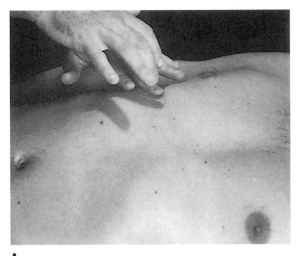 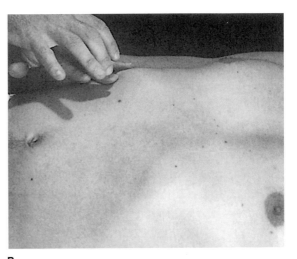

A   B

FIGURE 11-7 A and **B,** Manual percussion in the midclavicular line over the liver. (From Boissonnault W: *Examination in physical therapy practice, screening for medical disease,* ed 2, New York, 1995, Churchill Livingstone, p 111.)

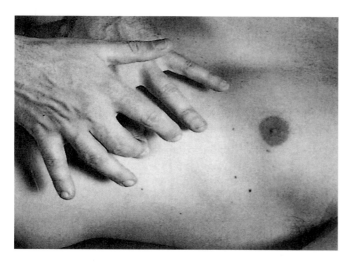

FIGURE 11-8 Manual percussion in the anterior axillary line over the spleen. (From Boissonnault W: *Examination in physical therapy practice, screening for medical disease*, ed 2, New York, 1995, Churchill Livingstone, p 112.)

often will provoke symptoms if the kidneys are inflamed or irritated.

- **Stomach** (gastric bubble): *Palpation* and *percussion* generally are performed over the epigastrium. Noting alterations of symptoms and tympany over this region is important.

After screening the structures and regions noted above, the PT generally palpates the four quadrants (left and right upper and lower quadrants, established by vertical and horizontal lines through the umbilicus) of the abdomen (Figure 11-9). This is a three-part process, palpating from superficial to deep.

First, the PT applies light pressure to an area in a circular fashion. If there is no major resistance and no complaint of symptoms, the PT continues with deeper pressure. If pain is provoked, then the PT performs a quick release of the tissue, assessing for the presence of *rebound tenderness* (exquisite

tenderness or pain provoked by the quick release, suggesting peritoneal irritation, possibly an internal bleed, or abscess). Suspicion of rebound tenderness should prompt the PT to contact the patient's physician to discuss the findings. If the patient does experience symptoms, the PT should note the location and the description of the symptoms as well as the location and depth of the palpation.

Another important structure to consider is the *abdominal aorta*. This arterial pulse is located halfway between the xiphoid process and the umbilicus, slightly left of center. Having the patient's hips and knees flexed tends to relax the abdomen and allow for easier palpation. The PT should first locate the pulse and assess it for intensity using the 0 to 4+ arterial scale (0 = absent; 2+ = normal; 4+ = bounding). The PT assesses the width of the aortic pulse by placing the index fingers of both hands side by side over the pulse and then slowly moving them apart until the borders of the pulsation are noted (Figure 11-10). If the PT suspects widening of the pulse (the normal width of the vessel is about approximately 2 cm) or if back pain is provoked, the PT should auscultate over the blood vessel, assessing for a bruit. If pain is provoked or if a bruit is noted, physician contact is warranted.

Neurologic Screening: Abdomen

Sensory testing. This screening tool includes sharp and dull testing over the abdominal region from the xiphoid process to just above the inguinal ligament (see Figure 11-6) to assess the sensory status of the T7 through T12 dermatomes.

Superficial abdominal reflex. The abdominal region is divided into four quadrants for this test (Figure 11-11). Using an object such as the end of a reflex hammer, lightly stroke each quadrant, moving the stimulus out and away from the umbilicus. In a normal response, the umbilicus moves in the direction of the stimulus.

Trunk Active Range of Motion (Double Knee to Chest). If standing-forward flexion of the trunk provokes symptoms (of the back

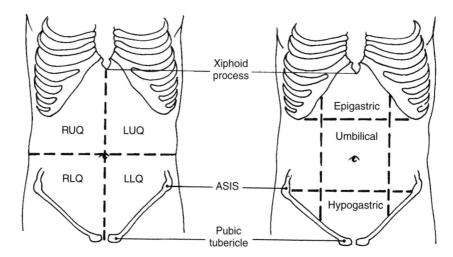

FIGURE 11-9 Terminology used to delineate the regions of the abdomen. *RUQ:* Right upper-abdominal quadrant; *LUQ:* left upper-abdominal quadrant; *RLQ:* right lower-abdominal quadrant; *LLQ:* left lower-abdominal quadrant. (From Boissonnault W: *Examination in physical therapy practice, screening for medical disease*, ed 2, New York, 1995, Churchill Livingstone, p 111.)

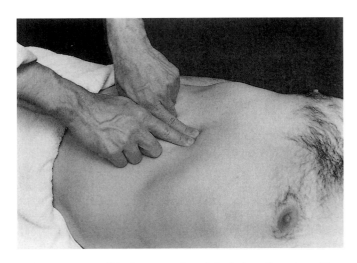

FIGURE 11-10 Palpation over the abdominal aortic artery. (From Boissonnault W: *Examination in physical therapy practice, screening for medical disease*, ed 2, New York, 1995, Churchill Livingstone, p 412.)

or lower extremity) the PT should assess this movement with the patient in a non–weight-bearing position. The PT may find that, although the standing-forward flexion worsens the symptoms, the *double-knee-to-chest* movement produces only a sensation of good stretch in the low back region. This finding would give the PT a method of attempting to normalize this important trunk movement.

Sacroiliac Joint Stress Tests. Two tests will help in implicating or ruling out the SI joint as a source of symptoms. For the compression and gapping test, the PT first makes contact just

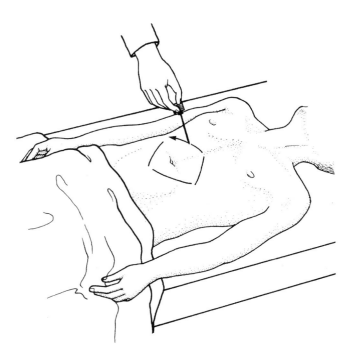

FIGURE 11-11 Superficial abdominal reflex testing. (From Magee DJ: *Orthopedic physical assessment*, ed 4, Philadelphia, 2002, WB Saunders, p 530.)

lateral to the anterior superior iliac spine (ASIS) of the iliac crests and applies pressure with both hands slowly in a medial direction. The PT should hold this pressure for about 5 seconds. Next, the PT's arms are crossed, the heels of the hands are placed on the medial aspects of the iliac crests (near the ASIS), and pressure is applied in a lateral direction bilaterally, again holding for about 5 seconds.

Another useful test is the ilial shear test described in Magee's textbook (see reference list). Stabilizing one ASIS with anteroposterior pressure, the PT applies an anteroposterior shear force to the opposite ASIS. The PT repeats this procedure on the opposite side, holding for about 5 seconds each time. The ilial shear test allows the PT to assess end feels, comparing the left side with the right side in addition to noting any change in symptoms.

LYMPH NODE PALPATION. The inguinal lymph nodes located in the femoral triangle (bordered by the inguinal ligament and the sartorius and adductor longus muscles) are divided into horizontal and vertical chains. The PT first locates the inguinal ligament, running between the ASIS and the pubic tubercle. Just caudal and running parallel to this ligament is the horizontal chain. In the medial third of the femoral triangle is the vertical chain, running parallel to the adductor longus. See Chapter 8 for normal and abnormal characteristics of lymph nodes.

Arterial Pulse: Lower Extremies. The PT should assess each of the lower extremity pulses for location, intensity, and symmetry, especially in patients presenting with complaints of intermittent claudication, symptoms of cold feet, or trophic or other changes in skin (see Chapter 8). The following landmarks can be used to locate the pulses:

- The femoral pulse is located in the femoral triangle.
- The popliteal pulse is found just cephalic to the popliteal crease. The patient's knee should be flexed to place the posterior soft tissues on slack, facilitating palpation of this deeply set artery. If this artery is difficult to locate with the patient in the supine position, the PT can assess the pulse with the patient in the prone position, again with the knee flexed.
- The posterior tibial pulse is located posterior to the medial malleolus.
- The dorsalis pedis artery is found on the dorsum of the foot over the first and second metatarsal bases.

Clearing the lower extremities. Clearing any joint implies examining the joint and related soft tissues to the point that the PT can confidently state that it is, or is not, a source of symptoms and that it is, or is not, involved from an impairment perspective. To reach these conclusions, the PT typically does not need to perform a complete detailed examination of the area. If symptoms are changed or if the PT notes significant impairments during the screening (clearing), the PT then should perform a detailed examination of the region. The PT began the clearing of the lower extremities with the posture and gait screening and the standing-squat maneuver. This joint clearing uses selected active range-of-motion and passive overpressures in a sequence similar to that used when clearing the upper extremities (see Chapter 10). Recommended movement tests for the lower extremities include:

Hip
- Flexion
- Internal/external rotation
- FABER (flexion, abduction, and external rotation) test
- FADIR (flexion, adduction, and internal rotation) test

Knee	Ankle	Toes
Flexion	Dorsiflexion	Flexion
Extension	Plantarflexion	Extension

The PT should clear the knee first because assessment of hip rotation will stress the knee joint. Next, the PT assesses hip flexion, then internal and external rotation, and if symptoms are not altered and the PT does not note significant impairments, the PT should carry out the combined-movement tests (FABER and FADIR). After finishing the test of hip range of motion, the PT moves to the ankles and feet and completes the movement testing. Performing the active ankle/foot movements bilaterally can save time, as can be done with the wrists and hands during the upper-quarter examination.

Straight leg raise. This is the second dural-tension test (after the head/neck flexion test) in the supine position. If the patient does not have acute symptoms, he or she first actively performs hip flexion with the knee extended (with the ankle and foot relaxed) while the PT monitors the range of movement and changes in symptoms. Next, the PT fully extends the patient's knee and then slowly flexes the hip passively until the patient complains of symptoms (typically of the posterior lower extremity). At this point, the patient is instructed to tell the PT when the symptoms begin to subside as the PT lowers the flexed hip. Finally, the ankle is passively dorsiflexed, and if the symptoms increase again, dural tissue may be implicated as the source of the symptoms.

Neurologic Screening: Lower Extremities Including Babinski Reflex. If the PT noted any positive neurologic findings during myotome or sensory testing with the patient in the weight-bearing positions (standing or sitting), those tests should be repeated now with the patient in the supine or non–weight-bearing positions for comparison. In addition, the PT should routinely assess the *Babinski reflex.* The PT firmly strokes the plantar aspect of the foot, starting at the heel and moving up the lateral side of the sole and eventually across the metatarsal heads medially. The patient often demonstrates a withdrawal response of the hip and knee (flexion), which is normal. An abnormal response or positive Babinski is extension of the great toe and abduction of the other toes. When this pathologic reflex occurs, it is indicative of upper-motor-neuron disease.

Prone

The PT again questions the patient about changes in symptoms during the final position change, as the patient moves into the prone position. The PT observes the trunk and lower extremities in this position, compares results with those of the standing position, and notes any differences.

ACTIVE RANGE OF MOTION: TRUNK AND LOWER EXTREMITIES. The PT should have the patient perform the *prone press-up* if standing, trunk-backward bending provokes symptoms of the back or lower extremity, for the same reasons noted during the supine double-knee-to-chest maneuver. The PT also can assess active hip extension, but the PT will encounter a challenge in controlling lumbar spine position and preventing lumbosacral backward bending and rotation during the assessment. Stabilizing over the ipsilateral ischial tuberosity will help localize the movement to the hip.

The patient next performs active knee flexion, followed by passive flexion. This test assesses several things. It brings the hamstring into play against gravity and places a tensile stress on both the femoral nerve and the rectus femoris muscle. The PT can identify the structure involved in symptom reproduction by end feel of the passive movement (rectus femoris) and through other neurologic tests germane to the femoral nerve previously performed.

NEUROLOGIC SCREENING: EXTREMITIES. If the PT noted any positive neurologic findings during myotome or sensory testing with the patient in the weight-bearing positions (standing or sitting), the PT should repeat the tests with the patient in a prone or non–weight-bearing position for comparison. As with the comparison of non–weight-bearing assessment of trunk ROM versus weight-bearing trunk ROM, positive neurologic findings may occur only in weight-bearing positions, giving guidance to the PT about body positions to be used in home exercise programs and about general patient education.

Summary

As with the upper quarter screening examination, the overall examination of the patient is not finished when the PT has completed the above tests, but at this point (after the history and lower quarter screening examination), the PT should have a strong hypothesis about the source of symptoms and the primary impairments related to functional limitations and disability, and should have identified red flags. In many instances, the collected information will give the PT sufficient guidance to initiate treatment. In addition, the PT will have decided which joint complexes may require more detailed assessment at subsequent visits.

As stated previously, when a patient presents with an acute injury, the PT's initial emphasis should be on the injured area, and then as the patient begins to recover, the PT should use the lower quarter screening examination to help identify any contributing factors (impairments) associated with the injury. Systematically proceeding through the screening examination will prevent the PT from being fooled by the location of symptoms. For example, primary hip conditions often present with a chief symptom of knee pain. When treatment focuses solely on the location of a patient's pain, a poor outcome to rehabilitation can occur.

PATIENT CASE

In the following case, the patient's chief symptom is pain in the left groin. This case summarizes the principles outlined earlier. The following symbols and abbreviations are used in the case:

- ↓ = decreased
- ↑ = increased
- WB = weight bearing
- mm = muscle
- n/c = no complaints
- c/o = complaint of
- sxs = symptoms

- EROM = end of range of motion
- OP = passive overpressure
- MSS = musculoskeletal system
- sl = slight
- abn = abnormal
- cc = chief complaint
- LB = low back
- LEs = lower extremities
- LLE = left lower extremity
- RLE = right lower extremity
- lt = light touch
- WNL = within normal limits

Tests	Findings	Analysis
PATIENT CC: LEFT HIP/GROIN PAIN		
Standing		
Observation/palpation, including postural assessment	↓ WB LLE; flat lumbar curve; sl. left hip flexed/knee flexed posture	Possible antalgic posture and/or structural abnormality of trunk/LEs. Possible weakness of LE mms; leg length difference.
	↑ mm tone of lumbar extensors and left hamstrings.	Possible mm guarding.
Gait	Slow, guarded; lists over to L during stance LLE, sl. c/o cc with WB on left side.	MSS problem. Possible antalgic gait. Possible weakness of LEs and/or trunk. Possible balance deficit.
Squat	Slow, difficult, limited by one third; deviation over RLE, sl. c/o cc upon rising.	MSS problem. Possible antalgia. Possible stiffness. Possible weakness. Possible trunk, hip or knee likely involvement.
Quick compression	↓ WB LLE, but n/c sxs.	Possible guarding/antalgia.
AROM (trunk)	Flexion: n/c sxs, limited to 8 inches from floor; OP n/c sxs; about 75 degrees of hip flex; trunk ROM okay; deviation to R on lowering.	Flexion: possibly limited, antalgic. Possible tightness; neural tension or hamstrings.
	Extension: n/c sxs, about 10 degrees of hip extension, one half trunk ROM; OP sl. L LB tightness.	Extension: Possibly limited; antalgia.
	Sidebending: good ROM, n/c sxs, OP n/c sxs, soft-tissue stretch at end range.	Sidebending: WNL. Sxs possibly not coming from trunk.
Heel raise	Okay for 5 repetitions RLE; more difficult (slower, guarded) on LLE, with trunk list to L.	Possible antalgia. Possible weak LLE. Possible disuse. Possible balance deficit.
Vertical trunk compression	Sl ↑ in cc.	WB tissues: help differentiate hip joint vs. LB.
Vertical trunk distraction	Patient reports "stretch feels good" to LB.	Decompress or unload WB tissues. Relax mms.
Sitting		
AROM (trunk)	Rotation: slightly limited to L; okay to R; n/c sxs.	Sxs possibly not coming from trunk.
LE neurologic screen: myotome and manual muscle test	Sl weakness of L hip flexors and abductors 4/5; all others 5/5, n/c sxs.	Slight weakness a contributing factor to symptoms and limitations?
LE neurologic screen sensory	Intact and equal to lt and pin LEs bilaterally.	No sensory deficit.
LE neurologic screen DTRs	2+ and equal at knees and ankles.	No motor/nerve root deficit.
Supine		
Neck flexion	N/c	No adverse neural tension.
Abdominal	Soft, nontender to palpation; abdominal aorta 2+ pulse and n/c sxs; abdominal reflexes intact and equal in all quadrants; sensory intact and equal in all quadrants.	Sxs not referred from non-MSS abdominal structures. Pulse amplitude normal.
Non-MSS	LE pulses 2+ and equal bilaterally; lymph nodes soft, nontender; mobile bilaterally.	Not referred from LE non-MSS structures. Pulse amplitude normal.
SI joint provocation tests	N/c.	Okay, possibly no SI involvement.
AROM (LEs)	L Hip:	MSS and coming from the hip.
	Flexion: 85 degrees, ** cc EROM.	Limited motions.
	ER: 40 degrees, ** cc EROM.	Inert > contractile tissues with sxs only at EROM.
	IR: 20 degrees, ** cc EROM.	
PROM (LEs)	Flexion: 85 degrees, spasm end feel after cc.	AROM/PROM findings are same, so possibly inert.
	ER: 40 degrees, mild spasm end feel after cc.	Possibly capsular pattern (need ABD information).
	IR: 20 degrees, spasm end feel after cc.	Abnormal end feels and not acute.

Continued

Tests	Findings	Analysis
AROM (LEs)	L hip: Abduction: 25 degrees, * cc EROM Adduction: 30 degrees, n/c sxs.	Moderate limitation in abduction: possible inert tissue.
PROM (LEs)	Abduction: 25 degrees, spasm end feel after cc. Adduction: 30 degrees, soft tissue end feel, n/c sxs.	Same as AROM: inert tissue, and now fits capsular pattern, chronic. Possible tight abduction/ITB by end feels.
Assessment of joint accessory movement	L hip: hypomobility with lateral and inferior distraction, posterior glide; ↓ cc with all movements.	L hip: inert tissue (joint).
SLR	75 degrees bilaterally, n/c.	No adverse neural tension; possible tight hamstrings.
Babinski test	Down-going great toe bilaterally.	Negative for neurologic upper motor neuron lesion.
Prone		
AROM (LEs)	L hip: Extension: 5 degrees, n/c sxs.	Moderate/marked limitation, possibly tight or weak.
PROM (LEs)	Extension: 5 degrees, ST stretch end feel, n/c sxs.	Hip flexor tightness likely given end feel.
LE neurologic screening	Sensory intact and equal posterior LEs bilaterally. Myotome hip extension 5/5, n/c sxs.	No neurologic deficit.

PATIENT CASE CLINICAL DECISION MAKING

I. Complete the Evaluation portion of the presented patient data (see above Analysis findings), including:

Develop an impairment list for this patient.

Determine a differential diagnosis for this patient.

Describe your initial treatment of this patient (be as specific as possible), and briefly describe your proposed treatment.

II. Significant Findings

Trunk/hip/knee postural dysfunction.

Altered and painful functional activities (squat and gait).

Limited trunk movements (extension and rotation [slight]).

Limited and/or painful active and passive physiological movements of the left hip (flexion, IR, ABD, extension).

Limited and/or painful accessory movements of the left hip (distraction and posterior glide).

Muscle tightness of the left hip (rectus, psoas, ITB).

Weakness of the left hip (psoas, gluteus medius, tensor fascia lata).

III. Differential Diagnosis

Musculoskeletal problem. Nonacute, inert, capsular problem (possibly osteoarthritis) of the left hip. This is based on limited and/or painful active and passive movements at the left hip in the same directions (symptoms at EROM), a capsular pattern of limited and painful movement of the hip, and no complaints of symptoms with resisted muscle wasting. The most likely source of symptoms is degenerative joint disease (DJD) of the hip. Patient also demonstrates secondary muscle tightness and weakness at the left hip joint.

IV. Plan of Care

Treat and do not refer.

V. Treatment at Initial Visit

The PT has several goals for the initial visit: help confirm the diagnosis, improve the patient's current condition, and possibly identify a maneuver that can be turned immediately into a home program. The PT must avoid doing too much to avoid irritating the condition. Frequent subjective and objective reassessment of the patient during the treatment portion of the visit will help prevent this. The treatment consists of the following:

Grade III + or IV + hip joint distraction and/or lateral distraction joint mobilization/manipulation. (This will help confirm the hip joint as a source of symptoms if it results in improvement and improves ROM; likely will make the patient feel better because symptoms improved with hip joint play assessment during the examination.)

Grade III or IV physiological hip abduction stretch. (This movement not only is painful and moderately limited, but is involved in gait and unilateral stance, which are functional limitations for this patient).

Modality (heat such as hot pack or diathermy). This may help alleviate some of the pain and also warms the tight tissues to allow for easier stretching.

Home program:

- Hip AROM abduction strengthening exercise
- Instruct in heat application if it improved the condition when used in clinic.
- Fit and instruct the patient in the use of a cane (assist in joint protection, the use in opposite hand) for gait if not already using one.

BIBLIOGRAPHY

1. Bickley LS: *Bates' guide to physical examination and history taking*, ed 8, Philadelphia, 2003, Lippincott Williams & Wilkins.
2. Boissonnault W: *Examination in physical therapy practice, screening for medical disease*, ed 2, New York, 1995, Churchill Livingstone.
3. Cyriax J. *Textbook of orthopaedic medicine: diagnosis of soft tissue lesions*, ed 8, London, 1982, Bailliere-Tindall.
4. Donatelli R, Wooden M: *Orthopaedic physical therapy*, ed 3, New York, 2001, Churchill Livingstone.
5. Goroll AH, Mulley AG: *Primary care medicine*, ed 4, Philadelphia, 2000, Lippincott Williams & Wilkins.
6. Magee DJ: *Orthopedic physical assessment*, ed 4, Philadelphia, 2002, WB Saunders.
7. Maitland G, Hengeveld E, Banks K, et al: *Maitland's vertebral manipulation*, ed 6, Oxford, 2001, Butterworth/Heinemann.
8. Meadows J: *Orthopedic differential diagnosis in physical therapy*, New York, 1999, McGraw-Hill.
9. Swartz MH: *Textbook of physical diagnosis: history and examination*, ed 4, Philadelphia, 2002, WB Saunders.

Epilogue and Patient Case

William G. Boissonnault, PT, DHSc, FAAOMPT

Chapters 5 through 11 present a process for collecting patient data, marked by many instances in which the physical therapist (PT) does more than one thing at a time during the examination process. For example, during the history-taking process, the PT also observes for skin lesions.

This principle of dual effort can carry over to the examination, where the PT can integrate interventions. For example, a patient says during the history that sitting increases the intensity of his low-back pain. While the patient is reporting this information, the PT notes that the patient is sitting in a slouched posture. The PT could stop the interview, place the lumbar cushion behind the patient's back, give quick instructions in posture, and then resume the interview. After a few minutes the PT could ask the patient how his back feels with the cushion compared with his earlier discomfort. If the PT is lucky, the patient will say that the intensity of pain has lessened. In this case, the patient's self-management and empowerment have begun.

The chapters in Sections Two and Three contained a variety of figures, tables, and boxes designed to help the reader. The reader also is directed to the textbook's website, which contains figures and illustrations that augment the material in these sections.

Next is a formal report of a patient case, reprinted with permission from the *Journal of Orthopaedic and Sports Physical Therapy*. This case summarizes several principles covered in Chapters 5 to 11 that lead to the decision to refer the patient to a physician. Both the *Journal of Orthopaedic and Sports Physical Therapy* and the *Physical Therapy Journal* have invited the submission of patient case reports. These reports can be very informative and educational, not only to the clinical community but also to the researchers of our profession. I encourage readers to contribute to the body of research in this way.

PATIENT CASE*

BACKGROUND

Sacral and sacroiliac (SI) joint pain, although not as common as low-back pain, occurs in all age groups. The pain may be a result of muscular, ligamentous, neurologic, mechanical, or bony dysfunction at or near the sacrum or SI joint. Many muscles, including the sacrospinalis (erector spinae), gluteus maximus, and piriformis, attach to the sacrum and potentially could become a source of pain if

strained or partially avulsed.[36] Ligamentous structures that attach to the sacrum and that could cause pain if injured include the sacroiliac, iliolumbar, sacrospinous, and sacrotuberous ligaments.[26] Pain near the sacrum also may be of neurologic origin, because the sacral plexus passes through the sacral foramina.[36]

Mechanical pain resulting from dysfunction of the SI joint may present as sacral pain and also may refer pain distally. In a study by Fortin et al[17], researchers studied pain-referral maps in 10 subjects without SI pain by injecting contrast material into the SI joint under fluoroscopy. They discovered that the SI joint referred pain to an area of 3×10 cm inferior and posterior to the superior iliac spine (primarily to the ipsilateral side) in all subjects. As with previous studies,[23,24] they found variability between subjects, as four subjects also experienced pain to the ipsilateral medial buttock, and two subjects experienced additional pain extending into the ipsilateral superior lateral thigh.[17]

Pain also may be referred to the sacrum from a distant structure. According to Kellgren, pain from the contralateral sacrospinalis muscle may produce pain around the sacrum,[23] as may the ipsilateral L3-S2 interspinous ligaments.[24] McCall et al[32] documented pain-referral patterns from lumbar facet joints after saline injections and found that ipsilateral, lateral sacral pain was provoked with injections at the L4-L5 facet joints.

Finally, pain in the sacral region may be of bony origin, such as a tumor, or may result from a fracture. Although primary tumors of the spine such as osteoid osteomas, chondrosarcomas, and osteosarcomas occur less often than metastatic disease,[25] they do occur. Brat et al[7] reported on a 30-year-old man with a 7-month history of mild sacral pain and intermittent sciatica. Plain radiographs revealed a lesion, and biopsy confirmed a chondromyxoid fibroma, which was surgically removed.[7] Primary breast, lung, and prostate cancers are among the most common cancers to metastasize to the axial skeleton, including the pelvic ring.[16,40] Cancer that has metastasized to the low-back region is more common in individuals aged 50 years and older.[3]

The other bony source of pain seen in all age groups is fractures, including stress fractures. Two types of stress fractures occur: *insufficiency fractures* and *fatigue fractures*.[9,13,14,30,35] Insufficiency fractures occur when normal muscular stress is applied to bone that is deficient in mineral content or elastic resistance.[9,13,14,35] Patients who sustain insufficiency fractures often have predisposing factors, such as osteoporosis, metabolic disorders, prolonged corticosteroid use, or Paget's disease.[8,30,38] The presence of these underlying conditions should alert the PT to the increased risk of bony lesions.

In contrast, fatigue fractures are caused by the application of abnormal muscular stress or mechanical torque to a bone that has normal elasticity and mineral content.[9,13,14,35] Bone, a dynamic structure, responds to the external forces placed upon it according to Wolff's law. However, this response in bone may be delayed compared with the response in muscle, because muscles typically adjust

---

*Reprinted from Boissonnault WG, Thein-Nissenbaum JM: Differential diagnosis of a sacral stress fracture, *J Orthop Sports Phys Ther* 32:613-627, 2002.

TABLE 1

Locations of Common Fatigue Stress Fractures and Related Activities*

Location	Activity
Lower limb	
Metatarsus	Marching, ballet, weight bearing after bunionectomy
Navicular bone	Marching, running
Calcaneus	Jumping
Tibia, proximal shaft	Walking, running
Tibia, mid and distal shaft	Running, leaping (basketball, aerobic dancing, ballet)
Fibula, distal shaft	Running
Patella	Hurdling
Femur, shaft	Ballet, running
Femur, neck	Ballet
Trunk	
Sacrum	Running, aerobics
Pelvis, obturator ring	Bowling, gymnastics
Lumbar vertebra (pars interarticularis)	Ballet, running, gymnastics
Upper limb	
Humerus, distal shaft	Throwing a ball
Ulna, shaft	Pitching a ball, propelling a wheelchair

*Reprinted from Boissonnault WG, Thein-Nissenbaum JM: Differential diagnosis of a sacral stress fracture, *J Orthop Sports Phys Ther* 32:614, 2002.

to increased demands at a faster rate than bone.[9,30] The athlete who has begun a running program or has recently increased the intensity of a program may be ready to increase the mileage or intensity from a muscular standpoint but not from a skeletal standpoint. Increasing the mileage or intensity of the workout will prolong the muscular pull and mechanical torque on bones that are not yet capable of accepting the added stress, putting the athlete at risk for fracture.[9]

Fatigue stress fractures often are observed in athletes and military recruits and account for 5% to 6% of overuse injuries.* Daffner and Pavlov[9] extensively reviewed the literature and correlated the location of various fatigue stress fractures with the causative activity (Table 1). Even though stress fractures do occur more often in the lower extremities than the upper extremities, fatigue fractures are not thought to occur often in the sacrum. In a longitudinal study by Matheson et al[31], only 1.7% (3 of 175 stress fractures) of the lower extremity were found to occur in the pelvis of female athletes.

Although there are case reports of sacral stress fractures,† few comprehensively explore the differential-diagnostic process.[10,41] Because stress fractures are a component of the very broad category of overuse syndrome and can be confused with many other medical conditions, PTs should thoroughly understand the etiology, clinical manifestations, and diagnosis of stress fractures.

This patient case describes a patient referred to physical therapy with sacral pain, which was subsequently diagnosed as a sacral stress fracture. The PT's differential diagnosis for this patient is explained.

DIAGNOSIS
History

A 34-year-old homemaker and long-distance runner was referred for physical therapy with a diagnosis of right sacral pain. She was a former elite collegiate runner and was currently training for interna-

tional competition. The referring physician explained to the PT his concern that a stress fracture may be responsible for the symptoms, but he preferred to attempt physical-therapy intervention, along with cessation of running, for at least 1 to 2 weeks before performing any diagnostic imaging. He had noted during his examination "significant asymmetry of the hip bones and a suspected sacroiliac joint injury." The physician reported that he had scheduled the patient for a magnetic resonance imaging (MRI) test in 10 to14 days, but would cancel the test if the patient showed improvement with the therapeutic intervention.

The patient reported a constant soreness and aching, and an intermittent "catch" sensation in the area of the right side of the sacrum as the sole symptoms (Figure 1). She reported that the intermittent catch was accompanied by her right hip feeling like it was "out of place." The pain had begun about 7 to 10 days before the initial visit to physical therapy while the patient was running a series of hills as part of her training regimen. The pain began suddenly and was intense (a 6 on a scale of 0-10, with 0 being pain free and 10 being the worst pain imaginable).

Within 24 hours of the onset of symptoms, the patient received chiropractic treatment consisting of chiropractic adjustments and ice, but this intervention did not reduce the patient's symptoms. Although the intensity of pain had decreased since the onset, the pain was still preventing her from running, which was the patient's sole goal of rehabilitation. The patient had not previously experienced right sacral pain but did report experiencing similar pain on the left side of the sacrum about 5 months before this initial visit. At that time, she had been diagnosed as having a stress fracture of the sacrum, left side.

At the initial visit, the patient rated the right sacral pain intensity between a 1 and a 4 on a scale of 0-10. Although she always experienced some discomfort, the sacral soreness and aching were most intense when the patient tried to run, when she walked more

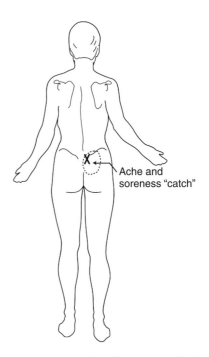

FIGURE 1 Location and description of symptoms at the time of the initial visit to physical therapy. The "X" designates where the patient experienced the catch sensation, and the circled area designates the area of the ache and soreness. (From Boissonnault WG, Thein-Nissenbaum JM: Differential diagnosis of a sacral stress fracture, *J Orthop Sports Phys Ther* 32:613-627, 2002.)

*References 1, 6, 8-10, 12, 14, 15, 20, 22, 30, 31, 33-35, 37, 39, 40.
†References 1, 6, 8, 10, 12, 14, 15, 30, 31, 33, 37, 38.

than a mile, or when she stood for more than 30 minutes. She experienced the "catch" sensation while riding a stationary bike, which she had been doing since she was told to refrain from running. The patient reported that since the physician visit, she had tried shallow water running in the pool but had to discontinue the activity because of intense right sacral pain. The sacral pain did not wake her from sleeping, but she always felt a low-intensity ache.

The patient reported that her overall health was "very good" and denied having any other symptoms, including numbness, tingling, weakness, fatigue, nausea, fever, chills, sweats, or unexplained weight change. She also denied having any symptoms associated with the review-of-systems checklists for the gastrointestinal and urogenital systems.[5]

The patient's medical history included a report of hypothyroidism (with a duration of about 12 months), for which she was taking levothyroxine sodium (Synthroid). She also reported taking ibuprofen (Advil; approximately 800 mg QD), daily calcium and iron supplements, and oral contraceptives. She denied tobacco and alcohol use, and reported that she avoided drinking beverages containing caffeine. The patient's surgical history was negative, and the two prior hospitalizations were associated with the births of her children (now 2 and 4 years old).

The patient's only report of significant injury was the left-sacral stress fracture, confirmed by MRI, sustained about 5 months before the onset of the right sacral pain. The patient reported that she had been unable to run for about 6 to 7 weeks after the left-sacral stress fracture had been diagnosed. She gradually returned to her running program and reported that during the 4 to 6 weeks before the onset of the right-sided sacral pain, her training program had been very intense. Finally, her family history (first-degree relatives) was negative for serious illness.

Impression from Patient's History

Based on the history collected, the first author was concerned about the etiology of the symptoms, considering that the patient recently had recovered from a stress fracture in the same general area, and that the onset of the right-sided symptoms was associated with a recent return to high-level running. The patient knew that the referring physician suspected a possible stress fracture but repeatedly said that the physician had found "asymmetry in the bony landmarks of her hip bones." Even though the patient acknowledged that the current right-sided sacral pain was similar to the pain she had experienced on the left, she did not believe that the current pain was due to a stress fracture. She frequently said during the interview that she felt as if "her hip bone was out of place" and that the pain was "right over the sacroiliac joint." In addition, the patient expressed concern during the interview that she could not miss many more weeks of running without jeopardizing her long-term goals for international competition. Because of the PT's concern about a possible stress fracture and because of the origin and location of symptoms, the PT determined that a detailed examination of the pelvic, lumbar, and hip regions was warranted.

Physical Examination

Observation revealed that the patient was of an ectomorphic body build. The physician's report noted that she was 170.2 cm tall and weighed 50.8 kg. During the standing postural assessment, the PT noted a slight decrease in the lumbosacral-junction lordotic curve. Palpation over the right sacral base provoked moderate tenderness, with the patient saying, "That is where my pain is." No other area of the pelvis, hips, or lumbar spine was painful or tender to palpation.

The right iliac crest, right posterior superior iliac spine, right anterior iliac spine, and right greater trochanter appeared to be elevated compared with the corresponding bony landmarks on the left side. The sacral pain did not increase or decrease during trunk active forward, backward, and side bending range-of-motion (ROM) or passive overpressures (of the same movements done actively) in standing, and the only active ROM deficit was a slight decrease in backward bending at the lumbosacral junction. At the end of the trunk-backward bending motion, the patient noted a slight pressure sensation at the midline of the lumbosacral junction.

Central and unilateral posteroanterior (PA) pressures of the lumbar spine and sacrum, as described by Maitland,[29] did not change the patient's symptoms, but unilateral pressures over the right side of L5 and of the sacrum revealed sight hypomobility (grade 2 on a 0-6 scale [0 = ankylosed, 3 = normal, and 6 = unstable]) as defined by Gonnella and Paris.[18] The patient reported local tenderness (and "that is where my pain is") during the PA pressures over the right side of the sacrum, but the aching did not increase during this maneuver. Good intertester reliability has been demonstrated for PA pressures of the lumbar spine in the provocation of pain, but poor reliability has been noted regarding accessory-motion testing.[28]

With the patient in a prone position, palpation over the sacral base (SB), right and left sides, and inferior lateral angles (ILA) of the sacrum revealed a slightly right-rotated position of the sacrum (the right SB and ILA appeared more posterior relative to the left SB and ILA). With the patient in a prone-on-elbows position, palpation over the same landmarks again revealed a right-rotated position of the sacrum, but with significantly increased asymmetry of the landmarks compared with the results when assessed with the patient in the prone position, and the right ILA also now appeared to be slightly inferior to the left ILA.

Finally, with the patient seated and in a forward flexed position of the trunk, palpation over the same landmarks did not reveal a rotated position of the sacrum. The ilial shear test, as described by Magee,[27] did not alter the patient's symptoms, and the end feel was symmetric.

Hip active and passive ROM testing, FABER, and the hip scour tests did not alter the patient's symptoms and revealed symmetric, normal mobility (per Magee[27]) with the exception of the combined movement of right hip flexion, medial rotation, and adduction. With the hip flexed to 90 degrees and in full medial rotation, adduction was limited to 25 degrees at the right hip, compared with 40 degrees at the left hip. During this maneuver, the patient experienced an intense deep "stretch" sensation in the right buttock, compared with a very mild stretch sensation that the PT noted in the left buttock when testing the left hip. A neurologic screening of the lower extremities including sensory and myotome testing and testing of quadriceps and Achilles tendon reflexes did not reveal any deficits, and lower extremity pulses were easily found and symmetric when extremities were compared. Finally, the straight-leg raise test was negative bilaterally.

Impression from the Physical Examination

The physical examination findings supported the physician's conclusion that the right sacral pain was local pain and not referred from another area. Symptoms were not changed during the assessment of the lumbar spine (palpation, active ROM, overpressures, PA pressures) nor during the assessment of the hip regions (palpation, active ROM, overpressures, FABER, and scour testing). Only palpation and pressure directly over the right sacral base area provoked any discomfort. Although the palpation and the PA pressures over the right sacral base did not make the patient's pain worse, the tenderness noted by the patient was "where my pain is." In addition, the most significant impairment noted was the right sacroiliac joint hypomobility. (Again, poor interrater reliability has been shown in the use of the PA techniques for mobility assessment, and reliability assessment has not been performed for palpation of sacral bony landmarks comparing position change with the patient prone, prone on elbows, and in seated trunk flexion.)

The asymmetric height of the ilial bony landmarks and greater trochanter suggested a possible leg-length discrepancy; this may have precipitated the sacroiliac joint injury while the patient was running hills, and the reduced mobility noted at the right hip could have developed secondary to the injury.

The author's one nagging concern was the inability to increase or decrease the patient's pain during the physical examination. If the pain had been of muscular origin, the patient's pain likely would have been reproduced with local palpation, passive stretching, or active contraction of the tissue. Ligamentous or joint pain likely would have been reproduced with stressing of the tissues with local palpation, active movements, overpressures, or special tests such as the hip FABER, scour test, and the ilial shear test. The neurologic exam was negative. Considering that the pain was severe enough to prevent running of any intensity and that the patient experienced a painful catch with biking, the author expected to be able to change the patient's symptoms at some point during the examination. This led to the question of whether the pain was truly associated with the right sacroiliac joint dysfunction and the reduced flexibility of the right hip, or, considering the patient's history, with a stress fracture.

COURSE OF INTERVENTION

During the initial visit, the PT used manual interventions to treat the right sacroiliac joint and the L5 dysfunction. The PT followed these techniques with passive stretching of the right hip into flexion, medial rotation, and adduction. After these interventions, the PT reassessed the sacral position with the patient positioned prone and prone on elbows, revealing symmetric sacral bony landmarks (SB and ILA). In addition, PA pressures over the right sacral base, although still eliciting tenderness, did not reveal the hypomobility as noted earlier in the examination. Right hip adduction (when measured with the hip flexed to 90 degrees, medially rotated) had improved to 35 degrees. The patient reported that her right hip generally felt much more flexible after the interventions and that walking was less painful.

The PT discussed the apparent leg-length discrepancy with the patient, and she reported that she had been given a heel lift for her left shoe after the diagnosis of the left sacral stress fracture. She reported that she never used the lift, even when she had resumed running. The patient was instructed to bring the heel lift to the next physical therapy visit, and to continue refraining from running. Finally, she was instructed in a home exercise to stretch the right hip.

The patient scheduled an appointment for 4 days after the initial visit. At that time, she reported that swimming and weight lifting were improving; she was able to increase the intensity of the workouts without an increase in pain. She also noted that she still felt pain with running in shallow water but felt the pain was not quite as intense. She reported that she had entertained the thought of land-based running, but the "catch" in her right hip stopped her. She reported at the start of this second visit that her right hip bone felt "out of place" and that she was concerned how that might have happened. She was unaware of anything that precipitated the sensation.

The physical examination again revealed moderate tenderness with palpation over the area of the right sacral base, but trunk backward bending was no longer limited at the lumbosacral junction, and only a

very slight right-rotated sacral position was noted in the prone-on-elbows position. In addition, as was seen after the initial intervention, the hypomobility of right L5 and the right sacral base was not noted with the PA pressures.

Finally, the right hip ROM deficit was significantly reduced; there was very little difference between the right and left hip combination of flexion, medial rotation, and adduction ROM. The PT expressed concern to the patient about the persistent "catch" in her hip, the continued pain with running in the pool (albeit reportedly less intense), and the moderate right sacral tenderness, despite the fact that the impairments noted during the initial visit apparently had improved. The patient agreed to keep the MRI appointment, which was scheduled for the next day, and to halt the physical therapy until the MRI results were known.

The next day, the referring physician contacted the PT and reported that the MRI revealed an abnormality in the right ala of the sacrum, and that the resultant diagnosis was an incomplete fracture of the right sacral ala (Figure 2). He stated the patient would continue to swim (laps only, no running) and participate in weight training at a clinic closer to her home for a month, after which a follow-up MRI would be done. The follow-up MRI (Figure 3) revealed that the amount of edema had worsened, and the fracture line was more visible compared with the first MRI. The patient admitted to a trial of land-based running during the previous 4-week period.

The physician instructed the patient to continue her current program of lap swimming and weight training without increasing either activity and to avoid running of any type. Finally, computed tomography (CT) was ordered 3 to 4 weeks after the second MRI (7 to 8 weeks after the original MRI). These films (Figure 4) revealed a linear sclerosis with a faint central lucency, consistent with a healing sacral stress fracture. The author was unsure why a CT scan was ordered this time instead of an MRI.

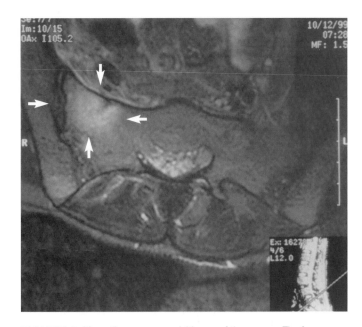

FIGURE 2 Magnetic resonance axial image of the sacrum. The four arrows identify the lesion of the right sacral ala; the zone of high signal intensity represents edema around the central area of decreased signal. This is consistent with an incomplete fracture of the right sacral ala. (From Boissonnault WG, Thein-Nissenbaum JM: Differential diagnosis of a sacral stress fracture, *J Orthop Sports Phys Ther* 32:613-627, 2002.)

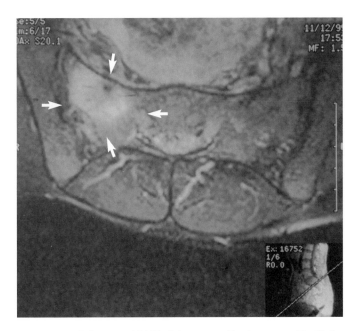

FIGURE 3 Follow-up axial MRI of the sacrum. The four arrows identify the lesion of the right sacral ala; the zone of high signal intensity represents an increase in the degree of edema compared with that noted in Figure 2, with the central area of decreased signal revealing a fracture line more visible than that noted in Figure 2. (From Boissonnault WG, Thein-Nissenbaum JM: Differential diagnosis of a sacral stress fracture, *J Orthop Sports Phys Ther* 32:613-627, 2002.)

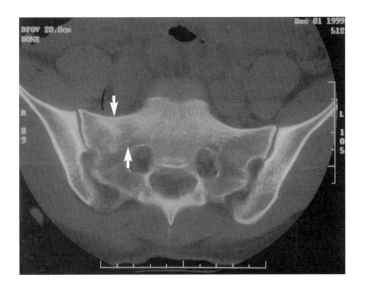

FIGURE 4 Follow-up CT scan of the bony pelvis, axial image. The two arrows identify an area of linear sclerosis with a faint central lucency in the right sacral ala, consistent with a healing stress fracture. (From Boissonnault WG, Thein-Nissenbaum JM: Differential diagnosis of a sacral stress fracture, *J Orthop Sports Phys Ther* 32:613-627, 2002.)

DISCUSSION

Sacral stress fractures present many screening, diagnostic, and management challenges to the PT. First, the development of stress fractures appears to be associated with a wide range of extrinsic and intrinsic risk factors. Second, multiple conditions, including soft-tissue strain, lumbar disk disease, SI joint sprain, sciatica, bony injury, metastasis,

osteogenic sarcoma, and Ewing's tumor can mimic the clinical presentation of stress fractures.[9,30,33,38] Third, several published case reports of sacral stress fractures describe a wide range of symptoms and signs (Table 2), many of which appear inconsistently and could be considered nonspecific. Finally, researchers disagree about the recommended sequence of diagnostic imaging modalities.

Thus a detailed history and thorough physical examination are essential to the development of an accurate diagnosis. As this case illustrates, however, the patient's response to treatment also can be an important factor that guides the practitioner's clinical decision making.

The literature suggests that the causes of stress fractures are multiple, and that athletes in particular can present with both extrinsic and intrinsic risk factors. Intrinsic factors, including gender, reduced aerobic fitness level, leg-length discrepancy, and diminished muscle strength, may play a role in the incidence of stress fractures. Women have a higher incidence of stress fractures than men; this is most likely due to a multitude of factors, including menstrual irregularities, lower bone density, and narrower bone width.[41] Extrinsic risk factors associated with stress fractures include a sudden change in the training regimen, improper footwear, and alterations in the training surface.[1,12,15,19,41]

This patient presented with both intrinsic and extrinsic factors, including female sex, a recent rapid increase in training intensity, and questionable footwear, considering that she was not wearing the recommended insert in the sole of her left shoe. In addition, she had recently recovered from a stress fracture in the same area, albeit on the opposite side.

Pain originating from a sacral stress fracture typically is described by patients as low-back pain, which is the symptom most often reported by patients seeking outpatient physical therapy services.[2,4,11,21] Physical therapy intervention is provided for many of the conditions listed earlier (soft-tissue strains, lumbar disk disease, sciatica, and SI joint sprains), all of which can mimic the clinical presentation of sacral stress fractures. When any bony lesion is suspected, PTs also must be vigilant for warning signs of the other more serious diseases, including bony metastasis, osteosarcoma, and Ewing's tumor. Although one can never be certain that the patient does not have cancer based solely on a history and physical examination, this patient did not present with any of the classic findings associated with cancer of the musculoskeletal system[3] (no personal history of cancer, no family history of cancer, her age, 32, falling outside the ranges of <20 and >50 years, sacral pain that did not worsen with assumption of a supine position, and lack of symptoms of night pain).

The patient described in this case report had apparent dysfunctions of the right SI joint and L5-S1 that could have been responsible for her pain symptoms. This fact clouded the clinical decision-making process, preventing a definitive diagnosis during the initial examination. This hypothesis was rendered less likely upon follow-up examination, however, as examination procedures of the trunk and pelvis did not alter the patient's symptoms, and the originally noted impairments improved without a concurrent reduction in the patient's chief symptom.

Table 2 summarizes the symptoms and signs reported in published case reports of sacral stress fracture. Of those noted, only localized pain,[1,10,14,19,39] tenderness with palpation,* normal lumbar spine ROM,† normal hip ROM,[1,6,12,14,19] and a normal neurovascular status[1,12,33] were consistently reported in these cases.

---

*References 1, 6, 8, 12, 14, 15, 19, 33.
†References 1, 6, 10, 12, 14, 19, 39.

TABLE 2

Signs and Symptoms Associated and Not Associated with Sacral Stress Fractures as Reported by Various Authors*

Signs/Symptoms	Authors finding a correlation with stress fracture	Authors finding no correlation with stress fracture
Localized pain	Atwell[1], Delvaux[10], Featherstone[14], Holtzhausen[19], Volpin[39]	
Antalgic gait	Atwell[1], Delvaux[10], McFarland[33]	McFarland[33]
Tenderness with palpation	Atwell[1], Bottomley[6], Czarnecki[8], Eller[12], Featherstone[14], Fink-Bennett[15], Holtzhausen[19], McFarland[33]	Atwell[1], Delvaux[10]
Normal ROM of hip	Atwell[1], Bottomley[6], Eller[12], Featherstone[14], Holtzhausen[19]	Schils[37], Volpin[39]
Normal neurovascular status	Atwell[1], Eller[12], McFarland[33]	
Positive Patrick test	Atwell[1]	Delvaux[10], McFarland[33]
Groin pain	Atwell[1], Volpin[39]	Delvaux[10]
Normal lumbar spine ROM	Atwell[1], Bottomley[6], Delvaux[10], Eller[12], Featherstone[14], Holtzhausen[19], Volpin[39]	
Pelvic tilt	Bottomley[6], Featherstone[14]	
Pain with SLR to 60-70 degrees	Czarnecki[8]	
Leg-length discrepancy	Bottomley[6], Czarnecki[8]	Delvaux[10]
Previous stress fractures at the same site	Eller[12]	
Decreased bone mineral density	Eller[12], Bottomley[6]	
Ischial tuberosity pain	Fink-Bennett[15]	

*Reprinted with permission from Boissonnault WG, Thein-Nissenbaum JM: Differential diagnosis of a sacral stress fracture, *J Orthop Sports Phys Ther* 32:618, 2002.

The patient in this case had localized sacral pain, tenderness over the area with palpation, and a normal neurovascular examination. She did have a slight decrease in backward bending at the lumbosacral junction; this may have been associated with the noted sacral and L5-S1 dysfunctions and not secondary to the stress fracture. She also presented with reduced right hip ROM, which may or may not have been directly associated with the sacral stress fracture.

Examining the patient only after the onset of symptoms precluded the PT from comparing examination findings from before and after the onset of pain. Ruling out the hip as the source of symptoms was important, because this case could have been an atypical presentation of a stress fracture of the femoral neck. The diagnosis of a femoral-neck stress fracture carries a sense of urgency because this lesion could progress to a devastating fracture and require immediate surgical pinning. Based on the noted intrinsic and extrinsic factors and the above information, the PT was most concerned about the possibility of a bony lesion of the sacrum. See Box 1 for a summary of the examination findings that led the PT to suspect that the patient's chief symptom was associated with a bony lesion, with stress fracture being of greatest concern.

BOX 1

Examination Findings Leading to Suspicion that a Bony Lesion Was Associated with the Patient's Chief Symptom

- Female sex
- Recent history of stress fracture in same area as the current chief symptom*
- Rapid increase in training intensity (running) before the onset of symptoms*
- Localized pain symptom
- Marked tenderness with local palpation
- Apparent leg-length discrepancy
- No provocation of symptoms with anything but local palpation*
- Improvement of lumbar, SI joint, and hip dysfunctions with lack of symptom improvement*

*Findings that most concerned the author about the source of the patient's symptoms. Reprinted from Boissonnault WG, Thein-Nissenbaum JM: Differential diagnosis of a sacral stress fracture, *J Orthop Sports Phys Ther* 32:619, 2002.

When a bony lesion is suspected, physicians will order a complete blood count (CBC) and diagnostic imaging as part of the differential diagnosis. Any abnormality in the CBC requires further diagnostic testing; the CBC is found to be normal in patients with stress fractures.[1,10,37,39]

Diagnostic imaging is not always conclusive when a stress fracture is suspected. In fact, of the case reports reviewed, many subjects with a stress fracture were found to have normal findings on plain radiographs.* Although plain-film radiography is the initial test for most patients with low-back pain, the sacrum is a challenge to definitively image on plain films secondary to the overlying soft tissues and bowel gas.[12,33] Plain films detecting a stress fracture also depend on the amount of time between the injury and the imaging.[9] Holtzhausen[19] suggested that 2 to 12 weeks are required from the onset of pain before positive findings appear on plain radiographs. Considering this possible lag time, if the initial plain films are read as normal, taking follow-up radiographs 1 to 2 weeks later may be recommended.[9] Because of the urgent need to form a diagnosis in athletes, however, follow-up diagnostic testing, such as radionuclide bone imaging, is recommended.

Bone scans, once considered the gold standard for diagnosing stress fractures, have been identified as the recommended diagnostic tool for follow-up in many case reports.† Bone scans prove to have nearly 100% sensitivity and may show abnormalities early in the course of a stress fracture, as early as 6 to 72 hours after the onset of symptoms.[13,19,31,35] Eller et al[12] reported, however, that the image resulting from the increased uptake of radioactive tracer is fairly non-specific in identifying anatomic detail. Fanciullo and Bell[13] suggested using computed tomography (CT) scanning to improve specificity. CT scanning has been used in many published cases of sacral stress fractures.‡

As with bone and CT scans, MRI is often used in patients with suspected stress fractures,[9,12,14] but authors disagree about the level of specificity of the MRI findings. Several authors reported that, even

*References 1, 6, 8, 10, 12, 14, 15, 19, 33, 39.
†References 1, 6, 8, 10, 12, 15, 19, 30, 33, 34, 37, 39.
‡References 1, 8, 10, 12, 30, 33, 39.

though plain radiographs and bone scans have served as the primary modalities for imaging suspected stress fractures, MRI allowed a more specific initial or follow-up diagnosis.[12,13,35] Eller et al[12] believed MRI to be valuable, localizing the involved area and enabling a clear distinction from other common problems, such as dysfunction of the SI joint. According to Daffner and Pavlov,[9] the MRI image of a stress fracture will show low signal on the T1-weighted image and increased signal on the T2-weighted images with injection of gadopentetate dimeglumine. The authors also believed the results to be nonspecific and were concerned that the findings may be confused with osteoporosis or infection. Several other authors thought that signal changes caused by edema or hemorrhage on MRI may be misleading or may be interpreted as neoplasia.[13,14]

The diagnostic imaging sequence for the patient in this case study was two successive MRI scans (4 weeks apart) followed by a CT scan performed about 7 weeks after the initial MRI. All three tests were performed without contrast. As stated earlier, the author did not know why a CT scan was ordered after the first two follow-up tests were MRI.

SUMMARY

Determining whether a patient's symptoms are associated with a condition for which physical therapy is indicated is one of the important challenges facing PTs during an initial patient visit. As this case illustrates, the answer to this question may not be clear until after subsequent patient visits.

Sacral stress fractures, although relatively uncommon, are a potential source of back pain, which is a common symptom in patients seeking physical-therapy outpatient services. Because bony lesions can be associated with serious medical conditions, such as cancers and fractures, early detection and an accurate diagnosis are paramount to appropriate care. An important element in screening for such conditions is recognizing patients with the risk factors. The presence of the risk factors associated with insufficiency and fatigue fractures, as described in this case, should alert the PT to thoroughly scrutinize symptoms and signs suggestive of a bony lesion. As described, the symptoms and signs for many of the conditions causing back pain and those of sacral stress fractures have an unfortunate degree of overlap.

Another important element of this screening process is establishing a prognosis that allows for patient progress, both from a subjective viewpoint and from the standpoint of the physical examination.[4] If the patient does not meet these expectations, the PT must reconsider the original diagnosis, and, as in this case, ensure that the patient is referred to the physician for follow-up and the recommended diagnostic workup.

REFERENCES

1. Atwell EA, Jackson DW: Stress fractures of the sacrum in runners. Two case reports, *Am J Sports Med* 5:531-533, 1991.
2. Battie MC, Cherkin DC, Dunn R, et al: Managing low back pain: attitudes and treatment preferences of physical therapists, *Phys Ther* 74:219-226, 1994.
3. Bigos S, Bowyer O, Braen G, et al: Acute low back problems in adults. In: *Clinical practice guideline*, quick reference guide no 14, Rockville, MD, US Department of Health and Human Services, Agency for Health Care Policy and Research, AHCPR pub no 95-0643, December, 1994.
4. Boissonnault W: Prevalence of comorbid conditions, surgeries, and medication use in a physical therapy outpatient population: a multi-centered study, *J Orthop Sports Phys Ther* 29:506-519, 1999.
5. Boissonnault WG: *Examination in physical therapy practice; screening for medical disease*, ed 2, New York, 1995, Churchill Livingstone.
6. Bottomley MB: Sacral stress fracture in a runner, *Br J Sports Med* 4:243-244, 1990.
7. Brat HG, Renton P, Sandison A, et al: Chondromyxoid fibroma of the sacrum, *Eur Radiol* 9:1800-1803, 1999.
8. Czarnecki DJ, Till EW, Minikel JL: Unique sacral stress fracture in a runner, *Am J Roentgenol* 151:1255, 1988.
9. Daffner RH, Pavlov H. Stress fractures: Current concepts, *Am J Roentgenol* 159:245-252, 1992.
10. Delvaux K, Lysens R: Lumbosacral pain in an athlete, *Am J Phys Med Rehabil* 80:388-391, 2001.
11. DiFabio RP, Boissonnault WG: Physical therapy and health-related outcomes for patients with common orthopaedic diagnoses, *J Orthop Sports Phys Ther* 27:217-230, 1998.
12. Eller DJ, Katz DS, Bergman AG, et al: Sacral stress fracture in long-distance runners, *Clin J Sports Med* 7:222-225, 1997.
13. Fanciullo JJ, Bell CL: Stress fractures of the sacrum and lower extremity, *Curr Opin Rheumatol* 8:158-162, 1996.
14. Featherstone T: Magnetic resonance imaging in the diagnosis of sacral stress fracture, *Br J Sports Med* 33:276-277, 1999.
15. Fink-Bennett DM, Benson MT: Unusual exercise-related stress fractures. Two case reports, *Clin Nucl Med* 9:430-434, 1984.
16. Fornasier VL, Horne JG: Metastases to the vertebral column, *Cancer* 36:590-594, 1975.
17. Fortin JD, Dwyer AP, West S, et al: Sacroiliac joint: pain referral maps upon applying a new injection/arthrography technique, *Spine* 19:1475-1482, 1994.
18. Gonnella C, Paris SV, Kutner M: Reliability in evaluating passive intervertebral motion, *Phys Ther* 62:436-444, 1984.
19. Holtzhausen LM, Noakes TD: Stress fracture of the sacrum in two distance runners, *Clin J Sports Med* 2:139-142, 1992.
20. James SL, Bates BT, Osternig LR: Injuries to runners, *Am J Sports Med* 6:40-50, 1978.
21. Jette AM, Davis KD: A comparison of hospital-based and private outpatient physical therapy practices, *Phys Ther* 71:366-375, 1991.
22. Jones BH, Harris JM, Vinh TN, et al: Exercise-induced stress fractures and stress reactions of bone: epidemiology, etiology, and classification, *Exerc Sport Sci Rev* 17:379-422, 1989.
23. Kellgren JH: Observations of referred pain arising from muscle, *Clin Sci* (3-4):175-190, 1938.
24. Kellgren JH: On the distribution of pain arising from deep somatic structures with charts of segmental pain areas, *Clin Sci* 4:35-46, 1939.
25. Leone A, Costantini A, Guglielmi G, et al: Primary bone tumors and pseudotumors of the lumbrosacral spine, *Rays* 25:89-103, 2000.
26. Levangie PK, Norkin CC: *Joint structure and function*, ed 3, Philadelphia, 2001, FA Davis.
27. Magee DJ: *Orthopedic physical assessment*, ed 3, Philadelphia, 1997, WB Saunders.
28. Maher C, Adams R: Reliability of pain and stiffness assessments in clinical manual lumbar spine examination, *Phys Ther* 74:801-809, 1994.
29. Maitland GD: *Vertebral manipulation*, ed 5, London, 1986, Butterworth.
30. Major NM, Helms CA: Sacral stress fractures in long-distance runners, *Am J Roentgenol* 174:727-729, 2000.
31. Matheson GO, Clement DB, McKenzie DC, et al: Stress fractures in athletes. A study of 320 cases, *Am J Sports Med* 1:46-58, 1987.
32. McCall IW, Park WM, O'Brien JP: Induced pain referral from posterior elements in normal subjects, *Spine* 4:441-446, 1979.
33. McFarland EG, Giangarra C: Sacral stress fractures in athletes, *Clin Orthop Rel Res* 329:240-243, 1996.
34. Milgrom C, Chisin R, Giladi M, et al: Multiple stress fractures. A longitudinal study of a soldier with 13 lesions, *Clin Orthop Rel Res* 192:174-179. 1985.
35. Monteleone GP: Stress fractures in the athlete, *Orthop Clin North Am* 263:423-32, 1995.
36. Rohen JW, Yokochi C: *Color atlas of anatomy*, ed 2, New York, 1988, Igaku-Shoin.
37. Schils J, Hauzer JP: Stress fracture of the sacrum, *Am J Sports Med* 20:769-770, 1992.
38. Stafford SA, Rosenthal DI, Gebhardt MC, et al: MRI in stress fracture, *Am J Roentgenol* 147:553-556, 1986.
39. Volpin G, Milgrom C, Goldsher D, et al: Stress fractures of the sacrum following strenuous activity, *Clin Orthop Rel Res* 243:184-188, 1989.
40. Wong DA, Fornasier VL, MacNab I: Spinal metastases: the obvious, the occult and the imposters, *Spine* 15:1-4, 1990.
41. Zeni AI, Street CC, Dempsey RL, et al: Stress injury to the bone among women athletes, *Phys Med Rehabil Clin North Am* 114:929-947, 2000.

SECTION **FOUR**

Special Populations

The Adolescent Population

12

Kristine M. Hallisy, PT, MS, OCS

Objectives

After reading this chapter, the reader will be able to:

1. Comprehend the elements of the physical therapy model of patient management (evidence-based medicine) as it relates to adolescent patients.
2. Describe how population size, age, and sex affect the socioeconomic challenges our country will face in providing health care to adolescents.
3. Explain the multisystem effects of puberty on the developing individual.
4. Explain how the psychosocial issues of the adolescent may affect the development of an effective therapeutic alliance among the PT, the patient, and potential caregivers.
5. Comprehend the special features of bone growth and development in the area of pediatric and adolescent neuromusculoskeletal injuries.
6. Select the appropriate components of an examination for a child or adolescent with a neuromusculoskeletal injury.
7. Explain the role of, and make appropriate referral for, diagnostic imaging of pediatric or adolescent patients with musculoskeletal injuries.
8. Differentiate common neuromusculoskeletal conditions and injuries seen in children and adolescents.
9. Understand and implement interventions, including health-promotion strategies, for pediatric or adolescent patients.

If we do not care for the children, who will care for the world when we grow old?

Unknown

Physical therapy is a profession that focuses on the diagnosis and management of dysfunctional human movement throughout the lifespan. Many PTs currently are attempting to develop the skills needed to succeed in a primary care environment. These primary care PTs must be able to recognize signs and symptoms that require referral or consultation with a specialist. Furthermore, these PTs must be able to deliver interventions that alleviate impairments and functional limitations, thus minimizing disability.

The review of systems (ROS) checklist (see Chapter 7) asks the PT to develop explanations for findings that may indicate occult disease. Weight loss, numbness, and cognitive or emotional changes could be indicators for anorexia in a male high-school wrestler or an insecure female teenager striving to meet the unrealistic standards of their culture. General fatigue and night pain could indicate an osteosarcoma or could simply be symptoms of a male adolescent who has grown 6 inches in the past few months and changed his basketball-training schedule. Weight gain, nausea and vomiting, and emotional withdrawal may be indicators of an unwanted pregnancy. These are but a few of the issues that the outpatient PT working with the adolescent population as a primary care provider must be prepared to investigate and reconcile.

The societal role of the adolescent is to engage in family interactions, school, and community activities and possibly play roles within a workplace. Unlike the stereotyped vision of youth, not all youngsters enjoy carefree days of childhood. World, community, and family events profoundly affect the developing individual. Given these facts, the PT must consider some unique health needs and psychosocial factors when working with this population. The physical, emotional, and psychological state of the adolescent, along with the influence, or lack thereof, from caregivers or peers, can profoundly affect the therapeutic alliance between the health care provider and the adolescent. Failure to respect the adolescent's unique perspective on the world can damage the treatment outcome.

Adolescence is a time of unique psychosocial concerns, preferences, and expectations.[27] The teenager is literally in *transition* between the dependency of childhood and the responsibility of adulthood. This period of development is marked by major physiological, intellectual, and emotional changes. To effectively manage the adolescent patient, the outpatient PT must comprehend the effects of hormonal changes on growth, structure, and function, as well as understand and respect the effect of motor learning and motor control on function. The state of the injury, disease, or surgical procedure and its potential rate of recovery, complications, precautions, and contraindications also are crucial concerns.

The care of pediatric (0 to 20 years) patients is paramount to the overall health and well-being of our society. Teenagers often fall into the cracks of medical care, especially in the area of mental health. Adolescents as a group are the primary users of illicit drugs, tobacco, and alcohol and make up the largest group with unwanted pregnancies, abortions, and sexually transmitted diseases.[104]

Given the skyrocketing cost of health care, health care practitioners must empower their young patients to care for themselves by educating them in health promotion. Health promotion is not only the detection and prevention of disease but also the endorsement of well being in the physical, cognitive, emotional, social, and spiritual domains.[31] *Healthy People 2010*,[123] a subsidiary of the Department of Health and Human Services, is

BOX 12-1
Healthy People 2010

Every health care practitioner should consider *Healthy People 2010* a significant resource. *Healthy People 2010* constitutes the nation's health promotion agenda for the new millennium. It is designed to identify the most important preventable threats to health and to establish national goals to reduce these threats. The two overriding goals of *Healthy People 2010* are to: (1) increase quality and years of healthy life for all people of all ages, and (2) eliminate health disparities among different segments of the population.

The National Center for Health Statistics will monitor 467 health objectives in the first decade of the twenty-first century. These population-based objectives address health care needs according to variables such as age, race, gender, educational attainment, and socioeconomic status (income). The 10 leading health indicators of the *Healthy People 2010* project are:

- Physical activity
- Overweight and obesity
- Tobacco use
- Substance use
- Responsible sexual behavior
- Mental health
- Injury and violence
- Environmental quality
- Immunization
- Access to health care

Healthy People 2010 challenges individuals, communities, and health care professionals, indeed, all of us, to take specific steps to ensure that all can enjoy good health, as well as long life.

REFERENCE

Healthy People 2010, Office of Disease Prevention and Health Promotion, US Department of Health and Human Services. Available at: www.healthypeople.gov.

discussed in Box 12-1 as a blueprint for health promotion and counseling specific to adolescents. With the use of this health-promotion model, physical therapy has the potential, *and the responsibility*, to improve the quality of life of all members of our society, including this chapter's vulnerable target population—the youth of America.

Evidence-Based Medicine Across the Lifespan

Population size and composition together explain global challenges and national challenges.

United States Census Bureau, 2000

The size and composition of a population are important, as they reveal a nation's support burden. They indicate challenges a country will face in providing health care to its children and elderly, education to its youth, employment opportunities to its young adults, and support to its elderly.[172] At 281.4 million people (4.6% of the world's 6.1 billion inhabitants), the United States is the third-most-populated country on Earth.[237] In 2000, the United States ranked sixth among all countries in contributing to the growth in the number of youth in the world. Persons under the age of 15 now make up 21.4%, or one in five, of *all* Americans.[172]

In 2000, 11.6% of American youth under the age of 18 years were uninsured. Uninsured rates for children by race (regardless of socioeconomic class) were as follows: Hispanics, 24.9%; Asian/Pacific Islanders, 14.0%; African Americans, 13.5%; and

whites, 10.8%. When families fall below the poverty level, more than one in five (21.6%) children under 18 years of age did not have health insurance. Almost 27% of adolescents aged 12 to 18 years were uninsured, followed by 19.2% of children aged 6 to 11, and 19.6% of children younger than 6 years of age.[67]

These staggering facts, along with rising costs of health care, obligate health care practitioners to make conscientious choices when providing medical care to adolescents. This judicious and explicit process for making decisions about the care of individual patients has been labeled evidence-based medicine (EBM). In any medical setting, EBM is the integration of the best research evidence (i.e., scientific merit of the treatment) with clinical expertise and the patient's values (e.g., cultural and family values, patient goals, and insurance or financial capabilities).[208]

Regular preventive health care visits are integral to patient management. The American Academy of Pediatrics (AAP) has published age-appropriate guidelines for preventive health care visits for children (0 to 20 years of age). The partnership among the health care provider, the adolescent, and his or her family (whatever form that family takes) should provide and monitor:

- *Age-appropriate developmental achievement of the child* (e.g., physical maturation, gross and fine motor skills, cognitive achievements, emotional development, and social competence and appropriateness)
- *Health supervision visits that include periodic assessment of medical and oral health* (e.g., regular review of systems, height, weight, head circumference (0-24 months),[62] heart rate, respiratory rate, temperature, blood pressure (>3 years), vision, hearing, developmental assessment, physical examination, and age-appropriate immunizations)[2,9]
- *Screening and anticipatory guidance* (e.g., emotional and mental health, healthy habits, nutrition, oral health,[14] peer relationships, prevention or recognition of illness, prevention of risky behaviors and addictions, safety and prevention of injury, self-responsibility and self-efficacy, sexual development and sexuality, community interactions, and school and vocational achievement).[230]

Progression through the Tanner stages of sexual maturation identifies the adolescent as a unique subset of the pediatric population. Many somatic, sexual, cognitive, moral, and social (e.g., self-identity and relationship to society) issues central to the developing adolescent are shown in Table 12-1. Relevant issues of development, musculoskeletal growth, and biomechanics across the pediatric lifespan follow and are shown in Table 12-2.

Overview: Fetal Development to Birth

Efficient human movement is a complex, endless process that starts in utero and has psychomotor, physiological, biochemical, biomechanical, psychosocial, and even gender considerations.[162] Fetal development has three distinct stages: pre-embryonic period (0 to 3 weeks), embryonic period (3 to 8 weeks), and fetal period (8 weeks to full term).[48] The differentiation and proliferation of embryonic and fetal cells directly affect pediatric (0-20 years) growth and development. *Nelson Textbook of Pediatrics* is an essential text for information on fetal development, pediatric growth and maturation, and the hormonal

TABLE 12-1

Central Issues in Early, Middle, and Late Adolescence

Variable	Early Adolescence	Middle Adolescence	Late Adolescence
Age (yr)	10-13	14-16	17-20 and beyond
Sexual maturity rating*	1-2	3-5	5
Somatic	Secondary sex characteristics; beginning of rapid growth; awkward	Height growth peaks; body shape and composition change; acne and odor; menarche; spermarche	Slower growth
Sexual	Sexual interest usually exceeds sexual activity	Sexual drive surges; experimentation; questions of sexual orientation	Consolidation of sexual identity
Cognitive and moral	Concrete operations; conventional morality	Emergence of abstract thought; questioning mores; self-centered	Idealism; absolutism
Self-concept	Preoccupation with changing body; self-consciousness	Concern with attractiveness; increasing introspection	Relatively stable body image
Family	Bids for increased independence; ambivalence	Continued struggle for acceptance of greater autonomy	Practical independence; family remains secure base
Peers	Same-sex groups; conformity; cliques	Dating; peer groups less important	Intimacy; possibly commitment
Relationship to society	Middle-school adjustment	Gauging skills and opportunities	Career decisions (e.g., drop out, college, work)

From Behrman RE, Klingman R, Jenson HB, eds: *Nelson textbook of pediatrics*, ed 16, Philadelphia 2000, WB Saunders.
*Based on Tanner stages of development.

TABLE 12-2

Key Principles of Development Across the Pediatric Lifespan

Infancy (0-12 months)	Physical development is the most rapid of any age. Exploration of the environment is a key component of cognitive and language development. Social and emotional tasks include understanding of self and family, bonding, attachment to caregivers, and trust that physical needs will be met.
	Consequences: Delays in mapping of the sensorimotor cortex are created if physical, nutritional, social, and environmental needs are not met (i.e., the child is unable to appropriately interact with his or her environment).
Early childhood (years 1-4)	Physical development slows to half the rate of infancy, and growth spurts begin. Gross motor skills, followed by fine motor skills, are acquired via maturation of the neurologic system. Language develops at extraordinary speed. Cognitive development is preoperational and lacks sustained logical thought processes as the child strives toward increased social independence and begins to set personal boundaries. Children learn to be self-sufficient in many activities, including toileting, feeding, walking, and talking or to doubt their own abilities.
	Consequences: Exposure to human interaction and verbal language exchange (e.g., reading to children) is imperative to language development, psychosocial development, and the attainment of developmental milestones.
Middle childhood (years 5-10)	Physical growth is steady but at a slower rate than the preschool and adolescent time periods. Cognitively, children are concretely operational in their thought processes and begin to display goal-directed exploration of the world. Environmental factors (e.g., family, culture, school) affect learning, self-esteem, social independence, interaction, and the development of self-efficacy. Moral development remains simple, but a child should display a clear knowledge of "right and wrong."
	Consequences: Failure to develop self-esteem within the child's major social structures can lead to guilt and poor self-esteem. Children with physical disabilities and chronic illness begin to face more environmental challenges that may prevent learning and development.
Adolescence (years 11-20)	Physical transition from childhood to adulthood with extensive endocrine-mediated changes. The adolescent proceeds through the Tanner stages of development. Cognitive development progresses to formal operational thinking; adolescents acquire the ability to reason logically and abstractly, and consider future implications of current actions. Socially and emotionally this can be a tumultuous time marked by the transition from family-dominated influences to peer influence and increasing autonomy.
	Consequences: The struggle for identity, independence, and intimacy may lead to stress, health-related problems, and, often, high-risk behaviors. The struggle for self-identity and independence is usually completed by age 20, although for some, full social and emotional maturity takes longer. This struggle also gives the health care professional an important opportunity for health promotion.

Modified from Szilagyi PG: Assessing children: infancy through adolescence. In Bickley LS, Szilagyi PG, eds: *Bates' guide to physical examination and history taking*, ed 8, Philadelphia, 2003, Lippincott/Williams and Wilkins.

cascade that stimulates normal and abnormal adolescent development.[27] The reader is encouraged to review the evidence showing how fetal development and congenital and genetic disorders could affect the daily practice of the primary care outpatient PT working with adolescents.*

In the United States, patients with congenital disorders (i.e., present at birth) and genetic disorders (i.e., hereditary disorders transmitted by the genes that may not manifest at birth but develop over time) typically have entered the health care system before reaching adolescence. Multidisciplinary health care teams that feature pediatric and neurologic PTs most often manage congenital and genetic disorders. As a member of a management team in either a medical or educational setting, a PT assists in identifying and ameliorating impairments, functional limita-

---

*References 27, 28, 36, 48, 50, 64, 66, 101, 104, 159, 242, 251.

tions, and disabilities in pediatric patients (0-20 years). Select congenital and genetic conditions that may require interventions that continue into adolescence and therefore could be seen by the primary care outpatient PT are found in Table 12-3.

Overview: Birth to 4 Years

During the infant and toddler years, the exact rate of growth depends on the individual child. By 2 years of age, a child generally weighs 26 to 28 lb and stands 32 to 33 inches. By 2½ years, a child should quadruple his or her birth weight. Children in this age range require 1300 to 1700 calories per day. The child should have developed a complete set of teeth by 3 years of age.[200] Infants and young children develop the ability to sleep through the night and may need only one nap per day.[183]

Curiosity about the environment motivates the young child to move and learn. The child's acquisition of skills from birth

---

TABLE 12-3

Pediatric Physical Therapy: Select Congenital, Genetic, and Acquired Pediatric Conditions that May Be Seen During Adolescence by a Primary Care Outpatient Orthopedic PT[3,8,28,48,104]

Achondroplasia (dwarfism) Most common form of disproportionate short stature.	Persons with achondroplasia typically have delayed motor milestones, hip-flexion contractures, bowing of the knees, thoracolumbar gibbus, increased lumbar lordosis, otitis media, obstructive sleep apnea (sweating and snoring at night), speech problems, and abnormal head growth (increased risk for seizures). Physical therapy management of back pain (spinal stenosis) and hip and knee pathology is common. For more information on achondroplasia, see the American Academy of Pediatrics policy statement: Health supervision for children with achondroplasia (RE9514), March, 95 (3):443-451, 1995.
Cerebral palsy (CP) CP is a disorder of movement and posture caused by a prenatal, perinatal, or postnatal nonprogressive lesion of the immature brain. Low birth weight (less than 1.5 kg or 3.3 lb) is a significant risk factor for postpartum onset of cerebral palsy. The incidence of CP in the United States is 2 in every 1000 infants.	CP involves one or more of the limbs and often the trunk. The impaired control and coordination of voluntary muscles are often accompanied by: Mental retardation or learning disabilities (60%) Dysarthria (25%) Auditory impairments (6%-16%) Seizure disorders (20%-30%) Visional impairment, usually strabismus or refractory problems (40%-50%) Sensory impairments; visual-motor and perceptual deficits; oral-motor, behavioral, social, and family problems may occur secondary to the presence of these primary deficits Physical therapy interventions include family education, handling techniques, facilitation of optimal sensorimotor development, and orthopedic and neurologic management (ROM, stretching, strengthening, neuromuscular reeducation, positioning, gross motor function, gait, and orthotics). PTs usually are part of a multidisciplinary team involved in the management of the child throughout the lifespan.
Cystic fibrosis Cystic fibrosis (CF), the most common life-shortening genetic disease in the white population, occurs in the United States in about 1 of 3300 white births, 1 of 15,300 black births, and 1 of 32,000 Asian-American births; 30% of patients are adults. Median survival is age 31 years.	CF is an autosomal recessive disease of the exocrine glands, affecting primarily the GI and respiratory systems, and usually characterized by COPD, exocrine pancreatic insufficiency (secondary to blockage), and abnormally high sweat electrolytes. Persons with CF often require management by a multi-disciplinary team including physicians, nurses, nutritionists, PTs and respiratory therapists (daily chest physical therapy to clear lungs), counselors, and social workers. The goals of therapy are maintenance of adequate nutritional status, prevention of pulmonary and other complications, encouragement of physical activity, and provision of adequate psychosocial support (age-appropriate adjustment at home and school). Despite myriad problems, the occupational and marital successes of patients are impressive.
Down syndrome (DS) (trisomy 21) The incidence of DS is 1 in every 1000 live births. Maternal age is key determining variable. There is no association between Down syndrome any given culture, ethnic group, socioeconomic status, or geographic region.	Primary impairments include early feeding difficulties, mild to moderate mental retardation, delayed growth and sexual development, hearing loss, hypotonia, low muscle-force production, slowed postural reactions, ligamentous laxity (atlanto-axial instability [AAI] in 20% of cases), foot deformities, scoliosis, congenital heart disease, and lung hypoplasia with pulmonary hypertension. Persons with Down syndrome also have a predisposition for immune deficiency, leukemia, and thyroid disease. The exercise prescription for management of obesity includes dietary education, behavioral modification, and increased activity level. AAI tests are required for participation in exercise or Special Olympics.

TABLE 12-3

Pediatric Physical Therapy: Select Congenital, Genetic, and Acquired Pediatric Conditions that May Be Seen During Adolescence by a Primary Care Outpatient Orthopedic PT[3,8,28,48,104]—cont'd

Hemophilia

Hemophilia is an X-linked disorder of blood coagulation present in 1 in 10,000 males.

Impairment is due to spontaneous hemorrhaging into any of the tissues of the body.

Hemarthrosis (hallmark sign): pain, swelling, limited ROM of affected joint, with elbows, knees, and ankles the joints most often affected.

Hematoma: bleeding into muscles produces pain, swelling; may produce muscle atrophy.

Mucous membrane bleeding (gums, nasal passages, and alimentary tract).

Hemorrhaging risks include peripheral nerve lesions (compression); intracranial, intraspinal, retropharyngeal, and retroperitoneal bleeds.

Joint-protection strategies and joint rehabilitation after bleeds or after total joint arthroplasty are common.

Juvenile rheumatoid arthritis

JRA collectively refers to three forms of childhood arthritis: pauciarticular (few joints) JRA, polyarticular JRA, and systemic-onset JRA (Still's disease). Associated arthritic conditions include systemic lupus erythematosus, dermatomyositis, and scleroderma. About 30,000 to 50,000 children in the United States are affected by JRA.

Systemic clinical manifestations of Still's disease (systemic-onset JRA) include fever (102° F), rash, anemia, lymphadenopathy, polyarthritis, pericarditis, pleuritis, peptic ulcer disease, and hepatitis. Differential diagnosis includes Lyme disease. Musculoskeletal manifestations include polyarthritis, polyarthralgias, myalgia, myositis, tenosynovitis, and skeletal growth disturbances.

Physical therapy interventions for pain control, mobility, strength, endurance (muscular and aerobic), and functional tasks are key for children afflicted by JRA. Loss of joint motion is the strongest indicator of functional disability in children with JRA.

Joint-protection strategies (e.g., mobility assistive devices, body mechanics education) and daily activity pacing are important to children (and adults) with rheumatoid arthritis. Twenty percent of children with JRA will have moderate to severe joint limitations in adulthood.

Neural tube defect (NTD)

Congenital defect in neural tube that can occur at any level of the spinal cord. Physiologic variations of this condition are many and include sensory or motor loss. Occurs in 1 to 2 cases per 1000 live births. An estimated 6000 to 10,000 children are born with some sort of spina bifida each year in the United States.

Three most common NTDs:

Spina bifida occulta (incomplete fusion of the posterior vertebral arch)

Meningocele (external protrusion of the meninges)

Myelodysplasia (protrusion of the meninges and spinal cord

Contributing factors include genetics (chromosomal abnormalities), ethnicity (whites > blacks), teratogens (alcohol), and nutritional deficits (lack of folic acid). Women in their childbearing years are advised to take 0.4 mg of folic acid per day. Folic acid supplementation should begin at least 3 months before conception. Multivitamins containing folic acid during the first 6 weeks of gestation will prevent up to 86% of NTDs.

PT responsibilities include mobility and postural alignment via stretching to prevent contractures, orthotic and wheelchair management, skin and wound management, bowel and bladder programs, and functional training. The outpatient orthopedic PT should be aware that 40% to 50% of these children develop latex sensitivity because of the high level of medical exposure early in life.

Osteogenesis imperfecta (brittle bone disease)

OA is an inherited connective-tissue disorder with an incidence of 1 in 20,000 live births.

Fracture management: physical therapy to combat the effects of immobilization.

Pain management via a multidisciplinary approach (physician, physical therapy, and psychology) to reduce or remove the pain, assist in mental well-being, and improve physiological function.

Physical agents include: thermal modalities, transcutaneous electrical nerve stimulation (TENS), gentle myofascial techniques, relaxation training, biofeedback.

Pharmaceutical management includes: over-the-counter pain relievers, NSAIDs, topical pain relievers, narcotic medications, antidepressants, and nerve blocks.

Prader-Willi syndrome (PWS)

PWS is a chromosomal disorder that can affect people of both sexes and of any race or country. Genetic causes include deletion, imprinting error, translocation, or maternal disomy of chromosome 15.

Primary impairments include severe hypotonia and feeding problems in infancy, excessive eating and obesity in childhood, reduced strength, poor fine and gross motor coordination. Many of these children are involved in birth to three (0-3) programs. The exercise prescription for management of obesity includes diet education, behavioral modification, limited access to food, and increased activity level.

For more information on PWS, go to the PWS Association at: www.pwsausa.org.

Sickle cell disease (SCD)

An inherited blood disorder in which normally round red blood cells become misshaped like sickles and clog vessels. These blockages cause painful episodes known as sickle cell crises. An estimated 1 in 500 African Americans have the genetic condition, which occurs when someone inherits two copies of a mutated gene for hemoglobin, the oxygen carrier in red blood cells.

Clinical presentation includes jaundice in the first few weeks of life, organomegaly (spleen, liver), moderate to severe anemia, cardiac systolic flow murmur, and musculoskeletal distortion and growth disturbance, particularly in the skull, vertebrae, long bones, and maxilla (may require referral for orthodontics).

A multidisciplinary team focus is on caregiver education including physical assessment skills (i.e., vital signs: HR, RR, temperature), how to treat pain, and when to administer prophylactic antibiotics. Education in stroke prevention is key, as blood transfusions may prevent recurrent stroke in children with SCA. Lung function should be monitored as children with SCD often have abnormal pulmonary function tests (PFT).

Continued

TABLE 12-3

Pediatric Physical Therapy: Select Congenital, Genetic, and Acquired Pediatric Conditions that May Be Seen During Adolescence by a Primary Care Outpatient Orthopedic PT[3,8,28,48,104]—cont'd

For more information on SCA, refer to *Management of Sickle Cell Disease*, ed 4, NIH pub no 02-2117, May 28, 2002, National Institutes x recessive Heart, Lung, and Blood Institute Bethesda, Md.	Adolescent issues: Monitor growth, development, and nutrition. Adolescents and parents should be counseled about potential social problems related to frequent illness, stature, and delayed sexual development. Concern about issues such as body size, sexual short function, pain management, and death often is expressed as rebellion, depression, or refusal to heed treatment plans and medical advice. Adolescents should be advised not to use tobacco, alcohol, and illegal drugs. Postpubertal adolescents should be educated about sexuality, safe sex practices, and the use of condoms to prevent sexually transmitted diseases. Girls should be counseled about the risks of pregnancy in women with SCD, safe birth control practices, and the merits of pregnancy at the right age and social circumstances.
Spinal muscle atrophy SMA is an inherited autosomal recessive genetic defect of chromosome 5 characterized by loss and degeneration of the large anterior horn cells in the brainstem and spinal cord.	Childhood SMAs are divided into four types: Type I, acute infantile SMA (Werdnig-Hoffmann) causes death by age 18 months. Type II, chronic Werdnig-Hoffmann, causes hypotonia and results in a shortened lifespan. Type III, Kugelberg-Welander, is a juvenile-onset disease (at ages 2-10 years), has a slower onset and less impairment. Patients will present with progressive proximal-muscle weakness (pelvic girdle and paraspinals), followed by shoulder-girdle weakness and bulbar signs. Although most will be wheelchair bound by early adulthood, there is potential for a normal life expectancy. Type IV, adult forms of SMA, will manifest in the teen years and are typically marked by weakness of the distal legs, particularly the anterior tibial and peroneal compartments. Primary-impairment muscle weakness (lower motor neuron) results from progressive loss of anterior horn cells in the spinal cord. Treatment is directed at minimizing spinal deformity, maintaining joint-level mobility, maintaining functional mobility, and preventing contractures. Individuals who maintain ambulation skills have been found to have a lower incidence of scoliosis. For severe scoliosis (curves >45 degrees on the Cobb method), surgical intervention often is required to stabilize the spine, as without it, there can be progressive respiratory and swallowing compromise, as well as increased integumentary-system stress.

to 4 years (e.g., motor control for crawling, sitting, standing, walking, running, hopping, speaking, communicating with adults, and toileting, and early cognitive skills) is known as psychomotor development.[218] Failure to meet these developmental milestones in early childhood can have deleterious effects on the child's or adolescent's continued cognitive development (including academic achievement), motor function (fine and gross motor tasks), and peer socialization.[27,48,162]

Overview: Preschooler (4 to 6 Years)

The child usually doubles his or her birth height (length) by 4 years of age. At 5 years of age, height and weight are generally the same. Caloric intake is about 1300 to 1700 calories per day. During the preschool years, the child should begin to thin. The protruding abdomen of the toddler years begins to disappear, and body proportions change as the legs rapidly grow. Posture is more erect, and gait continues to mature. Gross motor tasks of running, hopping, and skipping develop during this period. Control of fine motor skills begins during this time.

Children begin to imitate their adult and older-sibling role models, and take initiative in learning. Role modeling, proper nutritional habits, adequate fluid intake, and exercise will reinforce life-long positive health habits.[27,48,200] Caregivers should reinforce the child's sleep hygiene, including 9 to 12 hours of sleep per night and possibly a daily nap.[183]

Overview: School Age (6 to 12 Years)

During the early school years, children continue to learn and grow. Weight typically increases by 5 to 7 lb per year, and height increases an average of 3 inches per year. The child may have growth spurts. The intake needed to support growth usually is about 1800 to 2000 calories by 8 to 10 years of age. When puberty starts (age 10 to 12 years), caloric needs vary by sex: 1500 to 3000 for girls and 2000 to 3700 for boys.[200] Sleep needs vary from 8 to 12 hours, and these children typically do not require a nap.[183]

The child's gait should be completely normalized to adult patterns by age 7.[184] Vision is 20/20 at 7 years of age. Strength, physical ability, and coordination increase in the school-age child. By 12 years of age, boys typically surpass girls in strength, endurance, and agility, while girls exceed boys in flexibility and coordination.[200] In general, both sexes should have high energy levels for gross motor activities. Skills of fine motor manipulation should approximate those of the adult. Children become acutely aware of their physical abilities and interests compared with their peers.[48,200] Developmental delay in this age group can be a predictor of long-term problems for the child.[48]

Overview: Adolescence (12 to 20 Years)

During puberty, hormones guide the development of the body in conjunction with social systems (e.g., school, church, family, community and cultural programs) designed to foster the transition from childhood to adulthood.[27] Between the ages of 10 and 20 years, children undergo rapid changes in body size, shape, physiology, and psychological and social functioning. Except for the first year of life, physical growth is more rapid in adolescence than in any other stage of development.[230]

Children are anatomically and physically different from adults, but there are still some principles of child development that the PT must heed (see Table 12-2). Caloric requirements during adolescence are 2200 calories (range of 1500 to 3000) for girls and 2800 calories (range of 2000 to 3700) for boys.[200] Proper sleep hygiene for adolescents is 8.5 to 9.25 hours per night, although growth spurts can cause teens to sleep longer.[183]

PSYCHOSOCIAL DEVELOPMENT. Key elements of psychosocial development across the lifespan, as originally outlined by Erik Erikson in 1963, still hold true today.[80] Psychosocial development from birth to the onset of puberty can profoundly affect the adolescent's development of self-esteem. Babies learn at a young age (less than 12 months) to either trust or mistrust that others will care for their basic needs. Infants and toddlers (1 to 3 years) learn to be self-sufficient in many activities, including toileting, feeding, walking, and talking, or to doubt their own abilities (autonomy vs. shame or doubt). Psychosocial development in the formative years can sway the cognitive and emotional capabilities of preschool (initiative vs. guilt), school-age (industry vs. inferiority), and adolescent (identity vs. role confusion) youth. If children are made to feel inferior and inadequate before puberty, the development of a stable self-identity in the tumultuous adolescent years can appear to be a monumental task.

Adolescents are trying to answer the age-old question, "Who am I?" Adolescents acquire the cognitive ability to reason logically and abstractly, and consider future implications of their current actions. The rites of passage of adolescence either help teenagers establish ethnic, cultural, gender, sexual, and career identities, or they confuse teenagers about their future roles. Erikson further proposed that after they have passed through adolescence, young adults either seek out love and companionship or become isolated from other people.

The ability to learn responsibility for self, others, and society in the teenage years determines whether a child will grow up to be a productive and competent member of society or a burden to society. Health care professionals can help adolescents on this road to maturity by promoting appropriate health behaviors, such as proper nutrition and physical activity, responsible sexual behavior, and intelligent choices about tobacco and alcohol. Given the amount of poverty, crime, and homelessness in America, issues of psychosocial development (i.e., mental health) in our youth should be of paramount concern to every health care professional, parent, and politician.

Puberty: The Approach to Maturity

When I was a boy of fourteen, my father was so ignorant I could hardly stand to have the old man around. But when I got to be twenty-one, I was astonished at how much the old man had learned in seven years.

Mark Twain

Puberty and Sexual Maturation

Puberty can be divided into five stages. The PT monitors puberty via sexual maturity ratings (SMR) based on the Tanner Stages of Sexual Development (Table 12-4). The Tanner stages are used as a *guide* to the usual progression of male and female sexual maturation.[27,168,169] The physical changes of puberty include rapid increases in height and weight, changes in body composi-

tion (i.e., musculoskeletal system), growth of pubic hair and axillary hair, changes in thermoregulation (i.e., integumentary system), changes in the circulatory and respiratory systems, and development of sexual organs and secondary sex characteristics.[27,168,169,226]

The range of normal development among teenagers is wide and varies chronologically by gender, with girls usually proceeding through puberty earlier than boys. On average, girls enter puberty at age 10 (range of 8 to 13 years) and boys at age 11 (range of 9.5 to 14 years).[27] After it is started, the process of puberty usually completes in 4.5 years. Girls typically end their pubertal development with a peak-velocity growth spurt by age 14 years, compared with age 16 for boys.[230] These growth spurts typically correlate to a Tanner SMR of 3 or 4.

In girls, the first visible sign of puberty is the appearance of breast buds, between 8 and 13 years of age.[169] Less obvious changes in the adolescent girl include enlargement of the ovaries, uterus, labia, and clitoris; thickening of the endometrium and vaginal mucosa; and increased vaginal glycogen, predisposing to yeast infections.[27] Menarche, or the first menstrual period, is a significant event in the life of the developing female. Menses typically begin 2 to 2½ years after the development of breast buds (normal range of 9 to 16 years), and around the peak velocity in height growth.[27] A critical weight (48 kg or 106 lb) and body fat (24%) appear to be needed to produce menarche.[92,93,196,219] Pubertal onset and menarche appear to have a genetic correlation between mother and daughter and between sisters. Black girls usually have an earlier onset of puberty (9 years of age) and menarche (12.2 years) compared with whites (age 10 and 12.8 years, respectively).[27,93]

In boys, the first visible sign of puberty is testicular enlargement, which may begin as early as 9½ years.[168] The seminiferous tubules, epididymis, seminal vesicles, and prostate enlarge under the influence of luteinizing hormone (LH) and testosterone. The left testis normally is lower than the right. Gynecomastia, or breast hypertrophy, occurs in 40% to 65% of pubertal boys as a result of a relative excess of estrogenic stimulation. Fewer than 10% of young boys develop gynecomastia sufficient to cause embarrassment and social disability. Breast swelling less than 4 cm in diameter has a 90% chance of spontaneous resolution within 3 years. For greater degrees of enlargement, hormonal or surgical treatment may be indicated. Obesity may exacerbate gynecomastia and should be addressed through diet and exercise.[27]

Parents, caregivers, and health care providers should understand that normal progression through the Tanner stages varies widely depending on the individual child, his or her nationality or ethnic group, and a host of other environmental and geographic factors.[27,196] Socioeconomic conditions, general health and nutrition, and increased body fat are environmental triggers for puberty. Children living at lower altitudes and lower latitudes tend to start puberty earlier. Contemporary children in the United States enter puberty somewhat earlier than the published norms, perhaps because of increased weight and adiposity.[27]

PRECOCIOUS PUBERTY. Early signs of sexual development, before the age of 8 in girls, and before the age of 9 or 9½ in boys, is known as *precocious puberty*.[27,71] Precocious puberty is more common in girls than boys. Early prognosticators for

TABLE 12-4
Tanner Stages of Sexual Development

Tanner Stages of Female Puberty		
Stage	**Breast**	**Pubic Hair**
1 (Preadolescent)	Only papillae are elevated.	Vellus hair only, and hair is similar to development over anterior abdominal wall (i.e., no pubic hair).
2	Breast bud and papilla are elevated, and a small mount is present; areola diameter is enlarged.	There is sparse growth of long, slightly pigmented downy hair or only slightly curled hair, appearing along the labia.
3	Further enlargement of breast mound; increased palpable glandular tissue.	Hair is darker, coarser, more curled, and spreads to the pubic junction.
4	Areola and papilla are elevated to form a second mound above the level of the rest of the breast.	Adult-type hair; area covered is less than that in most adults; there is no spread to the medial surface of thighs.
5 (Adult)	Adult mature breast; recession of areola to the mound of breast tissue, rounding of the breast mound, and projection of only the papillae are evident.	Adult-type hair with increased spread to medial surface of thighs; distribution is as an inverted triangle.

From Marshall WA, Tanner JM: Variations in pattern of pubertal changes in girls, *Arch Dis Child*, 44(235):291-303, 1969.

Tanner Stages of Male Puberty		
Stage	**Genital Stage**	**Pubic Hair Stage**
1 (Preadolescent)	Testes, scrotum, and penis are about the same size and proportion as in early childhood.	Vellus hair over the pubis is no further developed than that over the abdominal wall (i.e., no pubic hair).
2	Scrotum and testes have enlarged, and there is a change in the texture of scrotal skin and some reddening of scrotal skin.	There is sparse growth of long, slightly pigmented, downy hair, straight or only slightly curled, appearing chiefly at base of penis.
3	Growth of the penis has occurred, at first mainly in length but with some increase in breadth. The testes and the scrotum have grown further.	Hair is considerably darker, coarser, and more curled and spreads sparsely over junction of pubes.
4	The penis is further enlarged in length and breadth, with development of glans. The testes and the scrotum are further enlarged. There is also further darkening of scrotal skin.	Hair is now adult in type, but the area it covers is smaller than that in most adults. There is no spread to the medial surface of the thighs.
5 (Adult)	Genitalia are adult in size and shape. No further enlargement takes place after stage 5 is reached.	Hair is adult in quantity and type, distributed as an inverted triangle. There is spread to the medial surface of the thighs but not up the linea alba or elsewhere above the base of the inverted triangle.

From Marshall WA, Tanner JM: Variations in the pattern of pubertal changes in boys, *Arch Dis Child* 45:13-23, 1970.

precocious puberty include physical changes, such as the appearance of genital hair (pubarche), onset of growth in breast tissue (thelarche), and increased growth rate and skeletal maturity (bone age) relative to chronological age. The child's physician (or other appropriate health care provider) should monitor the child's growth rate compared with sexual maturation using pediatric growth charts.[62] Determining actual bone age as it relates to sexual maturation requires radiographic evaluation of the ossification centers of the hand and wrist and/or iliac crest (Risser sign; refer to Fig. 12-6).[101,110]

Accurate differential diagnosis of precocious puberty requires sensitive hormone screening tests, including testing for gonadotropin-releasing hormone (GnRH) and the gonadotropins (i.e., luteinizing hormone and follicle-stimulating hormone). Because of the underlying disorders that can be associated with precocious puberty (e.g., central nervous system [CNS] disease, trauma, tumors, McCune-Albright syndrome, and chronic primary hypothyroidism), suspicion of this condition necessitates referral to an endocrinologist.[27]

DYSMENORRHEA. A girl who has reached Tanner stage 5 (i.e., the breasts are fully formed and pubic hair resembles adult quantity, texture, and an upside-down triangle form) should have a regular menstrual cycle. Late onset of menarche (after chronological age of 16) is an indication for referral to either a gynecologist or an endocrinologist. Many factors may contribute to a delay in menarche. The evaluating health care practitioner should consider endocrine disorders that cause effects opposite from precocious puberty, along with low overall body fat, eating disorders, and athletic amenorrhea[235] as possible causes. A delay in menarche or menstrual dysfunction is not uncommon among young athletic females, but these delays can have long-term effects on bone metabolism.[27,93,104,235]

NOCTURNAL EMISSIONS (WET DREAMS). When boys are going through puberty (usually ages 12 to 18), it is not uncommon or abnormal for them to experience nocturnal emission of sperm. Girls also can experience vaginal nocturnal secretion, but this normally is less noticeable than male emissions. Wet dreams are a totally normal function of the body and are not under voluntary control. This phenomenon usually stops when the individual begins masturbating or becomes sexually active.[27]

METABOLISM AND NUTRITION IN PUBERTY. Healthy growth and development of the body during puberty require adequate nutrition. Adequate nutrition encompasses proper caloric intake of carbohydrates, proteins, and fats, along with sufficient minerals, vitamins, and fluids. In 2000, the U.S. Department of Agriculture (USDA) published *Dietary Guidelines for Americans*.[245] Teenage girls should consume about 2200 calories per days, compared with 2800 calories for teenage boys. The guidelines recommend that Americans aim for a total fat intake of no more than 30% of their diet. Specifically, teenage girls should consume 73 grams of total fat, with 24 grams or less consisting of saturated fats. Boys may consume up to 93 grams of total fat, with 31 grams or less being saturated fats. Adolescents have a great need for phosphorus (1250 mg/day) and iron. Younger children require about 10 mg of iron each day. Adolescents require about 12 mg (males) to 15 mg (all menstruating females) of iron each day. The USDA recommends that all women capable of becoming pregnant consume 400 μg of folic acid daily throughout their childbearing years to reduce the risk of birth defects of the neural tube.[53]

Research suggests that 40% to 50% of skeletal calcium is established during the teenage years and peak bone mass (PBM) is reached between the ages of 25 and 35 years.[104] Adolescents and young adults between the ages of 11 and 24 years should get 1200 to 1500 mg of elemental calcium per day.[104] Some foods containing wheat bran or oxalic acid (e.g., cauliflower, rhubarb, beet greens, and brussel sprouts) can interfere with calcium absorption. Although many parents struggle to get their teenagers to eat their vegetables, chocolate, and caffeinated beverages (e.g., diet colas and coffee), which are also high in oxalic acid, are often staples of the American adolescent diet. Therefore choosing to drink diet colas and coffee not only are missing an opportunity to drink milk (which is high in calcium), but diet colas in particular have been hypothesized to reduce absorption of calcium from other foods.

Athletic endeavors that require high caloric intake, low body fat, or intense weight management can affect the adolescent's metabolism. Both male and female competitive athletes, particularly those involved in weight-oriented or appearance-oriented sports such as wrestling,[68] gymnastics, competitive dance, and figure skating, are at risk of osteoporosis because of their susceptibility to eating disorders.[171,235] The cultural drive to be thin likewise is dangerous to adolescents (girls more than boys) because it results in compromised skeletal health and an increased risk of osteoporosis in adulthood.[27,104,171,235] The combination of disordered eating, amenorrhea, and osteoporosis is known as the female athlete triad.[235]

Osteoporosis is the most common metabolic bone disease, affecting about 10 million people in the United States.[104] Primary idiopathic osteoporosis is most common in postmenopausal white females of Northern European ancestry, especially if they have an associated period of inactivity or depression.[104] Secondary osteoporosis may be caused by prolonged use of corticosteroids, heparin, anticonvulsants, laxatives, and other medications; low body weight and low body

mass index; smoking, alcoholism, malnutrition, malabsorption, or lactose intolerance; endocrine disorders (e.g., hyperthyroidism, hyperparathyroidism, type 2 diabetes mellitus, Cushing's disease, or male hypogonadism); and other medical conditions (e.g., medications associated with organ transplantation, cancer treatment medications, juvenile rheumatoid arthritis, osteogenesis imperfecta, or spinal cord injuries).[104]

Health care professionals working with adolescents should scrutinize for proper nutritional habits, behaviors, or personality changes that may indicate distorted eating habits, or abuse of nutritional supplements or illicit drugs. Table 12-5 discusses eating disorders, excessively low body mass index (BMI), and clinical features of anorexia nervosa and bulimia nervosa. Females tend to have more serious and devastating forms of eating disorders. In most cases, the drive to lose weight by males tends to be seasonal and transient as males attempt to achieve low body weight to remain competitive in sports such as gymnastics and wrestling.[68]

The PT can evaluate adolescent eating habits via the Eating Attitudes Test (EAT-26).[97] In 1998, the EAT-26* was selected as a screening instrument for the National Eating Disorders Screening Program, making it the most widely used standardized measure of symptoms and concerns characteristic of eating disorders. The PT should evaluate the entire context of the therapeutic situation, and referral to a nutritionist or qualified mental health professional who has experience in treating eating disorders is warranted.[96,97]

Poor nutritional guidance by the family, ethnic considerations, and inadequate finances (socioeconomic variables) also can lead to poor food selections among both male and female adolescents. In our fast-paced, fast-food society, the lack of family meal time and the prevalence of vending machines and advertisements for high-fat, high-calorie foods are but a few of the societal influences contributing to poor food choices by Americans. These variables together are more likely to lead to childhood and adolescent obesity, a topic that will be addressed further in the health promotion section of this chapter. The reader is encouraged to visit the USDA web page (www.nal.usda.gov/fnic/) for updated gender-specific dietary guidelines across the lifespan.

Puberty and the Musculoskeletal System

The development and health of the musculoskeletal (MS) system are a primary focus of the outpatient orthopedic PT working with adolescent patients. The MS system is one of four preferred patterns of practice (i.e., musculoskeletal, neuromuscular, cardiovascular/pulmonary, and integumentary) found in *The Guide to Physical Therapist Practice*, ed 2.[205] Many connective tissues collectively make up the MS system (e.g., bony skeleton, ligament, tendon, joint capsule and fascia, fibrocartilage, hyaline [articular] cartilage, and the striated

---

*The original publication of the EAT-26 can be found at Garner DM, Olmsted MP, Bohr Y, et al: The eating attitudes test: psychometric features and clinical correlates, *Psychol Med* 12:871-878, 1982. A copy of the EAT-26 can be obtained from the following publication: Garner DM: Psychoeducational principles in treatment. In Garner DM, Garfinkel PE, eds: *Handbook of treatment for eating disorders*, New York, 1997, Guilford Press.

TABLE 12-5

Eating Disorders and Excessively Low Body Mass Index

In the United States an estimated 5 to 10 million women and 1 million men suffer from eating disorders. These severe disturbances of eating behavior often are difficult to detect, especially in teens wearing baggy clothes, or in individuals who binge then induce vomiting or evacuation. Be familiar with the two principal eating disorders, *anorexia nervosa* and *bulimia nervosa*. Both conditions are characterized by distorted perceptions of body image and weight. Early detection is important, because prognosis improves when treatment occurs in the early stages of these disorders.

Clinical Features	
Anorexia Nervosa	**Bulimia Nervosa**

• Refusal to maintain minimally normal body weight (or BMI above 17.5 kg/m^2)
• Fear of appearing fat
• Frequent starving but denial; lack of insight
• Often brought in by family members
• May present as failure to make expected weight gains in childhood or adolescence, amenorrhea in women, loss of libido or potency in men
• Associated with depressive symptoms such as depressed mood, irritability, social withdrawal, insomnia, reduced libido
• Additional features supporting diagnosis: self-induced vomiting or purging, excessive exercise, use of appetite suppressants or diuretics
• Biological complications
  • *Neuroendocrine changes*: amenorrhea, increased corticotropin-releasing factor, cortisol, growth hormone, serotonin; reduced diurnal cortisol fluctuation, luteinizing hormone, follicle-stimulating hormone, thyroid-stimulating hormone
  • *Cardiovascular disorders*: bradycardia, hypotension, arrhythmias, cardiomyopathy
  • *Metabolic disorders*: hypokalemia, hypochloremic metabolic alkalosis, increased BUN, edema
  • *Other*: dry skin, dental caries, delayed gastric emptying, constipation, anemia, osteoporosis
	• Repeated binge eating followed by self-induced vomiting, misuse of laxatives, diuretics, or other medications; fasting; or excessive exercise
	• Overeating at least twice a week during 3-month period; large amounts of food consumed in short period (~2 hr)
	• Preoccupation with eating; craving and compulsion to eat; lack of control over eating; alternating with periods of starvation
	• Dread of fatness but may be obese
	• Subtypes of
	  • *Purging*: bulimic episodes accompanied by self-induced vomiting or use of laxatives, diuretics, or enemas
	  • *Nonpurging*: bulimic episodes accompanied by compensatory behavior such as fasting, exercise but without purging
	• Biological complications
	See changes listed for anorexia nervosa, especially weakness, fatigue, mild cognitive disorder; also erosion of dental enamel, parotitis, pancreatic inflammation with elevated amylase, mild neuropathies, seizures, hypokalemia, hypochloremic metabolic acidosis, hypomagnesemia

From Bickley LS: *Bates' guide to physical examination and history taking, ed 8,* Philadelphia, 2003, Lippincott/Williams and Wilcott, p 88.
Sources: World Health Organization: *The ICD-10 classification of mental and behavioral disorders: diagnostic criteria for research,* Geneva, 1993, World Health Organization. American Psychiatric Association: DSM-IV-TR: *Diagnostic and statistical manual of mental disorders,* ed 4, Washington, DC, 1994, American Psychiatric Association. Halmi KA: Eating disorders. In Kaplan HI and Sadock BJ, eds: *Comprehensive textbook of psychiatry,* ed 7, Philadelphia, 2000, Lippincott Williams and Wilkins, pp 1663-1676.

---

muscles of the body). A competent nervous system (afferent and efferent pathways and central nervous system modulation) is necessary for control of normal patterns of movement, while healthy cardiovascular and pulmonary systems supply the energy to run the human machine.

Skeletal modeling begins in the fifth week of gestation, when the hyaline-cartilage skeletal model first appears, and continues until the end of skeletal ossification, as late as age 25 years. Skeletal modeling is the process by which agents external to a growing tissue affect its growth and direction in ways that fashion its microscopic and gross architecture.[64] Collectively, the skeletal modeling process prepares the growing MS system to endure the demands of adult daily life.

The skeleton of the newborn contains 350 bones that fuse together to form the 206 bones found in the adult skeleton.[211] Symmetry and rate of growth of the *axial skeleton* (i.e., cranium, spine, thorax) and *appendicular skeleton* (i.e., pelvic girdle, shoulder girdle, and limbs) should be monitored across the pediatric lifespan (0 to about 25 years). The major clinical implications of skeletal modeling are: (1) the younger the child, the more pliable the skeletal system and (2) children and adolescents are at risk for traumatic epiphyseal injuries.[64,104,211]

VERTEBRAL COLUMN DEVELOPMENT. The primary curves of the spine, the kyphotic curves, are present at birth. The secondary curves, lordotic curves of the cervical and lumbar spine, develop as a result of accommodation to upright posture and continue to develop until growth stops in late adolescence or early adulthood. The bipolar neurocentral joints of the vertebral column fuse by age 7 to 8 years, while the annular (ring) epiphyses are activated just before puberty (age 7 to 9 years) and close between the ages of 14 and 24 years.

THORAX DEVELOPMENT. Babies usually are born with a barrel-shaped chest (i.e., round thorax) and horizontally oriented ribcage. Within a few years of birth, the ribs drop into their normal downwardly sloped position. By 6 years of age, the thorax develops into the more adult-like elliptical shape with an anteroposterior/transverse ratio of 1:2 or 5:7.[143] In general, the chest maintains this configuration well into adulthood. Persistence of a barrel-shaped chest after 6 years of age is abnormal and typically associated with respiratory diseases that cause hyperinflation of the lungs (e.g., asthma and cystic fibrosis).[104,143,167] A widening and flattening of the ribcage also is a normal physiological and relatively permanent response to pregnancy. Pregnant adolescent females should be educated about changes in the ribcage and respiratory rate, dyspnea, and the many other physiological changes associated with pregnancy (see Chapter 13).

Pectus excavatum (funnel chest) and pectus carinatum (pigeon chest) are two abnormal congenital chest configurations that are usually asymptomatic.[143] The latter is less common. Severe depression of the sternum in pectus excavatum can reduce the anteroposterior dimension of the chest, displace the heart, and reduce tidal volume.[167] These configurations may create a negative self-concept and embarrassment for the developing adolescent, particularly during school-related gym activities or sports activities or as they begin sexual experimentation.

LONG BONE DEVELOPMENT. The functional divisions of the long bones are displayed in Figure 12-1, *A*. The diaphysis, or the shaft of the long bone, is the portion of bone formed by the primary ossification center. The epiphysis, or the end of the long bone, is formed by the secondary ossification centers. The metaphysis is the wider part of the shaft of a long bone adjacent to the epiphyseal plate. The metaphysis consists of cancellous bone during development, and in adulthood the metaphysis becomes continuous with the epiphysis. The epiphyseal plate represents the bone's growth zone. The two types of epiphyses, pressure and traction, are shown in Figure 12-1, *B*. These regions of growth are common sites of injury in the adolescent.

The pubescent MS growth spurt usually begins distally, with enlargement of the hands and feet, and continues with the arms and legs and finally the trunk and chest. Body weight is increased in several ways, including increased height (length of bones), increased bone density, increased lean muscle mass in boys, and a higher fat/muscle ratio in girls (breasts, hips, and thighs).[27] Asymmetric growth patterns can give young adolescents a gawky appearance. Akin to the other growth spurts of childhood, adolescence often brings muscle imbalances and issues of coordination or motor control that may predispose to epiphyseal injuries. During periods of adolescent skeletal growth, flexibility exercises should be emphasized to prevent injury to muscles, tendons, joints, and apophyses. Exercise and diet are important to control increased fat mass, whereas strength training will improve bone density and muscle mass, which contributes to overall lean (fat-free) body mass.[50]

Puberty and the Nervous System

The overall function of the nervous system (NS) is well established before adolescence. At puberty, the brain releases hormones directing other body systems to change. Outpatient PTs should be skilled in testing the integrity of the *entire* nervous system across the lifespan because its function can be compromised by a variety of conditions (e.g., space-occupying lesions of the cranium, systemic disease, traumatic brain injuries, peripheral nervous system [PNS] disease, and trauma).

At birth, the brain is one fourth the weight of the adult brain, while the head is already 70% of its adult size.[50] By 6 months of age, the brain has doubled its weight. Glial cell formation is at its peak growth between the ages of 15 and 24 months.[195] The brain reaches 90% of its adult mass by 6 years of age, and at the onset of puberty (age 10 to 12 years), the brain reaches 100% of adult weight. Dendritic branching reaches levels of adult complexity during early and middle adolescence (from 12 to 16 years).[50] Abstract language concepts are possible, and the corticospinal tract is morphologically mature (but not electrophysiologically mature). By 13 years of age, low-frequency electroencephalographic rhythms typically change to adult high-frequency rhythms.

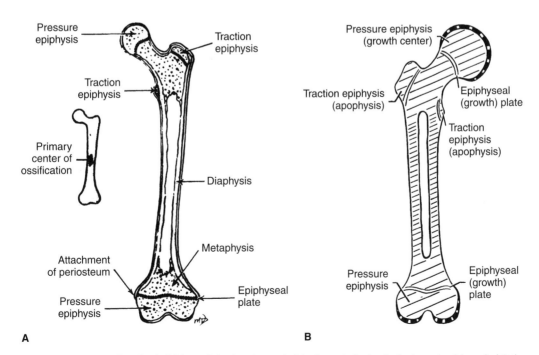

FIGURE 12-1 A, Functional divisions of the long bones (epiphysis, metaphysis, diaphysis, and epiphyseal plates). **B,** Types of epiphyses. (From Salter RB: *Textbook of disorders and injuries of the musculoskeletal system*, ed 3, Baltimore, 1999, Williams & Wilkins, p 340.)

Myelination of the PNS is largely complete at birth, giving the newborn sensory access to environmental surroundings (through touch, smell, motion, and taste). All cranial nerves (with the exception of the optic nerve [CN II]) are completely myelinated at birth. Formation of glial cells, unexcitable support tissues of the CNS including astrocytes, oligodendroglial cells, ependymal cells, and microglia continues within the brain into young adulthood. Myelination of association cortices (e.g., frontal, parietal, temporal lobes, along with reticular formation, internal capsule, and the association fibers) persists into adulthood.[50,108]

Brain metabolism (i.e., utilization of glucose) changes with CNS maturation. Tracking of the brain's glucose utilization via positron emission tomography (PET) is a mechanism for monitoring functional maturation.[50] Glucose utilization is closely linked to synaptogenesis, or synaptic proliferation, which occurs primarily between birth and 4 years of age. Synaptogenesis levels off during middle childhood, then declines in adolescence because of synaptic elimination that occurs within the cortex. The brain further diminishes its energy requirements into adulthood.[61]

A review of the adolescent's dietary history and current nutritional status can lend insight into overall NS and other body systems function. Nutritional habits, environmental quality, socioeconomic variables, and contextual factors (e.g., family, school, and peer-group influences) are key determinants of overall health and have been found to correlate to physical dysfunction, disease, and illness behavior.[228] Children who are malnourished before 3 years of age (including the gestational period) reportedly have impaired motor ability.[50] The number of children born to adolescent women who have poor prenatal care, poor nutritional habits, and poor societal support is a significant long-term health concern for the United States (see the information on teenage pregnancy in the Health Promotion section).

Puberty and the Cardiovascular and Pulmonary Systems

The health of the cardiovascular and pulmonary (CVP) systems affects the amount of oxygen that can be delivered to the various tissues and systems of the body. Whether we are discussing muscular endurance (peripheral), the cardiovascular pump (central), or the ventilation and gas-exchange capabilities of the lungs, the CVP system is literally the engine that allows the body to perform work. There are distinct physiological issues (e.g., of circulation, ventilation, and muscular metabolism) that PTs should consider when managing clients across the lifespan.

Heart rate, respiratory rate, and blood pressure are age dependent (Table 12-6). The CVP system of the developing child responds differently to metabolic load (exercise), and the atypically developing youngster adds further concern.[22,121] During the adolescent growth spurt, gender differences in cardiovascular and pulmonary function become apparent.[50] Only the skeletally mature adolescent will have vital signs and cardiopulmonary responses comparable with those of the adult.

AEROBIC METABOLISM. When maximal aerobic power is expressed as VO_2 (milliter per kilogram of body weight per

TABLE 12-6

Vital Signs, Caloric Needs, and Sleep Requirements Across the Pediatric Life Span

Age	HR (beats/min)	HR range (beats/min)	RR (breaths/min)	BP (mm Hg)	Calories	Sleep Needs
Newborn	120	70-190	30-40	NA	1300	Child develops the ability
1 year	120	80-160	20-40	NA	1300	to sleep through the night.
2 years	110	80-130	25-32	NA	1300-1500	May need only one nap
4 years	100	80-120	23-30	100 to 110 60 to 70	1300-1700	per day.
6 years	100	75-115	21-26		1300-1700	9 to 12 hours. May or may not require a nap.
8-10 years	90	70-110	20-26		2000-2400	8 to 12 hours. Does not require a nap.
12 years			18-22	100 to 120		
Female	90	70-110		60 to 80	1500 to 3000	
Male	85	65-105			2000 to 3700	
14 years			18-22			8.5 to 9.25 hours
Female	85	65-105			1500 to 3000	
Male	80	60-100			2000 to 3700	
16 years			16-20			
Female	80	60-100			1500 to 3000	
Male	75	55-95			2000 to 3700	
18 years			12-20			
Female	75	60-100			1500 to 3000	
Male	70	55-95			2000 to 3700	
Adults >20 years	70	60-100	12-20		2000-3000	6.5 to 8 hours
Well-conditioned athletes	55-70	50-100	10-20			6.5 to 8 hours

Data from references 104, 143, 183, and 200.
BP, Blood pressure; HR, heart rate; RR, respiratory rate.

minute), children are similar to adults. However, absolute VO_2 max is lower in children because children have smaller bodies and thus smaller hearts, lungs, and lung capacity. Overall, cardiac output (stroke volume × heart rate) is 1 to 3 L/min lower in prepubescent children compared with older adolescents and adults.[162,173]

During adolescence, the peak height velocity of teens leads to a rapid increase in height, allowing for a larger thorax and thus greater potential of the cardiopulmonary system. Between 6 and 12 years of age, the overall physical working capacity of children increases about eightfold.[162] Adolescent males have a greater advantage in height growth, develop larger hearts and lungs, and have higher blood pressure and lower resting heart rates than females.[27,200]

ANAEROBIC METABOLISM. When adjusted for body weight, young children have about 65% to 70% the total anaerobic capacity of mature adolescents and adults. Children appear to have equal concentrations of adenosine triphosphate (ATP) and creatine phosphate (CP) compared with adults. However, their ability to utilize glucose for anaerobic activity is reduced because they have lower concentrations of phosphofructokinase, the rate-limiting enzyme in glycolysis.[162,173,200] As a result of their lower rate of glycolysis, children demonstrate slower production and accumulation of lactate.

At 85% VO_2 max, adults rapidly begin to show negative side effects of elevated blood levels of lactic acid (e.g., increase in H^+ concentration, decrease in available energy, and decreased muscle contractile force during exercise) and quickly fatigue. Conversely, prepubescent children do not demonstrate elevated levels of lactate accumulation until they reach VO_2 max of 93%. This literally lets young children push the anaerobic threshold further, but they have less of an anaerobic reserve compared with adults. This explains why small children are able to go at high levels of intensity but then suddenly fatigue.[162]

The hormonal changes of puberty are so broad that they affect energy utilization systems literally down to individual cellular metabolism. By late adolescence, a teenager will have an exercise response that is similar to adults (i.e., lactate accumulation at 85% VO_2 max). The adolescent's apparently sudden change in tolerance of anaerobic exercise could be disconcerting to the observer who does not understand the exercise physiology of the developing individual.

According to investigations by the American Academy of Pediatrics, pediatric athletes have superior cardiac functional capacity, greater cardiac volume, and greater chamber size than nonathletes.[9] In general, studies support the theory that the effects of sustained submaximal exercise on cardiac function are similar in children and adults.[9,173,200] Careful assessment of cardiovascular status, including blood pressure and the possible presence of heart murmurs or abnormal rhythms, remains necessary in ongoing medical care of the young person. PTs also should consider thermoregulation when prescribing exercises for patients across the developmental years (see discussion of Integument).

CORONARY ARTERY DISEASE. Assessing for signs and symptoms of coronary artery disease (CAD) and its risk factors is an essential skill of the PT. The American Medical Association (AMA) considers CAD, the leading killer of adults, to be a *pediatric* disease. CAD has three periods of development: (1) incubation period (infancy to adolescence), (2) latent period (adolescence and early adulthood), and (3) clinical manifestation period (adulthood).[200]

Risk factors (both nonmodifiable and modifiable) of CAD are indicators of overall health, and several are relevant to teenagers. Nonmodifiable risk factors for CAD include age (women over 55 years and men over 45 years of age), male gender, family/genetic determinants, ethnicity, and infection (viral or bacterial).

Modifiable risk factors (listed hierarchically according to the efficacy of interventions in reducing the incidence of CAD) include cigarette smoking, high cholesterol, hypertension, malnutrition, obesity, physical inactivity, diabetes, altered hormonal status (e.g., oral contraceptives, hysterectomy, or oophorectomy), psychological stress, alcohol consumption (excessive or complete abstinence), and sleep-disordered breathing.[104] Among teens, cigarette smoking remains high and continues to be a major contributor to future CAD in America. Serum cholesterol levels, obesity, physical inactivity, diabetes, and environmental stress are all on the rise in American children.[34,200,214] As many as 40% of school-aged (6 to 12 years) children currently display at least one risk factor for heart disease.[200]

Puberty and the Integumentary System

Skin is the largest organ of the body and performs many vital functions. The PT always should assess the skin during observational and palpatory examinations because it can tell us much about the general health of our patients. The integumentary system, which houses hair follicles, apocrine and eccrine units (thermoregulation via perspiration), and sebaceous glands (production of sebum [oil] for lubrication), undergoes significant changes during puberty.

The endocrine system regulates changes in patterns of hair growth and the output of sebaceous and sweat glands. Tanner's stages of sexual development (see Table 12-4) delineate the specific changes in growth of pubic hair. In girls and boys, growth of axillary hair typically begins 2 years after growth of pubic hair. For boys, facial hair also begins 2 years after the onset of puberty.[27] In middle adolescence, activation of hair growth of the sebaceous and sweat glands can lead to issues with acne and body odor (i.e., hygiene). Given their stage of psychosocial development, adolescents are naturally concerned with how changes in their integumentary system affect their self-identity and relationships.

ACNE. Acne is a problem of the sebaceous glands, which are stimulated by the hormonal changes of adolescence. Facial acne can be a significant emotional stressor for the adolescent. Almost all adolescents (ages 11 to 20) have at least occasional breakouts of whiteheads, blackheads, or pimples. Most teens manage their acne with over-the-counter treatments, but more than one in every three (35%) will consult a physician for treatment of severe acne.[115] Acne is believed to affect young men slightly more than young women, and males are more likely to have severe, longer-lasting forms of acne. Hormonal changes associated with the menstrual cycle and the use of cosmetics may make some young women more susceptible to acne problems.

TABLE 12-7

Heat Stress Disorders, Clinical Features, and Treatment for Adolescents/Adults[13,40,117]

Heat Stress Disorder	Clinical Features	Treatment
Heat illness Weight loss via sweat, less than 5% body weight	Thirst, chills, clammy skin, cramps, nausea, muscle twitches, weakness, and fatigue	Drink ½ cup of water every 15-20 min. During breaks, rest in the shade when possible. Remove extra clothes.
Heat exhaustion Weight loss via sweat, 5% to 10% body weight	Reduced sweating, dizziness, headaches, SOB, lack of saliva, extreme fatigue, weak and rapid pulse, lack of coordination, and thirst	*Stop* activity and move to a cool place. Drink 2 cups of water for every pound lost. Remove wet clothes and sit in a chair in a cold shower.
Heat stroke Weight loss via sweat, more than 10% body weight	Lack of sweat, dry, hot skin, lack of urine, hallucinations, swollen tongue, deafness, aggression, ataxia, high temperature, seizures, vomiting, rapid HR, diarrhea	**Medical emergency** *Stop* activity and move to a cool place; place ice bags on head and back until help arrives. Do not attempt to give water (aspiration possible).

From American College of Sports Medicine: Position stand: exercise and fluid replacement, *Med Sci Sports Exerc* 28:i-vii, 1996; Burke LM and Hawley JA: Fluid balance in team sports: guidelines for optimal practices, *Sports Med* 24:38-54, 1997; Hallisy KM: *Sports injury prevention for the high school athlete*, Detroit, 1994, proceedings from Henry Ford Health System Sports Medicine Symposium.

Recalcitrant (unmanageable) acne is often treated with pharmaceuticals. Isotretinoin (Accutane) has been marketed in the United States since 1982. The drug is an effective treatment for acne that is refractory to other therapies, but it is a teratogen with serious side effects.[132,262] This drug should never be taken during pregnancy or even 1 month before a *planned* pregnancy. Unfortunately, 71% of teenage pregnancies are unintended.[128] Despite being a known teratogen, the number of dispensed prescriptions for isotretinoin increased 2.5-fold (250%) in the United States from 1992 to 2000. Of these prescriptions, 51% were written to female patients between the ages of 15 and 24.[262]

THERMOREGULATION. The hormones of puberty activate apocrine and eccrine units, increasing sweating mechanisms that aid in thermoregulation of the body. Prepubescent individuals differ from adolescents and adults in their thermoregulatory responses to exercise and heat. Despite the fact that young children have the same number of sweat glands, they produce 2.5 times less sweat per gland compared with adults.[162] Children also have limited blood flow to the skin that further limits their cooling potential. As a result, children create more heat per body mass, can experience a greater rise in core body temperature, and acclimatize more slowly to warm environments.[162] Given the fact that pubertal onset varies among individuals, coaches, parents, and young athletes must watch for signs of heat injury and dehydration (Table 12-7). Limiting the time spent playing and training for sports in hot, humid conditions and ensuring adequate fluid intake can prevent heat injury.[13,40,117]

Examination Schema

> The process of obtaining a history, performing a systems review, and selecting and administering tests and measures to gather data about the patient/client.
> *Guide to Physical Therapist Practice*[205]

Setting the Stage for Adolescent Management

The examination of the adolescent follows the sequence used with the adult (refer to sections One, Two, and Three).

Communication skills (see Chapter 4) and an appreciation of adolescent culture (see Chapter 3) are critical to the development of a therapeutic alliance between health care provider and the young patient. Examination of the adolescent includes a focus on issues unique to this population: puberty, growth, and development; family and peer relationships; sexuality; and decision-making and risk behaviors.[230]

The cognitive development of the adolescent affects the format of the history and physical examination. Subjective data can be gathered directly from the patient or with the assistance of a primary caregiver, teacher, coach, or employer. This can make subjective interviewing a potentially delicate situation in which health care practitioners must balance individual patient rights with the caregiver's desire to protect and influence the child.

Adolescent health care needs change as the child progresses through puberty (i.e., early, middle, and late years). During early adolescence, the physical changes of sexual maturation make modesty during interactions with others paramount. Keep the patient dressed during the subjective history, and leave the room when the patient gowns. Most adolescents prefer to be examined without a parent or caregiver in the room, but this depends on the patient's developmental level, familiarity with the examiner, relationship with the caregiver or parent, and medical issues.[230] For younger adolescents, ask the child and the caregiver their preferences. Respectfully allow all adolescents to have control and input into the examination and treatment process. Reassurance and nonjudgmental interaction between the adolescent and health care provider are crucial not only to the development of the youth's social identity but also to the youth's long-term perception of the importance and value of health care.

Overview of the Adolescent Examination Model

PTs working with the adolescent population should strongly, and appropriately, emphasize examination of the developing neuromusculoskeletal system.[202,205,228,242] Sullivan and Markos' Evaluation Model (1995) reminds the PT to go beyond the

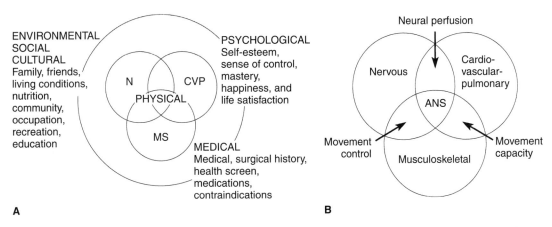

FIGURE 12-2 A and **B,** Evaluation model categorizing interaction of many factors that affect physical capability. (From Sullivan PE, Markos PD: *Clinical decision making in therapeutic exercise,* Stanford, CT, 1995, Appleton and Lange, pp 2, 4.)

physical systems and examine the other factors (e.g. medical, environmental, social, cultural, and psychological variables) that affect a patient's overall physical capabilities (Fig. 12-2, *A*).[228]

The central interlocking rings (see Fig.12-2, *B*) of Sullivan and Markos' evaluation model depict the areas most affected by the practice of physical therapy (physical systems). These three rings represent three of the four preferred practice patterns (PPP) of physical therapy: (1) musculoskeletal [MS], (2) nervous (i.e., neuromuscular) (N), and (3) cardiovascular-pulmonary (CVP) systems. The fourth PPP (integumentary system) (I) could be symbolized by simply encircling the physical systems with a "layer of skin." The development of these four systems and key adolescent issues were previously discussed.

The overlap of the musculoskeletal and nervous systems denotes the *control of movement.* PTs routinely measure areas related to the control of movement, and work to restore, maintain, or promote not only optimal physical function, but also optimal wellness, fitness, and quality of life as it relates to movement.[205] All health care practitioners should recognize that the anthropometric changes of puberty can alter neuromuscular control and predispose the adolescent to musculoskeletal injury.

The intersection of the cardiovascular-pulmonary and musculoskeletal systems designates the patient's *capacity for movement.* A patient's capacity for movement largely depends on bioenergetics. Bioenergetics, or the flow of energy in a biological system, is concerned primarily with the conversion of food—large carbohydrates, protein, and fat molecules—into biologically useful forms of energy.[20] Bioenergetics requires proper nutrition and healthy functioning of several large body systems: (1) gastrointestinal tract (including enzymes of digestion and absorption), (2) endocrine system (hormones of metabolism), (3) circulatory and respiratory systems (energy-delivery system), (4) musculoskeletal system (the conversion of chemical energy into mechanical energy), and (5) excretory

system (management of waste products by sweat mechanisms and kidneys).

The overlap of the nervous and cardiovascular/pulmonary systems is known as *neural perfusion.* An uninterrupted vascular supply to the nervous system (including the central nervous system [CNS], peripheral nervous system [PNS] and autonomic nervous system [ANS]) is required for normal sensory function and the planning and execution of all motor and autonomic functions.

Table 12-8 summarizes key adolescent health care issues by individual body systems. This table highlights signs and symptoms (S/S) of key adolescent diseases and outlines tests and measures per the *Guide to Physical Therapist Practice.*[205]

Medical and Psychological Factors

"To treat, or not to treat, that is the question."
                                   Shakespeare, modified

As with all patients, the initial clinical decision in the patient-management process is to determine whether the adolescent: (1) can be safely treated by the PT, (2) can be managed by a PT in consultation with another health care practitioner, or (3) needs medical referral.

Because adolescence is a time of unique physical, emotional, and social development, identifying risks to the patient's health (see Chapter 5), investigating presenting symptoms (see Chapter 6), and thoroughly reviewing body systems (see Chapter 7) require a different thought process compared with other age groups. The PT must know the common adolescent health conditions (e.g., respiratory conditions or cancers), relevant teenage lifestyle factors (e.g., illicit drug or alcohol abuse, unsafe sexual practices, or drunk driving), and causes of injury and death (e.g., accidents specific to adolescents).

Age, gender, race, ethnicity, and socioeconomic status all play important roles in the development of disease. In the

TABLE 12-8

Adolescent Health Care Issues by Body System

Circulatory system

Per the *Guide to Physical Therapist Practice*, measures of circulation include arterial, venous, and lymphatic circulation and aerobic capacity.

Examination of the adolescent's circulatory system mirrors the adult physical examination.

Examination items include:
Heart rate
Heart rhythm
Heart sounds
Blood pressure
Peripheral circulation including skin color, skin texture, skin temperature, hair growth, nails, and distal pulses
Peripheral edema
Response of the body to positional changes, movement, and exercise

There are currently eight preferred practice patterns (PPPs) specific to the CVP system in the *Guide to Physical Therapist Practice*, ed 2.

This age group is not typically at risk for acquired diseases of the circulatory system (arteriosclerosis, arrhythmias, CAD, and PVD). Children, adolescents, and young adults often have an innocent systolic murmur, often called a *flow murmur*, that is thought to reflect pulmonary blood flow.[31] Murmurs should be monitored by the adolescent's primary care physician (pediatrician), particularly as part of preparticipation sports physicals.

HR norms (see Table 12-6)
Red flags in adolescents:
Bradycardia in a thin adolescent may be due to anorexia nervosa.
HR > 180-200 beats/minute indicates supraventricular tachycardia.
Bradycardia or tachycardia in a noncooperative patient could be a sign of drug overdose.
Blood pressure (see Table 12-6)
Using average (readings on at least three separate occasions) systolic and/or diastolic pressure for age, sex, and height, adolescent blood pressure is defined as follows:

Normal	<90th percentile
High-normal	90th-95th percentile
High	≥95th percentile

For more details on adolescent BP, see: Update on the 1987 task force report on high blood pressure in children and adolescents: a working group report from the National High Blood Pressure Education Program, *Pediatrics* 98:649, 1996.

Cholesterol screening: Everyone age 20 and older should have his or her blood cholesterol measured at least once every 5 years. Screening is recommended for persons under 20 years of age if one parent presents with high blood cholesterol or a parent or grandparent has premature cardiovascular disease (before age 50). The presence of other risk factors, such as diabetes, smoking, high blood pressure, obesity/overweight, a family history of early heart disease, and birth control medication (for females), is an indication to monitor cholesterol levels.

LDL cholesterol	<100 mg/dL
Total cholesterol	<200 mg/dL
HDL cholesterol	<40 is low; ≥60 is high

Endocrine system

Per the *Guide to Physical Therapist Practice*, measures of endocrine system include specific questioning in the subjective interview.

Examination items include:
Objective tests of the endocrine system are disease specific.

The functions of the body are regulated by the endocrine and nervous systems.
Important glands and hormones of the endocrine system include:
Adrenal cortex (cortisol and aldosterone)
Anterior pituitary (growth hormone, adrenocorticotropin, thyroid-stimulating hormone, follicle-stimulating hormone, luteinizing hormone, and prolactin)
Islets of Langerhans of the pancreas (insulin and glucagon)
Ovaries (estrogen and progesterone)
Parathyroid (parathyroid hormone)
Placenta (human chorionic gonadotropin, estrogens, progesterone, and human somatomammotropin)
Posterior pituitary (vasopressin and oxytocin)
Testes (testosterone)
Thyroid (thyroxine, triiodothyronine and calcitonin)

Puberty brings extensive physical changes via the endocrine system. Health care providers should monitor adolescents for normal progression through the Tanner Stages of Sexual Development (see Puberty discussion).

Most common adolescent diseases specific to the endocrine system:
Cystic fibrosis
Diabetes (thirst or polydypsia, nocturia)
Precocious puberty
Thyroid (adenoma, cancer hypofunction or hyperfunction)

Gastrointestinal system

Per the *Guide to Physical Therapist Practice*, measures of GI system include specific questioning in the subjective interview.

Gastrointestinal signs and symptoms (S/S): Abdominal pain, achalasia, appetite changes, bowel movements (change in control, color, size, and bowel habits), constipation, disordered eating habits, diarrhea, dysphagia, excessive belching, excessive flatulence, food intolerance, GI bleeding (hematemesis, hematochezia, and melena), heartburn, hemorrhoids, jaundice, and nausea or vomiting.[31,104]

Review of systems questioning specific to GI system (see Chapter 7).

TABLE 12-8

Adolescent Health Care Issues by Body System—cont'd

Examination items include: Objective tests of the GI system are disease specific but may include height, weight (anthropometrics), inspection, palpation, auscultation, and percussion of organs.

Most common adolescent diseases specific to the GI system:
Crohn's disease
Disordered eating patterns (anorexia nervosa, bulimia)
Gastric ulcer
Inflammatory bowel disease (IBD)
Obesity
Peptic ulcer disease
Ulcerative colitis

Integumentary system

Inspection and palpation of the integumentary system gives the evaluating therapist insight into the overall health of the adolescent. Examination of the adolescent's skin mirrors the adult physical examination.

Skin lesions can result from a wide variety of etiologic factors.[104] Causes of skin lesions include: physical trauma; contact with injurious agents (e.g., chemical toxins) and infective organisms; reaction to medication, allergens, or radiotherapy; systemic origin (e.g., diseases with cutaneous manifestations; arterial insufficiency); hereditary factors, burns (thermal, electrical, chemical, inhalation); and neoplasm. Signs and symptoms of skin injury or disease include bleeding, pruritus (itching), urticaria (hives), rash, blisters, xeroderma (dryness).[104]

Areas of specific interest for the integumentary system of the adolescent:
Acne is a key disorder of this age group as sebaceous glands become more active with endocrine changes (see Puberty discussion).

Five PPPs currently are dedicated to the integumentary system in the *Guide to Physical Therapist Practice*, ed 2.

Thermoregulation changes as the child enters and advances through puberty (see Puberty discussion).

Burn injuries, especially to the face, have a profound effect on self-esteem and self-identity. Given adolescents' stage of psychosocial development, burns can be psychologically taxing to the adolescent.

Wound healing: Delayed wound healing can be a sign of local or systemic disease or even mental illness. Suspicion of self-mutilation (self-injury) should be a red flag for psychological disorder.

Chronic regional pain syndromes (reflex sympathetic dystrophy)

Musculoskeletal system (MS)

Per the *Guide to Physical Therapist Practice*, measures of MS system include muscle performance (strength, power, and endurance), joint integrity and mobility, ROM (including muscle length), and functional tasks like gait and body mechanics.

Musculoskeletal S/S: Loss of AROM or PROM, weakness, or myofascial pain symptoms (lower-back pain, neck pain) and joint pain are common MS symptoms. Joint pain is a common symptom in persons seeking health care. Joint pain with systemic symptoms (fever, chills, rash, anorexia, weight loss, or weakness) or other organ symptoms should be referred for medical evaluation.

Adolescence is a time marked by skeletal growth, increased muscle mass, and sexual development and maturation. It is not unusual to hear a child complain of growing pains and to require increased sleep. Growth and development produce changes in posture, flexibility, strength, and motor control (neuromuscular coordination).

Examination of the adolescent's MS system mirrors the adult physical examination, with special attention to growth factors.

For detail, please refer to the chapter sections entitled Puberty and the Musculoskeletal System, and Musculoskeletal Disorders of Adolescence.

There are currently 10 PPPs specific to the MS system in the *Guide to Physical Therapist Practice*, ed 2.

Nervous system

Per the *Guide to Physical Therapist Practice*, measures of neuromuscular system include: arousal, attention, cognition, cranial-nerve and peripheral-nerve integrity, motor function, neuromotor development and sensory integration, pain, reflex integrity, and sensory integrity.

Nervous system S/S: changes in mood, attention, or speech; changes in orientation, memory, insight or judgment; headache, dizziness, or vertigo; generalized proximal or distal weakness, numbness, abnormal sensation, or loss of sensation; abnormal muscle tone; loss of consciousness; syncope or near-syncope; seizures or tremors.

Lower motor neuron (LMN) lesion:
Ipsilateral flaccid paralysis
Reduced tone and deep tendon reflexes; muscle atrophy
Sensory disturbances and fasciculation

Upper motor neuron (UMN) lesion:
Spastic paralysis
Increased tone, hyperreflexia, and minimal muscle atrophy
Possible sensory disturbances

Continued

TABLE 12-8

Adolescent Health Care Issues by Body System—cont'd

Examination of the adolescent's nervous system mirrors the adult physical examination.

Examination items include:
CNS, PNS, and ANS
Mental status
Appearance/behavior
Cognitive functions
Mood
Speech and language
Thought and perception

There are currently nine PPPs specific to the neuromuscular system in the *Guide to Physical Therapist Practice*, ed 2.

Cranial Nerve Functions: refer to Chapter 7 screening

Autonomic nervous system considerations:
The ANS regulates the viscera, overall metabolism, secretions, body temperature, reproduction, and blood flow in the viscera, muscle, and periphery. Many chronic-pain syndromes (e.g., complex regional pain syndrome [CRPS], fibromyalgia, myofascial trigger points) and mental conditions (e.g., depression, anxiety, attention deficit hyperactivity disorder) can be intensified by the influences of the sympathetic nervous system. The treatment approach for these conditions should be multidisciplinary, including patient education; physical, occupational, and behavioral therapy; and pharmacologic treatment with antiepileptic, psychiatric, and/or analgesic drugs.[71]

For details, please refer to the chapter section entitled Puberty and the Nervous System.

Psychological system (an extension of the nervous system)

Mental disorders seen in children and adolescents (and adults).

The World Health Organization (WHO) predicts that by the year 2020, childhood neuropsychiatric disorders will rise by over 50% internationally to become one of the five most common causes of morbidity, mortality, and disability among the world's youth.

Mental health screening:
In addition to screening for nervous-system function, the PT must screen adolescents for behavior changes caused by mental illness, substance abuse (drugs or alcohol), and suicidal tendencies. Up to a third of all primary care visits involve mental health, including depressed mood, anxiety, somatic concerns, and more serious disorders of mood and mental function.[31,33]

Risk factors for suicide include: psychiatric illness, substance abuse, personality disorder, previous suicide attempt or family history of suicide, and gender-identity crisis or persecution.

Most common neuropsychiatric disorders seen in adolescents:
Anxiety disorders (generalized anxiety disorder [GAD]; obsessive-compulsive disorder [OCD]; panic disorder; posttraumatic stress disorder [PTSD]; phobias, including specific and/or social phobia; separation anxiety; selective autism)
Attention deficit hyperactivity disorder (ADHD)
Autism and other pervasive developmental disorders
Depressive disorders
Disruptive behavior disorders
Eating disorders (anorexia nervosa, bulimia nervosa, and binge-eating disorder; 35% of those affected are male)
Learning disabilities
Manic/bipolar disorder
Mood disorders
Schizophrenia
Tics and Tourette's syndrome

Current estimates are that 1 in 10 American children and adolescents suffers from mental illness severe enough to impair daily functioning. The National Institute on Mental Health estimates that only 1 in 5 of these youth receives needed treatment.[182]

Respiratory system (thorax and lungs)

Per the *Guide to Physical Therapist Practice*, measures specific to the respiratory system include aerobic capacity, ventilation and respiratory/gas exchange, joint integrity, and mobility specific to the thorax.

Examination of the adolescent's respiratory system mirrors the adult physical examination.

Respiratory S/S: Chest pain or discomfort, cough, dyspnea, hemoptysis, sputum (color, quantity), and wheezing could be signs and symptoms of asthma, bronchitis, emphysema, pneumonia, and tuberculosis.
This age group is not typically at risk for chronic pulmonary diseases. Smoking in adolescence is a risk factor for future pulmonary and cardiovascular disease.

Examination of this system mirrors the adult physical examination:

Age	Normal respiratory rate of adolescents
10 years	20 to 26
12 years	18 to 22
14 years	18 to 22
16 years	16 to 20
>18 years	12 to 20

Common adolescent concerns specific to the respiratory system:
Asthma: 66.2 per 1000 persons under age 18 have asthma.

CHAPTER 12 **The Adolescent Population** **193**

TABLE 12-8

Adolescent Health Care Issues by Body System—cont'd

Examination items include: Thorax contour Respiratory rate Respiratory rhythm Breathing pattern Rib cage expansion Joint mobility (T-spine and rib cage) Percussion auscultation (breath sounds) Aerobic capacity	Asthma is a complex disorder involving biochemical, autonomic, immunologic, infectious, endocrine, and psychological factors. Asthma is a long-term, often progressive, disease in which swelling of the lining of the airways and narrowing of the passageways make breathing difficult. It has been described as "arthritis of the airways." *Cystic fibrosis*: Cystic fibrosis (CF), the most common life-shortening genetic disease in the white population, occurs in the United States in about 1 of 3300 white births, 1 of 15,300 black births, and 1 of 32,000 Asian-American births. CF is an autosomal recessive disease of the exocrine glands, affecting primarily the GI and respiratory systems, and usually characterized by COPD, exocrine pancreatic insufficiency (secondary to blockage), and abnormally high sweat electrolytes. The median survival is to age 31 years.
Reproductive system (genital system) The reproductive system undergoes significant changes during adolescence (puberty). Knowledge of normal sexual maturation (Tanner stages) is pertinent to recognizing delayed development or precocious puberty (see Puberty discussion).	Females: age of menarche; menstrual regularity, frequency, duration, and amount of bleeding; dysmenorrhea; amenorrhea; sexual habits; bleeding with or after intercourse; vaginal discharge; sores; itching; and exposure to sexually transmitted diseases (STDs) are all part of the reproductive-system health history and examination. Males: hernias, discharges from the penis or sores on the penis, testicular pain or masses, sexual habits, and exposure to STDs are all part of the genital-system health history and examination. Although this system generally is not the domain of the PT, function of sacral nerve roots (S2-S4) is part of the lower quarter screening examination. *Common adolescent concerns specific to the reproductive system*: Sexual habits, preference, interest, and function, sexual satisfaction, birth control methods, condom use, and unprotected sex. Is the adolescent at risk of STDs, pregnancy, or being victimized? Issues of confidentiality and privacy laws.
Urinary system Examination of the adolescent's urinary system mirrors the adult physical examination. Examination items include: Subjective questions regarding urinary function (e.g., output, control, color) Inspection of external organs (as needed) Palpation of the abdomen Percussion of the kidneys	Urinary and renal S/S: color changes (clear, concentrated yellow, reddish, or brown); dysuria (urgency, frequency, or hesitancy and/or reduced stream); glucouria; hematuria; kidney, flank, or groin pain; nocturia; polyuria; stress incontinence; suprapubic pain or ureteral colic. The urogenital system is located primarily within the midline of the abdomen. It has extensive connections to the endocrine system in regard to regulation of overall function. The urinary system consists of the kidneys, ureters, bladder, and urethra. Common adolescent concerns specific to the urinary system: Screening for alcohol or drug abuse Chronic urinary tract infections (UTIs) or bladder infections could be a sign of unsafe sexual practices, putting the adolescent at greater risk for sexually transmitted diseases. Untreated pelvic inflammatory disease (PID) can have serious ramifications, including female (>male) sterility, tubal pregnancies, and congenital infant conditions (e.g., prematurity, eye disease, and pneumonia) and systemic illness (see STD discussion).

United States, the leading causes of death vary across the lifespan (Fig. 12-3). Heart disease and stroke, cancer, and chronic obstructive pulmonary disease are the leading causes of death in all Americans, while unintentional injuries are the leading cause of death among young people ages 1 to 19 (41% of all deaths).[91,197] Behavioral and lifestyle factors such as diet, exercise, smoking, and substance abuse cause more than half of all deaths in the United States.[104]

These statistics underscore the importance of environmental factors in the rates of death and disease in pediatric patients. Asking teenagers questions about their environmental and personal safety habits is statistically more important than looking for the signs and symptoms of CAD or cancer. From the perspective of overall management, education in health promotion and prevention should be the *primary focus* of the adolescent-intervention process (see the discussion of Health Promotion and *Healthy People 2010*).

Medical and Psychosocial Risks of Chronic Health Conditions in Adolescence

Screening for chronic illnesses and diseases, and their impairments, functional limitations, and potential disability is a component of any medical interaction. As a group, adolescents present with different chronic illnesses compared with other age groups. The National Center for Health Statistics (www.cdc.gov/nchs/) regularly compiles data on select chronic conditions per 1000 persons, by age, sex, race, and income.[4]

Observers currently estimate that 10 to 20 million U.S. children and adolescents (16.6% to 33% of all U.S. children and adolescents) have some type of chronic health condition. At least one in five children has a chronic condition severe enough to affect his or her daily life. This effect may result from persistent symptoms, required treatments, limitations of activity or mobility, or interference with school, recreation, work, and

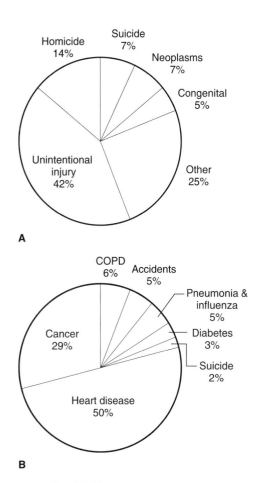

A

B

FIGURE 12-3 A and **B,** Mortality rates: the major causes of death for all Americans vs. persons younger than 20 years of age. (**A** from Friedrich MJ: Report documents causes of child death. Health and the American child, part 1: a focus on mortality among children: risks, trends, and priorities for the 21st century, Public Health Policy Advisory Board (PHPAB), *JAMA* 282:1903-1905, 1999. **B** from Goodman CC, Boissonnault WG, Fuller KS: *Pathology: implications for the physical therapist,* ed 2, Philadelphia, 2003, WB Saunders.)

family activities.[11] These conditions often require extended medical attention across multiple domains of health care practice (e.g., inpatient or outpatient therapies, school-based therapy, home-health).[225] Overall, children with special health needs account for four fifths of all children's health costs.[74]

An estimated 5 million children in the United States now suffer with asthma (66.2 per 1000 persons compared with 55.2 per 1000 among all other age groups). Asthma is the most common chronic illness in children of color (e.g., African-American, Hispanic) in the United States, with Latino children the most afflicted. The incidence of other chronic allergic diseases is: chronic bronchitis, 57.3 per 1000: hay fever and allergic rhinitis without asthma, 58.7 per 1000; chronic sinusitis, 63.9 per 1000; and chronic disease of tonsils and adenoids, 20.2 per 1000. In 1995, children with asthma alone missed an estimated 10 million days of school and were hospitalized 170,000 times, costing the U.S. health care system $387 million.[74]

The number of children in the United States with insulin-dependent diabetes and cardiovascular disease (or CAD) is growing as obesity and physical inactivity grow as societal health care problems.[34,74,123,200] Children with diabetes are

three times more likely to be hospitalized as their classmates.[74] Diabetes and CAD carry many long-term systemic ramifications (e.g., neuropathy, retinopathy, increased risk of amputation and disability) that will affect the quality of life of these young Americans as they age as well as increase society's overall economic and health care burdens.

These conditions (asthma, diabetes, and CAD) are but a few of the chronic conditions (see Table 12-3) found in children and adolescents in the United States. Recent medical and surgical advances have markedly reduced the mortality rates of children and adolescents with chronic conditions. Given this change in survival, outpatient PTs likely will provide health care to the adolescent who has a specific musculoskeletal condition and a co-morbid chronic illness. Physical therapy interventions should maximize the adolescent's functional abilities and sense of well being, improve overall health-related quality of life, and improve development into healthy and productive adults.

Screening for Childhood Cancer

Each year in the United States, about 12,400 persons under 20 years of age are diagnosed with cancer. Almost 2,300 (18.5%) of these juveniles die from their illness, making cancer a leading cause of disease-related mortality for children 1 to 19 years of age.[104,144,197] Fortunately, over the past 2 decades, advances in diagnosis and treatment have dramatically improved the survival of pediatric cancer. Now almost 65% of all children younger than 20 years of age survive 5 years or more, an increase of almost 40% since the early 1960s.[104,197] Furthermore, because of the variation in cancers common to adolescents (15 to 19 years), the overall 5-year survival rate for this age group has improved to 77%.[197]

The leading risk factors for cancer are advancing age, lifestyle and personal behaviors (e.g., smoking, poor diet or nutrition, excessive alcohol use, and high-risk sexual habits), exposure to viruses, geographic location, environmental variables, gender, ethnicity, socioeconomic status, occupation, heredity, presence of precancerous lesions, and stress. Given that adolescents are young patients (12-20 years), most of their cancers are the result of genetic or heredity factors. A compendium of statistical trends and risk factors associated with childhood cancers is available from the United States SEER (Surveillance, Epidemiology and End Results) Program, 1975-1995[197] and the American Cancer Society.[144]

Cancers vary across the lifespan by histology, site of disease origin, race, and gender. In 1995, the International Cancer Institute classified childhood cancers into four distinct 5-year age groups (Table 12-9). The incidence of cancer per million is highest in adolescents age 15-19 years (202.2 per million), followed by the under-5-years age group (199.9 per million), the 10- to 14–year age group (117.3 per million), and finally children 5 to 9 years of age (110.2 per million).[197]

The adenocarcinomas (e.g., lung, breast, prostate, and colorectal cancers) common in adults are rarely seen in children.[104] The embryonal cancers that predominate among young children less than 5 years of age (e.g., neuroblastoma, Wilms' tumor, retinoblastoma, and hepatoblastoma) are distinctly uncommon among 10-to-19–year olds. Children

TABLE 12-9

Age-specific Cancer Incidence Rates per Million and Percentage of Total Cases by International Classification of Childhood Cancer (ICCC) Category and Age Group, All Races, Both Sexes, SEER 1986-1995, Table XIII.1

Tumor category	Age (in years) at Diagnosis				
	<5 Rate	5-9 Rate	10-14 Rate	15-19 Rate	% of Total Cancers Affecting 15-19 Group
All sites	199.9	110.2	117.3	202.2	100.0%
Acute lymphoblastic leukemia (ALL)	58.2	30.3	17.8	12.9	6.4%
Acute myeloid leukemia (AML) (Ib)	10.1	4.5	5.7	8.5	4.2%
Hodgkin's disease (IIa)	0.8	3.9	11.7	32.5	16.1%
Non-Hodgkin's lymphoma (NHL) (IIb, c, e)	5.9	8.9	10.3	15.3	7.6%
CNS tumors (III [total])	36.0	31.9	24.6	20.2	10.0%
Ependymoma (IIIa)	5.6	1.6	1.3	1.1	0.5%
Astrocytoma (IIIb)	15.0	15.9	15.1	12.3	6.1%
Medulloblastoma/PNET (IIIc)	9.6	7.3	4.0	2.5	1.2%
Neuroblastoma and ganglioneuroblastoma (IVa)	27.4	2.6	0.8	0.5	0.2%
Retinoblastoma (V [total])	12.5	0.5	0.0	0.1	0.0%
Wilms', rhabdoid, clear cell sarcoma (VIa)	18.0	5.8	0.6	0.4	0.2%
Hepatic tumors (VII [total])	4.8	0.4	0.4	1.0	0.5%
Hepatoblastoma (VIIa)	4.6	0.2	0.1	0.0	0.0%
Osteosarcoma (VIIIa)	0.3	2.8	8.3	9.4	4.6%
Ewing's sarcoma (VIIIc)	0.3	1.9	4.1	4.6	2.3%
Soft-tissue sarcoma (IX [total])	10.9	8.3	10.9	15.9	7.9%
Rhabdomyosarcoma and embryonal sarcoma (IXa)	6.5	4.4	3.5	3.9	1.9%
Non-rhabdo soft-tissue sarcoma (IXb-e)	4.4	4.0	7.4	11.9	5.9%
Germ cell, trophoblastic, and other gonadal tumors (X [total])	6.9	2.4	6.7	30.8	15.2%
Thyroid carcinoma (XIb)	0.1	1.0	4.1	14.6	7.2%
Malignant melanoma (XId)	0.8	0.6	2.8	14.1	7.0%
Other and unspecified carcinomas (XIf)	0.4	0.8	2.8	10.5	5.2%

From Age-specific cancer incidence rates per million and percentage of total cases by International Classification of Childhood Cancer (ICCC) category and age group, all races, both sexes, SEER 1986-1995, Table XIII.1

younger than 14 years of age also are more likely to contract acute lymphoblastic leukemia (ALL) and CNS tumors, the more deadly of the childhood cancers. The top seven adolescent (15 to 19 years) cancers, their prevalence, and key diagnostic and prognostic factors are discussed in Table 12-10.

Rates of specific cancers vary not only by age, but also by gender and race. Adolescent females are more prone to Hodgkin's disease (36.5 female to 28.8 male cases per million; F/M ratio 1.3:1), thyroid cancer (26.2 female to 3.7 male cases per million; F/M ratio 7:1), and melanoma (17.9 female to 10.5 male cases per million; F/M ratio 1.7:1). Males are more susceptible to acute lymphoblastic leukemia (17.5 male to 8.0 female cases per million; M/F ratio 2.2:1), non-Hodgkin's lymphoma (19.4 male to 11.0 female cases per million; M/F ratio 1.8:1), CNS cancer (23.0 male to 17.3 female cases per million; M/F ratio 1.3:1), bone cancer (17.3 male to 10.4 female cases per million; M/F ratio 1.7:1), and soft tissue tumors (17.4 male to 14.3 female cases per million; M/F ratio 1.3:1).

Black adolescents age 15 to 19 years have an overall lower incidence of childhood cancers than whites (W/B ratio of 1.5 to 1). Soft tissue sarcoma is the only cancer more common in blacks than whites (20.5 black cases to 14.5 white cases per million; B/W ratio 1.4:1). Adolescent whites, age 0 to 14 years, have a substantially higher rate of leukemia than their black counterparts (45.6 white cases per million versus 27.8 black cases per million; W/B ratio 1.64:1). Likewise, whites have a much higher incidence of Ewing's sarcoma (W/B ratio 18:1), testicular germ cell tumors (W/B ratio 2.5:1), and melanoma (W/B ratio 53.7:1); and a moderately higher incidence of acute lymphoblastic leukemia (W/B ratio 2.2:1) and thyroid cancers (W/B ratio 2.3:1).[197]

Observers currently estimate that 1 in 1000 people between the ages of 20 and 29 is a survivor of childhood or adolescent cancer. The exact late effects of these diseases and their treatments (surgery, radiation, and chemotherapy) on non-malignant tissues as well as the social, emotional, and economic consequences are not yet known. Late effects have been identified in almost every organ system, and children and adolescents who have received chemotherapy have a tenfold greater chance of developing a second malignancy compared with a child who has never had cancer.[104,197] Patient and family education and support are crucial to the long-term physical and emotional recovery from childhood and adolescent cancer. The Cancer Information Service (http://cis.nih.gov) is the National Cancer Institute's link to the public, offering current scientific information in understandable language for health care professionals, the general public, patients, and their families.[197]

Screening for Infection in Adolescents

Clinical manifestations and prognoses for infectious diseases are many and vary with the etiological agent (e.g., virus, bacteria, fungus, tuberculosis, or parasite) and the body system affected. Systemic symptoms of infectious disease include fever, chills,

---

TABLE 12-10

Common Adolescent Cancers: Prevalence and Key Diagnostic and Prognostic Factors for Teenagers

Neoplastic Disease Source	Diagnostic and Prognostic Factors
Hodgkin's disease: cancer of lymphoid tissue	Ann Arbor Staging System: 70% to 80% of persons are diagnosed in stage II or III.
	I Involvement of one lymph node or a single lymphoid structure
Represents 16.1% of all adolescent cancers	II Involvement of two or more lymph nodes on the same side of the diaphragm
	III Involvement of lymph nodes on two sides of the diaphragm
	IV Diffuse extralymphatic disease
	Absence or presence of fever (more than 38° C or 102° F), night sweats, or weight loss (more than 10% of body weight in the last 6 months).
Germ cell, trophoblastic, and gonadal tumors	Linked to hormonal changes of puberty; representing 15.2% of adolescent tumors
	White males > black males (testicular)
Represents 15.2% of all adolescent cancers	Black females > white females (ovarian)
Central Nervous System Tumors	The number-two cancer-related killer of children under the age of 20.
Medulloblastoma: ages 0-9 years	Presentation depends on the topographic distribution of the tumor (check for CN I-XII
Astrocytoma: ages 10-14 years	competency, coordination, mental-status changes, neurologic changes).
Pilocytic astrocytoma: ages 15-19 years	Temporally dependent headache occurs in 33% of cases (worse in morning and better later in the day).
Represents 10% of all adolescent cancers but is the most common solid tumor of childhood (0-14 years) and second-most-common malignancy of childhood.	Headaches are intensified by activities that increase intracranial pressure (e.g., stooping, Valsalva maneuver, and exertion/exercise).
	From 20% to 50% of adults develop seizures (first presenting sign).
Rhabdomyosarcoma: soft tissue carcinoma (same embryonic tissues that form striated muscle)	Males > females
	Blacks > whites, especially in the 15-19 age category
	Common sites: head and neck, genitourinary tract, and extremities
	Head and neck tumors can lead to CNS involvement, and 90% of these children die.
Represents 7.9% of all adolescent cancers	Correlation with growth spurts (#1 peak = 2 to 5 years, and #2 peak = 15 to 19 years).
	Congenital anomalies and genetic conditions are risk factors for soft tissue sarcomas.
Non-Hodgkin's lymphomas: solid tumors arising from the cells of the lymphatic system	Represents 15% of *all* childhood malignancies (Burkitt's and lymphoblastic lymphoma).
	May be associated with autoimmune disease, infection, and immunologic defects.
Represents 7.6% of all adolescent cancers	A wide variety of immunodeficiencies, including collagen vascular diseases, juvenile rheumatoid arthritis (JRA), and AIDS, have been associated with lymphomas.
Carcinomas and other malignant epithelial neoplasms: cancer of the thyroid, melanomas, adenocarcinomas, nasopharyngeal carcinomas, and other skin carcinomas	These carcinomas are very rare (<1%) *before* adolescence.
	Thyroid cancer: females > males
	Malignant melanoma is a disease on the rise in America. Among those 15-19 years, females > males; whites significantly > blacks.
	Risk factors include sun exposure and preexisting melanocytic and dysplastic nevi.
Thyroid cancer represents 7.2% of all adolescent cancers, while malignant melanoma is 7.0%.	Environmental damage to the ozone and sunburn at a young age are known contributors to the increase in skin carcinomas.
Leukemia: cancer of the blood forming cells	Number-one cancer-related killer of children under the age of 20.
ALL: acute lymphoblastic leukemia*	Manifestations: fever, bleeding, anemia, malaise, lymphadenopathy, bone pain, headaches, and increased susceptibility to infection (oral-pharynx, pulmonary, and gastrointestinal)
ANLL: acute nonlymphocytic leukemia	With aggressive treatment (chemotherapy and bone-marrow transplantation), about 60% of children will survive. If left untreated, all leukemias are fatal.
CML: chronic myelocytic leukemia	
CLL: chronic lymphocytic leukemia	White males are most affected.
ALL represents 6.4% of adolescent cancers but is the most common and deadly childhood leukemia.	

---

sweating, malaise, and nausea and vomiting (see Infection in Chapter 6). If the infection is specific to the central nervous system (CNS), symptoms also may include focal headache, nausea, vomiting, stiff neck and back; focal neurologic signs including hemiparesis, aphasia, ataxia, disorders of the limbs, and seizures; temporal-lobe disturbances such as memory loss and hallucinations; and a positive Kernig's or Brudzinski's sign (meningeal inflammation). Because the brain (and its network of cerebrospinal fluid) lacks an immune system to fight infection, it is highly susceptible to damage from infection.

In the United States, about 2600 people a year are infected by bacterial meningitis. About 10% to 15% die, and another 10% have long-term complications (e.g., deafness, seizures, retardation,

loss of limb use).[104] Fever, headache, and a stiff and painful neck are hallmark symptoms of meningitis. A lumbar puncture with bacterial culture is the only absolute means of diagnosing meningitis. Radiographs should be taken to rule out fracture, sinusitis, and mastoiditis, while computed tomography (CT) scan will reveal evidence of brain abscess or infarction.[104]

Encephalitis is an acute inflammatory disease of the brain caused by direct viral invasion. The herpes simplex virus (most often) and mosquito-borne or tick-borne virus are the most common infectious agents. Signs and symptoms of viral encephalitis are similar to bacterial CNS infection, but a lumbar puncture will be negative. Brain electroencephalogram (EEG) is always abnormal. Vascular studies and CT scan or magnetic resonance imaging will display cerebral edema and vascular damage. Brain biopsy is necessary to diagnose the herpes simplex virus.

With the exception of acyclovir (Zovirax), an antiviral medication for the treatment of a herpes simplex virus, treatment is targeted to prevent complication of cerebral edema and includes surgical decompression, hyperventilation, and mannitol (diuretic). The use of corticosteroids is controversial because of possible suppression of antibody protection within the CNS. Herpes simplex encephalitis has a 20% mortality rate and a 50% rate of neurologic sequelae.[104]

Brain abscess (local infection of the brain) is more likely with bacterial, fungal, or parasitic infections. A patient developing a brain abscess will present with fever, chills, headache, and focal neurologic signs that progress with time. These signs and symptoms, along with a recent history of infection or immunosuppression, lead to suspicion of brain abscess or neoplasm. A CT scan and MRI are required to differentiate a tumor from an abscess. Treatment of abscess can include antibiotics specific to the infectious agent, corticosteroids to control cerebral edema, and surgical drainage to reduce mass effect. Almost half of all persons with brain abscess are left with neurologic sequelae (e.g., focal signs, seizure activity).[104]

Although infections of the CNS are rare because of the protection of the blood-brain barrier, they have been seen in the adolescent population. Given the nature of their activities and environment (e.g., frequent exposure to large numbers of people through living in dormitories, by attending school activities and concerts), adolescents are more susceptible to CNS infections than other age groups. Many observers advocate vaccination of adolescents against meningococcal disease, particularly those living in dormitories (see Immunization discussion in Health Promotion section).[2,11,216]

Along with screening for systemic infection, health care professionals must monitor for signs and symptoms of local infection or injury. The four cardinal signs of local infection or inflammation include pain (dolor), erythema (rubor), heat (calor), and swelling (tumor). A fifth cardinal sign of inflammation, loss of function, should always be thoroughly appraised by the health care practitioner.[46]

Given the growth potential of pediatric patients, infections of synovial joints can be particularly harmful to long-term function. There are four types of infectious arthritis: (1) bacterial arthritis (e.g., gonococcal, infectious endocarditis, Lyme disease, septic arthritis, syphilis, tuberculosis; (2) fungal arthritis (e.g., *Candida*); (3) viral arthritis (e.g., Epstein-Barr virus [EBV], hepatitis, human immunodeficiency virus [HIV], mumps, and rubella; and (4) reactive arthritis (e.g., acute rheumatic fever, chlamydial infections, enteric infections, and Reiter's syndrome).[104] Lyme disease has been heralded as the fastest-growing infectious disease in the United States after AIDS.[247]

Adolescents also can develop infections from routine orthopedic surgeries (e.g., arthroscopy or peripheral joint ligamentous reconstruction), from open traumatic injuries (e.g., lacerations, abrasions), and occasionally from closed traumatic injury. Olecranon bursitis and prepatellar bursitis resulting from traumatic injury are the closed-space conditions most likely to develop an abscess.[164] Spinal infections are particularly rare in adolescents, given that most cases of diskitis are associated with postoperative complications of diskectomy (3% postoperative incidence in the 25-to-45 age group).[104]

Children and adolescents who develop an insidious limp or joint irritability with pain on active or passive motion, numbness, or tingling and weakness should be thoroughly examined (Fig. 12-4). Referral for first-order diagnostic imaging (i.e.,

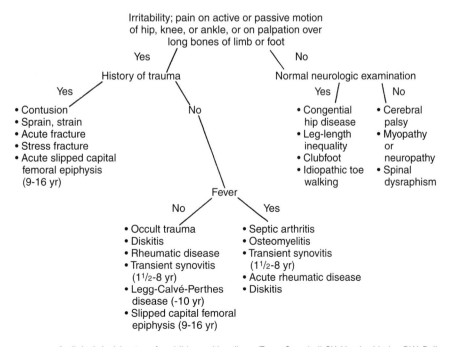

FIGURE 12-4 A clinical decision tree for children with a limp. (From Campbell SK, Vander Linden DW, Palisano RJ, eds: *Physical therapy for children*, ed 2, Philadelphia, 2000, WB Saunders, p 411. Originally from Scoles PA: *Pediatric orthopedics in clinical practice*, ed 2, St Louis, 1988, CV Mosby, p 21.)

radiograph) is *always* indicated for the pediatric patient with pain and loss of function about a joint, even in the absence of macrotrauma or prior surgical intervention.[166]

Screening for Sexually Transmitted Diseases in Adolescents

The PT also must be vigilant for sexually transmitted diseases (STDs), another source of infection in adolescents. STDs are hidden epidemics of enormous health and economic consequence in the United States.[6,55,86,140,241a,253] Currently 65 million Americans are living with an incurable STD, and an additional 15 million contract one or more new cases of STDs each year.[55]

Teens experimenting with sex are at a high risk for acquiring most STDs. Teenagers and young adults are more likely than any other age group to have multiple sex partners, to engage in unprotected sex, and for young women, to engage in sexual acts with persons older than themselves. Moreover, teenage women are biologically more susceptible to chlamydia, gonorrhea, and HIV.[55]

More than 25 diseases are spread primarily through sexual activity. Not including HIV, the most common STDs tracked by the CDC are chlamydia, gonorrhea, syphilis, genital herpes, human papillomavirus (HPV), hepatitis B, trichomoniasis and bacterial vaginosis, and chancroid. The CDC report, *Tracking the Hidden Epidemics: Trends in STDs in the United States (2000)*, gives an excellent analysis of STDs across race, ethnicity, gender, age, and geographic distribution.

Table 12-11 outlines key STDs, causal agents, incidence, and adolescent facts.

Consequences of untreated STDs include pelvic inflammatory disease (PID), sterility (females more than males), systemic illness and death, tubal pregnancies, and congenital conditions among infants (e.g., prematurity, eye disease, and pneumonia).[55] Chlamydia and herpes simplex virus type 2 (genital herpes)[86] increase the risk of contracting HIV. Females infected with chlamydia are three to five times more likely to get HIV. Genital herpes also can make HIV-infected persons more infectious and is believed to play a major role in the heterosexual spread of HIV in the United States.[55]

HIV/AIDS. The United Nations AIDS project estimates that 10 million of the 30 million people living with HIV worldwide are between the ages of 10 and 24 (33%). In the United States, 25% of all new HIV infections (between 27 and 54 per day) are estimated to occur in people under the age of 21.[188,236]

The National Centers for Disease Control and Prevention has reported gender, racial, and ethnic disparity in the prevalence

---

TABLE 12-11

Sexually Transmitted Diseases (STDs), Causal Agents, Incidence, and Effects Among Adolescents[55,86,140]

Sexually Transmitted Disease, Causal Agent	Incidence	Effects among Adolescents
Chlamydia: bacterial agent	The CDC estimates 3 million new cases each year (most common); the 660,000 reported are only the tip of the iceberg	Chlamydia is particularly dangerous to female teens; 40% of untreated females develop PID.
Easily *cured* with antibiotics		1 in 5 women with PID become sterile.
		Females are 3-5 times more likely to get HIV.
	Dangerous because 75% of women and 50% of men have no symptoms.	Infant complications (e.g., prematurity, eye disease, and pneumonia) are common.
Gonorrhea: bacterial agent	Overall rate of infection: 131.4 per 100,000 Female adolescents: 198.3	Only 50% of gonorrhea cases are reported per year.
Easily *cured* with antibiotics	Black: 802.4 to 848.8 Gay/bisexual males: up to 85%	Highest rate in the industrial world; 8 times Canada and 50 times Sweden.
Syphilis: bacterial agent	U.S. rate lowest since 1941: 2.5 per 100,000 Male/female ratio is 1.5 to 1.	Congenital syphilis rates were 14.3 per 100,000 live births in untreated women (1999).
Easily *cured* with antibiotics	Black/white ratio is 30 to 1.	
Herpes simplex virus type 2 (genital herpes)	The CDC reports 1 million new cases each year with1 in 5 Americans (45 million) infected.	Seroprevalence for adolescents (12-19 years): Black teenagers: 8.8%
		Mexican Americans: 5.4%
Noncurable		White teenagers: 4.5%
	Seroprevalence is race-specific and gender-specific.	Herpes can be transmitted between sexual partners and from mothers to newborns, and can increase a person's risk of contracting HIV.
	All races and ethic groups: 20.8%	
	All whites: 16.5%, with white women 18.7% and white men (14.1%)	
	All blacks: 47.6%, with black women 55.7% and black men (37.5%)	Symptoms (i.e., ulcer) are *flare-up* specific, but herpes can be transmitted while persons are with or without symptoms.
Hepatitis B: viral agent	5% of US population is infected: 40% through unsafe heterosexual sex	Adolescents second to 25-39 group in overall prevalence.
Noncurable. Symptoms can be acute or chronic liver disease, cirrhosis; affected persons have an increased risk of liver cancer	18% through unsafe homosexual sex 15% through injecting drug abuse 3% through household contact 2% through health care employment	Seroprevalence is race-specific: blacks, 12%; Mexican Americans, 4.4%; and whites, 3.0%.

of HIV/AIDS. Female teens now represent 49% of all adolescent HIV/AIDS cases reported in the United States.[51] African American and Latina teens accounted for 82% of the cumulative HIV/AIDS cases among young women age 13 to 19 years. Among males 13 to 19, 41% of AIDS cases were among young men who have sex with men (YMSM), and 52% were YMSM who also inject drugs.[188]

Many young people become infected in their teen years but do not manifest symptoms until their 20s. During these years, they unwittingly carry and spread the disease each time they engage in unprotected sexual behavior or intravenous drug use.[1] HIV infection is the leading cause of death among people 25 to 44 years of age and the sixth-leading cause among all people age 15 to 24. There is also a racial disparity in death rates among those 15 to 24 years. AIDS is the seventh-leading cause of death among white males and females, sixth among Latino males and females, fifth among black males, and third among black females.[18]

Although declining rates of sexual activity and increased condom use among sexually active youth sound a hopeful note, the HIV/AIDS epidemic among young people of color and YMSMs underscores the need for more focused, gender-appropriate and culturally appropriate prevention programs.[6,253] Currently about 50% of high-school students have sexual intercourse, and only 56.8% of these teenagers use a condom. Condom use varies by race among sexually active female teens, with 41.1% of black, 50.8% of white, and 60% of Latina females failing to use condoms at their last sexual intercourse. Unprotected sex among YMSMs is 28.7% for those age 17 to 19, and ranges from 34.3% to 55.3% in those age 20 to 22 years.[7,55] Females who have sex with older male partners are at greater risk for STDs and HIV.[55,241a,253]

Older male sexual partners are more likely to be infected than their younger male counterparts (because of increased potential for more sexual partners and more varied sexual and drug experiences).[76] Although the phenomenon of older men engaging in sexual relations with younger women is widespread, a disproportionately high percentage of adult men with minor partners are black and Latino.[253] Overall, the risk of HIV infection is higher among urban black and Latina women who are living in or near poverty because of high rates of injection drug use in these communities.[253] A small proportion of U.S. high-school students (about 2%) put themselves and their sexual partners at risk of HIV infection through injection drug use.[6,146]

Screening for Substance Abuse in Adolescents

Substance abuse is common in U.S. society among people of every age and every social, economic, professional, and educational status. Substance abuse includes a wide variety of mood-affecting chemicals: caffeine (e.g., coffee, black tea, chocolate, soft drinks), cannabis (marijuana), depressants (e.g., alcohol, sedatives, and tranquilizers), narcotics (e.g., heroin, opium, morphine, codeine), stimulants (e.g., amphetamines, cocaine, crack), anabolic androgenic steroids, and tobacco (e.g., cigarettes, cigars, chewing tobacco).[104] On an individual level,

substance abuse can impair judgment, delay wound healing, and slow the rehabilitation process. Its societal ramifications include violence, homicide, assault, accidental injury, suicide, sexually transmitted diseases, and 50% of all motor vehicle accidents.

Substance abuse in the formative years has long been a concern of parents, caregivers, teachers, coaches, and health care providers. Athletic associations at all levels of competition prohibit the use of performance-enhancing drugs, while youth associations also ban tobacco, alcohol, and illicit drugs. If ever there was a group of human beings susceptible to the traps and pitfalls of substance abuse, it is the adolescent age group. Trial-and-error learning, questioning of authority, and peer pressure all can lead to physical addiction and psychological craving and dependence.

Monitoring the Future (MTF), a long-term study of licit and illicit drug use, has been scrutinizing substance abuse among U.S. adolescents (eighth, tenth, and twelfth graders) since 1975.[146] Over time, this study has monitored trends in the use of drugs, perceived risk, availability, and personal disapproval. According to the latest version of the MTF study (December 2003), there has been an 11% decline in overall drug use by eighth, tenth, and twelfth graders over the first 2 years of the new millennium. This finding translates into 400,000 fewer teen drug users in the last 2 years and generates a more positive picture of American youth than was seen at the end of the last century.[146]

These declines were broad, with only two major classes of drugs (tranquilizers and barbiturates) showing any sign of increase in use. Two specific drugs in the narcotic classification (Oxycontin and Vicodin) were added to the MTF drug list in 2002. Oxycontin showed up in 2002 with a lifetime prevalence of 1.3% in eighth graders, 3.0% in tenth graders, and 4.0% in twelfth graders, while Vicodin registered at 2.5%, 6.9%, and 9.6% respectively.

In 2003, MTF reported that 22.8% of all eighth graders, 41.4% of all tenth graders, and over half of all adolescents (51.1%) had tried some sort of illicit drug by the time that they finished high school.[146] Drugs on the rise among teenagers in the early years of the new millennium included the "club drugs" (e.g., LSD, MDMA [ecstasy], methamphetamine, ketamine [special K]); the "date rape" drugs (e.g., Rohypnol and GHB [gamma-hydroxybutyrate], but all of these drugs dropped in prevalence except for anabolic steroids by twelfth graders (2.5% in 2000 to 3.5% in 2003). Given their availability, inhalants have historically been the only drug abused more by younger teens. Heroin use (injected or without a needle) currently is stable across all age groups (approximately 1.5%), with younger persons using a needle more frequently and older persons using without a needle. Box 12-2 shows the lifetime prevalence rates for key drugs used by adolescents in 2003.

ANABOLIC ANDROGENIC STEROIDS. *Anabolic androgenic steroids* (AAS) is the name for synthetic substances related to the male sex hormone, testosterone. Anabolic steroids are abused by approximately 2.5% of eighth graders, 3.5% of tenth graders, and 4.0% of twelfth graders.[146] These drugs have medical uses, such as treating delayed puberty, some types of impotence, and

Trends in Lifetime Prevalence of Use of Various Drugs in Eighth, Tenth, and Twelfth Graders

	Grade Level		
Drug Use	**8**	**10**	**12***
Any illicit drug	22.8	41.4	51.1
Alcohol	45.6	66.0	76.6
Been drunk[†]	20.3	42.4	58.1
Amphetamines	8.4	13.1	14.4
Cigarettes	28.4	43.0	53.7
Cocaine	3.6	5.1	7.7
Crack	2.5	2.7	3.6
Hallucinogens	4.0	6.9	10.6
Heroin	1.6	1.5	1.5
Inhalants	15.8	12.7	11.2
LSD	2.1	3.5	5.9
Marijuana/Hashish	17.5	36.4	46.1
MDMA (Ecstasy)	3.2	5.4	8.3
PCP	—	—	2.5
Sedatives	—	—	8.8
Smokeless tobacco	11.3	14.6	17.0
Steroids	2.5	3.0	3.5
Tranquilizers	4.4	7.8	10.2

From The Monitoring the Future Study, the University of Michigan. Available at: www.monitoringthefuture.org.
*2003 Data; entries listed as percentages of students who have used the substance.
†Subgroup of alcohol users.

wasting of the body caused by HIV infection or other diseases. However, when abused, AAS can have serious health consequences. In boys and men, the abuse of AAS can reduce sperm production, shrink the testicles, and cause impotence and irreversible breast enlargement. Girls and women can develop more masculine characteristics, such as laryngeal growth with deepening of the voice and excessive body hair. Both sexes run the risk of cranial hair loss, increased incidence of acne, and aggression.[35] In addition, the abuse of AAS can stunt bone growth in adolescents and result in potentially permanent damage to the heart, liver, and kidneys.[27,104] Individuals who inject anabolic steroids with nonsterile needles also risk developing HIV, hepatitis, and other blood-borne infections.[72]

Given the adolescent's preoccupation with appearance and society's emphasis on athletic performance, it is not surprising that teens, both male and female, have turned to the use of AASs and other performance enhancers. Studies have reported that teenagers viewed AAS as a harmless way to "bulk up," to achieve athletic goals, and to improve appearance.[72,102,141] Among male adolescents, steroid abuse is associated with worse self-esteem and higher rates of depressed mood and attempted suicide, worse knowledge, worse attitudes about health, greater participation in sports that emphasize weight and shape, greater parental concern about weight, and higher rates of disordered eating and substance use.[72,101,141]

Among females, a similar but less consistent pattern of results also emerged.[141] Work by Goldberg and Elliot substantiates the benefits of a gender-specific, sport-team-centered approach to adolescent health risks and behaviors. For males, refer to the program entitled *Adolescents Training and Learning*

to Avoid Steroids (ATLAS), and for females, *Athletes Targeting Healthy Exercise and Nutrition Alternatives* (ATHENA).[102] Scientific information on AAS is readily available on the NIDA website (www.steroidabuse.org).

MARIJUANA/HASHISH. Marijuana has been the most widely used illicit drug for the 27 years of the MTF study. Annual marijuana use peaked at 51% among twelfth graders in 1979, after a rise that began during the 1960s.[146] Currently, nearly half (46%) of high school seniors, slightly less (36%) of tenth graders, and nearly one in five eighth graders (17.5%) have tried marijuana. It continues to be easily accessible to students, with nearly half (45%) of eighth graders, three quarters (74%) of tenth graders, and 87% of high school seniors stating they could easily obtain marijuana if they so desired. Eighty percent of teens disapprove of "regular use" of marijuana, and about 60% of teens perceive it as carrying a risk of leading to other behaviors. Of the 7.1 million Americans who need drug treatment, 19% are youth age 12 to 17 years (1.35 million), and more than 60% (4.26 million) need treatment for marijuana.[146]

ALCOHOL. Alcohol abuse and alcohol dependence are not only adult problems. They affect a significant number of adolescents between the ages of 12 and 20, even though the legal drinking age is 21 years. According to the National Institute on Drug Abuse (NIDA), the average age when juveniles first try alcohol is 11 years for boys and 13 years for girls. Four of every five students have consumed alcohol by the end of high school, with nearly half getting started by eighth grade, and nearly three fourths in tenth grade. In 2003, almost two thirds of the twelfth graders, nearly one half of tenth graders, and over one fifth of eighth graders reported having been drunk at least once in their life.[146]

Adolescents who begin drinking before age 15 are four times more likely to develop alcohol dependence than those who begin drinking at age 21. More than 3 million teenagers are outright alcoholics, and several million others have serious drinking problems that will require professional help.[181] Dependence on alcohol (and other drugs) also has been associated with psychiatric problems such as depression, anxiety, oppositional defiant disorder, and antisocial personality disorder. Alcohol is a leading contributor to death in those 15 to 24 years old and is linked to the vast majority of young-adult automobile crashes, homicides, suicides, and bicycle crashes.[32,131,181] As with any addictive behavior at any age, self-help groups with advice and support from a health care professional are the best way to address the addiction. Treatment also should involve family members (and peers) because family history may play a role in the origins of the problem, and treatment cannot succeed in isolation.[180]

SMOKELESS TOBACCO. Smokeless tobacco (e.g., snuff and chew) has been associated with halitosis, tooth loss, gum disease, and oral and esophageal cancers (Box 12-3). Thankfully, the use of smokeless tobacco by teens has fallen substantially from its all-time high of 32.4% of twelfth graders in 1992. The current lifetime rate of smokeless tobacco use is approxmately 11% for eighth graders, 15% for tenth graders, and 17% for twelfth graders. It is almost exclusively a male behavior, with 30-day prevalence rates of 5.4%, 9.9%, and 12.2% in grades 8, 10, and 12 respectively, versus 1.3%, 2.1%, and 1.2% among

---

BOX 12-3

Dangers of Tobacco

Addictiveness: The addictive potential of nicotine is similar to that of heroin. Some believe it is more difficult to stop smoking than to stop any other addiction.

Back pain: Smoking is a major risk factor in recovery from back pain, because poor oxygen levels of those who smoke prevent lumbar disks from being adequately oxygenated.

Bladder cancer: Smoking causes 40% of all cases of bladder cancer.

Breast cancer: Women smokers are 75% more likely to develop breast cancer than are nonsmoking women.

Cervical cancer: Women who smoke are four times more likely to develop cancer of the cervix than are nonsmoking women.

Childhood respiratory ailments: Children exposed to their parents' tobacco smoke have six times more respiratory problems (such as colds, ear infections, tonsillitis, bronchitis, asthma, and pneumonia) than children of nonsmoking parents.

Diabetes: Smoking reduces the body's absorption of insulin.

Drug interactions: Smokers need higher-than-normal dosages of certain drugs.

Ear infections: Children of smokers face an increased risk of otitis media.

Emphysema: Smoking causes about 85% of all deaths from emphysema.

Esophageal cancer: Smoking causes about 80% of all throat cancer. Snuff and chewing tobacco cause many cases.

Fires: Smoking is the leading cause of fire in homes, hotels, and hospitals.

Gastrointestinal cancer: Smoking doubles the risk of cancer of the stomach and duodenum.

Heart disease: If you smoke, you are about four times more likely to develop cardiovascular disease than those who do not smoke.

Infertility: Couples in which at least one member smokes are more than three times more likely to have trouble getting pregnant than nonsmoking couples.

Kidney cancer: Smoking causes 40% of all kidney cancers.

Laryngeal cancer: If you smoke more than 25 cigarettes daily, you are almost 30 times more likely to develop cancer of the voicebox than those who are nonsmokers. In addition, many cases of cancer of the larynx are caused by snuff or chewing tobacco.

Leukemia: Tobacco smoke contains several cancer-causing chemicals, some of which are known to cause leukemia.

Low birth weight: Women who smoke as few as 5 cigarettes per day during pregnancy have a significantly greater risk of giving birth to an unnaturally small, lightweight baby.

Mouth cancer: Tobacco (whether dipped, chewed, or smoked) causes almost every case of cancer of the mouth, lips, cheek, tongue, salivary glands, and tonsils.

Nutrition: Smokers tend to have poorer nutrition than nonsmokers. Smoking causes lower levels of HDL cholesterol.

Osteoporosis: Women smokers tend to have menopause 5 to 10 years earlier than expected, causing increased bone thinning at an earlier age, which increases the later risk of hip fracture and vertebral compression fractures.

Pharyngeal cancer: Most of those who are killed by cancer of the pharynx are smokers.

Premature aging: Constant exposure to tobacco smoke prematurely wrinkles facial skin and yellows teeth and fingernails.

Recovery from injury or surgery: People who smoke have delayed healing of wounds and bones. They are also at greater risk of complications from surgery and anesthesia.

Stroke: Smoking doubles the risk of stroke.

Tooth loss: Use of snuff or chewing tobacco causes gum recession and tooth abrasion, which contribute to tooth loss.

REFERENCE

American Cancer Society: The dangers of tobacco, *Patient Medical Assistant*, August 23, 1999.

---

females.[146] An estimated 38% to 47% of teens perceive smokeless tobacco as dangerous, while 71% to 80% of teens disapprove of smokeless tobacco.

CIGARETTES. The greatest preventable cause of disease and mortality in the United States is cigarette smoking (see Box 12-3).[146] While adult smoking rates have been steadily falling in recent years, teenage smoking rates remain high, with only modest declines.[146] According to the Centers for Disease Control and Prevention, 3000 American adolescents between 13 and 17 years begin smoking each day, and the average age for smoking onset is 14. In 2003, more than half (54%) of twelfth-grade adolescents had tried cigarettes, and almost a third were current smokers. Nearly half of tenth graders and 28% of eighth graders have tried cigarettes. Sadly, one in eight eighth graders (12%) already has become a regular smoker.[181]

Children who experiment with cigarettes can become physically addicted to tobacco rapidly.[44,45,73] Teenage girls took an average of 3 weeks to become addicted to tobacco, even if they smoked only occasionally (two cigarettes, one day per week). Half of all boys hooked on tobacco were firmly addicted within 6 months.[73] The Center for Addiction and Substance Abuse (CASA) reports that teenagers who smoke are less likely to engage in sports or other after-school activities, have less dynamic relationships with parents, and are more likely to get poor grades. Teens who smoke are 5½ times more likely to have tried marijuana, 6 times more likely to get drunk at least once a month, and three times more likely to try an illegal drug in the future than teens who do not smoke.[44,45]

Screening the Mental Health of Adolescents

One in every 10 American youths currently has mental-health problems that interfere with normal development and functioning.[88,217] The mental-health problems affecting children and adolescents include depressive disorders, anxiety disorders, attention deficit hyperactivity disorder (ADHD), eating disorders, autism, other pervasive developmental disorders (PDD), and schizophrenia.

DEPRESSIVE DISORDERS. Depressive disorders (e.g., major depressive disorder, dysthymic disorder, and bipolar disorder) adversely affect mood, energy, interest, sleep, appetite, and overall functioning. Primary clues for depression include: low self-esteem, anhedonia (failure to find pleasure in daily activities), sleep disorders, and difficulty concentrating or making decisions. Depressive disorders are associated with an increased risk of suicidal behavior. In 1999, suicide was the third-leading cause of death in those 15 to 24 years old and the fourth-leading cause of death among those 10 to 14 years old. Evidence suggests that depressive disorders emerging early in life often continue into adulthood, and that early-onset depressive disorders may predict more severe illnesses in adult life.[217]

Screening for depressive disorders in the adolescent (and all patients) is recommended as a component of routine health maintenance assessment.[33] The second edition of the *Beck Depression Inventory (BDI-II)* is an invaluable tool for depression screening and diagnosis.[24] This 21-item tool assesses the intensity of depression in clinical and normal individuals in an age range of 13 to 80 years. The BDI-II takes just 5 minutes to complete and also is used extensively to monitor therapeutic progress. Early diagnosis and treatment of depressive disorders in children and adolescents are critical in enabling young people to live up to their full potential.[182]

ANXIETY. Adolescents are not immune to stress. Environmental, social, cultural, and psychosocial stresses can potentially lead to anxiety for adolescents.[31,217] Anxiety disorders, including generalized anxiety disorder, obsessive-compulsive disorder (OCD), panic disorder, posttraumatic stress disorder (PTSD), phobias, separation anxiety, and selective autism, are the most common mental illnesses in children and adolescents.[41,182] Researchers estimate that in any 6-month period, 13% of American children and adolescents will have an anxiety-related disorder.[182] Up to 30% of children and 25% to 40% of adults with attention deficit hyperactivity disorder (ADHD) also have an associated anxiety disorder.[58,182]

Symptoms of anxiety, stress, and depression can be expressed in three primary modes: somatic, psychological, and behavioral (Table 12-12).[190] These expressions of stress differ slightly across the lifespan and also depend somewhat on the individual and his or her level of psychosocial development. Conversely, relaxation is a positively perceived state of mind and body in which a person feels relief from tension/strain.

The three aims of relaxation training are: (1) to protect the organs of the body from unnecessary wear, (2) to help relieve stress in conditions such as anxiety, essential hypertension, tension headache, insomnia, asthma, immune deficiency, and

panic, and (3) to create coping skills to calm the mind and allow thinking to be more clear and effective.[238] Various forms of psychotherapy, including cognitive-behavioral therapy and family therapy, as well as certain medications, particularly selective serotonin reuptake inhibitors (SSRIs), are used to treat anxiety disorders in children and adolescents. Research on the safety and efficacy of these treatments is ongoing.[182]

ATTENTION DEFICIT HYPERACTIVITY DISORDER. From 1.7% to 16.7% of school-age children and adolescents have attention deficity hyperactivity disorder (ADHD), which can reduce their ability to learn.[37,58] ADHD's core symptoms include developmentally inappropriate levels of attention, concentration, activity, distractibility, and impulsivity.[37] Children with ADHD usually have impaired functioning in peer relationships and in multiple settings, including home and school. Most hyperactive children will continue to meet the criteria for ADHD as adolescents and adults.[74] Untreated ADHD also has been found to have long-term adverse effects on academic performance, vocational success, and social-emotional development.[182]

Psychostimulant medications, including methylphenidate (Ritalin) and amphetamine (Dexedrine and Adderall), are by far the most widely researched and most-prescribed treatments for ADHD. Many short-term studies have established the safety and efficacy of stimulants and behavioral psychosocial treatments in alleviating the symptoms of ADHD. Research suggests that treating ADHD in children and adolescents may reduce the likelihood of future drug and alcohol abuse.[103]

EATING DISORDERS. *Eating disorders* (refer to Table 12-5) entail serious disturbances in eating behavior, such as extreme and unhealthy reduction of food intake or severe overeating, as well as feelings of distress or extreme concern about body shape or weight. Eating disorders often co-occur with other

---

TABLE 12-12

Modes of Anxiety Expressed by Body System and Recommended Treatment[198]

Body System	Modes of Anxiety Expression	Treatment Methods
Somatic: physiological changes	Increased HR (palpitations), BP, RR Increased sweating Reduced blood flow to the periphery (cold hands and feet) Raised blood coagulation rate Raised blood glucose level Muscle tension (headaches; neck, shoulder, and low-back pain) GI: indigestion, constipation, and diarrhea	Progressive relaxation techniques (Jacobson) Diaphragmatic breathing Physical interventions including stretching, aerobic exercise, yoga, tai chi, Feldenkrais, Alexander technique Biofeedback
Cognitive (mental): symptoms reported by the patient	Tiredness or difficulty in sleeping Headache Difficulty concentrating, worry Impatience; feeling irritable; easily angered (Patient also may report any of the above somatic changes)	Cognitive restructuring via self-statements and self-awareness activities Imagery Meditation
Behavioral: observable actions	Increased consumption of alcohol, tobacco, food Loss of appetite or excessive eating Restlessness Loss of sexual interest A tendency to experience accidents Acting-out behaviors (e.g., hitting, yelling)	Behavioral relaxation training Social and coping skills Autogenics: teaching the body and mind to relax (combines with cognitive)

Modified from Payne RA: Relaxation techniqies: a practical handbook for the health care professional, New York, 1995, Churchill Livingstone.

illnesses such as depression, substance abuse, and anxiety disorders. Eating disorders are associated with a wide range of other health complications, including neuropathies, serious heart arrhythmias, and kidney failure, which may lead to death. Because of their complexity, eating disorders require a comprehensive treatment plan involving medical care and monitoring, psychotherapy, nutritional counseling, and, when appropriate, medication management.[96,182]

AUTISM AND OTHER PERVASIVE DEVELOPMENTAL DISORDERS. *Autism and other pervasive developmental disorders (PDDs),* including Asperger's disorder, Rett's disorder, childhood disintegrative disorder, and pervasive developmental disorder-not otherwise specified (PDD-NOS), are brain disorders that occur in an estimated 2 to 6 per 1000 American children. PDDs usually develop by 3 years of age and typically affect the ability to communicate, to form relationships with others, and to respond appropriately to the outside world.[182]

Recent research has made it possible to identify earlier those children who show signs of developing a PDD and thus to initiate early intervention. While no single treatment program is best for all children with PDDs, both psychosocial and pharmacologic interventions can help improve their behavioral and cognitive functioning. The National Institute of Mental Health (NIMH) is funding studies of behavioral treatments and medications to determine the best time to start treatment, the optimum intensity and duration of treatment, and the most effective methods to reach both high-functioning and low-functioning children.[182]

SCHIZOPHRENIA. *Schizophrenia* is a chronic, severe, and disabling brain disorder that affects about 1% of the population during their lifetime. Symptoms include hallucinations, false beliefs, disordered thinking, and social withdrawal. Schizophrenia typically emerges in late adolescence or early adulthood. Researchers are just beginning to make headway into understanding the origins of schizophrenia (i.e., genetic factors combined with developmental disturbances and environmental stressors).[182]

Treatments that help manage schizophrenia have improved significantly in recent years. Antipsychotic medications are especially helpful in reducing hallucinations and delusions in children and adolescents. The newer-generation "atypical" antipsychotics, such as olanzapine and clozapine, also may help improve motivation and emotional expressiveness in some patients. Children with schizophrenia and their families also can benefit from supportive counseling, psychotherapies, and social-skills training aimed at helping them cope with the illness. Special education or other accommodations may be necessary to help children with schizophrenia to succeed in the classroom.[182]

Musculoskeletal Disorders of Adolescence

The first step toward cure is to know what the disease is.

Latin proverb

Disorders and injuries of the musculoskeletal (MS) system are many and of paramount concern to the orthopedic practitioner.[211] There are six major categories of MS, or orthopedic, disease: (1) congenital (see Table 12-3), (2) inflammatory, (3) metabolic, (4) vascular, (5) neoplastic, and (6) traumatic.[174]

Age, gender, and race of the patient are important predictive variables in the differential diagnosis of musculoskeletal disease.[48,104,211] Other variables include behavior of the lesion (osteoblastic or osteolytic), locus of the lesion (epiphysis, apophysis, metaphysis, diaphysis, or articular surface), shape and margins of the lesion, and a history of trauma.[174]

Radiologic evaluation, which requires a systematic approach, is absolutely essential to the management of these six categories of pediatric orthopedic conditions.[160,166,174] Radiographic diagnosis of orthopedic trauma and disease in the maturating skeleton can be a complicated process. First, only the ossified portions of bone have sufficient radiographic density to be imaged. Second, differentiation of fractures is complicated by the presence of epiphyseal plates, dense growth plates, dense growth lines, secondary centers of ossification, and large nutrient foramina, all of which may be confused with fracture lines. Comparison films of the uninvolved side often are obtained to assist in differential diagnosis.[166,174,211] Advanced diagnostic imaging techniques, including contrast-enhanced radiography, conventional tomography, computed tomography (CT), nuclear imaging (i.e., bone scan), and magnetic resonance imaging (MRI), often are required in distinguishing osteocartilaginous and soft tissue structures located about a joint (see Chapter 17, Diagnostic Imaging).[160,174]

Neoplastic and nonneoplastic (e.g., inflammatory, metabolic, and vascular) diseases characteristically manifest at specific bones or specific sites within bones and joints across the lifespan.[104,174,211] During the growth years, nearly all bone neoplasms, both benign and malignant, avoid the epiphysis. Epiphyseal growth plates are vulnerable to idiopathic necrosis (osteochondrosis), local growth disorders (dysplasias and osteochondritis dissecans), and a variety of traumatic conditions (e.g., apophysitis, epiphyseal fractures).[174,211] By contrast, the epiphyses tend to resist other afflictions. Hematogenous osteomyelitis, for example, never begins at the epiphysis and rarely spreads into it through the epiphyseal plate.[211]

Osteochondrosis (Avascular Necrosis of the Epiphyses)

The osteochondroses are idiopathic disorders seen in the immature skeleton, usually involving a secondary epiphyseal center or pressure epiphysis at the end of the long bone. They occasionally involve the primary epiphyseal center of a small bone (e.g., Kohler's disease, Kienböck's disease). Knowledge of the blood supply of epiphyses and their epiphyseal plates (physes) is pivotal to understanding these growth-plate disorders. The epiphyses covered by the most articular cartilage are the most vulnerable (i.e., they have the most precarious blood supply; see Figure 12-5).

Increased intracapsular joint pressure resulting from repetitive trauma, transient synovitis, infection, or granulation tissue is thought to disrupt blood flow and lead to the various conditions known as avascular necrosis, aseptic necrosis, and ischemic necrosis. In some of the osteochondroses (particularly Legg-Calvé-Perthes disease), there is a likely association with parental smoking during pregnancy, exposure to secondhand smoke in childhood, and hypofibrinolysis and thrombophilia (a deficiency

TABLE 12-13

Epiphyseal Disorders: Disorders of Epiphyseal Growth

Epiphyseal Disorder	Incidence	Clinical Features and Diagnosis	Treatment and Outcome
Slipped capital femoral epiphysis (SCFE) (Adolescent coxa vara) By far the most significant of the lower-limb epiphyseal-plate disorders. It is the most common hip disorder seen in adolescents.	Males (13 to 16 years of age) are 2-5 times more likely to be affected than females (11 to 14 years of age) 25%-33% bilateral, especially in boys <12 years More common in blacks	Obesity (75% of cases) Mild hip pain referred to the medial aspect of the knee Slight limp that increases with fatigue; positive Trendelenburg sign Posture: lower extremity unloaded into flexion, ER, and abduction to avoid impingement of metaphysis on the anterior lip of acetabulum Reduced hip flexion, IR, abduction Diagnosis is confirmed with x-ray. AP and lateral views helpful, but frog view with positive Kline's line is definitive	Prescription: prevent further slip, maintain ROM, prevent OA, immobilize via a hip spica and NWB status. If slip is <1 cm, screw/pin in situ, cast and WB after surgery.
Blount's disease (tibia vara) Growth suppression with premature closure of the medial portion of the upper tibial epiphyseal plate.	Girls > boys Type in infants <2-3 years is the most common Juvenile type: 4-10 years Adolescent: 11 + years Finland and Jamaica have the highest incidence of disease	Often seen in obese children who are early ambulators Lateral thrust during stance Tibial varum Early x-ray is essential as it displays the defective ossification on the medial side of the tibia, beaked appearance of the underlying metaphysis, and obvious longitudinal growth disturbance	Prescription: prevent progression of the varus deformity. If unilateral infantile form (<3 yr) hip, knee, ankle, foot, orthosis (HKAFO) 23 hr/day or night splints to correct varus deformity. If >4 years: splinting usually fails and osteotomy of the tibia is required (often must be repeated). Black girls have the worst prognosis.
Madelung's deformity Localized epiphyseal dysplasia on the medial (ulnar) side of the distal radial epiphysis.	Adolescent onset Girls > boys Usually bilateral	Insidious onset of wrist pain Loss of forearm/wrist ROM (wrist flexion and supination) Prominence of the distal end of the ulna on the dorsum of the wrist and forward displacement of the hand in relation to the forearm	Correction of the deformity via surgical excision of the distal portion of the ulna and osteotomy of the deformed end of the radius.

in antithrombotic factor C or S, with an increased tendency toward thrombosis).[164,211,255]

Osteochondroses are most common in the middle years of growth, ages 3 to 10 years. They affect boys more than girls (a 4:1 ratio), affect lower limbs more than upper limbs, and have a bilateral presentation at any given epiphysis about 10% to 15% of the time.[211] These disorders are self-limiting (i.e., heal spontaneously) and follow four distinct stages:
- *Avascularity phase*: involves obliteration of the blood vessels to the epiphysis (variety of causes) and kills the osteocytes and the bone-marrow cells within the epiphysis.
- *Revascularization phase*: represents the vascular reaction of the surrounding tissues to dead bone and is characterized by revascularization of the dead epiphysis.

- *Bone healing phase*: bone resorption ceases and bone deposition continues so that the fibrous and granulation tissue is slowly replaced by new bone.
- *Residual deformity phase*: when bony healing of the epiphysis is complete, its contours remain relatively unchanged.
  Scheuermann's disease (i.e., adolescent kyphosis or vertebral epiphysitis) is the most significant of the adolescent spinal osteochondroses. It involves the ring epiphysis of the thoracic vertebra. It is more common in males age 12 to 16 (and up to 19) years. Clinical manifestations include: exaggerated kyphosis with possible compensatory lumbar lordosis, prominent vertebral spinous process with or without pain, local musculoskeletal pain, tenderness, and fatigue; stiffness on joint play assessment (JPA) of the spine; and possible Schmorl's nodes

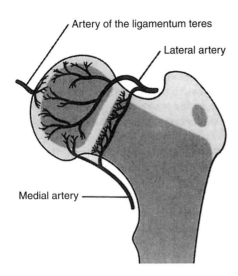

FIGURE 12-5 Blood supply of the femoral head in a child. (From Goodman CC, Boissonnault WG, Fuller KS: *Pathology: implications for the physical therapist*, ed 2, Philadelphia, 2003, WB Saunders, p 937. Originally from Bullough PG: *Orthopaedic pathology*, ed 3, London, 1997, Mosby-Wolfe, p 263.)

(vertically displaced nuclear material secondary to end-plate degradation).[104,165,167] The treatment goal of this self-limiting disease is prevention of progressive deformity. Treatment includes therapeutic exercise (e.g., postural exercises, stretching, thoracic hyperextension), soft tissue and joint mobilization, traction, and occasionally thoracic extension orthoses if the deformity advances rapidly (greater than 60 degrees).[48,104]

LEGG-CALVÉ-PERTHES DISEASE (LCP). LCP is by far the most significant, most common, and most serious of the lower-extremity osteochondroses. LCP disease involves the pressure epiphysis of the proximal femur, strikes boys more than girls (a 5:1 ratio) and whites more than blacks (10:1 ratio), and is bilateral 10% to 15% of the time.[48,211] The treatment goal is containment of the femoral head in the acetabulum via abduction casting. Prognosis is inversely related to age of onset and to gender (boys worse than girls). Fifty percent of all patients have disabling osteoarthritis by the age of 50 years, and total hip arthroplasty is a typical long-term outcome.

FREIBERG'S DISEASE. Forefoot pain on weight bearing caused by osteochondrosis of the pressure epiphysis of the metatarsal heads (second more than third metatarsal) occurs most often in adolescent females. A congenitally long second metatarsal or short first metatarsal is a contributing factor. Shoe modifications (e.g., avoidance of heels and a stiff rocker-bottom sole) will redistribute weight, but occasionally surgical excision of the distorted portion of the metatarsal head is required.[211]

UPPER EXTREMITY OSTEOCHONDROSES. The upper extremity osteochondroses include *Panner's disease* (capitellum of the humerus) and *Kienböck's disease* (lunate). Panner's disease should be ruled out in children age 3 to 11 years who present with pain, swelling, and limited range of motion in the elbow joint. Conservative treatment via immobilization (sling during symptomatic period) usually leads to a good prognosis given the non–weight-bearing nature of the elbow joint.

Kienböck's disease has an inferior prognosis, and progression to degeneration of the wrist is common. Aching in the wrist, tenderness over the lunate, and swelling secondary to repetitive microtrauma (occupations with vibration and wrist impact) in late adolescence and young adulthood characterize Kienböck's disease. The healing process is slower and often incomplete in adults compared with children and adolescents. Treatment is excision of the lunate before degenerative changes develop in the perilunar carpals.

Epiphyseal Dysplasia, Disorders of Epiphyseal Growth

Epiphyseal dysplasias begin during the growing years and tend to progress as long as the child is still growing. These disorders include: slipped capital femoral epiphysis (SCFE or adolescent coax vara), Blount's disease (tibia vara), Madelung's deformity (epiphyseal dysplasia at the elbow), and idiopathic scoliosis. SCFE is the most significant epiphyseal-plate disorder of the lower extremity, and the most common hip disorder seen in adolescents.[211] The incidence, clinical features, treatment, and prognosis of the extremity epiphyseal disorders are discussed in Table 12-13.

IDIOPATHIC SCOLIOSIS, A DIAGNOSIS OF EXCLUSION. The pediatric spine is susceptible to growth-plate interruption and external stresses that can cause abnormal skeletal modeling. MS injury also can cause nonstructural lateral deviation of the spine (scoliosis). Idiopathic scoliosis (75% to 80% of cases) is a *diagnosis of exclusion*, meaning all other sources of curvature have been ruled out.[101,165]

Nonstructural scoliosis (no inherent osseous change in the vertebral column) can be caused by habitual posturing, pain or muscle hypertonicity (i.e., sciatic scoliosis often seen with LBP), leg length discrepancy (LLD) (e.g., bony anomaly, slipped capital femoral epiphysis, Blount's disease, or growth retardation secondary to a prior epiphyseal injury), lower quarter biomechanical or pathoanatomical deformity (e.g., hyperpronation, internal-rotation deformity [IRD], or external-rotation deformity [ERD]), or pelvic-girdle lesion (e.g., anterior or posterior innominate lesion or innominate upslip).[150,165,210,212] Treatment for nonstructural scoliosis is always directed at the precipitating cause.[15,16] Pelvic-girdle lesions can be addressed via muscle energy techniques (MET) and direct mobilization or manipulation.[139,212,252] Other interventions include postural re-education, treatment of back pain and tone issues, treatment of muscular imbalances and orthopedic conditions in the lower kinetic chain, and compensation for a true bony LLD. Depending on the amount of LLD and the age and growth potential of the patient, treatment could range from a simple shoe lift or corrective foot orthosis to surgical osteotomy or a long-bone lengthening procedure via an Ilizarov external fixator.

Structural scoliosis may be neuromuscular, osteopathic, or idiopathic. Neuromuscular causes of scoliosis (15% to 20% of cases) include cerebral palsy, myelomeningocele (spina bifida), neurofibromatosis, spinal cord injury, neuromuscular disorders (e.g., muscular dystrophy and spinal muscle atrophy), and myopathic diseases (e.g., amyotonia congenita or arthrogryposis).[48,101,165,211] Congenital osteopathic scoliosis (5% of cases) is due to in-utero vertebral maldevelopment (e.g., wedge vertebrae, hemivertebrae, congenital bar or block vertebrae). Acquired osteopathic scoliosis can be due to Scheuermann's disease, osteomalacia, nutritional deficits, rickets, traumatic sports-related conditions (e.g., compression fractures, spondylolysis, spondylolisthesis, end-plate fractures, or Schmorl's nodes), or infections (e.g., diskitis, spondylitis, spondyloarthropathy).[48,101,104,167]

Structural scoliosis (regardless of type) is always accompanied by specific osseous changes in the vertebral column:

Convex side	Concave side
Vertebral body rotation	Spinous process deviation
Posterior rib cage hump	Posterior rib cage hollow
Thoracic cage AP narrowing	Thoracic cage AP widening

It is named by the shape (**C** shape or **S** shape), location, and convexity of the curve. Severity of curve is determined through radiographs (lateral and AP views of the spine) and the *Cobb method* of measurement.[101,104,110,167] Management is based on etiology, gender, shape, location, and degree of curve.

Infantile idiopathic scoliosis strikes from birth to 3 years of age, typically creates a left thoracic curve, and is more common in boys. Juvenile idiopathic scoliosis develops between the age of 3 and the onset of puberty (mean age 6 years) and typically creates a right thoracic curve. The incidence of juvenile scoliosis is 1.3%, and there is an equal distribution among males and females.[48] Idiopathic adolescent scoliosis has an overall prevalence of 2% to 4% in children 8 to 16 years of age.[30,48,104] The overall female/male ratio for adolescent idiopathic scoliosis is 3.6:1. It is significantly more common in females, especially as the magnitude of the curve increases.

In curves of about 10 degrees, the female/male ratio is 1.4:1, while curves of 20 degrees or greater have a female/male ratio of 6.4:1.[48]

The *Adam's forward bending test* (specificity, 0.64; sensitivity, 0.56) is used as a screening tool to identify children and adolescents with idiopathic scoliosis.[264] Its lack of reliability makes its general use in grade-school screenings controversial at best.[110,264] Youngsters suspected of having idiopathic scoliosis should be referred for medical examination. Monitoring of the curves via radiographs through growth spurts is crucial. The Risser sign (Fig. 12-6), or degree of iliac crest ossification (stages 1 to 5), is customarily used to determine chronological bone age.[101,110]

The prognosis for idiopathic adolescent scoliosis is based on age of onset, gender, and shape, location, and degree of curve. Younger patients, especially females before menarche, will have more growth potential and thus a greater risk of curve progression. Curves will progress in 19.3% of females compared with 1.2% of males. Double-curve patterns (S-curve) carry a greater risk for progression than single-curve patterns (C-curve). Curves with greater initial magnitude are always at risk to progress. A progressive curve is defined by a continued increase of 5 degrees or more on two or more consecutive examinations occurring at 4-month to 6-month intervals.[48,101,119] The PT should obtain magnetic resonance imaging in patients with an onset of scoliosis before age 8, rapid curve progression, an unusual curve pattern, neurologic deficit, or pain.[110]

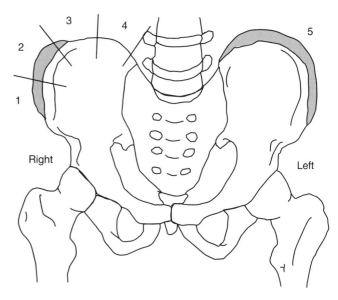

FIGURE 12-6 Risser sign, a predictor of scoliotic progression in adolescence. (From Greiner KA: Adolescent idiopathic scoliosis: radiologic decision-making, *Am Fam Phys* 65:1817-1822, 2002.)

Mild deformities (curves of 10 to 20 degrees) are generally asymptomatic and respond well to conservative treatment.[119] Conservative therapy must address flexibility, strength, and muscle imbalance of the trunk, shoulder girdle, and pelvic girdle. Pelvic derotation (posterior pelvic tilt), proprioceptive exercises (pelvic clock), postural stabilization, and selective stretching are considered standard protocol.[48,104,119,150] Respiratory exercises should be added as necessary for thoracic mobility. Global-movement programs such as yoga, Pilates, tai chi, and Feldenkrais all may prove useful, but more research is needed in this area.

Moderate deformities (curves of 25 to 40 degrees) typically create musculoskeletal pain as well as cosmetic issues for the adolescent. Biomechanical bracing with end-point control and redundant three-point pressure systems should be implemented when the apex of the curve is between 25 and 40 degrees, or when the curve appears progressive.[83,119] Goals of orthotic management include halting curve progression, gaining some permanent correction, and allowing for continued spinal growth.[48] Custom-molded total-contact thoracolumbosacral orthoses (TLSO) are the current industry standard. Bracing requires strict compliance on the part of the patient (23 hours per day) and should be employed in conjunction with a customized exercise program.[119]

Surgical correction of scoliosis is reserved for progressive curves of more than 45 to 50 degrees that compromise cardiovascular-pulmonary function, impair musculoskeletal function, or result in intractable pain.[30,48,83,119] Spinal fusion, or arthrodesis, is achieved via internal fixation with Luque rods (L-rods) or Harrington rods. The need for postoperative TLSO depends on the type of curve that was fused, the type of instrumentation, the postoperative alignment of the trunk, and the surgeon's discretion.[30,48,83] A less invasive surgery, video-assisted thoracoscopic anterior spine fusion, is now available at a handful of hospitals across the country.[30,178]

Osteochondritis Dissecans, Tangential Avascular Necrosis of a Pressure Epiphysis

The convex surfaces of certain pressure epiphyses are susceptible to avascular necrosis of a small tangential segment of subchondral bone that may become separated, or "dissected," from the remaining portion of the epiphysis by reactive fibrous and granulation tissue; thus the name, *osteochondritis dissecans* (OCD).[211] Although a relatively uncommon disorder, OCD is seen most often in older children, adolescents, and young adults, and in boys more than girls. It is seen most often in the medial femoral condyle, undersurface of the patella, femoral head, dome of the talus, and capitulum of the humerus (Panner's disease).[211] In most cases, the cause of the initial avascular necrosis is unknown. Rotational or shearing trauma to a joint often is an aggravating variable in adolescents and adults.

The tangential area of avascular necrosis on the convex surface of the joint usually is no larger than 2 cm in diameter and is often smaller. The overlying articular cartilage, which is nourished by movement of synovial fluid, remains alive over the necrotic subchondral bone defect. The necrotic segment is eventually revascularized by a combination of bone resorption (osteoclasts) and bone deposition (osteoblasts). This can take up to 2 to 3 years. Juvenile-onset forms (i.e., with epiphyseal plates still open) have the best prognosis.[211]

The patient usually presents with little restriction in range of motion, pain (particularly during the revascularization phase), moderate effusion, and disuse atrophy or reflex inhibition of the muscles crossing the joint of interest. Because these symptoms mirror other joint symptoms, tangential view radiographic imaging is imperative. MRI is a more powerful imaging tool to determine continuity of the overlying articular cartilage, while arthroscopy of the joint is considered the most definitive diagnostic tool for OCD.[129,164,211]

The success of healing and the subsequent congruency of the joint surfaces depend on the size of the lesion, joint compressive forces, and the presence of concomitant joint-destabilizing forces (e.g., obesity, ligamentous laxity, muscle imbalances, muscle tightness, or poor proprioceptive control).[211]

Physical impairments (e.g., loss of ROM, muscle weakness, and poor proprioceptive awareness) should be treated with physical therapy. Gross rotational ligamentous laxity or meniscal lesions should be addressed surgically.

Activity modification may be necessary to prevent fragment separation ("joint mouse") and subsequent abrasive wear inside the synovial joint. The knee and elbow joints are very susceptible to fragment separation. Detached loose bodies causing intermittent locking or catching should be surgically removed. Loose fragments greater than 2 cm in diameter, particularly in weight-bearing surfaces, should be fixated internally if feasible. If this is not possible, autogenous periosteal grafting followed by continuous passive motion may be required to preserve the articular surface. Ligamentous stability of the joint and thorough postoperative rehabilitation are imperative if autogenous periosteal grafting is to be successful over the long term.[100,129]

Neoplastic Disorders (Bone Tumors and Soft Tissue Tumors)

Primary tumors of the musculoskeletal system are rare, but this does not negate their importance. The childhood, adolescent, and young-adult years show a predilection for malignant, as well as benign, bone tumors.[174] During the pediatric years, bone tumors tend to predominate in the ends of long bones that undergo the greatest growth and remodeling and have the greatest amount of cell activity.[104] Prevalence of bony tumor is as follows: distal end of the femur (53%), proximal tibia (26%), humerus (12%), fibula (5%), scapula (1%), ileum (1%), and other (2%) (Fig. 12-7).[255]

There are many tumors of cartilaginous origin. Most are asymptomatic unless located in proximity to a nerve, tendon, or bursa. Their prognosis is favorable, as they usually cease their growth as the skeleton reaches full maturity at the end of adolescence. Osteochondroma, the most common primary benign neoplasm of bone, is common in the growing skeleton of teenagers (males more than females). It is often an incidental finding on radiographs and rarely converts to malignant form.[104]

Benign tumors usually do not cause the constant severe pain that is associated with progressive malignant disease. Indeed, pain is the hallmark of malignant tumor development and progression.[104] Local signs such as soft tissue swelling, tenderness, joint pain, or the presence of a mass without incident of trauma should raise a red flag for the health care practitioner. Systemic

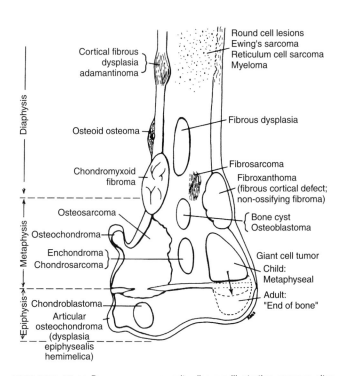

FIGURE 12-7 Bone cancer: composite diagram illustrating common sites of bone tumors. (From Goodman CC, Boissonnault WG, Fuller KS: *Pathology: implications for the physical therapist*, ed 2, Philadelphia, 2003, WB Saunders, p 908. Originally from Madewell JE, Ragsdale BD, Sweet DE: Radiologic and pathologic analysis of solitary bone lesions. I. Internal margins, *Radiol Clin North Am* 19:715, 1981.)

warning signs of occult disease (e.g., night pain, pain unrelated to position, fever, weight loss, night sweats, and fatigue) require referral for medical evaluation for potential bone tumor (infection or inflammatory condition).[36,104,174,211] Bony tumors sometimes manifest via a pathologic fracture during childhood or adolescent sporting events. If the lytic process affects a significant portion of the bone cortex (more than 50%) or occupies 60% of the bone diameter, the risk for fracture increases.[104]

Because sarcomas can readily metastasize to lung, liver, and other bone sites by hematogenous routes, early detection and treatment are warranted. Medical management of bony tumors and neoplasms includes several goals: (1) complete and permanent control of the primary tumor (amputation and limb-sparing procedures), (2) control and prevention of microstatic (radiation therapy) and metastatic (chemotherapy) disease, and (3) preservation of function.[48]

Fifteen percent of all childhood amputations are disease-related (e.g., cancer, vascular, neurologic), whereas trauma (e.g., vehicular accidents, gunshot wounds, and power or farm machinery) accounts for the remaining 85% of all adolescent-acquired amputations. Osteosarcoma and Ewing's sarcoma account for half of all disease-related amputations.[48] Amputation is decreasing as a result of early detection, reconstructive surgery, and improved cancer treatments.[165,197]

Persons caring for those undergoing radiation or chemotherapy treatments for malignant musculoskeletal tumors must use a comprehensive treatment approach to address the physical and psychosocial needs of the young patient.[104] Chemotherapy drugs, radiation therapy, and amputation will compromise the physical endurance of the patient, necessitating pacing strategies and/or assistive technology to aid with functional activities. Young men should be told that most chemotherapy drugs will have no long-term effect on fertility, but some may reduce the number of spermatozoa. Young females should be taught that menses may become irregular or stop during chemotherapy, but that most often menses will return to normal after the treatment finishes. Long-term follow-up of women treated for bone cancer during childhood and adolescence indicates that the risk of permanent ovarian damage is very low.[255]

Traumatic Musculoskeletal Disorders

Traumatic injuries in childhood and adolescence are common. These injuries are either intrinsic or extrinsic in origin. Intrinsic injuries arise from the patient's own physical activity (e.g., violent muscle contraction, an awkward movement, fall, deceleration or pivot, or inadequate physical conditioning or skill to tolerate the activity). Falls or blows from external forces or objects result in extrinsic injuries in which the adolescent "gets hurt" by something or someone else. Many accidents, as well as sports-related injuries, are preventable with common-sense principles, adequate training and conditioning, and properly fitting protective equipment (refer to Box 12-7 in the Health Promotion section).

Grade-school and middle-school students participating in sports are less likely to suffer from severe injury because they are smaller and slower than older athletes (i.e., less inertia and momentum at impact). High-school athletes are bigger, faster, stronger, and capable of delivering tremendous forces in contact sports, especially to younger, smaller athletes who are skilled enough to play at the same competitive level. Traumatic injuries tend to be most common in organized and unorganized contact sports (e.g., football, basketball, soccer) and roller sports (Box 12-4), whereas overuse injuries (e.g., tendonitis, stress fractures) are seen in repetitive impact loading sports (e.g., running, basketball, gymnastics) and the throwing or racquet sports.

BOX 12-4

Roller Sports, Adolescent Injuries, and Safety Recommendations

The rate of injuries from roller sports (e.g., roller blades, skateboards, and foot-powered scooters) has exploded in recent decades. While roller blades and skateboards grew in popularity through the late 1980s and 1990s, the foot-powered scooter is clearly the toy of the new millennium. In 2000, 5 million foot-powered scooters were sold in the United States, and related emergency-room injuries increased 700%.

Those under 15 years of age account for 90% of injuries from roller sports, with the most injured age group being young adolescents 10 to 14 years of age. Males have a higher incidence than females. One third of injuries happen in first-time participants. Nearly 50% of all injuries occur in the after-school hours of 4 PM to 7 PM in residential and public places. One out of every two injurious falls results in a fracture (49% fracture; 51% soft tissue injuries), creating an increased risk for growth-plate injury. The vast majority (85%) of fractures are wrist or elbow fractures from a fall-on-an-outstretched-hand (FOOSH injury). Seventy percent of soft tissue injuries also occur in the upper extremity. Head injuries occur almost exclusively to those participants *not* wearing a helmet.

TIPS FOR PREVENTING INJURIES ON SKATES AND SKATEBOARDS
- Learn to fall safely.
- Wear specially designed wrist guards, elbow guards, kneepads, and helmets, regardless of age, experience, or skating site. Wrist and elbow guards help prevent common arm and wrist fractures. Helmets that fit properly help prevent less common, but more severe, head injuries.
- Avoid skating in the road, the most common setting of skating-fall injuries.
- Avoid skating on streets with traffic, never skate against traffic, and be very careful at intersections. Pay attention to traffic lights, enter intersections cautiously, and watch out for vehicles, pedestrians, other skaters, and bicyclists.
- Keep speed consistent with experience, with the condition of the skating surface, and with the speed of other travelers.
- Do not skate at night because it is difficult to see and be seen.
- Check equipment often to make sure it is in good working condition.
- Children under the age of 8 should be supervised.

REFERENCES
Hassan I, Dorani BJ: Rollerblading and skateboarding injuries in children in northeast England, *Emerg Med J* 16:348-350, 1999.
Heller DR, Routley V, Chambers S: Rollerblading injuries in young children, *J Pediatr Child Health* 32(1):35-38, 1996.
Ross M: *CPSC reports as scooter sales skyrocket, injuries soar*, September 5, 2000, US Consumer Product Safety Commission, release 00-178; (301) 504-0580.

Traumatic Brain Injury

Traumatic brain injury (TBI) is a public-health problem in the United States (Fig. 12-8). One million people are treated and released from hospital emergency rooms and an average of 50,000 Americans die as a result of TBI each year. An estimated 5.3 million survivors of TBI (about 2% of the U.S. population) currently live with neuropsychological impairments that result in disabilities affecting work or social activity.[5] The monetary costs associated with TBI in the United States have been estimated at $37.8 billion per year.[5]

In 2002, the CDC reported the major causes of TBI-related deaths across the lifespan as firearm related (40%), motor-vehicle related (34%), and fall related (10%). Among youths age 0 to 19, motor-vehicle–related TBIs were the leading cause of death.[5] Firearm-related TBI death rates were highest among persons age 20 to 24, followed by those age 15 to 19. In youths 0 to 20 years, the rate of TBI injuries and deaths from falls decreases with increasing age. Adolescents (15 to 19 years) have the highest percentage of TBI-related fatal outcomes (17.1%), followed by those 10 to 14 (9.2%), and those age 5 to 9 and 0 to 4 (7.5% for each age group). TBI-related death rates for males were higher than for females across all age groups.

TBI can occur during adolescent sports activities. A classification of concussions, along with common signs, symptoms, and return-to-play guidelines, is displayed in Box 12-5. The Glasgow Coma Scale (GCS) is widely used for the assessment and ongoing management of patients with TBI.[104,156,167] Unless depressed skull fractures are suspected, skull x-rays in children with minor brain injury are not useful because skull x-rays rarely affect clinical management (i.e., do not necessarily correlate with the severity of brain injury). Children (and adults) with moderate or severe brain injuries must be hospitalized, have CT brain scans, and be managed by or in consultation with intensive care physicians or neurosurgeons.[156]

Instructions to parents and caregivers for home observation of children after TBI include: (1) observe your child carefully for 24 hours, (2) attempt to wake your child briefly every 2 hours, and (3) call your physician or bring your child promptly to the emergency room if the child develops any of the following: weakness of any arm or leg, seizures, worsening headache, unequal pupils, unusual behavior, or disorientation or confusion, or if the child will not waken (coma).[104,156,167] Problems with memory, attention, behavior, and academic performance can occur after mild brain injuries, but studies show that most children 1 year after mild brain injury have no increased incidence of cognitive or behavioral problems.[156] Children with moderate to severe TBI often have an increased need for general medical services and rehabilitation services. About 7% of persons who have had severe TBI develop posttraumatic epilepsy.[156]

Spinal Cord Injuries

Spinal cord injuries (SCIs) can be classified into traumatic (more than 80% of cases) and nontraumatic (e.g., tumor, infection) categories. A SCI is a catastrophic event of low incidence and high cost and predominantly occurs in young persons between the ages of 15 and 30 years (median age is 18 years).[104] Adolescent and young males (15 to 24 years) sustain about 80% of all spinal cord injuries. The leading causes of SCI are motor-vehicle accidents (44%), acts of violence (24%), falls (22%), sports (8% with two thirds from diving), and other (2%).[224] About 30 to 40 new cases occur per 1 million people per year, with an additional 6 to 8 deaths occurring before hospitalization.[104] Currently about 183,000 to 230,000 Americans are living with SCIs.[104] The number of deaths and severity of injury are decreasing as a result of improved delivery of initial urgent medical care.

Acute spinal cord injury is accompanied by a phenomenon called *spinal shock*. Signs of spinal shock include flaccid paralysis, absence of deep tendon reflexes, loss of anal wink, and lack of response to plantar stimulation of the feet.[104,242] Classification of SCI is based on the American Spinal Injury Association (ASIA) classification system. A complete spinal cord lesion will result in bilateral loss of all sensory modalities and motor function. Incomplete cord injury may have a confusing presentation, but knowledge of spinal cord anatomy and function will help with differential diagnosis. Specific incomplete SCI lesions include: (1) *Brown-Sequard syndrome* (hemi-section of the spinal cord); (2) *central cord syndrome* (associated with hyperextension injuries of the cervical spine); (3) *anterior cord syndrome* (associated with flexion mechanism of injury); (4) *posterior cord syndrome* (rare and characterized by proprioceptive loss and ataxia); and (5) *cauda equina syndrome*.

Patients suspected of having an SCI should be hospitalized in an intensive care unit and receive neurosurgical consultation.[156] Careful neurologic examination, spinal radiographs to look for bony injury that may require stabilization, and magnetic resonance imaging (MRI) are essential to defining the extent of SCI. Administration of high-dose methylprednisolone for 1 to 2 days after injury is now advocated in an attempt to minimize secondary injury after traumatic cord injury.[156]

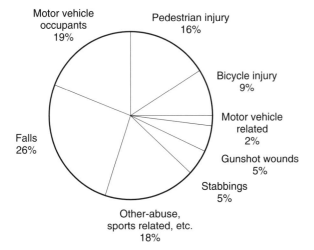

FIGURE 12-8 Children and adolescents with disability due to traumatic injury. (From National Pediatric Trauma Registry (NPTR): *Children and adolescents with disability due to traumatic injury: a data book*, Boston, 1996, Research and Training Center in Rehabilitation and Childhood Trauma, Tufts University School of Medicine.)

BOX 12-5

Concussion: Classification, Common Signs and Symptoms, and Return-to-Play Guidelines

SIGNS AND SYMPTOMS OF CONCUSSIONS

Acute	Late (Delayed)
Lightheadedness	Persistent low-grade headache
Delayed motor and/or verbal responses	Easy fatiguability
Memory or cognitive dysfunction	Sleep irregularities
Disorientation	Inability to perform daily activities
Amnesia	Depression/anxiety
Headache	Lethargy
Balance problems/incoordination	Memory dysfunction
Vertigo/dizziness	Lightheadedness
Concentration difficulties	Personality changes
Loss of consciousness	Low frustration tolerance/irritability
Blurred vision	Intolerance to bright lights, loud sounds
Vacant stare (befuddled facial expression)	
Photophobia	
Tinnitus	
Nausea	
Vomiting	
Increased emotionality	
Slurred or incoherent speech	

From Magee DJ: *Orthopedic physical assessment*, ed 4, Philadelphia, 2002, WB Saunders.

SIGNS AND SYMPTOMS OF CONCUSSION (TORG CLASSIFICATION)

	Grade 1	Grade 2	Grade 3	Grade 4	Grade 5
Confusion	None or momentary	Slight	Moderate	Severe	Severe
Amnesia	No	Posttraumatic amnesia <30 min	Posttraumatic amnesia <30 min	Posttraumatic amnesia >30 min	Posttraumatic amnesia >24 hours
			Retrograde amnesia	Retrograde amnesia	Retrograde amnesia
Residual symptoms	No	Perhaps	Sometimes	Yes	Yes
Loss of consciousness	No	No	No	Yes (<5 min)	Yes (>5 min)
Tinnitus	No	Mild	Moderate	Severe	Often severe
Dizziness	No	Mild	Moderate	Severe	Usually severe
Headache	No	May be present (dull)	Often	Often	Often
Disorientation and unsteadiness	None or minimal	Some	Moderate	Severe (5-10 min)	Often severe (>10 min)
Blurred vision	No	No	No	Not usually	Possible
Postconcussion syndrome	No	Possible	Possible	Possible	Possible
Personality changes	No	No	No	Possible	Possible

From Vegso, IJ and JS. Torg: Field evaluation and management of intracranial injuries. In Torg JS. *Athletic injuries to the head, neck and face.* St Louis, 1991, Mosby-Year Book, pp 226-227.

GUIDELINES FOR RETURNING TO SPORTS AFTER TRAUMATIC BRAIN INJURIES[159]

	First concussion	Second concussion	Third concussion
Grade 1 (transient confusion without loss of consciousness, resolves <15 min)	Return when asymptomatic for 15 min	Return when asymptomatic for 1 week	Return when asymptomatic for 1 month
Grade 2 (same as grade 1, resolves >15 min)	Return after a physician has examined and after asymptomatic for 1 week	Wait at least 2 weeks after asymptomatic. Consider terminating season	Return next season if asymptomatic
Grade 3 (any loss of consciousness)	Needs immediate medical examination, consider transport to emergency department. Wait at least 1 month, after which may return if asymptomatic for 1 week	Wait at least 2 weeks after asymptomatic. Consider waiting until next season.	Terminate the sport

*No headache, dizziness, or impairment of concentration or memory either at rest or with exertion.
From Kriel RL, Krach LA: Traumatic brain and spinal cord injuries in children. In Maria BL: *Current management in child neurology*, Boston, 1999, Blackwell Sciences.

Physical therapy intervention is critical to the overall management of the patient with SCI and is typically performed by neurologic PTs. Rehabilitation includes psychosocial adjustment, physical skills training appropriate to the level of injury (e.g., survival skills, bed mobility, transfers, locomotion), health maintenance, and vocational adjustments. Given the fact that most SCIs involve young people, caregiver and external long-term support will need to be established.[104,242]

Peripheral Nerve Injuries

Figure 12-9 shows the pathway of the peripheral nervous system (PNS) from spinal cord to muscle and the types of peripheral neurologic injuries (PNIs).[167] The more central the injury (i.e., closer to the spinal cord), the worse the prognosis. The PNS can be damaged by (1) disease (e.g., anterior-horn-cell degradation in poliomyelitis or ALS, demyelinating disease)[90]; (2) repetitive entrapment or compression syndromes (e.g., carpal tunnel syndrome, sciatica, thoracic outlet syndrome, double-crush syndromes); (3) tensile or traction injuries; and (4) trauma (e.g., lacerations, burns, or adolescent sports-related injury).[104,240,241]

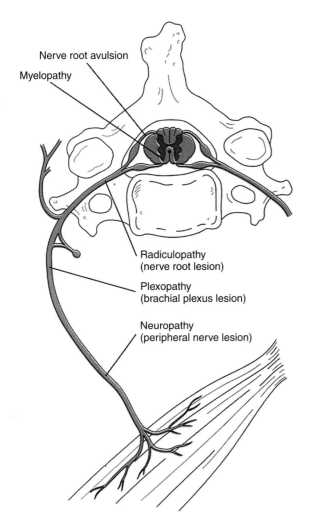

FIGURE 12-9 PNS lesions: Path of neurologic tissue from spinal cord to muscles, showing sites of neurologic lesions. (From Magee DJ: *Orthopedic physical assessment*, ed 4, Philadelphia, 2002, WB Saunders, p 20.)

Nerve root avulsion
Myelopathy
Radiculopathy (nerve root lesion)
Plexopathy (brachial plexus lesion)
Neuropathy (peripheral nerve lesion)

BRACHIAL PLEXUS INJURIES ("BURNERS" AND "STINGERS"). Whereas neonatal brachial plexus injuries (BPIs) occur at a rate of 0.5 to 2.5 per 1000 live births,[251] 2.2% of U.S. football players suffer BPIs per year.[19] About 50% of all collegiate football players have sustained a *stinger*. Of these, 30% suffered their first BPI while playing high-school football. Participants in other contact sports such as wrestling, rugby, and hockey also are susceptible to this neurovascular injury.[7] BPIs also can be caused by repetitive trauma (carrying a backpack that is too heavy), macrotrauma (car accidents), or incidental injuries (cradling a telephone under the neck while reaching for something). The aforementioned activities all apply to the adolescent population.

The signs and symptoms of acute BPI are immediate, sharp, burning or stinging pain that radiates from the clavicular region down the involved upper extremity, associated numbness, and tingling or weakness of the arm ("flail arm") that may last for a few seconds to several minutes to months.[7,241] The musculature of the proximal upper trunk of the brachial plexus (C5 and C6) is most often involved (e.g., the deltoid, rotator cuff, biceps), and rarely the brachioradialis, supinator, and pronator teres (C5, C6, and C7) are involved. True neck pain should not appear with this injury, and if it is present, one should suspect a cervical-spine injury. Bilateral upper extremity burning should be considered a major red flag for a significant cervical spine injury, and the victim should be treated with spinal precautions (i.e., cervical spine immobilization via spine board).[241,255]

BPIs are classified by the degree or length of motor weakness. The worst possible scenario involves a proximal-nerve-root avulsion, axonotmesis, or neurotmesis (see Fig. 12-9). The most common level of nerve root avulsion is C7, characterized by frank elbow extension weakness.[7] In severe cases, a concomitant Horner's syndrome, caused by disruption of the sympathetic nerve fibers, can be seen on the affected side. The classic signs are a drooping eyelid (ptosis), constricted pupil (miosis), and lack of sweat (anhidrosis) on the affected side. This situation is also a medical emergency.[265]

Many professionals in sports medicine believe that a physician should examine *all* athletes after their first stinger, and that a complete cervical radiograph series should be taken.[7,240,241,265] The greatest concern is the presence of a Torg ratio (size of the vertebral canal relative to the vertebral body) of less than 0.80. Those with a Torg score less than 0.80 are three times more likely to suffer recurrent BPIs, especially if the mechanism of injury is extension-compression of the cervical spine.[240,241,265]

Sports-specific treatment for BPIs includes strengthening of the neck and shoulder-girdle musculature, proper sports techniques (heads-up tackling, avoidance of spearing), protective equipment (neck-rolls and built-up or elevated shoulder pads), and prohibition of contact if there is persistent strength loss. Return to normal sports is allowed when the athlete demonstrates normal strength and endurance in the affected shoulder.[241]

Fractures: Discontinuity of Osseous and/or Cartilaginous Structures

Fractures constitute a low 5% to 6% of all musculoskeletal sports-related injuries. Most adolescent fractures occur in the extremities. Rarely are the skull and spine fractured, and forceful hyperextension represents the most common mechanism of adolescent spinal fracture (e.g., spondylolysis with or without spondylolisthesis).

A *fracture*, whether of a bone, an epiphyseal plate, or a cartilaginous joint surface, is simply a *structural break in continuity*.[221] A fracture will always produce some degree of concomitant soft tissue injury (e.g., pain, tenderness, deformity, edema, ecchymosis) and loss of mobility and function.[104,113,185] The extent of injury depends on several factors, including: (1) type of bone fractured (cortical or cancellous), (2) location within the skeleton (intra-articular, extra-articular, or at a growth zone), (3) type of load (tension, compression, bending, shear, torsion, or combined loading), (4) amount and frequency of load (stress-strain or fatigue-curve of the structure), (5) metabolic and disease status of the bone, and (6) overall fitness level and age of the individual.[104,113,174,185,211]

A bending force on a long bone causes a compressive failure on the concave side of the bone and an explosive tension failure (e.g., transverse or oblique fracture) on the convex side. In children and young adolescents, cortical bone is much more pliable (like green wood in a living young tree), and bending moments tend to create one of three incomplete fractures: greenstick, plastic bowing, or torus (buckling) fracture (Fig. 12-10).

A twisting (torsional, rotational) force creates a spiraling tension fracture in long bones. Shear loads in children can create severe epiphyseal-growth-plate injuries, avulsion fractures, or ligamentous injuries depending on skeletal maturity. A fracture that involves the articular cartilage of a joint is called an intra-articular fracture. The radiographic method used most often for the classification of pediatric epiphyseal fractures is the *modified Salter-Harris classification system* (Box 12-6). Because 15% to 20% of pediatric fractures involve the epiphyseal region, up to one in five children has the potential for interrupted growth if these injuries go undetected.[174]

Fracture Management

Medical management of fracture depends on: (1) location of the fracture, (2) type of fracture, (3) need for reduction, (4) presence of instability after reduction, (5) extent of concomitant connective or neurovascular injury, and (6) functional requirements of the injured patient.[36,78,104,220] Fracture reduction is achieved through either closed-reduction (e.g., traction, reduction, and immobilization) or open-reduction methods. Surgical intervention (open reduction) includes bone grafts or bone substitutes (e.g., ceramic materials), internal fixation (e.g., metal plating, wiring, screws), or external fixation (e.g., Ilizarov external fixator). With or without surgical intervention, after bone fracture a period of immobilization usually is employed to prevent longitudinal or shear stresses. Failure to stabilize the fracture site can result in pain, nonunion, or malunion.

Fractures in children usually heal in 4 to 6 weeks; in adolescents in 6 to 8 weeks; and in adults in 10 to 18 weeks.[78,104] Many factors, both local and systemic, affect healing. Local factors include type, size, and location of fracture, postinjury infection or retained foreign body, movement or excessive pressure that compromises local blood supply, and electromagnetic energy or ultrasound (used when physicians anticipate healing problems).[46,78,104] Systemic factors affecting healing include age, metabolic status, general health (e.g., presence of comorbid conditions, medications that impede healing), nutrition, and avoidance of substances that inhibit bone formation (e.g., nicotine, corticosteroids, alcohol).[46,78,104]

Osseous Overuse Injuries

Osseous stress fractures and ligament-bone disruptions caused by continual overuse of a joint are fairly common in adolescents.[185] The main symptom of a stress fracture is pain. Initial x-rays often do not reveal signs of a stress fracture, and radionuclide bone scan is the most sensitive and specific

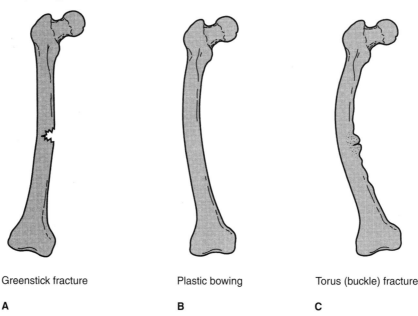

Greenstick fracture

Plastic bowing

Torus (buckle) fracture

A   **B**   **C**

FIGURE 12-10 A-C, Classification of incomplete fractures often seen in children. (From McKinnis LN: *Fundamentals of orthopedic radiology*, Philadelphia, 1997, FA Davis, p 82.)

BOX 12-6

Modified Salter-Harris Classification System for Epiphyseal Fractures

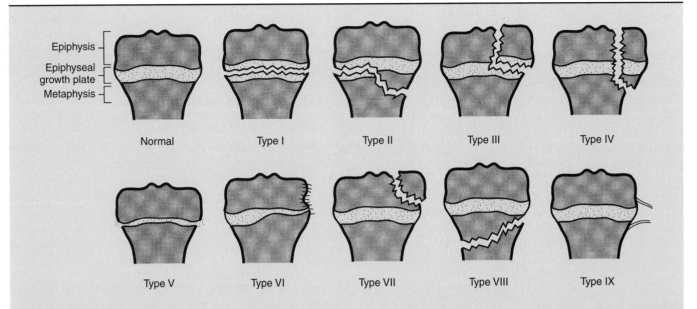

Epiphysis
Epiphyseal growth plate
Metaphysis

Normal   Type I   Type II   Type III   Type IV

Type V   Type VI   Type VII   Type VIII   Type IX

Type I: The fracture line extends through the physis, separating and displacing the epiphysis from the normal position. This is common in younger children and is associated with birth injuries. Prognosis is good for normal growth.

Type II: The fracture line extends through the physis and exits through the metaphysis, creating a triangular wedge of metaphysis that displaces with the epiphysis. This is the most common type and occurs most often in children over 10 years of age. Prognosis is good for normal growth.

Type III: The fracture line extends from the joint surface through the epiphysis and across the physis, resulting in a portion of the epiphysis becoming displaced. Partial growth arrest is a possibility, and surgical fixation is warranted.

Type IV: The fracture line extends from the joint surface through the epiphysis, physis, and metaphysis, resulting in one fracture fragment. Partial growth arrest is possible, and surgical fixation is necessary.

Type V: The fracture is a crush-type injury that damages the physis by compression forces. It is difficult to diagnose this injury in acute stages. Eventual growth arrest may be the only clue that this injury has occurred. Two nontraumatic causes of this type of injury are infection and epiphyseal avascular necrosis, which may cause dissolution of cartilage cells with resultant growth arrest.

Rang's type VI: This injury involves the *perichondral ring* or the associated periosteum of the physis. While little or no damage occurs directly to the physes, the reparative process at the periosteum may cause an osseous bridge to develop between the metaphysis and the epiphysis, arresting growth and leading to angular deformity.

Ogden's type VII, VIII, and IX: These fractures do not directly involve the physis but may later disrupt growth. Type VII is an osteochondral fracture of the articular portion of the epiphysis, type VIII is a fracture of the metaphysis, and type IX is an avulsion fracture of the periosteum.

From McKinnis LN: *Fundamentals of orthopedic radiology*, Philadelphia, 1997, FA Davis, p 84.

---

test.[25,164,185,211] Nearly all (95%) stress fractures are in the lower extremity. Jumping and impact-loading athletes in their late teens are most susceptible. The incidence of stress fracture is tibia (33% to 66%), metatarsals (0% to 35%), fibula, and proximal femur.[25] Normally, 6 to 8 weeks (range, 2 to 24 weeks) of relative rest (rest from impact but not training) is required to heal stress fractures adequately. During this time, contributing factors (inflexibility, proximal weakness [gluteus medius, quadriceps], and overpronation) should be addressed before the patient begins a graduated return to activity.[15,16,24,60,231]

Because of their biomechanical make-up and relationship to external loads, the developing peripheral joints are particularly susceptible to overuse injury.[8,161,166,184,185] The most susceptible pediatric joints and potential differential diagnoses are displayed in Figures 12-11 (knee), 12-12 (ankle), and 12-13 (elbow).[166] The increase in physeal injuries during adolescence is believed to be due to biomechanical and structural weakness of the physeal cartilage during this stage of rapid musculoskeletal growth. Long-bone growth surges, muscle inflexibility, and increases in muscle mass and torque-generating capacity of

muscle (because of the surge in testosterone), may explain why there are so many growth-plate injuries. Young boys incur more physeal injuries as a result of four developmental factors: (1) males have a greater propensity for impact sports, (2) males have a higher overall rate of traumatic injury, (3) males have a greater percentage of increase in muscle mass, and (4) male growth plates remain open longer than those of girls.[174]

Apophysitis, or posttraumatic avulsion of the traction epiphysis, is a benign but annoying malady affecting the growing skeletons of active youngsters.[7] The symptoms of these growth-plate conditions usually begin at 8 to 15 years of age. Clinical features of apophysitis include: activity-related pain and swelling at the insertion site, associated loss of flexibility resulting from pain or secondary to growth spurts, reflex inhibition of the muscle secondary to pain and swelling, and functional limitations specific to the joint. The pain usually does not awaken the adolescent at night. The tenderness is well localized, and there are no other significant abnormalities of the joint.[164,166]

Osgood-Schlatter's disease is a partial avulsion of the patellar ligament at the tibial tubercle. It is most common in boys

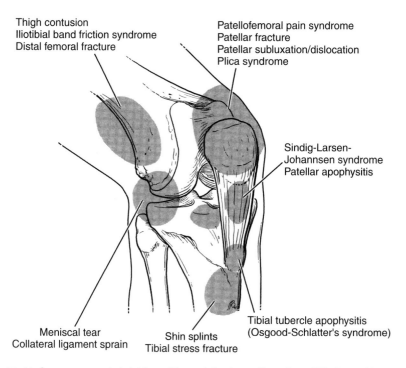

FIGURE 12-11 Common musculoskeletal conditions of the knee. (From Lyon RM, Street CC: Pediatric sports injuries, *Pediatr Clin North Am* 45:221-244, 1998.)

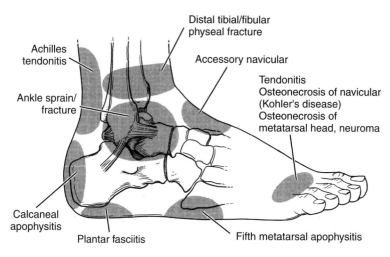

FIGURE 12-12 Common musculoskeletal conditions of the ankle. (From Lyon RM, Street CC: Pediatric sports injuries, *Pediatr Clin North Am* 45:221-244, 1998.)

10 to 15 years of age and girls 10 to 11 years of age, with a boy/girl ratio of 3:1. Like all osteochondroses, activity-related anterior knee pain is the presenting problem (e.g., kneeling, direct blow, forceful quadriceps contraction). Radiographs (AP and lateral) show irregular tibial tuberosity (fragmentation) and are necessary to rule out tumor. Treatment consists of activity modification (rest), stretching, quadriceps strengthening, ice, iontophoresis, knee orthoses, and taping for comfort. While usually self-limiting (heals in less than 2 years), débridement of avulsion bone fragments is sometimes required.[164,266]

Sindig-Larsen-Johannsen disease is a partial avulsion of the inferior pole of the patella and is most common in boys age 10 to 15 years. No long-term disability is expected, and treatment is for symptoms only (see treatment of Osgood-Schlatter's disease).[164]

Sever's disease is a partial avulsion of the calcaneal apophysis. It is characterized by posterior heel pain (possibly bilateral), tenderness and swelling at the insertion of the Achilles, and calcaneal-gait deviation (poor control of tibial advancement in midstance). It is most common in girls of 5 to 10 years of age and often seen in boys of 10 to 12 years. Radiographs are *not* diagnostic. Usually self-limiting (heals in less than 1 year), Sever's disease responds to rest, ice, stretching of 1-joint and 2-joint plantar flexors, iontophoresis, and 1-cm heel lift to reduce stress on the tendon insertion.[164]

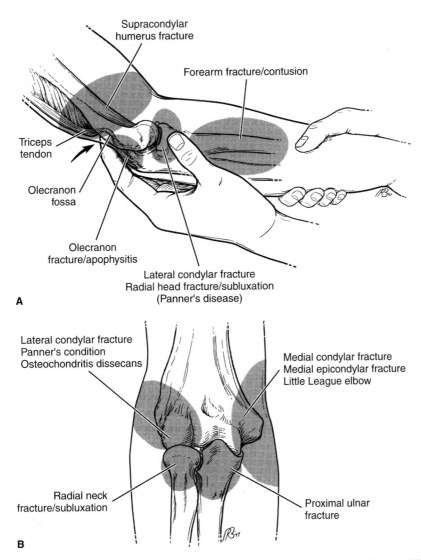

FIGURE 12-13 A and **B,** Common musculoskeletal conditions of the elbow. (From Lyon RM, Street CC: Pediatric sports injuries, *Pediatr Clin North Am* 45:221-244, 1998.)

Sudden onset of anterior or posterior hip pain is most common in older adolescents and males more than females. Ballistic trauma (usually from sprinting) can cause avulsion of the rectus femoris at the anterior inferior iliac spine (AIIS) or a traction injury of the hamstring origin at the ischial tuberosity. For acute treatment, these injuries respond best to rest, ice, and gentle stretching of the involved one-joint and two-joint hip muscles. Postinjury strengthening is crucial after the initial healing phase. An elastic hip spica orthosis or neoprene sleeve to warm tissues and bias (protect) the muscle of interest also can offer the athlete postinjury protection.[164] Long-term care of *all* lower-extremity injuries should include proximal stabilization exercises (abdominals, gluteal musculature, and quadriceps) to create muscular balance to control lower kinetic chain forces. Foot orthoses also may be indicated to control ground reaction forces.[7,79,220] Neural mobilization techniques may be indicated for chronic conditions.

Pain and inability to extend the elbow fully after a trivial injury or repetitive microtrauma in boys 5 to 10 years old (boys more than girls) could be *Panner's disease*. Radiographs are diagnostic, and rest via a sling and restriction of strenuous activity for the elbow are critical. If repetitive elbow trauma continues, a true osteochondritis dissecans of the elbow can develop (usually in early teen years; boys more than girls). If a fragment of bone from the capitellum loses its blood supply, loosens, and becomes a loose body in the joint, surgery often is required to correct the problem. Radiographs are diagnostic, and strict rest via a sling and avoidance of *all* strenuous activity for the elbow are essential to prevent long-term dysfunction (loss of elbow extension).

Overhand-throwing athletes (boys more than girls) occasionally develop a stress fracture of the proximal humeral epiphysis (Little Leaguer's shoulder). This condition must be differentiated from the many impingement-related conditions that can occur about the shoulder (rotator-cuff tendonitis, biceps tendonitis, multidirectional instability, bursitis). Radiographs are diagnostic. Rest is essential for healing of stress fractures and to prevent further damage.

Most adolescent shoulder and elbow overuse injuries are self-limiting and respond well to relative rest (avoidance of the precipitating mechanism), ice, and analgesics (acetaminophen or NSAIDs), followed by a comprehensive rehabilitation program.[23] The best way to prevent upper extremity (UE) overuse injuries is to strengthen proximal musculature (scapular stabilizers) and core body muscles (abdominals and hip extensors and abductors).[70,138,147,257,258] Learning proper pitching technique, avoiding specialty pitches at a young age, and limiting the number of pitches (less than 350 per week) allowed in Little League baseball is crucial.[23,138,257-259]

Connective Tissue Injuries

A comprehensive list of common lower-extremity (LE) and upper extremity (UE) musculoskeletal injuries in the adolescent is presented in Tables 12-14 (LE) and 12-15 (UE). Integument and soft tissue injuries (contusions) represent minor sports injuries that occur more often in physical-education classes and free-play sports than in organized team sports. For the most part, little time is lost from sports or general activities as a result of these injuries.[7] Injuries to other connective tissues (e.g., ligaments, tendons, menisci, and articular cartilage) of the maturing skeleton, however, can constitute a more serious injury, with potential long-term consequences if improperly managed.

Integument Injuries (Lacerations and Abrasions)

When tissue injury has occurred, basic goals of wound management include: (1) protecting the wound and surrounding tissue from additional trauma; (2) reducing strain on the tissues near the wound; (3) protecting the tissue in the area of the wound from mechanical stress or movement; (4) reducing the number of pathogenic microorganisms in and around the wound; (5) expediting the healing process; and (6) reducing the formation of scar tissue.[81,151,191]

All open wounds run the risk of contamination from the environment. Likewise, the presence of blood necessitates the use of universal precautions to protect the health care provider and other persons in the vicinity of the injury from blood.[149,191] Universal precautions are the use of barriers such as gloves, gowns, masks, and eyewear when working with blood and other potentially infectious material (i.e., any and all body fluids, secretions, and excretions, except sweat) that pose the risk of bloodborne pathogens (e.g., human immunodeficiency virus [HIV], hepatitis B, and hepatitis C).[191] Young athletes and parents should be reassured that to date there have been no reported cases of HIV transmission in football, basketball, or wrestling, where abrasions are common.[149]

Contusions

Contusions (bruises) are the most common sports injury and rarely cause a student-athlete to be sidelined.[8] Contusions also are a common consequence of non–sports-related accidents (e.g., vehicular accidents, falls). A contusion occurs when blunt trauma causes bleeding in the underlying muscle or other soft tissues. No break occurs in the skin, and ecchymosis develops in the area.[116] Contusions may be graded as mild, moderate, or severe. If the range of motion (ROM) in the adjacent joint is two thirds that of normal, the contusion is considered mild.

TABLE 12-14

Common Lower-Extremity (Hip, Thigh, Knee, Lower Leg, Ankle, and Foot) Injuries in the Adolescent[7,166,174,220]

General Category	Specific Entities, Proximal LE	Specific Entities, Knee	Specific Entities, Lower Leg, Ankle, and Foot
Instability	Sacroiliac joint (SIJ) instability	Patellar subluxation/dislocation	Ankle mortise dislocation and/or dislocation of any of the foot/toe joints
Ligamentous and/or capsular injury at the joint of interest	Pubic symphysis instability	Femoral-tibial subluxation/ dislocation (with associated ligamentous damage)	Ligamentous sprain (key ligaments of the ankle: anterior talo-fibular (ATF), posterior talo-fibular (PTF), calcaneo-fibular (CF), and deltoid)
	Hip dislocation	Ligamentous sprain (key ligaments of the knee: ACL, MCL, PCL, and LCL)	Tendon rupture (e.g., Achilles, tibialis posterior)
		Tendon rupture (hamstrings, patellar tendon/ligament rupture)	
Impingement and/or nerve injuries	Hip labrum impingement (rare)	Peroneal nerve entrapment (complication of short leg casting)	Tarsal tunnel syndrome (tibial nerve)
	Lumbosacral plexus injuries from trauma		Nerve entrapment at the ankle retinaculum status post (s/p) trauma (peroneal, sural, or tibial branches)
	Lumbar radiculopathy from HNP (rare in adolescents)	Fat pad impingement	
		Plica syndrome	
	Piriformis syndrome		

TABLE 12-14

Common Lower-Extremity (Hip, Thigh, Knee, Lower Leg, Ankle, and Foot) Injuries in the Adolescent[7,166,174,220]—cont'd

Fractures	Pelvis (ischium, ilium, and pubis, and acetabular fractures) Sacrum Intracapsular (e.g., femoral head, subcapital and femoral-neck fractures) Extracapsular (e.g., intertrochanteric, subtrochanteric, and femoral-shaft fractures) Apophyseal avulsion fractures Iliac crest: abdominals ASIS: sartorius AIIS: rectus femoris Ischial tuberosity hamstrings	Distal femoral-shaft fractures Supracondylar fractures (e.g., displaced, nondisplaced, impacted, comminuted, condylar, and intercondylar) Tibial avulsion fracture (mimics ACL instability) Patellar fractures (e.g., vertical, transverse, comminuted, or avulsion, all of which can be displaced and nondisplaced) Tibial plateau fractures (described on the Hohl classification system as type I-VI) Fractures of the proximal fibula Osteochondritis dissecans (OCD)	Bimalleolar and trimalleolar fractures, including a *Tillaux fracture* (juvenile triplane fracture with intraarticular anterolateral ankle mortise fracture) Calcaneus fractures (Rowe classification system type I-V) Talus fractures (described by location, i.e., body, dome, neck, or head) Navicular fracture Tarsometatarsal (LisFranc) Metatarsal and phalangeal fractures
Soft tissue injuries (including overuse)	Muscle strain/tendonitis (any muscle about the hip) Contusion with potential complication of myositis ossificans (quads) Delayed-onset muscle soreness (DOMS) of the proximal thigh musculature	Muscle strain/tendonitis (any muscle about the hip) Patellar tendon/ligament "tendonitis" Meniscus tears (e.g., vertical, horizontal, cleavage, bucket-handle) ITB tendonitis (runner's knee) Osgood-Schlatter's disease (jumper's knee) Sindig-Larsen-Johanssen disease Patello-femoral pain syndrome (PFPS)	Tibialis anterior and posterior tendonitis ("shin splints") Achilles tendonitis Sever's disease Plantar fasciitis Contusions of the foot/toes Nail bed injuries Compartment syndrome
Referred pain	L-spine and knee referral (one joint above and below the joint of interest) GI system referral Reproductive-system referral Urinary-system referral	Lumbar spine, pelvis, hip referral to the knee	Lumbar spine, pelvis, hip, and knee referral to the LLAF
Other	Degenerative joint disease (hip) Rheumatoid arthritis (hip) Avascular necrosis of the hip Slipped femoral capital epiphysis Congenital dislocation of the hip	Degenerative joint disease (knee) Rheumatoid arthritis (knee)	Degenerative joint disease (ankle) Rheumatoid arthritis (ankle) Gout (rare in children)

Rehabilitation note: The PRICE principle is the focus of acute injury management. During the inflammatory phase of healing (days 0-6), connective-tissue injuries should be treated with edema control, icing, and protection (i.e., motion control). Weight bearing with an orthosis (brace or taping) is allowed as tolerated (as long as the athlete does *not* have a limp). Athletes should use assistive devices when and if a normal gait pattern cannot be tolerated. Protected motion with progressive strengthening and closed-kinetic-chain balance training are advanced individually, with return to sports allowed as early as a few days to 4 weeks for lesser sprains. Protection of ruptured ligaments during the first 3 weeks (proliferation phase) to 6 weeks (maturation phase) is crucial for optimal stabilization.[220] Strengthening and balance programs (i.e., closed-kinetic-chain training), impact loading, and sport-specific training are recommended for optimal return to sport function.[234] Prophylactic use of braces for ankle injuries is useful but controversial for the knee joint.[49,155,220,232,234,265,266]

TABLE 12-15

Common Upper-Extremity (Shoulder, Elbow, Wrist, and Hand) Injuries in the Adolescent[7,23,166,174]

General Category	Specific Entities, Shoulder	Specific Entities, Elbow	Specific Entities, Wrist and Hand
Instability	SC joint instability	Radial head subluxation/dislocation	Triangular fibrocartilage complex (TFCC)
	AC joint instability	Ulnar collateral ligament tear	Collateral ligaments of the PIP proximal interphalangeal (PIP) and distal interphalangeal (DIP) joints
	GH dislocation/ subluxation		Ulnar collateral ligaments of the thumb
	GH unidirectional, bidirectional, and multidirectional instability (MDI)		Dislocations of the fingers and thumb
	Labral tears		
Impingement and/or nerve injuries	Rotator-cuff tendonitis	Cubital-tunnel syndrome (ulnar nerve)	Carpal-tunnel syndrome (median nerve)
	Biceps tendonitis		De Quervain's tenosynovitis
	Subacromial bursitis	Pronator teres syndrome (median nerve)	Guyon tunnel syndrome (ulnar nerve)
	Impingement: primary or secondary caused by multidirectional instability (MDI)	Ligament of Struthers (median nerve)	Gymnast wrist
	Brachial plexus injury (BPI)	Radial-tunnel syndrome: arcade of Frohse in the supinator (posterior interosseous branch of the radial nerve)	
Fractures	Clavicle (described by location and including physeal fracture)	Distal fractures of the humerus (supracondylar, transcondylar, intercondylar, condylar, articular, and epicondylar classifications)	Distal radius/ulna (Colles' fracture)
			Scaphoid (vulnerable blood supply)
	Humerus: proximal shaft, neck, or avulsion fracture of tuberosity		Hook of the hamate
		Olecranon fractures (extraarticular and intraarticular groups)	Metacarpal fractures (head, neck, shaft, or base)
	Scapula: rare; glenoid labrum rim fracture associated with traumatic GH dislocation	Radial head (Mason classification types I-IV)	Bennett's fracture: intra-articular avulsion fracture and subluxation of the base of the first metacarpal
			Rolando's fracture: comminuted fracture of the base of first metacarpal
		Radial and ulnar shaft (Monteggia's, Galeazzi's, and Colles' fractures)	Phalangeal fractures (stable, unstable, or intraarticular)
		Osteochondritis dissecans (OCD) of the elbow	Mallet finger (avulsion of the extensor tendon of the distal phalanx)
		Panner's disease	Jersey finger (rupture of the flexor digitorum profundus; ring finger most often)
Soft tissue injuries (overuse)	Contusion (watch for complication of myositis ossificans in the biceps brachii)	Tennis elbow (lateral epicondylitis)	Nail bed injuries
		Golfer's elbow (medial epicondylitis)	Subungual hematoma
	Muscle strain		Contusion
	Brachial plexus injuries	Olecranon bursitis (and/or infection)	
	Peripheral nerve injuries		
	Delayed-onset muscle soreness (DOMS)		

TABLE 12-15

Common Upper-Extremity (Shoulder, Elbow, Wrist, and Hand) Injuries in the Adolescent[7,23,166,174]—cont'd

General Category	Specific Entities, Shoulder	Specific Entities, Elbow	Specific Entities, Wrist and Hand
Referred pain	C-spine and elbow referral (one joint above and below the joint of interest)	Cervical spine, shoulder, and wrist/hand referral to the elbow	Cervical spine, shoulder, and elbow referral to the wrist/hand
	Cardiac and pulmonary referral		
	GI referral Gallbladder to right shoulder Spleen to left shoulder		
Other	Thoracic-outlet syndrome	Arterial injuries (Volkmann's ischemia as a complication of peri-elbow fracture)	Swan-neck deformity (PIP joint hyperextension with metacarpophalangeal (MCP) and DIP flexion caused by rupture of the volar plate)
			Boutonnière deformity (extension of the MCP and DIP and flexion of the PIP caused by rupture of the central tendinous slip of the extensor hood)
			Rheumatoid arthritis

Rehabilitation note: Proximal stability is a prerequisite for distal mobility and UE function. Full active and passive range-of-motion and joint mobility are imperative. Joint mobilization can be useful in gating pain (grades I and II) or in stretching (grades III, IV, and V [thrust]) contributory joint-hypomobility dysfunction.[258] Scapulohumeral rhythm must be restored. Suggested scapulothoracic muscles to target include: serratus anterior, all fibers of the trapezius, levator scapulae, rhomboids, latissimus dorsi, and pectoralis major and minor. Rotator-cuff and arm/forearm exercises also are advocated.[138,147,138,257,258] Closed-kinetic-chain (proprioceptive) exercises should be incorporated (pushups with emphasis on protracting scapula). The objective of a kinesthetic rehabilitation program is to facilitate the shoulder's performance of a complicated skill without conscious guidance.[70] Gradual return to functional activity via a variety of interval training programs is warranted for any of these UE injuries. Finally, improper technique, insufficient conditioning, or unsafe biomechanical practices must be addressed. Weakness, inflexibility, and poor proprioceptive control (lack of skill) in the lower quarter and/or trunk also can be contributory in sports that require repetitive overhead activity (e.g., throwing and racquet sports).

One third to two thirds of normal ROM constitutes a moderate contusion, while less than one third is classified as severe.[95] Prompt treatment for contusion, and indeed *all* connective-tissue injuries, incorporates the PRICE principle.[7,36,46,116,158,265]

P   Protect the injured part (may include protective orthoses or assistive devices)
R   Rest the injured part
I   Ice application during the inflammation phase of injury
C   Compression with elastic bandages to minimize soft tissue bleeding and edema
E   Elevation of the injured part

Myositis ossificans (MO), or the formation of heterotopic bone within muscle, can be a complication of severe or poorly managed contusions.[116,158,265] In adolescent athletes, common sites for contusion and MO are the quadriceps and biceps brachii muscle bellies. Warning signs of severe contusion include a marked decrease in range of motion, significant pain, a sympathetic associated joint effusion, and decreased function (loss of weight-bearing or anti-gravity muscle force production). If after several days of PRICE treatment a palpable mass develops at the site of injury, one should suspect myositis ossificans. Initial radiographs will be negative. Bone scintigraphy, magnetic resonance imaging (MRI), and ultrasonography have been reported to reveal myositis ossificans before it is visible on conventional plain radiographs, but the utility of these techniques for early cases has yet to be confirmed.[118,154,158,222]

After 3 to 6 weeks, radiographs will reveal any heterotopic ossification, typically deep within the muscle and adjacent to the bone.[158]

Larson et al[158] describe three phases for the treatment of muscle contusions (and myositis ossificans). Phase I consists of pain control through (1) rest, compression, cooling, and elevation algorithm for 24 to 48 hours regardless of injury severity (avoid or limit direct application of ice over superficial nerves to avoid potential injury); (2) positioning of the extremity so that the injured muscle is held out to length without additional pain; (3) 2 to 6 weeks of naproxen (750 mg qd) or indomethacin (50 mg bid) for moderate and severe contusions, and (4) analgesics such as acetaminophen (or hospitalization as needed) for pain control. Corticosteroids should be avoided, but nonsteroidal antiinflammatory drugs may reduce edema and the risk of heterotopic bone formation.[130,152,158,249,250]

Phase II encompasses restoration of mobility via gentle active and passive range-of-motion exercises with a focus on regaining flexion. Rehabilitation protocols that include early flexion exercise can hasten recovery and reduce the likelihood of myositis ossificans.[158] The patient initiates low-intensity exercise in functional movement patterns (e.g., walking, biking, upper-body ergometer, aquatic activities) during the second phase of healing. Compression wraps are advocated to stabilize the muscle and improve comfort of the athlete.

Phase III consists of functional rehabilitation (i.e., sports-specific activity). Protective padding is recommend for the injured muscle for 3 to 6 months after the injury.[158]

Rehabilitation typically is not altered if myositis ossificans develops. If the disorder persists but remains asymptomatic, as is most common, no additional treatment is needed. Excision of the heterotopic bone is advocated if the mass is symptomatic with continued muscle atrophy, limited joint motion, and pain after conservative treatment. Bone scan must confirm that the lesion is mature (usually 6 to 12 months) before excision. After excision, NSAIDs (naproxen or indomethacin) should be taken for 6 weeks to inhibit bone growth, and patients should follow the three-step recovery protocol described earlier.[158,220]

Strains: Disorders of Contractile Tissue

Contractile tissue (i.e., the musculotendinous unit) is composed of four elements: muscle, musculotendinous junction (MTJ), tendon, and the tendon's interface with the bone. A strain is an injury (a partial or complete tear) to any portion of the musculotendinous unit, from an abrupt, excessive, or repeated muscle contraction that exceeds the tissue's tensile capability. The transition zones, tendon insertion (traction epiphysis or apophysis) and MTJ, are most susceptible to injury. Strains, like ligamentous sprains, are classified as mild (grade I), moderate (grade II), or severe (grade III).[36,46,104,116,167] Clinical findings include pain, edema, loss of motion, tenderness upon palpation, protective muscle spasm or cramping, and possible weakness.

MTJ injuries are diagnosed by active or resistive contraction of the muscle (i.e., Cyriax's[65] resisted motions in neutral [RMIN] classification system), passive elongation (stretching of the muscle), and palpation.[46,65,164,167] Radiographic imaging of muscle strain in adolescents is essential to rule out avulsion fractures.[222]

Contact or ballistic sports such as soccer, football, hockey, boxing, wrestling, and track put people at risk for strains. Gymnastics, tennis, rowing, golf, and other sports that require extensive gripping can increase the risk of hand, forearm, and elbow strains. Strains of both the upper and lower extremity sometimes occur in children and adolescents who lack proximal stability and kinesthetic control to participate in repetitive overhead activity (e.g., racquet sports, volleyball, baseball) or repetitive lower quarter impact-loading sports (e.g., basketball, soccer, track).[7]

Sprains: Disorders of Ligaments or Joint Capsules

Ligaments and joint capsules connect bone to bone, stabilize joints, restrict and guide joint movement, and allow for conscious kinesthesia.[113,161,184] Signs and symptoms of sprain include the sound or feeling of a "pop" when the injury occurs, the feeling that a joint is "loose" or unstable, an inability to bear weight because of pain, loss of motion, and joint swelling with possible reflex muscle inhibition and loss of function.[7,116,167,185] The American Academy of Orthopedic Surgeons (AAOS) classifies sprains on a three-point scale.[116]

- Grade I (mild) sprains occur when fibers are stretched without loss of continuity (i.e., damaged microscopically via intrasubstance rupture of cross-links).

- Grade II (moderate) sprains result when some fibers are stretched and some are torn (i.e., plastic deformation has occurred on the stress-strain curve). These tears produce some joint laxity and often are very painful given the fact that the remaining fibers and related soft tissues experience more stress because of the resultant joint instability.

- Grade III (severe) sprains are a complete or nearly complete ligament rupture with resultant joint laxity, associated joint effusion, reflex inhibition, and loss of function.[116,185] After the initial injury, grade III sprains may not produce pain, as the ligaments and their stretch-sensitive receptors can no longer transmit noxious mechanical signals to the sensory cortex.

Disorders of Fibrocartilage

Three types of fibrocartilage (FC) are found in the body: (1) white (menisci, intervertebral disks (IVD), glenoid labrum, acetabular labrum, and pubic symphysis), (2) yellow (ears and epiglottis), and (3) hyaline articular cartilage.[161] The healing potential of FC depends on age, extent of injury, potential blood supply, and, for articular cartilage, nutrition via low-compressive-load joint movement.[38,42,100]

The most pertinent FC structures include the knee menisci, shoulder glenoid labrum, and hyaline cartilage of all synovial joints. A report of locking or clicking with movement, joint effusion, loss of active and passive range of motion, springy block end-feel, joint line pain, and positive special tests implicates FC injury.[135,153,163,175,187,221] MRI is the diagnostic imaging tool of choice for FC injuries.[174] Plain radiographs may expose joint effusion, but they will not expose muscle, fat pads, fat lines, joint capsules and ligaments, periosteum, and menisci like MRI will, especially given the confusion of the epiphyseal growth plates in the immature skeleton.[104,167,174,220]

Knee meniscal injuries in children younger than 10 years of age are rare, and indeed children under the age of 15 account for only 5% of all meniscal injuries.[42,174,229] In late adolescence (15 to 19 years), decreased vascularity and resiliency of the knee menisci coupled with increased sports participation make meniscal injuries a common occurrence.[42,220,229]

In the 13- to 18-year-old group, nearly 50% of all knee injuries involve the menisci.[42,94] Medial meniscus injuries are more common (88%) because of the medial meniscocapsular junction and the stress of closed-kinetic-chain pronation during pivoting and cutting activities. Thirty-six percent of patients also display a concomitant ACL injury. In children, longitudinal tears parallel to the periphery account for 50% to 90% of meniscus tears.[94] The lateral meniscus is more prone to injury if the developmental abnormality often called a *discoid meniscus* is present. An abnormally wide lateral radiographic joint space is evident on the AP knee projection if discoid meniscus is present.[174]

The long-term health of synovial joints depends on FC tissues.[38,107,220] The patient's age, site of injury, and blood supply (e.g., white zone [inner third], red-white zone [middle third], and red zone [outer third]) dictate whether selective resection (partial meniscectomy) or meniscal repair is performed.[107,220] The October and November 1998 issues of the *Journal of*

Orthopedic and Sports Physical Therapy (JOSPT) are an excellent resource on the surgical interventions for articular cartilage (e.g., débridement, abrasion chondroplasty, autologous osteochondral transplantation [OATS], autologous chondrocyte implantation, and total joint replacement). Gross ligamentous instability or directional instability resulting from weak musculature must be surgically addressed before or in conjunction with fibrocartilaginous repair or transplant. Use of continuous passive-motion devices, unweighting systems, and aquatic therapy is advocated for the treatment of articular cartilage, meniscus, and other lower-kinetic-chain injuries that require selective weight-bearing progression.[100,113,116,137,184,185]

Lower Quarter Musculoskeletal Injuries

Lower quarter musculoskeletal injuries (see Table 12-14) can be the result of macrotrauma or microtrauma. Proximal injuries (i.e., pelvic ring, hip, and femur) typically are the result of high-energy trauma (e.g., motor vehicle or bicycle accidents, sports-related collisions, or falls from a height). Rotational or pivoting forces in the lower limb are a significant contributor to injuries at both the knee and ankle.

ANKLE INJURIES. Across all ages, the most common foot and ankle injuries are sprains of the lateral ligaments (e.g., talofibular and calcaneofibular ligaments), Achilles' tendonitis (strain), and plantar fasciitis. Eighty-five percent of ankle sprains are due to inversion (and planter flexion) forces and involve the anterior talofibular ligament.[61,220] Eversion sprains of the deltoid ligament (15% of sprains) typically are more painful and slower to heal given the stresses of closed kinetic-chain pronation during weight-bearing. Syndesmotic, or high ankle sprains, may result from an abduction and external rotation force on a planted foot.[77,220] The syndesmotic (interosseous) membrane stabilizes the tibia and fibula of the leg and the mortise joint of the ankle. These sprains tend to be serious, and athletes can take twice as long (more than 2 months) to return to sports. If the medial stabilizing structures (deltoid ligament) also are injured, a distal syndesmotic stabilization screw is required. A variant of this more severe injury is associated with a fracture of the fibula just proximal to the distal tibiofibular syndesmosis (Maisonneuve fracture).[77,220]

KNEE INJURIES. An oversimplification of the knee joint's relationship to ligamentous injury says, "The knee joint—it bends and straightens, and gets injured frequently."[79] The long contributing levers (femur and tibia) predispose this joint to injury from direct extrinsic blows as well as intrinsic pivoting, cutting, and deceleration injuries. Knowledge of the mechanism of injury is extremely useful in differential diagnosis. Figure 12-14 denotes major knee instabilities and ligamentous special tests often performed on the knee.[167]

In isolation, the medial collateral ligament (MCL) is the knee ligament most often sprained.[7,36,220,263] Most MCL sprains, including complete tears (grade III), can be treated conservatively. A bundle of the MCL is intimate with the medial joint capsule, posterior oblique ligament, and meniscotibial fibers, making the medial meniscus (along with the anterior cruciate ligament [ACL]) susceptible to forceful valgus rotation loads. The resultant injury—the terrible triad (MCL, ACL, and medial

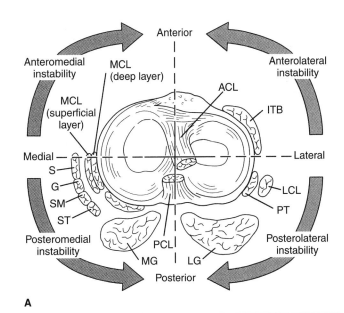

Ligamentous Tests Commonly Performed on the Knee

One-plane medial instability:	Valgus stress at 0° and 30° Hughston valgus stress at 0° and 30°
One-plane lateral instability:	Varus stress at 0° and 30° Hughston varus stress at 0° and 30°
One-plane anterior instability:	Lachman test or its modifications Drawer test Active drawer test
One-plane posterior instability:	Posterior sag Drawer test Active drawer test Godfrey test
Anteromedial rotary instability:	Slocum test
Anterolateral rotary instability:	Pivot shift test Losee test Jerk test of Hughston Slocum ARLI test Crossover test Noyes flexion-rotation drawer test
Posteromedial rotary instability:	Hughston's posteromedial drawer test Posteromedial pivot shift test
Posterolateral rotary instability:	Hughston's posterolateral drawer test Jakob test External rotation recurvatum Loomer's posterolateral rotary instability test Tibial external rotation test

FIGURE 12-14 A and **B,** Knee instabilities and ligamentous tests (special tests) commonly performed on the knee. (From Magee DJ: *Orthopedic physical assessment,* ed 4, Philadelphia, 2002, WB Saunders, p 696.)

meniscus)—is best handled surgically to prevent long-term mechanical degradation of the knee (osteoarthrosis).

The severity of MCL injury determines the aggressiveness of rehabilitation. All persons with MCL injuries should be treated with early range of motion (ROM) and strengthening of musculature that stabilizes the knee joint.[6,36,229,263] Weight-bearing after injury depends on the severity of the sprain:

- Grade I: Short-term use of crutches may be indicated, with weight-bearing-as-tolerated (WBAT) ambulation.
- Grade II: A short-hinged brace that blocks 20 degrees of terminal extension but allows full flexion should be used. The patient may ambulate WBAT. Closed-chain exercises allow for strengthening of knee musculature without putting stress on the ligaments.
- Grade III: The patient initially should be non–weight-bearing (NWB) on the affected lower extremity. A hinged brace should be used with gradual progression to full weight-bearing (FWB) over 4 weeks. Grade III injuries may require 8 to 12 weeks to heal.[6]

The lateral collateral ligament (LCL) is part of a complex of ligaments collectively named the posterolateral corner (PC). The structures in the PC include the LCL, popliteofibular ligament, popliteus ligament, arcuate ligament, short lateral ligament, and posterolateral joint capsule.[167] The LCL is the primary restraint against varus (lateral gapping) of the knee, and along with the MCL and popliteus corner checks lateral rotation of the tibia.[155,167]

LCL injuries are the rarest form of athletic knee injuries. Athletes will report a varus force to the knee but usually will be able to ambulate after the acute injury. Pain, stiffness, swelling, and erythema are localized to the lateral aspect of the knee, and concomitant injury of the lateral meniscus is rare. Instability or mechanical symptoms (e.g., locking or popping sensation) are uncommon. Isolated tenderness at the proximal or distal insertion sites may indicate an avulsion-type injury, especially in the young population.[6]

Grade-I and grade-II sprains of the LCL typically are braced for protection for 4 to 6 weeks and treated with a regimen similar to that of other ligamentous injuries (e.g., PRICE for acute treatment, ROM, strengthening, progressive loading, and proprioceptive training). LCL injuries heal more slowly than MCL injuries because of the difference in collagen density.[6] Severe LCL injuries (grade III) with concomitant posterolateral corner knee injury typically are treated surgically because of rotational instability. Patients may require bracing and physical therapy for up to 3 months to prevent later instability.[6,229,263]

The ACL is the primary restraint (85%) on anterior translation of the tibia. It is supplemented by the MCL, LCL, middle third of the mediolateral capsule, popliteus corner, semimembranous corner, iliotibial band,[167] and dynamic synergistic muscle activity from the quadriceps, and hip external rotators and abductors (chiefly gluteus medius). Tear of the ACL is the most problematic of the ligamentous knee injuries.

Most ACL injuries (78%)[186] are the result of a sudden cut (pivot) or deceleration injury (i.e., noncontact, intrinsic injury). The ACL also is susceptible to extrinsic blows to the posterolateral portion of the tibiofemoral joint and forced hyperextension. In the younger adolescent, avulsion of the tibial eminence must be differentiated from true ACL sprain via radiographs. In the case of mid-substance ACL tears, the PT must differentiate between the child with significant growth potential and the adolescent with minimal growth potential. In the skeletally immature athlete (i.e., with open physes), there is at least a theoretical risk for growth disruption if surgical management is undertaken.[220]

The PT should take care to assess the stability of the medial and lateral knee structures if valgus or varus mechanisms were part of the mechanism of injury. Valgus stress can result in MCL injury or a Salter I separation (see Box 12-6), distal femoral physeal injury, or meniscal injury.[220] Distal femoral physeal fractures are about 10 times as common as proximal tibial fractures. They can occur at any age but are seen most often in boys age 10 to 14. This age range is a time of significant growth, when the physis is weakest.[223] Joint-line tenderness may be indicative of a meniscal injury.[167,220] The PT should assess stability of the patella to rule out a patellofemoral dislocation or subluxation. Standard knee radiographs include anteroposterior, lateral, tunnel, and sunrise (skyline) views. Varus and valgus stress views can differentiate between collateral-ligament tears and physeal separations. MRI is considered the gold standard for differential diagnosis of ACL and other associated knee injuries.[174,211,220]

In children age 8 to 11, anterior drawer laxity with the aforementioned signs and symptoms is most likely a tibial avulsion fracture.[223] Classification and treatment of tibial eminence avulsion fractures are as follows:

- Type I: Minimal to no displacement treated via casting or bracing in full extension for 10 to 14 days.[223]
- Type II: Anterior displacement with a beak-like appearance on the lateral radiograph of the knee treated via closed reduction (or open reduction internal fixation [ORIF] if necessary) and casting or bracing in full extension for 4 weeks.
- Type III: Fragment is completely lifted off and displaced from the tibia and requires ORIF with casting or bracing in full extension for 3 to 4 weeks.[220,223] It is usually 2 to 3 months before the patient returns to full athletic activity after an open reduction.

The long-term function of these patients is variable, with 74% having persistent anterior laxity, but only a small portion of these persons complain of clinical instability.[220,223]

The treatment of mid-substance ACL tears in the adolescent is somewhat more complex. If the physeal plates are near closure (Tanner stage IV or V), treatment is similar to that of an adult, with intraarticular reconstruction using a graft of the surgeon's preference (e.g., middle third of the patellar tendon, hamstrings, allograft [cadaver]). In the child who is obviously skeletally immature, extraarticular reconstruction (iliotibial band tenodesis) may be attempted. This procedure may reduce the pivot-shifting phenomenon but does not normalize the anterior translation, and long-term results are poor. Most observers advocate protective bracing and *strict* modification of activity (no pivoting, cutting, or impact sports) to prevent secondary instability, meniscus, or articular-cartilage injury until the child is physically mature enough to have a more definitive intraarticular reconstruction. Nonsurgical treatment of ACL tears in the young population is unsuccessful.[220] The failure rate of rehabilitation and bracing is nearly 100% if the patient returns to pivoting sports. The incidence of meniscal tears increases with chronic instability.[105,186]

The posterior cruciate ligament (PCL) functions as the knee's central axis of rotation, assists in the "screw home" mechanism of the knee, and acts as a secondary restraint of valgus and varus rotation (rotary stabilizer).[167] Common mechanisms of PCL injury include a fall onto a flexed knee with the ankle plantar flexed, direct blow on the tibial tuberosity (i.e., a motor-vehicle dashboard injury), hyperextension, and a combination of rotation and lateral force directed at the medial side of the knee.[177,206]

PCL injuries have attracted far less attention than ACL injuries because they occur less often (only 3% to 20% of all knee injuries implicate the PCL) and create much less functional disability. Persons with PCL instability report vague symptoms such as unsteadiness or insecurity of the knee and usually do not have incapacitating pain. Undiagnosed and untreated PCL injuries may result in disability years later (e.g., 80% to 90% report patellofemoral pain, and 40% to 50% have degenerative changes on long-term follow-up).[99,111,177,233]

Upper Quarter Musculoskeletal Injuries (see Table 12-15)

A fall onto an outstretched hand (FOOSH) is the most common mechanism of upper extremity traumatic injury. Depending on the angle and speed of impact (compression load), a variety of upper quarter injuries are possible (e.g., fractures, dislocations, sprains, strains, contusions). Forceful traction (tensile) or rotational (shear) loads to the extremities typically will result in soft tissue damage (e.g., brachial plexus stretch, muscle strain, ligament sprain, glenohumeral subluxation or dislocation, and radial-head dislocation [nursemaid's elbow]).

STERNOCLAVICULAR JOINT SPRAIN. Traumatic posterior dislocation of the sternoclavicular (SC) joint is rare but constitutes a *medical emergency*. Complications include respiratory distress, venous congestion or arterial insufficiency, brachial plexus injury, and myocardial conduction abnormalities. A myriad of reconstructive procedures have been recommended, but some authors advocate resection of the medical clavicle given that failure of the fixation devices also can cause serious injury and even death.[261]

ACROMIOCLAVICULAR SEPARATION (SPRAIN). Acromioclavicular (AC) separation involves damage to the AC ligament and the two divisions of the coracoclavicular (CC) ligament—the trapezoid ligament (lateral portion of the CC ligament) and the more medial conoid ligament.

AC sprains (separation) are graded via bilateral anteroposterior (AP) radiographic views of the AC joint, with and without weights in the upper extremities:

- Grade I (mild sprain): Minimal widening of the AC joint space with CC distance within normal limits.
- Grade II (moderate sprain): Widening of the AC joint space to 1.0 to 1.5 cm with a 25% to 50% increase in the CC distance.
- Grade III (severe sprain): Widening of the AC joint space 1.5 cm or more with a 50% or more increase in the CC distance. The AC joint is dislocated, and the clavicle is displaced superiorly.[174]

- Grade IV: Tearing of all three AC ligaments with posterior displacement of the clavicle (occasionally through the trapezius).[23]
- Grade V: Severe superior clavicle displacement, disrupting the deltoid and trapezius attachments on the clavicle.[23]
- Grade VI: Severe inferior clavicle displacement with potential damage to the underlying brachial plexus and subclavian vessels.[23]

Acute management of AC sprains consists of protection from further injury via a sling, ice, and pain medication. In the milder cases (grades I and II), the shoulder becomes relatively pain free within 3 weeks (or by the end of the proliferation phase of healing).[23,46,265] If there is no danger of making the condition worse, activity can be determined by the symptoms. Grade-III AC separation usually is treated conservatively except in those patients who are unwilling to accept cosmetic deformity or who continue to have pain and dysfunction despite adequate conservative rehabilitation. Grade-IV through grade-VI separations often require operative treatment.[23,259]

GLENOHUMERAL INJURIES. Glenohumeral (GH) or shoulder-joint problems are common in the adolescent population (see Table 12-16).[22,136,259] The GH joint is an inherently unstable joint and exhibits the greatest amount of motion of any joint in the body. From 90% to 97% of all shoulder dislocations are anterior. The primary mechanism of anterior dislocation is forceful shoulder external rotation and abduction via traumatic collision or a FOOSH mechanism. Posterior dislocations of the GH joint are rare (3% to 10%) and usually are the result of posteriorly directed force through a flexed humerus. The patient with posterior dislocation will present with a forward flexed, adducted, and internally rotated position.

Relocation can be spontaneous or can require emergency department care. The PT should rule out axillary nerve damage, which fortunately is rare, via sensory testing of the lateral shoulder (dermatome) and resisted testing (myotome) of the shoulder abductors (deltoid). Routine radiographs (AP with internal rotation and AP with lateral rotation) should be taken after traumatic GH dislocation to rule out glenoid chip fractures, Hill-Sachs lesion (fracture of the posterolateral portion of the humeral), damage to the acromioclavicular arch, or acute supraspinatus rupture (may require contrast to be visualized). Specialty views, including the axillary and oblique views, are useful for shoulder dislocations, while the tangential view visualizes the bicipital groove. Fractures of the scapular body are best viewed on the lateral view of the scapula, while fractures of the glenoid fossa are best found via the AP view of the scapula.[174] An MRI will rule out associated injuries to the glenoid labrum. Surgical stabilization (e.g., Bankart repair with or without capsular shift) often is indicated for the management of recurrent dislocation.[23]

Traumatic GH dislocation or subluxation is rehabilitated in a fashion similar to that of overuse injuries after the initial phase of inflammation and repair has been addressed.[70,95] Treatment of acute anterior dislocation consists of 1 to 2 weeks of GH immobilization with shoulder-girdle and distal-joint mobility exercises. Treatment of posterior GH dislocation is controversial, with both surgical and nonoperative methods being reported.[23] Recurrence of GH dislocation among young athletes is high and *necessitates* aggressive physical therapy.[70]

ELBOW/WRIST/HAND INJURIES. Figure 12-13 and Table 12-15 present the differential diagnoses that should be considered when the patient has areas of pain, swelling, tenderness, deformity, or loss of function in the distal upper extremity. Persistent symptoms or a history of trauma make radiographic evaluation imperative. Referral to an orthopedic specialist (physician), occupational therapist, or certified hand therapist may be necessary to optimize the young patient's long-term UE function.

Management of Musculoskeletal Conditions in the Adolescent

The successful treatment of MS conditions depends on early and accurate differential diagnosis and implementation of an appropriate rehabilitation program.[138,164,234] Safe and efficacious exercise prescription integrates the three elements of evidenced-based-medicine. The PT's *clinical expertise* ensures that the goals of therapy are directed at specific pathology, impairments, functional limitations, or disabilities. The PT also screens for specific contraindications and precautions (e.g., growth variables, injury and disease limitations, soft tissue healing constraints). The *scientific merit* for the intervention in the face of the presenting condition or medical history must be considered. Finally, *patient values* and motivation for physical therapy intervention, as well as caregiver or parental and peer support must be incorporated into treatment planning. Cost, convenience, and availability of exercise equipment, and the safety of the exercise environment, always must be a priority.

The exercise prescription goes beyond differences in growth and maturation as they affect trainability (i.e., measurable physiological changes in a body system resulting from training). It must include the adolescent's cognitive ability to comprehend training dosage, adolescent temperament, and attention span.[27,194] The PT should devote additional deliberation to adolescents with chronic diseases, because they may differ from their healthy peers in their level and pattern of spontaneous activity, physical capabilities, attitudes towards exercise and sports, and motivation for changing lifestyle behaviors.* Table 12-16 illustrates the importance of disease-specific factors that may limit exercise tolerance.[121]

The PT working with the adolescent population (and with all patients) should readily be able to adjust these exercise parameters:

- Posture: position of the patient (e.g., standing, sitting, quadruped)
- Mode: method of exercise (e.g., biking, walking, swimming)
- Movement pattern of the exercise: precise description of the activity is imperative to specificity of training (e.g., part versus whole training, single plane or tri-planar activity, isolated pattern of movement versus functional task).
- Speed of movement pattern (e.g., deliberate and slow, self-selected speed, or fast motion)
- Frequency (e.g., times per day, times per week, or times per year for periodization)
- Repetitions: the number per training set or session
- Duration: the length or time of treatment session
- Type of muscle contraction (e.g., isometric, concentric, eccentric)
- Sequence: the order in which exercises are performed
- Method of muscular training (e.g., isometric, isotonic, isokinetic, open versus closed kinetic chain, impact loading, and plyometrics)
- Intensity and repetitions for muscle performance exercises (i.e., strength or power training versus endurance, percentage of 1 rep max)

---

*References 3, 10, 22, 27, 28, 34, 47, 48, 57, 64, 66, 74, 90, 101, 121, 159.

TABLE 12-16

Physiologic Functions that Limit Physical Performance and Exercise Tolerance in Children and Adolescents with Chronic Diseases[121]

Function	Diseases
Low maximal heart rate	Beta blockers, congenital complete atrioventricular block, anorexia nervosa, artificial pacemakers (fixed and variable rate), postsurgical period after Mustard operation for transposition of the great arteries
Low maximal stroke volume	Aortic stenosis, cardiomyopathy, detraining, Ebstein's anomaly of the tricuspid valve (also postoperatively), severe hypohydration, pulmonary stenosis, tetralogy of Fallot (also postoperatively), postsurgical period after Mustard operation for transposition of the great arteries, ventricular septal defect
Low oxygen-carrying capacity of arterial blood	Anemia, cyanotic heart defects, hemoglobinopathies, 2, 3-diphosphoglycerate deficiency
Low peripheral oxygen extraction	Detraining, severe malnutrition, muscle atrophies and dystrophies, spina bifida, 2, 3-diphosphoglycerate deficiency
Low lung diffusion capacity	Cystic fibrosis
Low maximal alveolar ventilation	Cystic fibrosis, muscle atrophies and dystrophies, extreme obesity, advanced kyphoscoliosis
High submaximal oxygen cost	Arthritis, cerebral palsy, muscle atrophies and dystrophies, advanced obesity, leg prosthetics (e.g., after amputation)
Low muscle strength	Cerebral palsy, muscle atrophies and dystrophies, storage diseases, Prader-Willi syndrome
Low muscle endurance and peak power	Advanced anorexia, advanced cystic fibrosis, cerebral palsy, McArdle's disease, muscle atrophies and dystrophies

From Bar-Or O: Training considerations for children and adolescents with chronic disease. In Hasson SM, ed: *Clinical exercise physiology*, St Louis, 1994, Mosby, p 267.

- Intensity of aerobic and anaerobic exercise (e.g., perceived exertion or heart-rate prescription via the Karvonen formula)
- Environment of practice (e.g., closed versus open environment; indoors or outdoors; and clinic, home, school, or community location)

Control of the exercise prescription will be much easier in the confines of a clinic compared with the home, school, or community. Biofeedback—visual, auditory (verbal feedback), and kinesthetic (manual) inputs—will affect the patient's ability to train and learn.[218] Periodization principles (including pre-season, in-season, post-season, and off-season components) should be used to maximize the effect of year-round training programs for adolescent athletes.[20,85,87] The reader is encouraged to review the evidence about the specifics of exercise physiology and exercise prescription.*

Environmental Factors Affecting Adolescents

> Human diversity makes tolerance more than a virtue; it makes it a requirement for survival.
>
> Rene Dubos (1901-1982)

Many researchers say that hormonal changes affect adolescent emotional and social development.[56,88,194,226] Changes in adolescent moods, attitudes, and behaviors (i.e., mood lability, mood intensity, irritability, and conflict with parents and caregivers) historically were presumed to be the negative result of biological factors (hormones).[56] To *blame* adolescent behavior on the raging hormones of puberty is far too simplistic. The prevailing culture surrounding the young child and adolescent can lead to a wide range of attitudes, beliefs, and behaviors. Relevant environmental, social, and cultural factors must be considered by the health care professional (see Fig. 12-2).[228]

Environmental quality (e.g., exposure to ozone pollution and tobacco smoke, unsafe living conditions, location, and geography); socioeconomic variables (e.g., race, ethnicity, family composition, income, and access to education and health care); and contextual factors (i.e., family, school, and peer-group influences) are key determinants of adolescent behavior.[194,226] Relevant psychological variables include the adolescent's self-esteem, gender-role orientation, sense of mastery and control, and level of anxiety versus happiness and life satisfaction.[80,98,226,228,230] In early adolescence, the trend toward separation from family with increasing involvement in peer activities accelerates.[27] All of these factors have the potential to affect overall health and have been found to correlate to physical dysfunction, disease, and illness.[228]

Poverty in America: Our Children at Risk

The U.S. Census Bureau uses poverty data to evaluate the nation's economic status and national challenges, such as health care needs, educational needs, and employment opportunities. Children growing up in poverty may be at double jeopardy because they face increased biological risk factors such as prematurity, lead poisoning, and malnutrition as well as increased social risk factors such as overcrowding, lower maternal education, exposure to violence, and lack of access to health care.[63,67,109,192]

Because poor people in the United States are too diverse to be categorized along any one dimension, poverty rates are stratified by age, race, Hispanic origin, nativity, family composition, work experience, and geography.[67] Persons under 18 years of age have the highest poverty rate (16.2%) of any age group in America.[67] Observers estimate that more than 2500 babies are born into poverty every day. More than one in five (22.7%) children under 6 years of age is living in poverty and may grow to be an adolescent with health problems.[63,67,199]

Children, those younger than 18 years of age, living in households headed by a female with no husband have an overall poverty rate of 39.8%, which is five times the rate of their counterparts in married-couple families (8.2%). White children in families headed by women fare best, with a poverty rate of 20% to 25%, followed by black (40%) and Hispanic (50%) children.[67]

Poverty rates are stratified by race and ethnicity factors. In 2001, nonwhites had the following poverty rates: American Indians and Alaska Natives, 25.9%; Hispanics, 22.8%; blacks, 22.1%; and Asian and Pacific-Islander Americans, 10.8%.[67] Ironically, noncitizens living in the United States actually have a lower poverty rate (19.4%) than black, Hispanic, and Native-American citizens. Contrast all of these numbers with the white nonHispanic poverty rate of 7.5%, and one realizes that strong discriminatory influences are still at work in the United States. The effects of this poverty carry over to access to health care (see Health Promotion section).[63,67,109,123]

Homelessness in America: Lost Educational Opportunities

Observers estimate that children under the age of 18 account for 25% of all homeless people in the United States.[243] Homeless children have poor educational role models and insufficient access to educational, technological, and health care opportunities.[143,209,243] Homeless children transfer among schools at 16 times the rate of the typical American child. They are more likely than non-homeless children to repeat a grade and to be placed in special-education classes. Furthermore, observers estimate that 20% to 25% of the single-adult homeless population suffers from some form of severe and persistent mental illness. This means that homeless children in the United States not only confront a lack of food, shelter, clothing, and educational opportunities, but up to one in four persons they meet on the streets has a mental disorder.[199,243]

Crime in America: Vulnerability of the Adolescent

Vulnerability to violent crime (e.g., homicide, rape, sexual assault, robbery, and aggravated assault) varies across the age spectrum. The victimization rate increases through the teenage years, crests at around age 20, and steadily decreases through the remaining years. This pattern, with some exceptions, holds across all race, sex, and ethnic groups (Fig. 12-15).[192]

---

*References 7, 9, 10, 17, 20, 22, 36, 60, 82, 84, 85, 87, 89, 114, 116, 121, 133, 159, 173, 189, 201, 210, 212.

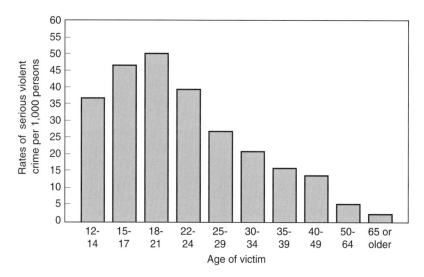

FIGURE 12-15 Age patterns of victims of serious violent crime. (From Perkins CA: Age patterns of victims of serious violent crimes, *Bureau of Justice Statistics: special report* [NCJ-162031], Washington, DC, July 1997, US Department of Justice.)

American adolescents and young adults (12 to 24 years) make up 35% of all murder victims and almost 50% of all victims of violent crime (e.g., rape, robbery, and assault).[39,192] Adolescents are most often victimized by people they know.[199] Teens are three times more likely to be murdered by an adult than a peer, and a school-aged youth is a dozen times safer from being murdered at school than at home.[209]

Adolescent victimization has distinct differences in gender and race. Late-adolescent males (18 to 21 years old) are more likely than females to be victims of violent crime, with black males being victimized at a rate of 72 incidents per 1000 compared with 50 per 1000 young Hispanic males and 46 per 1000 young white males. Males are much more likely to be victims of violence inflicted by strangers, whereas females are as likely to be hurt by family members and close associates as by strangers. The victims of 55% of all *reported* rapes and sexual assaults were females younger than 25 years, with the following age distributions: 12 to 14 years, 8%; 15 to 17 years, 12%; 18 to 21 years, 21%; and 22 to 24 years, 14%.[192] Most of them knew their assailants.

Young people living in the presence of substance abuse, alcoholism, homelessness, or poverty are at greatest risk.[67,106,199,227,243] Teens struggling with chronic illness or disability,[148] intellectual handicap,[203] or sexual orientation[98,198,213] are often victimized at higher rates than other children. This victimization ranges in severity from peer and public alienation to physical isolation and culminates in violent crimes such as robbery, physical abuse and neglect, sexual abuse, and even death.[246] Sadly, teenagers are the age group *least likely* to report a crime.[207]

Many Americans believe today's youth are uniquely criminal, violent, and out of control. California's crime rates (which in many cases mirror national trends), however, suggest that today's children and teenagers are considerably less crime-prone, and today's middle-aged adults are far more so, than their counterparts of the past.[43] Youth crime appears to be strongly related to socioeconomic status and *not* race. In U.S. counties where poverty is high, the crime rate is higher regard-less of race. Nonwhite persons are statistically more likely to be burdened by poverty. The high homicide rate among nonwhite youth is a direct result of industrial abandonment and jobless-ness, which forces young people into more dangerous alternatives, such as gangs. Where youths, regardless of race, have the same socioeconomic status as adults, youths display murder and other crime rates lower than those of adults.[43] A health care provider is statistically more likely to care for a youth who has been a victim of a violent crime than to be a victim of a violent crime himself or herself.[192,246]

Health Promotion and Counseling for Adolescents

> An ounce of prevention is worth a pound of cure.
> Benjamin Franklin (1706-1790)

Nowhere in health care is this sentiment more applicable than in the developing patient. Prevention at a young age can improve health for many decades. Current medical literature is strewn with accounts of unhealthy children growing up to be unhealthy adults with multisystem health care problems.[34,123] Physical inactivity and obesity are becoming endemic to the U.S. culture. Overweight and obesity substantially raise the risk of illness from high blood pressure, high cholesterol, type-2 diabetes, heart disease, stroke, gallbladder disease, arthritis, sleep disturbances, breathing problems, and certain types of cancers.[34] Obese individuals, especially children, also may suffer from social stigmatization, discrimination, and lowered self-esteem.[123]

Our society is currently at war against the ominous enemy of chronic disease.[34] Roughly 20 million of the nation's children suffer from at least one chronic illness.[74] Health care professionals should view every interaction with an adolescent as an opportunity to advocate wellness. The adolescent's intelligence mandates that the health care provider form a *direct* therapeutic alliance with the client.[230] Caregivers, schoolteachers, coaches, and community leaders who interact with adolescents should be considered agents of change and appropriately educated by the health care team.

Health promotion has three fundamental components: primary, secondary, and tertiary prevention. Primary health prevention means preventing disease in a susceptible or potentially susceptible population via general health promotion and education. Secondary health prevention means reducing the duration of illness, severity of disease, and sequelae of disease via early diagnosis and prompt intervention. Tertiary health prevention means limiting the degree of disability and promoting rehabilitation and restoration of function in clients with chronic or irreversible conditions.[104,205] Health promotion for adolescents is not only the detection and prevention of disease, but also the promotion of well being that spans physical, cognitive, emotional, social, and spiritual domains.[230]

Health Promotion Topics Specific to Adolescents*

BACKPACK GUIDELINES. A backpack and its contents should not exceed 10% to 15% of a child's body weight. Individual levels of fitness may affect this recommendation.[193] Extra weight can result in musculoskeletal strain or pain in the back, shoulders, and neck. Parents and teens should look for the following features in a backpack:

- Wide, padded, and contoured shoulder straps. Avoid single-strap bags and slinging the backpack over one shoulder only.
- A padded back (contoured back a plus) to protect the vertebral spinous processes.
- A suspension bar in the backpack to distribute load more evenly.
- A padded waist belt to distribute some load to the pelvis.
- Compression straps that, when tightened, compress the pack's contents to stabilize them.
- A size appropriate for the size of the child.

Look for signs of musculoskeletal strain: struggling to don or doff the backpack, pain, red marks from straps, poor posture, and numbness and tingling in the upper extremities. These are signs that a backpack fits poorly or is overloaded.

CANCER: GENERAL PREVENTION GUIDELINES. Primary care health care providers, including PTs, should teach adolescents to take control of their health at a young age. Teach family members, teens, and the general public to recognize the signs and symptoms of occult disease (see Medical Screening information in Section Two). Know which cancers are specific to the adolescent population (see Medical Conditions above). Fifty percent of all adult cancers can be prevented by following seven recommendations outlined in national public health policies.[4,12,18,34,123] These seven cancer-prevention tips also can lower the long-term risk for heart disease, stroke, and diabetes.[34,123]

- Do not smoke.
- Eat a healthy diet.
- Maintain a healthy weight.

- Protect yourself from the sun.
- Drink less than one alcoholic beverage a day.
- Get at least 30 minutes of physical activity every day.
- Protect yourself and your partner(s) from sexually transmitted infections.

COMPUTER ERGONOMIC GUIDELINES. Computers are an integral part of American culture. At the turn of the twentieth century, 40% of U.S. children age 2 to 17 (more than 25 million) were on the Internet. Currently, 70% of teenagers access the Internet regularly. By 2005, almost 44 million children age 2 to 17 will be using the Internet.[112] While computers and the Internet certainly will have a profound effect on children's learning and development worldwide, they likewise bring the consequences of repetitive strain and poor posture and ergonomics. The risk of long-term musculoskeletal overuse injuries in young bodies is greater than ever. The primary care PT has an opportunity to make a difference in the general health of society, starting with its youngest computer-using members.

The "Top 10 Ways to Monitor Kids' Computer Health" is available on the American Physical Therapy Association website (www.apta.org).[260]

DENTAL HEALTH GUIDELINES. The American Dental Association offers many tips for better dental health. These tips apply across the lifespan. A balanced diet is essential, including foods from each of the five major food groups: (1) breads, cereals, and other grain products, (2) fruits, (3) vegetables, (4) meat, poultry, and fish, and (5) milk, cheese, and yogurt. Limiting snacks, a difficult task for all ages in our culture, is a wise dental-health tip. After consumption of food that contains sugars or starches, the teeth are attacked by acids for 20 minutes or more. Therefore, healthy snacks, such as cheese, raw vegetables, plain yogurt, or a piece of fruit, are safer for the teeth. At a minimum, one should brush twice a day with fluoride toothpaste, and, if possible, brush after all meals. One should floss daily to clean between the teeth and visit a dentist regularly.[14]

SEXUALITY AND GENDER IDENTITY. Gay, lesbian, bisexual, transgender, and questioning (GLBTQ) youth often face rejection from their families after coming out. While some observers believe that peers tend to be more accepting of sexual ambiguity, the 1995 Safe Schools Coalition Study of Seattle public schools found that GLBTQ youth were more than five times more likely than their heterosexual peers to be targets of violence or harassment.[209] Many young people are thrown out of their homes, are mistreated, or become the focus of the family's dysfunction.[213] Several studies have shown evidence that GLBTQ youth are at a higher risk (up to 7 times higher) of suicide than are their heterosexual peers.[198,213]

Health care practitioners have an obligation to meet the health care needs of adolescents by practicing nonjudgmental acceptance and encouragement of individual social and sexual identity.[209,230] In conjunction with the federal government's *Healthy People 2010* project, the Gay and Lesbian Medical Association (GLMA), with involvement of dozens of experts in lesbian, gay, bisexual, and transgender (LGBT) health and the recently formed National Coalition for LGBT Health, has yielded the first-ever comprehensive document on the state of LGBT health. The *Healthy People 2010* Companion Document for GLBT Health is a

---

*__Disclaimer__: This alphabetized list of adolescent health care topics is not meant to be all-inclusive or hierarchical in terms of health issues important to this age group.

comprehensive look at the multicultural LGBT community. It is written by and for health care consumers, providers, researchers, educators, government agencies, schools, clinics, advocates, and health professionals in all settings.[98]

SPORTS INJURY PREVENTION. The American Academy of Pediatrics' Committee on Sports Medicine and Fitness updated its policy statement regarding "Intensive Training and Sports Specialization in Young Athletes," in July 2000 (http://aap.org/policy/re9906.html). This document is a recommended reference for anyone working with highly competitive youngsters. Although intense sports competition among children raises many concerns, little scientific information is available to support or refute these risks.[10]

Health care providers must assist young athletes in avoiding the risks of early, excessive training and competition. Young athletes must obtain preparticipation physicals yearly before the start of practice and competition.[134] Coaches should strive for prevention, early recognition, and treatment of overuse injuries. Children should be encouraged to participate in sports at a level consistent with their abilities and interests. Pushing children beyond their limits is discouraged, as is specialization in a single sport before adolescence. Parents and health care providers should ensure that coaches know proper training techniques, signs of heat stress (see Table 12-7), biomechanics of the sport, safety equipment, and the unique physical, physiological, and emotional characteristics of young competitors.

Given the underlying demands of adolescence for growth and development, young athletes should be monitored for adequate nutritional intake and growth. The intensely trained, specialized young athlete needs ongoing assessment of nutritional intake, with particular attention to total calories, a balanced diet, and intake of iron and calcium. Pediatric visits should focus on serial measurements of body composition, weight, and stature; cardiovascular findings (blood pressure, heart rate, and rhythm); sexual maturation; and evidence of emotional stress (psychosocial development). The pediatrician should watch for signs and symptoms of overtraining, including decline in performance, weight loss, anorexia in females and males, amenorrhea (in females), and sleep disturbances.

In 1997, the American Red Cross and the U.S. Olympic Committee joined forces to develop a *Sport Safety Training Course* to teach coaches the basic first-aid skills and knowledge needed to care for athletic injuries.[17] The American Red Cross also offers a full line of texts and courses on water and swim safety, CPR, and first aid. Health care providers should be proficient and certified (depending on state practice act guidelines and employer specifications) in infant, child, and adult CPR (Box 12-7). Competence in the use of the automated external defibrillator (AED) for cardiac arrest is now standard protocol for all health care providers.

Healthy People 2010

Healthy People 2010 should be a significant resource for the health care practitioner (see Box 12-1). Ten objectives have been identified as leading health indicators for the new millennium, and these objectives will serve as an ongoing federal blueprint for public health in America.

Physical Activity, Overweight, and Obesity

Age-specific and sex-specific charts are available to assess body mass index (BMI) of children and adolescents. BMI has three important categories: (1) youth below the 5th percentile, who are considered *underweight*, (2) children above the 95th percentile,

---

BOX 12-7

Pediatric and Adolescent Considerations in Sports Medicine

Juvenile participation in organized interscholastic and recreational athletics has steadily risen in the United States in the last 30 years. Since the advent of Title IX in 1972, women's participation in physical activity and sports has increased dramatically (700%).[239] Fifty percent of boys and 25% of girls between the ages of 8 and 16 compete in organized sports programs at sometime during each year. Three fourths of junior high schools and middle schools have competitive interscholastic sports program. At the high-school level, there are 32 male and 27 female competitive sports, with 7 million high-school students participating.[239] Beyond organized sports, millions compete and participate in physical-education classes, community intramural programs, church programs, and other recreational sporting activities.[7,265] Studies show that 30% to 50% of all juvenile sports injuries are considered overuse (repetitive microtrauma) injuries. The American College of Sports Medicine estimates that 50% of overuse injuries in children and adolescents are avoidable.[211]

COMMON SENSE PRINCIPLES OF SPORTS INJURY PREVENTION[8,10,17,20]
- Obtain medical clearance for participation (including subjective history and a preparticipation physical examination [PPE]).[134]
- Immediately stop participation of any athlete with a sudden change in weight-bearing status or persistent pain, numbness, tingling, weakness, or altered function.
- Use and maintain proper protective equipment (cover the head to toe spectrum).[244]
- Evaluate field or court conditions before practice and competition.

- Study and apply the appropriate biomechanics of the sport (requires adequate coaching of technique).
- Enforce specific rules of safety (e.g., no spearing or clipping in football).
- Avoid the "No Pain—No Gain" mentality (many injuries are the result of fatigue).
- Promote psychological preparation in the athlete (visual practice, mental preparation, and training in stress management and relaxation).
- Foster high-quality communication on and off the field (recognize risks).
- Practice sound total conditioning principles (e.g., proper warm-up and cool-down, proper nutrition and fluid intake).[13,40]
- Prevent athlete burnout and susceptibility to overuse injuries via total conditioning principles (periodization).[20,85]
- Periodization: year-round training principles for the adolescent athlete. The off-season is a key time to work on the fundamental skills of the sport.

Activity	Post-season	Off-season	Pre-season	In-season
Flexibility	Maintain	Increase	Increase	Maintain
Strength		Increase	Increase	Maintain
Cardiovascular endurance		Increase	Maintain	Maintain
Sport skills		Increase	Increase	Increase
Total rest	Increase			Maintain
Active rest		Increase		Maintain
Visualization	Increase	Increase	Increase	Increase

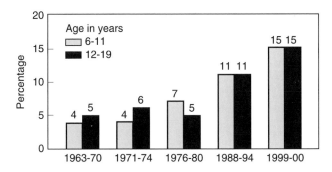

FIGURE 12-16 Prevalence and trends of overweight among US children and adolescents; data for 1999 to 2000. (From Ogden CL, Flegal KM, Carroll MD, et al: Prevalence and trends of overweight among US children and adolescents 1999-2000, *JAMA* 288;1728-1732, 2002. Modified from National Center for Health Statistics, Division of Data Services, Hyattsville, MD.)

who are considered *overweight*, and (3) children above the 85th percentile, who are considered *at risk for being overweight*.[245]

More than half of adults in the United States are estimated to be overweight or obese.[123] Fifteen percent of children age 6 to 19 are overweight. The proportion of adolescents from poor households who are overweight or obese is twice that of adolescents from middle-income and high-income households.[123] Figure 12-16 shows a historical perspective (last 40 years) of the percentage of children (6 to 12 years) and adolescents (12 to 19 years) who are overweight.

In modern society, declines in work-related physical activity and increases in sedentary behavior have tended to drive down the daily expenditure of energy among Americans. Conversely, energy intake is up. High-fat, energy-dense foods and large portion sizes in the fast-foods industry have increased American caloric intake. These changes are having widespread ill effects on the health of Americans, including our children and adolescents.

Obesity in adolescence, as at any age, is difficult and discouraging to treat and is one of the most common presenting conditions in adolescent clinics.[26] Primary endocrine or metabolic disorders are uncommon, and most cases are due to the habit of eating more than is needed to meet normal demands of the basal metabolic rate and activity. Secondary medical problems (e.g., low back pain, knee pain, hypertension, diabetes) seen in overweight and obese adults also are found in pediatric patients. The obese adolescent often has a poor self-image and becomes more sedentary and socially withdrawn.[26]

Treatment should include: (1) education in proper nutrition (for the adolescent, caregivers, and food providers); (2) behavior modification, including reduction and control of caloric intake (i.e., permanent changes in eating habits); and (3) increased physical activity (aerobic activities coupled with strength training to burn calories and increase lean body mass).[20,26,173] Physical activity counseling by primary care providers is a key objective of the *Healthy People 2010* project. PTs have the requisite knowledge and expertise to address issues related to physical inactivity (Box 12-8). Activities that improve muscular strength, endurance, flexibility, and fitness (e.g., worksite, community, and school physical education) all have the potential to reduce the prevalence of obesity, coronary heart disease, and other chronic conditions.

BOX 12-8

Health Promotion and Physical Activity: Strategies to Create Successful Exercise Programs and Biopsychosocial Benefits of Regular Activity and Exercise

STRATEGIES TO CREATE SUCCESSFUL EXERCISE PROGRAMS

- Ask the client if he or she is currently exercising regularly (or was before illness or injury). Briefly describe the benefits that the person could achieve from such a program.
- Emphasize exercise benefits of improving health rather than achieving weight loss.
- Allow the person to respond to the recommendation for an exercise program. Encourage the person to verbalize any thoughts or reactions to your suggestions.
- Determine whether the person believes that an exercise program will benefit him or her personally. Help the individual to set personal goals for exercise.
- Elicit from the client a statement accepting an exercise program.
- Be aware of any cultural or philosophical beliefs the person may have about exercise.
- If resistance to the idea of an exercise program is encountered, give the person an opportunity to list potential barriers to exercise. Ask the person to suggest ways to overcome potential barriers.
- Whenever possible, provide a written description (preferably just pictures because of the potential of undisclosed illiteracy) of the proposed exercise program. Review progress and reward attempts, successes, and progression of the exercise program.
- Make it fun to foster a lifestyle approach characterized by long-term adherence.

BIOPSYCHOSOCIAL BENEFITS OF REGULAR ACTIVITY AND EXERCISE

Reduce/prevent functional declines associated with aging Maintain/improve cardiovascular function; improve submaximal exercise performance; reduce risk for high blood pressure; decrease myocardial oxygen demand

Aid in weight loss and weight control

Improved function of hormonal, metabolic, neurologic, respiratory, and hemodynamic systems

Alteration of carbohydrate/lipid metabolism resulting in favorable increase in high-density lipoproteins

Strength training helps to maintain muscle mass and strength, especially in the aging group.

Reduces age-related bone loss; reduction in risk for osteoporosis

Improved flexibility, postural stability, and balance; reduction in risk of falling and associated injuries

Psychologic benefits (e.g., preserves cognitive function, alleviates symptoms/behavior of depression, improves self-awareness, promotes sense of well-being)

Reduction in disease risk factors

Improves functional capacity

Improves immune function (excessive exercise can inhibit immune function)

Reduces age-related insulin resistance

Reduces incidence of some cancers (e.g., colon, breast)

Contributes to social integration

Improves sleep pattern

From Goodman CC, Boissonnault WG, Fuller KS: *Pathology: implications for the physical therapist*, ed 2, Philadelphia, 2003, WB Saunders, pp 33, 36.
From American College of Sports Medicine (ACSM): Position stand: exercise and physical activity for older adults, *Med Sci Sports Exerc* 30(6):992-1008, 1998.

Tobacco Use

Tobacco, in smoked or chewed form, has pervasive multiple-system effects (refer to Box 12-3). Tobacco is the most common cause of cancer in the United States, accounting for 30% of all diagnosed cancers.[12] It is the strongest modifiable risk factor for coronary artery disease and significantly complicates the ramifications of other diseases (e.g., diabetes, low back pain, osteoporosis).[104] Preventing a teen from smoking today will pay off in the long run. According to research, if teens have not started smoking by age 20, chances are that they never will.[73] Prevention of tobacco use in adolescents is paramount, considering the serious health consequences of addiction, not to mention its monumental financial burden on the American health care system.

Substance Abuse

Substance abuse is common in U.S. society among people of every age, social, economic, professional, and educational status. In recent years, health and human-services organizations have emphasized the importance of developing adult-to-child mentoring programs to help children make better choices about drugs, alcohol, and tobacco. "Talk to your Kids"[231] television advertisements and Drug Abuse Resistance Education (DARE)[75] programs are two of these beacons of public information for children. Given the sheer scope of the substance-abuse problems in U.S. culture, health care workers should take advantage of any opportunity to deter a child from harmful addictions.

According to the National Institute on Drug Abuse (NIDA), successful drug-abuse-prevention programs embrace the following nine criteria: (1) target the most critical age groups; (2) provide multiple years of intervention; (3) include a well-tested, standardized intervention with detailed lesson plans and student materials; (4) teach drug-resistance skills through interactive methods; (5) foster positive social bonding to the school and community; (6) contain appropriate content (e.g., teach social competence and drug-resistance skills that are culturally and developmentally appropriate); (7) promote positive peer influence and promote antidrug social norms; (8) emphasize skills-training teaching methods and include an adequate dosage (10 to 15 sessions in the first year and another 10 to 15 booster sessions); and (9) retain core elements of the effective intervention design (implementation fidelity), training, and monitoring; and undergo periodic evaluation.[181]

Responsible Sexual Behavior

The American Medical Association believes that reducing the nation's rate of teen pregnancy is one of the best strategic means of improving overall child well-being in America.[54] Since the 1990s, birth rates have been declining nationwide regardless of age, marital status, race, and ethnicity.[69,170,176] Still, the United States holds the dubious honor of having one of the highest rates of teen pregnancy and birth in the industrialized world.[69,176,254]

Teen pregnancy and out-of-wedlock birth are a function of the early initiation of sex and the practice of unprotected sex.[69] A sexually active teenager who does not use contraception has a 90% chance of pregnancy within 1 year.[128,176] Among the most important factors contributing to the initiation of sex are going steady with a girlfriend or boyfriend who is 3 or more years older, having sexually active peers, having a parent or older sister who gave birth as a teen, and living in a poor community with high unemployment.[176] Conversely, when students do well in school, participate in extracurricular activities, do not drop out of school, or have plans for education beyond high school, they are more likely to use contraception if they have sex and are less likely to become pregnant.[54,176]

Many social issues are associated with teen pregnancy, including access to birth control and sexual education, welfare dependency, poverty, lack of medical prenatal and postpartum care, infant mortality rates (IMRs), services for mother and child, and irresponsible fatherhood. Children under 12 months of teenage mothers have high IMRs. In the United States, IMRs range from 4.5 to 15.4 infant deaths per 1000 live births (mean of 6.76), depending on race, ethnicity, and geographic distribution.[122,237] Individual variables contributing to IMRs include birth to a teenage mother (less than 18 years old), late or no prenatal care, low maternal education (less than 12 years), and maternal race or ethnicity (blacks, 13.9 deaths per 1000; whites, 6.4 deaths per 1000; and Hispanics, 5.9 deaths per 1000). Community-level variables that affect IMRs include population size of a city, segregation within a city, median household income, and childhood poverty.[29,122]

Responsible sexual behavior education for adolescents spans a wide continuum of topics: (1) abstinence as an option, (2) education in safe-sex practices (condom use), (3) contraceptive education and use, (4) education on sexually transmitted diseases, (5) prevention of unwanted pregnancy, and (6) identification and prevention of sexual abuse.[35,54,55,63] U.S. health care professionals reluctant to address sexual-health issues with adolescents may be considered negligent in providing comprehensive health care. However, these professionals are caught between the individual patient rights and confidentiality and the rights of caregivers and parents to know about the health of the minors in their care.

Homophobia, religious restrictions, and cultural attitudes about gender roles and condoms continue to hamper efforts to improve education about contraceptives and encourage consistent condom use in this country.[145] Health care providers and researchers agree that youth must be educated about drug-use behaviors and safe-sex practices for both same-sex and opposite-sex relationships. In a review of 35 programs around the world, the World Health Organization found that programs that teach only abstinence were less effective than programs that promote the delay of first sexual intercourse and teach about safer sex practices (i.e., contraception and condom use).[21] Peer-based interventions can reduce risk-associated behavior, increase condom acquisition and use, and reduce unprotected sexual intercourse, frequency of sexual intercourse, and the number of sexual partners.[145,253] Family factors, including a teens' perception of receiving warmth, love, and caring from parents and parental disapproval of teen sexual activity, are protective in delaying initiation of sexual intercourse.[199]

Mental Health (More than Just a U.S. Problem)

The future of our country, indeed of the world, depends on the mental health and strength of its youth. What is most worrisome is that the World Health Organization (WHO) predicts that by the year 2020, childhood neuropsychiatric disorders will rise by more than 50% internationally, to become one of the five most common causes of morbidity, mortality, and disability among the world's youth.[182] The inclusion of mental health in the *Healthy People 2010* project indeed represents a shift in this government's concern for mental health as compared with previous decades.[41] The Child and Adolescent Mental Health division of the National Institute of Mental Health (NIMH) has made research on diagnosis, early intervention, and treatment of children an absolute priority.[182]

Unfortunately, our society has insufficient resources to adequately address this issue, and fewer than 1 in 5 children who are mentally ill receive treatment.[41] There is politically heated debate about the finances and proper roles of medications and psychotherapies for children at risk and children already suffering from mental illness. However, one thing is clear: Children who go untreated suffer, cannot learn, cannot form healthy relationships with peers and family, and are at increased risk of unemployment, homelessness, trouble with the law, and imprisonment.[125-127,215,217,246,248]

Injury and Violence

UNINTENTIONAL INJURY. Unintentional injury accounts for about 60% of adolescent deaths from injury, while violence (e.g., homicide and suicide) accounts for the remaining 40% (see Fig. 12-3).[207] Alcohol abuse and irresponsible behavior play a significant role in a variety of adolescent deaths and injuries.[52] Adolescents are far less likely to use seat belts than any other age group. Males are more likely than females to die of any type of injury. Males age 15 to 19 years, are about 2.5 times more likely to die of any unintentional injury and 5 times more likely to die of homicide or suicide.[52] The gender difference is most pronounced in drowning, where males are 10.6 times more likely to die than females of the same age.

CHILD ABUSE AND NEGLECT. In 1998, about 3.1 million reports of child abuse were received by child-protective-services agencies. This correlates to 45 abuse cases per 1000 children, and one child-abuse report every 11 seconds. These troubling numbers do not include the thousands of unreported cases. Types of child abuse included: neglect (51%), physical abuse (25%), sexual abuse (10%), emotional abuse (3%), and other child maltreatment (11%). About three children died each day in the United States from abuse or neglect.[246] One half of all Americans believe child abuse and neglect is the most important public-health issue facing the United States (compared with other public-health issues like drug and alcohol abuse, heart disease, cancer, and HIV/AIDS).[4]

Given these facts, the health care provider working with adolescents must be vigilant for signs of injury resulting from physical or emotional abuse. The PT should suspect physical abuse in the following situations:

- The patient has unexplained injuries that seem inconsistent with his or her story.
- The patient conceals injuries and appears embarrassed by them.
- The patient has delayed seeking medical care.
- The patient has a history of repeated injuries or accidents.
- A caregiver or person close to the patient has a history of substance abuse.[230]

In a national survey of more than 2000 U.S. families, about 50% of the men who frequently assaulted their wives also frequently sexually abused their children.[227] The intimate physical signs that may indicate sexual abuse in children and adolescents (e.g., torn, stained, or bloody underclothing; pain or itching in the genital area; bruises or bleeding in external genitalia, vaginal, or anal regions; sexually transmitted disease or pregnancy) are not typically within the domain of the physical examination by the PT. Any child with a concerning history or physical signs should be referred to a sexual-abuse expert for a complete history and sexual-abuse examination.[230]

The effects of substance abuse and violence against children and adolescents are well documented.[59,106,246,248] Almost one half of substantiated cases of child neglect and abuse are associated with parental alcohol or drug abuse.[59] Observers estimate that one in every four children in the United States (28 million) is living in a household with an alcoholic adult.[106] Men and women serving time in the nation's prisons and jails report a higher incidence of abuse as children than the general population. More than a third of women in prison or jail reported abuse as children, compared with 12% to 17% of women in the general population. About 14% of male inmates reported abuse as children, compared with 5% to 8% of men in the general population.[248]

Caregiver neglect constitutes more than half (51% to 53%) of childhood abuse cases.[63,246] Nearly 35% of all 12-year-olds take care of themselves outside of school, and overall, youngsters 10 to 14 years of age spend 40% of their time without responsible adult companionship or supervision.[63] Unsupervised youngsters are most at risk during after-school hours (3 to 8 PM). Although many people believe that unsupervised adolescents with poor influences from the media and peers are the perpetrators of crime, statistics show that unsupervised children are 10 times more likely to become victims of crime than they are to be arrested as perpetrators.[39,63,248]

Further complicating the plight of children is the fact that families today have fewer support resources.[63] In March, 1996, 28% of children lived in one-parent families, contrasted with the 12% who lived in such families in 1970.[63] In 1996, 22.8 million U.S. women (21%) who had never been married had given birth to at least one child. Each year, more and more children enter the foster-care system or live with their aging grandparents.

Currently, more than 650,000 children will spend all or part of the year in government-run foster care, either in foster homes (75%), or in group homes, children's shelters, and other institutions (25%). Of these, in 1998, 32% were adolescents (13 years or older), 32% were 6 to 13 years of age, 31% were ages 1 to 5, and 5% were under the age of 1 year. Of these children, 39% were white, 40% were black, 12% were Hispanic, and the rest (9%) were of other backgrounds.[63] Factors contributing to foster care and adoption in the United States include a parental history of child abuse and neglect, domestic violence, substance abuse, and criminal offenses.

Environmental Quality

Allergic diseases affect more than 38 million people in the United States and result in more than 20 million visits to physicians' offices annually.[4,104] The number of pediatric patients (persons under 18 years of age) visiting physician offices for respiratory problems is *dramatically* rising.[4,123] Environmental quality is a key determinant of airway disease.

Environmental quality encompasses six major areas within the *Healthy People 2010* project: (1) outdoor air quality (including exposure to ozone pollution), (2) water quality, (3) toxins and wastes, (4) healthy homes and healthy communities, including indoor air quality (i.e., exposure to second-hand smoke and allergens), (5) infrastructure and surveillance, and (6) global environmental health.

Recommendations of the National Asthma Education and Prevention Program for addressing environmental allergens and irritants include:

- *Air pollution*: Consider limiting outdoor activities when levels of air pollution are high.
- *Animal dander*: Permanently remove pets from the house or, at least, keep pets away from the bedroom, carpeted areas, and upholstered furniture.
- *Cockroaches*: Use chemical measures and remove sources of food and water.
- *Dust mites*: Encase mattresses and pillows in vinyl or semipermeable covers; wash all bedding every 1 to 2 weeks in hot water of at least 54.4° C (130° F); other desirable measures include: reduce indoor humidity to less than 50%; remove carpet from the bedroom and carpet over concrete; avoid lying or sleeping on upholstered furniture.
- *Indoor mold*: Eliminate water leaks and damp areas associated with mold growth; consider reducing indoor humidity to less than 50%.
- *Pollens and outdoor molds*: Avoid outdoor activities when pollen and spore counts are high.
- *Tobacco*: Avoid exposure to active and passive tobacco smoke.[180]

Immunization

Immunization against diphtheria, tetanus, pertussis, poliomyelitis, measles, mumps, rubella, and hepatitis B is an effective method for preventing these diseases. These diseases are associated with birth defects, paralysis, brain damage, hearing loss, and liver cancer.[2] In 2002, the American Academy of Pediatrics (AAP) published their latest policy statement on the recommended childhood immunization schedule.[9]

If a second dose of *measles, mumps, and rubella (MMR)* has not been given, it should be given during adolescence. Adolescent females should be advised to avoid becoming pregnant within 3 months of vaccination. *Varicella* vaccine is recommended for susceptible adolescents (i.e., those who lack a reliable history of chicken pox or who have not been previously immunized). Booster doses of *tetanus and diphtheria (Td)* are recommended at 10-year intervals. All adolescecents should be immunized against *hepatitis B virus*. Adolescents (and adults) who plan to travel or work in a country with a high or intermediate rate of endemic *hepatitis A*, or who live in a community with a high rate of hepatitis A, are among those for whom vaccine should be considered. All adolescents should be immunized against *hepatitis B* virus. Those at high risk of influenza and anyone who requests an immunization should receive an annual *influenza immunization*.

The Advisory Committee on Immunization Practices (ACIP) and the AAP recommend informing parents of college students about *meningococcal disease* and the vaccine, and administering the vaccine if requested. The American College Health Association (ACHA) recommends *Neisseria meningitis* vaccine for all college students. Most insurers currently will reimburse for routine meningococcal immunization for college freshmen. Some college health services offer meningococcal immunization at no cost or reduced cost for entering freshman. Healthy adolescents do not require *pneumococcal* immunization until age 65.

Access to Health Care

Access to health care is the last of the 10 leading health care indicators of the *Healthy People 2010* project. Education, poverty, race, ethnicity, unemployment, and rising health care insurance premiums all adversely affect access to health care.[67] In the new millennium, the American tragedy of September 11, 2001, the dip in the economy, unemployment, and crises among federal and state budgets are likely to reduce health care coverage for all age groups.

Given these facts, the *Healthy People 2010* project identified four objectives in the delivery of health care in order to improve access to comprehensive, high-quality health care services for *all* Americans:

- *Primary Care Objective*: Increase the proportion of people who have a specific source of ongoing care
- *Clinical Preventive Care Objective*: Increase the proportion of people with health insurance
- *Emergency Services Objective*: Reduce the proportion of people who delay or have difficulty in getting emergency medical care (because delayed care typically causes increased cost in the long run)
- *Long-Term Care and Rehabilitative Services Objective*: Increase the access to the continuum of long-term care services for a greater proportion of people with these needs.

Strong predictors of access to quality health care include having (1) health insurance, (2) a higher income level, and (3) a regular primary care provider or other source of ongoing health care. Adults with health insurance are twice as likely to receive routine health check-ups as are adults without health insurance.

Adults can serve as important role models for children, demonstrating the importance of having a primary care provider, receiving appropriate preventive care (e.g., cancer screening, blood pressure, immunization, and early prenatal care), and advocating wellness concepts. With health costs skyrocketing, PTs likely will have an opportunity to play a vital role in providing primary care services and preventive-care services to patients of all ages.

Summary

> When I look upon a child I am filled with admiration—not so much for what that child is today as for what it may become.
>
> Louis Pasteur

The aforementioned topics affect not only the overall health and welfare of adolescents but also the future health of the United States. When talking to teens about health care issues, create an open, nonjudgmental environment that fosters safe, honest, and continuing dialogue. Juveniles are at a pivotal point in their physical, psychological, and psychosocial development, and health habits that start in adolescence can have long-lasting effects.

Adolescents face many potential barriers to participating in health-promotion activities and a healthy lifestyle. Cultural, family, and peer influences and self-esteem issues are the primary deterrents for adolescents.[142] Adolescents may cite variables such as cost, access, time, family opposition, or job or school constraints. Indeed, studies show that socioeconomic factors such as low income, low education, a difficult living environment, and lack of exposure to proper health promotion are key factors in failure to participate in health-promotion activities.[123,207]

The child with disability or disease (e.g., diabetes, arthritis, Down syndrome, cerebral palsy) also faces increased environmental barriers, increased costs, and access constraints. PTs should readily refer at-risk or uninsured children and their families to state and federal agencies to see whether they qualify for federal or state aid for health care. Information on the Children's Health Insurance Program (CHIP) can be accessed at the Health Care Financing Administration (www.hcfa.gov). Many national and international organizations offer research, educational materials, and health-promotion guidelines for children and adolescents (refer to Appendix 12-1).

This chapter is intended to be the PT's first step in developing the communication, technical, and clinical decision-making skills needed to provide safe, effective, and efficacious health care to adolescents. It is the first step in meeting the challenge of autonomous practice set forth by the Primary Care Special Interest Group of the Orthopedic Section of the American Physical Therapy Association. But it is only the first step. The ever-changing health care environment demands that all health care providers make a commitment to life-long learning. Just as the youth of America grow and change, so must we as health care professionals.

REFERENCES

1. Reference deleted in proofs.
2. Abbotts B, Osborne LM: Immunization status and reasons for immunization delay among children using public health immunization clinics. *Am J Dis Child* 147:965-968, 1993.
3. Adams RC: Spina bifida: life span management. In:Wadsworth C, ed: *Orthopedic interventions for pediatric patients, APTA orthopaedic section: home study course 10.2.2,* LaCrosse, WI, 2002.
4. Adams PF, Hendershot GE, Marano MA: Current estimates from the National Health Interview Survey, 1996, National Center for Health Statistics, *Vital Health Stat* 19(200):1-212, 1999.
5. Adekoya N, Thurman DJ, White DD, et al: Surveillance of traumatic brain injury deaths, 1989-1998, *MMWR Morb Mortal Wkly Rep* 51:SS-10, 2002.
6. Alford S, Linnen G: The facts: Adolescents, HIV/AIDS and other STDS, *Advocates for Youth,* November, 1998.
7. American Academy of Orthopedic Surgeons: The young athlete, *AAOS Online Services,* February 2002.
8. American Academy of Pediatrics: Policy statement: health supervision for children with achondroplasia (RE9514), *Pediatrics* 95:443-451, 1995.
9. American Academy of Pediatrics: Policy statement: intensive training and sports specialization in young athletes (RE9906), *Pediatrics* 106:154-157, 2000.
10. American Academy of Pediatrics: Policy statement: psychosocial risks of chronic health conditions in childhood and adolescence (RE9338), *Pediatrics* 92:876-878, 1993.
11. American Academy of Pediatrics: Policy statement: recommended childhood immunization schedule—United States, 2002, *Pediatrics* 109:162, 2002.
12. American Cancer Society: The dangers of tobacco, *Patient Medical Assistant,* August 23, 1999, p 1.
13. American College of Sports Medicine: Position stand: exercise and fluid replacement, *Med Sci Sports Exerc* 28:i-vii, 1996.
14. American Dental Association. Available at: http://ada.org.
15. American Physical Rehabilitation Network: *When the feet hit the ground everything changes, 1986,* Toledo, OH, 1986, American Physical Rehabilitation Network.
16. American Physical Rehabilitation Network: *Taking the next step, 1992,* Toledo, OH, American Physical Rehabilitation Network.
17. American Red Cross Sport Safety Training Handbook and Course. Available at: www.redcross.org/services/hss/courses/sports.html.
18. Anderson RN: Deaths: leading causes for 2000, *National Vital Statistics Reports* 50(16):1-88, 2002.
19. Andrews JR, Wilk KE: *The athlete's shoulder,* Philadelphia, 1994, Churchill Livingstone.
20. Baechle TR, Earle RW, eds: *Essentials of strength training and conditioning,* ed 2, Champaign, IL, 2000, Human Kinetics.
21. Baldo M, Aggleton P, Slutkin G: *Does sex education lead to earlier or increased sexual activity in youth?* Presented at the Eleventh International Conference on AIDS, Berlin, June 6-10, 1993, Geneva, Switzerland, World Health Organization, 1993.
22. Bar-Or O: Training considerations for children and adolescents with chronic disease. In Hasson SM, ed: *Clinical exercise physiology,* St Louis, 1994, Mosby.
23. Barrett J, Anderson MA, Palmer P, et al: Upper extremity injuries and rehabilitation of the pediatric athlete. In Wilk K, ed: *APTA sports physical therapy section pediatric home study course* 2000-2, *sports section,* LaCrosse, WI.
24. Beck AT, Steer RA, Garbin MG. Psychometric properties of the Beck Depression Inventory: Twenty-five years of evaluation, *Clin Psych Rev* 8:66-100, 1988.
25. Beck BR: Tibial stress injuries. An etiological review for the purposes of guiding management, *Sports Med* 26:265-279, 1998.
26. Beers MH, Berkow R, Burs M, eds: Obesity, *Merck manual of diagnosis and therapy,* ed 17, Rathway, NJ, 1999, Merck & Co.
27. Behrman RE, Klingman RM, Jenson HB, eds: *Nelson textbook of pediatrics,* ed 17, Philadelphia, 2004, WB Saunders.
28. Bertoli DB: Cerebral palsy life span management. In: *Orthopedic interventions for pediatric patients, orthopedic section, APTA orthopaedic section home study course 10.2.4,* LaCrosse, WI, 2000.
29. Best Start: *Community action for healthy babies,* Toronto, Ontario, Canada, 1999, Best Start Resource Centre [e-mail: beststart@beststart.org].
30. Betz RR, Harms J, Clemens DH, et al: Comparison of anterior and posterior instrumentation for correction of adolescent thoracic idiopathic scoliosis, *Spine* 24:225-239, 1999.

31. Bickley LS: *Bates' guide to physical examination and history taking*, ed 8, Philadelphia, 2003, Lippincott/Williams and Wilkins.

32. Bicycle Helmet Safety Institute. Available at:: www.bhsi.org/stats.html.

33. Boissonnault WG: Prevalence of comorbid conditions, surgeries, and medication use in a physical therapy outpatient population: a multi-centered study, *J Orthop Sport Phys Ther* 29:506-519, 1999.

34. Booth FW, Chakravarthy MV, Gordon SE, et al: Waging war on physical inactivity: using modern molecular ammunition against an ancient enemy, *J Appl Physiol* 93:3-30, 2002.

35. Borowsky IW, Hogan M, Ireland M: Adolescent sexual aggression: risk and protective factors, *Pediatrics* 100:E7, 1997.

36. Brotzman SB, Wilk KE: *Clinical orthopaedic rehabilitation*, ed 2, St Louis, 2003.

37. Brown TE, ed: *Attention deficit disorders and comorbidities in children, adolescents and adults*, Washington, DC, 2000, American Psychiatric Press.

38. Buckwalter JA: Articular cartilage: injuries and potential for healing, *J Orthop Sport Phys Ther* 28:192-202, 1998.

39. Bureau of Justice Statistics, US Department of Justice: *Special report on teenage victims*, Washington, DC, 1986, US Department of Justice.

40. Burke LM, Hawley JA: Fluid balance in team sports: guidelines for optimal practices, *Sports Med* 24:38-54, 1997.

41. Burns BJ, Costello EJ, Angold A, et al: Data watch: children's mental health service use across service sectors, *Health Affairs* 14(3):147-159, 1995.

42. Busch MT: Meniscal injuries in children and adolescents, *Clin Sports Med* 9:661-680, 1990.

43. California Criminal Justice Statistics Center: *Crime and delinquency in California, 1975-98; California Criminal Justice Profiles, Statewide, 1978-98*, Sacramento, California Department of Justice.

44. Califono JA: *National survey of American attitudes on substance abuse VII: teens, parents and siblings*, New York, 2002, National Center for Addiction and Substance Abuse at Columbia University.

45. Califono JA, Booth A: *National survey of American attitudes on substance abuse IV: teens, teachers and principals*, New York, 1998, National Center for Addiction and Substance Abuse at Columbia University.

46. Cameron MH: *Physical agents in rehabilitation: from research to practice*, ed 2, Philadelphia, 2003, WB Saunders.

47. Cameron JR, Bar-Or O: *New horizons in pediatric exercise science*, Champaign, IL, 1995, Human Kinetics Publishers.

48. Campbell SK, Vander Linden DW, Palisano RJ, eds: *Physical therapy for children*, ed 2, Philadelphia, 2000, WB Saunders.

49. Cawley PW: *Is knee bracing really necessary? A review of current research on brace function, the natural history of graft remodeling and physiologic implications*, Carlsbad, CA, 1989, Smith & Nephew Donjoy Biomechanics Research Laboratory.

50. Cech DJ, Martin S: *Functional movement development across the lifespan*, ed 2, Philadelphia, 2002, WB Saunders.

51. Centers for Disease Control and Prevention: *HIV/AIDS surveillance report* 9:1-39, 1997.

52. Centers for Disease Control and Prevention: *Injury mortality: national summary of injury mortality data 1984-1990*, Atlanta, 1993, Centers for Disease Control and Prevention.

53. Centers for Disease Control and Prevention: Knowledge and use of folic acid by women of childbearing age—United States, 1995, *MMWR Morb Mortal Wkly Rep* 44:716-718, 1995.

54. Centers for Disease Control and Prevention: Surveillance summaries: teenage pregnancy, *MMWR Morb Mortal Wkly Rep* 47(SS-3), 1997.

55. Centers for Disease Control and Prevention: Tracking the hidden epidemics: trends in STDs in the United States, 2000.

56. Cheng Mei-Fang: The ABCs of the hormones and behavior, *Bioscience* 14:214-215, 1996.

57. *Children and adolescents with disability due to traumatic injury: a data book*, Department of Physical Medicine and Rehabilitation, National Pediatric Trauma Registry (NPTR), 1996.

58. Children and adults with attention-deficit/hyperactivity disorder (CHADD), 8181 Professional Place, Suite 201, Landover, MD 20785. Available at: www.chadd.org.

59. Child Welfare League of America: *Alcohol and other drug survey of state child welfare agencies*, Washington, DC, 1998, Child Welfare League of America.

60. Chu D: *Jumping into plyometrics*, Champaign, IL, 1998, Human Kinetics.

61. Chugani HT: A critical period of brain development: studies of cerebral glucose utilization with PET, *Prev Med* 27:184-188, 1998.

62. Clinical growth chart, National Center for Health Statistics, *National Center for Chronic Disease Prevention and Health Promotion, May 30, 2000*. Available at: www.cdc.gov/growthcharts.

63. Collins AQ: Our children at risk: children and youth issues, *YMCA Report*, 1998.

64. Cusick B: Lower extremity musculoskeletal development. In: Wadsworth C, ed: *Orthopedic interventions for pediatric patients, Orthopedic Section, APTA Orthopaedic Section: Home Study Course* 10.2.2, LaCrosse, WI, 2002.

65. Cyriax J: *Textbook of orthopedic medicine*, ed 6, Baltimore, 1975, Williams & Wilkins.

66. Dabelstein J: Lower-leg orthoses and casts. In: *Orthopedic interventions for pediatric patients*, APTA orthopaedic section: home study course 10.2.3, 2000.

67. Dalaker J: United States Census Bureau, current population reports, series P60-214, *Poverty in the United States: 2000*, US Government Printing Office, Washington DC, 2001.

68. Dale KS, Landers DM: Weight control in wrestling: eating disorders or disordered eating? *Med Sci Sports Exer* 31:1382-1389, 1999.

69. Darroch JE, Singh S: *Why is teenage pregnancy declining? The roles of abstinence, sexual activity and contraceptive use*, Alan Guttmacher Institute, occasional report no 1, 1999.

70. Davies G, Dickoff-Hoffman S: Neuromuscular testing and rehabilitation of the shoulder complex, *J Orthop Sport Phys Ther* 18:449-458, 1993.

71. Diaz A, Danon M: Recent advances in the diagnosis and treatment of precocious puberty, *Indian J Pediatr* 67:211-215, 2000.

72. Dickinson BP, Mylonakis E, Strong LL, et al: Potential infections related to anabolic steroid injection in young adolescents (letter), *Pediatrics* 103:694, 1999.

73. DiFranza JR, Savageau JA, Rigotti NA, et al: Development of symptoms of tobacco dependence in youths: 30 month follow-up data from the DANDY study, *Tobacco Control* 11:228-235, 2002.

74. Dougherty D: *Children with chronic illness and disabilities*, pub no 02-M025, Rockville, MD, 2002, Agency for Healthcare Research Quality.

75. Drug Abuse Resistance Education (DARE). Available at: www.dare.com.

76. Duberstein-Lindberg L, Sonenstein FL, Ku L, et al: Age differences between minors who give birth and their adult partners, *Fam Plann Perspect* 29:61-66, 1997.

77. Ebraheim NA, Mekhail AO, Gargasz SS: Ankle fractures involving the fibula proximal to the distal tibiofibular syndesmosis, *Foot Ankle Int* 18:513-521, 1997.

78. Eiff PM, Hatch RL, Calmbach WL: *Fracture management for primary care*, Philadelphia, 2002, Saunders.

79. Erickson ME (oral communications): Knee kinesiology and injuries. In: *Physical therapy 677: physical agents in rehabilitation* [course packet], University of Wisconsin-Madison Physical Therapy Program, 2003.

80. Erikson E: *Childhood and society*, ed 2, New York, 1963, Norton.

81. Euhardy M: Wound care: In: *Physical therapy 521: physical agents in rehabilitation* [course packet], University of Wisconsin-Madison Physical Therapy Program, 2003.

82. Faigenbaum AD, Wescott W: *Strength and power for young athletes*, Champaign, IL, 2000, Human Kinetics Publishers.

83. Flanagan P, Gavin TM, Gavin DA, et al: Spinal orthoses. In Lusardi MM, and Nielson CC: *Orthotics and prosthetics in rehabilitation*, Boston, 2000, Butterworth-Heinemann.

84. Fleck SJ, Kraemer WJ: *Designing resistance training programs*, ed 2, Champaign, IL, 1997, Human Kinetics.

85. Fleck SJ, Kraemer WJ: *Periodization breakthrough: the ultimate training system*, Ronkonkoma, NY, 1996, Advanced Research Press.

86. Fleming DT, McQuillian GM, Johnson RE, et al: Herpes simplexvirus type 2 in the United States, 1976 to 1994, *N Engl J Med* 337:1105-1111, 1997.

87. Foster TB, Tippett S: Resistance training in the adolescent athlete, In Wilk K, ed: *APTA sports physical therapy section pediatric home study course*, pp 2000-2002.

88. Frances A, Pingus HA, First MB, eds: *Diagnostic and statistical manual of mental disorders*, ed 4, Washington, DC, 1994, American Psychiatric Association.

89. Franklin BA, ed: *American College of Sports Medicine (ACSM) guidelines for exercise testing and prescription*, ed 6, Philadelphia, 2000, Lippincott/Williams & Wilkins.

90. Fredericks CM, Saladin LK: *Pathophysiology of the motor systems: principles and clinical presentations*, Philadelphia, 1996, FA Davis.

91. Friedrich MJ: Report documents causes of child death, *JAMA* 282:1903-1905, 1999.

92. Frisch RA, Barbier RL: *Female fertility and the body fat connection*, Chicago, 2002, University of Chicago Press.

93. Frisch RE, Revelle R: Height and weight at menarche and a hypothesis of critical weights and adolescent events, *Science* 169:397-399, 1979.

94. Fu FH, Baratz M: Meniscal injuries. In DeLee J, Drez D, eds: *The knee*, Philadelphia, 1994, WB Saunders.

95. Fu FH, Stone DA, eds: *Sports injuries: mechanisms, prevention, treatment*, Baltimore, 1994, Williams & Wilkins, pp 758-759.

96. Garner DM: Psycho-educational principles in treatment. In Garner DM, Garfinkel PE, eds: *Handbook of treatment for eating disorders*, New York, 1997, Guilford Press.

97. Garner DM, Olmsted MP, Bohr Y, et al: The eating attitudes test: psychometric features and clinical correlates, *Psych Med* 12:871-878, 1982.

98. Gay and Lesbian Medical Association and LGBT health experts: *Healthy People 2010 companion document for lesbian, gay, bisexual, and transgender (LGBT) health*, San Francisco, CA, 2001, Gay and Lesbian Medical Association.

99. Geissler WB, Whipple TL: Intraarticular abnormalities in association with posterior cruciate ligament injuries, *Am J Sports Med* 21(6):846-849, 1993.

100. Gillogly SD, Voight M, Blackburn T: Treatment of articular cartilage defects of the knee with autologous chondrocyte implantation, *J Orthop Sport Phys Ther* 28:241-251, 1998.

101. Godfried DH: Scoliosis and pediatric spinal deformity. In: Orthopedic interventions for pediatric patients, *APTA orthopaedic section: home study course* 10.2.6, LaCrosse, WI, 2000.

102. Goldberg L, Elliot D: The adolescents training and learning to avoid steroids program: preventing drug use and promoting health behaviors, *Arch Pediatr Adolesc Med* 154:332-338, 2000.

103. Goldman LS, Genel M, Bezman RJ, et al: Diagnosis and treatment of attention-deficit/hyperactivity disorder in children and adolescents, *JAMA* 279:1100-1107, 1998.

104. Goodman CC, Boissonnault WG, Fuller KS: *Pathology: implications for the physical therapist*, ed 2, Philadelphia, 2003, Saunders (Elsevier Science).

105. Graf BK Lange RH, Fujisake CK, et al: Anterior cruciate ligament tears in skeletally immature patients: meniscal pathology at presentation and after conservative treatment, *J Arthroscopy Rel Surg* 8:229-233, 1992.

106. Grant B: Estimates of US children exposed to alcohol abuse and dependence in the family, *Am J Pub Health* 90:112, 2000.

107. Gray JC: Neural and vascular anatomy of the menisci of the human knee, *J Orthop Sport Phys Ther* 29:24, 1999.

108. Green E: Developmental neurology. In Stokes M, ed: *Neurological physiotherapy*, St Louis, Mosby, 1998, pp 215-228.

109. Greenberg LJ: Globalization and unequal access to health care: resources for people with AIDS and other life-threatening illnesses, *The Health GAP Coalition White Paper*, March 23, 2002.

110. Greiner KA: Adolescent idiopathic scoliosis: radiologic decision-making, *Am Fam Phys* 65:1817-1822, 2002.

111. Gross ML, Grover JS, Bassett LW, et al: Magnetic resonance imaging of the posterior cruciate ligament: clinical use to improve diagnostic accuracy, *Am J Sports Med* 20:732-737, 1992.

112. Grunwald Associates: Children, families and the internet 2002 (survey), 1793 Escalante Way, Burlingame, CA.

113. Guitong Y, Hayashi K, Woo SLY, et al: *Biomechanics: proceedings of 4th China-Japan-USA Singapore conference on biomechanics*, River Edge, NJ, 1995, World Scientific Publishing.

114. Guyton AC: *Textbook of medical physiology*, ed 10, Philadelphia, 2000, WB Saunders.

115. Campbell JL, Quitadomo MJ, Zug KA, et al: Acne. In Habif TP, ed: *Skin disease: diagnosis and treatment*, St Louis, 2001, Mosby, pp 72-83.

116. Hall C, Thein-Brody L: *Therapeutic exercise: moving towards function*, Philadelphia, 1999, Lippicott/Williams & Wilkins.

117. Hallisy KM: *Sports injury prevention for the high school athlete*. In: Proceedings from Henry Ford Health System Sports Medicine Symposium, Detroit, MI, 1994, Henry Ford Health System.

118. Hanquinet S, Ngo L, Anooshiravani M, et al: Magnetic resonance imaging helps in the early diagnosis of myositis ossificans in children, *Pediatr Surg Int* 15:287-289, 1999.

119. Harrigan TM: Orthotics and exercise in the management of scoliosis. In: Lusardi MM, Nielson CC: *Orthotics and prosthetics in rehabilitation*, Boston, 2000, Butterworth-Heinemann.

120. Hassan I, Dorani BJ: Rollerblading and skateboarding injuries in children in northeast England, *Emerg Med J* 16(5):348-350, 1999.

121. Hasson SM, ed: *Clinical exercise physiology*. St Louis, 1994, Mosby.

122. Haynatzka V, Peck M, Sappenfeld W, et al: Racial and ethnic disparities in infant mortality rates—60 largest US cities, 1995-1998, *MMWR Morb Mortal Wkly Rep* 51(15):329-332, 343, 2002.

123. *Healthy People 2010*, Office of Disease Prevention and Health Promotion, Washington, DC, 2002, US Department of Health and Human Services. Available at: http://healthypeople.gov.

124. Heller DR, Routley V, Chambers S: Rollerblading injures in young children, *J Ped Child Health* 32:35-38, 1996.

125. Henggeler SW, Schoenwald SK, Borduin CM, et al: *Multisystemic treatment of antisocial behavior in children and adolescents*, New York, 1998, Guilford Publications.

126. Henggeler SW, Rowland MD, Randall J, et al: Home-based multisystemic therapy as an alternative to the hospitalization of youths in psychiatric crisis: clinical outcomes, *J Am Acad Child Adol Psych* 38:1331-1339. 1999.

127. Henggeler SW, Schoenwald SK, Pickrel SG: Multisystemic therapy: bridging the gap between university- and community-based treatment, *J Consult Clin Psychol* 63:709-717, 1995.

128. Henshaw SK: US teenage pregnancy statistics, with comparative statistic for women aged 20-24, New York, 1998, Alan Guttmacher Institute.

129. Hixon Al, Gibbs LM: Osteochondritis dissecans: a diagnosis not to miss, *Am Fam Phys* 61:151-156, 158, 2000.

130. Hoffmann S, Trnka HJ, Metzenroth H, et al: General short-term indomethacin prophylaxis to prevent heterotopic ossification in total hip arthroplasty, *Orthopedics* 22(2):207-211, 1999.

131. Holder HD, Gruenewald PJ, Ponicki WR, et al: Effect of community-based interventions on high-risk drinking and alcohol-related deaths, *JAMA* 284:2341-2347, 2000.

132. Honein MA, Pualozzi LJ, Erickson JD: Continued occurrence of Accutane-exposed pregnancies, *Teratology* 64:142-147, 2001.

133. Hopkins WG, Hawley JA, Burke LM: Design and analysis of research on sport performance enhancement, *Med Sci Sports Exer* 31:472-485, 1999.

134. Hunter S, Rich BSE, Smith DM, et al: *Pre-participation physical evaluation*, ed 2, Minneapolis, 1997, American Academy of Family Physicians, American Academy of Pediatrics, American Medical Society for Sports Medicine, American Orthopaedic Society for Sports Medicine, American Osteopathic Academy of Sports Medicine.

135. Hurley JA, Anderson TE: Shoulder arthroscopy: its role in evaluating shoulder disorders in the athlete, *Am J Sports Med* 18:480-483, 1990.

136. Ireland M, Hutchinson M: Upper extremity injuries in young athletes, *Clin Sports Med* 14:533-569, 1995.

137. Irrgang JJ, Pezzello D: Rehabilitation following surgical procedures to address articular cartilage lesions of the knee, *J Orthop Sport Phys Ther* 28:232-240, 1998.

138. Irrgang JJ, Whitney SL, Harner CD: Non-operative treatment of rotator cuff injuries in throwing athletes, *J Sport Rehab* 1:197-222, 1992.

139. Isaacs ER, Bookout MR: *Bourdillon's spinal manipulation*, ed 6, Woburn, MA, 2002, Butterworth-Heinemann Publications.

140. Institute of Medicine's summary report, *The hidden epidemic: confronting sexually transmitted diseases*, Washington DC, 1997, National Academy Press.

141. Irving LM, Wall M, Neumark-Sztainer D, et al: Steroid use among adolescents: findings from Project EAT, *J Adolesc Health* 30(4):243-252, 2002.

142. Jackson A, Davis GA, Abeel M, et al: *Turning points 2000: educating adolescents in the 21st century*, New York, 2000, Teachers College Press.

143. Jarvis C: *Physical examination and health assessment*. Philadelphia, 1992, WB Saunders.

144. Jemal A, Murray TA, Thun M: A cancer journal for clinicians, *Cancer Stat* 52(1), 2002.

145. Jemmott JB, Jemmott LS: Behavioral interventions with heterosexual adolescents. In: *NIH consensus development conference on interventions to prevent HIV risk behaviors*, Bethesda, MD, 1997, National Institutes of Health.

146. Johnston LD, O'Malley PM, Bachman JG: *Monitoring the future national survey results on adolescent drug use: overview of key findings, 2002*, NIH pub no 03-5374, Bethesda, MD, 2003, National Institute on Drug Abuse.

147. Kamkar A, Irrgang JJ, Whitney SL: Nonoperative management of secondary shoulder impingement syndrome, *J Orthop Sport Phys Ther* 17(3):212-224, 1993.

148. Kaye S: Disability watch: the status of people with disabilities in the US, San Francisco, 1998, Disability Statistics Center, University of California, San Francisco.

149. Kell R, Jenkins AP: HIV transmission and athletics: realities and recommendations, *National Strength Conditioning Aassociation Journal* 20:1, 1998.

150. Kendall FP, McCreary EK, Provance PG: *Muscles—testing and function*, ed 4, Baltimore, 1993, Williams and Wilkins.

151. Kerstein MD, Bensing KA, Brill LR, et al, eds: *The physiology of wound healing (monograph)*, Philadelphia, PA, 1998, Oxford Institute for Continuing Education, Allegheny University of The Health Sciences.

152. Kienapfel H, Koller M, Wust A, et al: Prevention of heterotopic bone formation after total hip arthroplasty: a prospective randomised study comparing postoperative radiation therapy with indomethacin medication, *Arch Orthop Trauma Surg* 119(5-6):296-302, 1999.

153. Kim S-H, Kwon-Ick H, Kye-Young, H, et al: Biceps load test: a clinical test for superior labrum anterior and posterior lesions in shoulders with recurrent anterior dislocation, *Am J Sports Med* 27:300-303, 1999.

154. Kirkpatrick JS, Koman LA, Rovere GD: The role of ultrasound in the early diagnosis of myositis ossificans: a case report, *Am J Sports Med* 15179-181, 1987.

155. Knecht JF: Knee orthoses. In Lusardi MM, Nielson CC, eds: *Orthotics and prosthetics in rehabilitation*, Boston, 2000, Butterworth-Heinemann.

156. Kriel RL, Krach LA: Traumatic brain and spinal cord injuries in children. In Maria BL: *Current management in child neurology*, Boston, 1999, Blackwell Sciences.

157. Langlois JA, ed: Traumatic brain injury in the United States: assessing outcomes in children. In: *Summary and recommendations from the expert working group*, Atlanta, October 26-27, 2000, National Center for Injury Prevention and Control of the Centers for Disease Control and Prevention.

158. Larson CM, Almekinders LC, Karas SG, et al: Evaluating and managing muscle contusions and myositis ossificans, *Phys Sports Med* 30:2, 2002.

159. Leach J: Pediatric musculoskeletal disorders. In: *Orthopedic interventions for pediatric patients, APTA Orthopaedic Section: home study course* 10.2.5, LaCrosse, WI, 2000.

160. Leonard JW: Diagnostic imaging of the bones and joints. In: *APTA orthopaedic section: home study course*, LaCrosse, WI, 1999, p 9.1.2.

161. Levangie PK, Norkin CC: *Joint structure and function*, ed 3, Philadelphia, 2001, FA Davis.

162. Lewis C: Physiological response to exercise in the child: considerations for the typically and atypically developing youngster. In: *Proceedings from the American Physical Therapy Association combined sections meeting*, San Antonio, TX, 2001.

163. Liu SH, Henry M, Nuccion S, et al: A prospective evaluation of a new physical examination in predicting glenoid labrum tears, *Am J Sports Med* 24B:721-725, 1996.

164. Loth TS, Wadsworth CT: *Orthopedic review for physical therapists*, St Louis, 1998, Mosby.

165. Lusardi MM, Nielsen CC: *Orthotics and prosthetics in rehabilitation*, Boston, 2000, Butterworth-Heinemann.

166. Lyon RM, Street CC: Pediatric sports injuries, *Ped Clin North Am* 45(1):221-244, 1998.

167. Magee DJ: *Orthopedic physical assessment*, ed 4, Philadelphia, 2002, Saunders.

168. Marshall WA, Tanner JM: Variations in the pattern of pubertal changes in boys, *Arch Dis Child* 45:13-23, 1970.

169. Marshall WA, Tanner JM: Variations in the pattern of pubertal changes in girls, *Arch Dis Child* 44:291-303, 1969.

170. Martin JA, Hamilton BE, Venture SJ, et al: Births: final data for 2000, *NVSS: National Vital Statistics Reports* 50(5)1-102, 2002.

171. Massachusetts Osteoporosis Awareness Program: *Adolescents with eating disorders are significantly increasing their risk of osteoporosis*, Boston, July 13, 1998, Massachusetts Department of Public Health.

172. McDevitt TM, Rowe PM: *The United States in international context: 2000*, Washington, DC, 2002, US Census Bureau. Available at: www.census.gov/ prod/cen2000/doc/sfl.pdf.

173. McArdle WD, Katch FI, Katch VL: *Exercise physiology: energy, nutrition, and human performance*, ed 5, Philadelphia, 2001, Lippincott/Williams & Wilkins Publishers.

174. McKinnis LN: *Fundamentals of orthopedic radiology*, Philadelphia, 1997, FA Davis.

175. Mimori K, Muneta T, Nakagama T, et al: A new pain provocation test for superior labral tears of the shoulder, *Am J Sports Med* 27:137-142, 1999.

176. Moore KA, Driscoll A, Duberstein-Lindberg L, et al: *A statistical portrait of adolescent sex, contraception, and childbearing*, Washington, DC, 1998, The National Campaign to Prevent Teen Pregnancy.

177. Morgan EA, Wroble RR: Diagnosing posterior cruciate ligament injuries, *Phys Sports Med* 25, 1997.

178. Morgenstern WA, Metz-Stavenhagen PJ, Seidel T, et al: The results of selective anterior thoracic fusion for King II/Lenke type CL adolescent idiopathic scoliosis, *ISIS*, published online March 30, 2001.

179. Murphy SL: Deaths: final data for 1998. *Natl Vital Stat Rep* 48:1-105, 2000. National Clearinghouse for Alcohol and Drug Information (NCADI) web site. Available at: www.health.org/.

180. National Asthma Education and Prevention Program, *J Allergy Clin Immunol* 110(5), 2002.

181. National Institute on Alcohol Abuse and Alcoholism: *Youth drinking: risk factors and consequences, alcohol alert no 37*, Bethesda, MD, July, 1997, subsidiary of National Institute on Drug Abuse. Available at: www.nida.nih.gov or www.drugabuse.gov.

182. National Institute of Mental Health: *Brief notes on the mental health of children and adolescents*, Bethesda, MD, 2003, NIMH. Available at: *www.nimh.nih.gov/publicat/childnotes.cfm*.

183. National Sleep Foundation, 1522 K Street, NW, Suite 500, Washington, DC 2005; NSF@sleepfoundation.org.

184. Neumann DA: *Kinesiology of the musculoskeletal system: foundations for physical rehabilitation*, St Louis, 2002, Mosby.

185. Norkin M, Frankel VH: *Basic biomechanics of the musculoskeletal system*, ed 3, Philadelphia, 2001, Lippincott, Williams & Wilkins.

186. Noyes FR, Mooar PA, Matthews DS, et al: The symptomatic anterior cruciate-deficient knee. Part I: the long-term functional disability in athletically active individuals, *J Bone Joint Surg* (Am) 65:154-162, 1983.

187. O'Brien SJ, Pagnini MH, Fealy S, et al: Active compression (O'Brien) test for labral abnormality, *Am J Sports Med* 26:5, 1998.

188. Office of National AIDS Policy: *Youth and HIV/AIDS: an American agenda. A report to the president*, Washington, DC, 1996.

189. O'Sullivan SB, Schmitz TJ: *Physical rehabilitation laboratory manual: focus on functional training*, Philadelphia, 1999, FA Davis.

190. Payne RA: *Relaxation techniques: a practical handbook for the health care professional*, NewYork, 1995, Churchill Livingstone.

191. Pierson FM, Fairchild SL: *Principles and techniques of patient care*, ed 3, Philadelphia, 2002, Saunders.

192. Perkins CA: *Age patterns of victims of serious violent crime, Bureau of Justice Statistics: special report*, July 1997, NCJ-162031.

193. *For your health, back pack guidelines, PT Magazine* 17(Sept):13, 2001.

194. Pruitt D, ed: *Your adolescent: emotional, behavioral, and cognitive development from early adolescence through the teen years*, ed 2, New York, 2000, HarperCollins.

195. Rabinowicz T, de Courten-Myers G, McDonald-Comber Petetot J, et al: Human cortex development: estimates of neuronal numbers indicate major loss late in gestation, *J Neuropathol Exp Neurol* 55:320-328, 1996.

196. Rao S, Joshi S, Kanade A: Height velocity, body fat and menarcheal age of Indian girls, *Indian Pediatrics* 35:619-630, 1998.

197. Reis LAG, Smith MA, Gurney JG, et al, eds: *Cancer incidence and survival among children and adolescents: United States SEER program 1975-1995* [NIH publ No. 99-4649], Bethesda, MD, 1999, National Cancer Institute, SEER Program.

198. Remafedi G, French S, Story M, et al: The relationship between suicide risk and sexual orientation: results of a population-based study, *Am J Pub Health* 88:57-60, 1998.

199. Resnick MD, Bearman PS, Blum RW, et al: Protecting adolescents from harm: findings from the national longitudinal study on adolescent health, *JAMA* 278:823-832, 1997.

200. Robergs RA, Roberts SO: *Exercise physiology: exercise, performance, and clinical applications*, St Louis, 1997, Mosby.

201. Roberts S, Weider B, Demayo P: *Strength and weight training for young athletes*, 1994, McGraw-Hill/Contemporary Books.

202. Robinson LR: Role of neurophysiologic evaluation in diagnosis, *J Am Acad Orthop Surg* 8:190-199, 2000.

203. Roeher Institute. Vulnerable: sexual abuse and people with an intellectual handicap, New York, 1988, The Roeher Institute.

204. Ross M: *CPSC reports as scooter sales skyrocket, injuries soar* [Consumer Product Safety Commission, release 00-178;(301) 504-0580] Washington, DC, US Consumer Product Safety Commission.

205. Rothstein JA, ed: *Guide to physical therapist practice*, ed 2, Alexandria, VA, 2001, American Physical Therapy Association.

206. Rubinstein RA Jr, Shelbourne KD, McCarroll JR, et al: The accuracy of the clinical examination in the setting of posterior cruciate ligament injuries, *Am J Sports Med* 22:550-557, 1994.

207. Runyan CW, Gerken EA: Epidemiology and prevention of adolescent injury: a review and research agenda, *JAMA* 16:2273-2278, 1989.

208. Sackett DL, Straus SE, Richardson WS, et al: *Evidence-based medicine: how to practice and teach EBM*, ed 2, Edinburgh, 2000, Churchill Livingstone.

209. Safe Schools Coalition of Washington: *Safe schools anti-violence documentation project: third annual report*, Seattle, WA, 1996, Safe Schools Coalition.

210. Sahrmann S: *Diagnosis and treatment of movement impairment syndromes*, St Louis, 2001, Mosby.

211. Salter RB: *Textbook of disorders and injuries of the musculoskeletal system*, ed 3, Baltimore, 1999, Williams and Wilkins.

212. Saunders HD, Saunders R: *Evaluation, treatment and prevention of musculoskeletal disorders*, vol 1 (spine), ed 3, Chaska, MN, 1995, The Saunders Group.

213. Savin-Williams RC: Verbal and physical abuse as stressors in the lives of lesbian, gay male, and bisexual youths; associations with school problems, running away, substance abuse, prostitution and suicide, *J Consult Clin Psychol* 62:261-269, 1994.

214. Schoenborn CA, Adams PF, Barnes PM: *Body weight status of adults: United States, 1997-98. Advance data from vital and health statistics, #330*, Hyattsville, MD, 2002, National Center for Health Statistics.

215. Schoenwal SK, Ward DM, Henggeler SW, et al: MST treatment of substance abusing or dependent adolescent offenders, costs of reducing incarceration, inpatient, and residential placement., *J Child Fam St* 4: 431-444, 1996.

216. Setswe G: A policy analysis of the childhood immunization initiative in Philadelphia, *Internet Med J* 6(1), 2002.

217. Shaffer D, Fisher P, Dulcan MK, et al: The NIMH diagnostic interview schedule for children version 2.3 (DISC-2.3): description, acceptability, prevalence rates, and performance in the MECA study. Methods for the epidemiology of child and adolescent mental disorders study, *J Am Acad Child Adolesc Psychiatr* 35:865-877, 1996.

218. Shumway-Cook A, Woollacott MH: *Motor control: theory and practical application*, ed 2, Baltimore, 2000, Lippincott, Williams and Wilkins.

219. Sizonenko PC: Pubertal development: the view of the pediatric endocrinologist. Zeist, Netherlands, 1997, Medical Forum International, BV. Available at: www.medforum.nl.

220. Slawski DP, Seip R, Dahlgren G: Lower extremity injuries in the young athlete. In Wilk K, ed: *APTA sports physical therapy section pediatric home study course* 2000-2, LaCrosse, WI, 2000.

221. Solomon DH, Simel DL, Bates DW, et al: The rational clinical examination. Does this patient have a torn meniscus or ligament of the knee? Value of the physical examination, *JAMA* 286:1610-1620, 2001 (review).

222. Speer KP, Lohnes J, Garrett WE Jr: Radiographic imaging of muscle strain injury, *Am J Sports Med* 21:89-95, 1993.

223. Stanitski C, Sherman C: How I manage physeal fractures about the knee, *Phys Sportsmed* 24:59-70, 1996.

224. *Statistics on spinal cord injury*, St Louis, 2000, Spinal Cord Injury Program, Washington University, School of Medicine.

225. Stein RE, Gortmaker SL, Perrin EC, et al: Severity of illness: concepts and measurements, *Lancet* 2:1506-1509, 1987.

226. Steinberg L, Levine A: *You and your adolescent: a parent's guide for ages 10 to 20*, Quill, New York, 1997, Harper Resource.

227. Straus MA, Gelles RJ: *Physical violence in American families: risk factors for adaptations to violence in 8,145 families*, New Brunswick, NJ, 1990, Transactions Books.

228. Sullivan PE, Markos PD: *Clinical decision making in therapeutic exercise*, Stamford, CN, 1995, Appleton & Lange.

229. Swenson TM, Harner CD: Knee ligament and meniscal injuries. Current concepts, *Orthop Clin North Am* 26(3):529-546, 1995.

230. Szilagyi PG: Assessing children: infancy through adolescence. In Bickley LS, Szilagyi PG, eds: *Bates' guide to physical examination and history taking*, ed 8, Philadelphia, 2003, Lippincott, Williams and Wilkins.

231. Talking with kids about tough issues: a national survey of parents and kids, New York, 2001, Nickelodeon. Available at: www.talkingwithkids.org.

232. Teitz CC, Hermanson BK, Kronmal RA, et al: Evaluation of the use of braces to prevent injury to the knee in collegiate football players, *J Bone Joint Surg* 69A:2-9, 1987.

233. Tewes DP, Fritts HM, Fields RD, et al: Chronically injured posterior cruciate ligament: magnetic resonance imaging, *Clin Orthop* Feb(335):224-232, 1997.

234. Thacker SB, Stroup DF, Branche CM: The prevention of ankle sprains in sports, *Am J Sports Med* 27:753-760, 1999.

235. Thein LA, Thein JM: The female athlete, *J Orthop Sport Phys Ther* 23:134-148, 1996.

236. The White House: *The national AIDS strategy*, Washington, DC, 1997, Office of the President.

237. *The world factbook*, Washington, DC, 2001, Central Intelligence Agency.

238. Titlebaum H: Relaxation. In Zahourek RP, ed: *Relaxation and imagery: tools for therapeutic communication and intervention*, Philadelphia, 1988, WB Saunders.

239. *Title IX at 30: report card on gender equity*, Washington, DC, June, 2002, National Coalition for Women and Girls in Education.

240. Torg JS, Naranja J, Pavlov H, et al: The relationship of developmental narrowing of the cervical spinal canal to reversible and irreversible injury to the cervical spinal cord in football players, *J Bone Joint Surg (Am)* 78:1308-1314, 1996.

241. Torg JS, Ramsey-Emrhein JA: Cervical spine and brachial plexus injuries: return-to-play recommendations, *Phys Sports Med* 25(7), 1997.

241a. Trends in sexual risk behaviors among high school students, 1991-1997, *MMWR Morb Mortal Wkly Rep* 47(36):749-752, 1998.

242. Umphred DA: *Neurological rehabilitation*, ed 4, St Louis, 2001, Mosby.

243. US Conference of Mayors: *A status report on hunger and homelessness in American cities 1998: a 30-city survey*, Washington, DC, December, 1998.

244. US Consumer Product Safety Commission (CPSC), Washington, DC, 20207.

245. US Department of Agriculture and US Department of Health and Human Services: *Nutrition and your health: dietary guidelines for Americans*. Washington, DC, 2000, USDA, USDHHS.

246. US Department of Health and Human Services and Children's Bureau: *Child maltreatment 1998: reports from the states to the National Child Abuse and Neglect Data System (NCANDS)*, Washington, DC, 2000, US Government Printing Office.

247. US Department of Health and Human Services, Centers for Disease Control and Prevention: *Lyme disease report*, July, 2002.

248. US Department of Justice, Bureau of Justice Statistics: Prior abuse reported by inmates and probationers: based upon several surveys of inmates and adults on probation (1995-1997), April, 1999, *NCJ* 172879. Available at: www.ojp.usdoj.gov/bjs.

249. Van der Heide HJ, Koorevaar RT, Schreurs BW, et al: Indomethacin for 3 days is not effective as prophylaxis for heterotopic ossification after primary total hip arthroplasty, *J Arthroplasty* 14:796-799, 1999.

250. Vielpeau C, Joubert JM, Hulet C: Naproxen in the prevention of heterotopic ossification after total hip replacement, *Clin Orthop* 369:279-288, 1999.

251. Volpe JJ: *Neurology of the newborn*, ed 4, Philadelphia, 2001, WB Saunders.

252. Wainner RS, Flynn TW, Whitman J: *Spinal and extremity manipulation: the basic skill set for physical therapists* [CD-ROM], Minneapolis, MN, 2001, Manipulations, Inc. Available at OPTP.com

253. Weeks MR, Schensul JJ, Williams SS, et al: AIDS prevention for African American and Latina women: building culturally and gender-appropriate interventions, *AIDS Educ Prev* 7:251-263, 1995.

254. *Whatever happened to childhood? The problem of teen pregnancy in the United States*, Washington, DC, 1997, National Campaign to Prevent Teen Pregnancy.

255. Wheeless CR: *Wheeless' textbook of orthopaedics*, Durham, NC, 2002, Duke University Medical Center. Available at: Orthopaedics Online, Belgian Orthoweb. http://wheelessonline.com.

256. Whiteside JA: Musculoskeletal overload problems in the immature recreational athlete. Part I: the lower extremity and spine, *Sports Med Update* (a publication of Healthsouth Sports Medicine Network & American Sports Medicine Institute) 9:20-30, 1994.

257. Wilk KE, Arrigo C: Current concepts in the rehabilitation of the athletic shoulder, *J Orthop Sport Phys Ther* 18:365-378, 1993.

258. Wilk KE, Arrigo C, Andrews JR: Rehabilitation of the elbow in the throwing athlete, *J Orthop Sport Phys Ther* 17:305-317, 1993.

259. Wilkins K: Shoulder injuries. In Stanitski CL, Delee JC, Drez D, eds: *Pediatric and adolescent sports medicine*, Philadelphia, 1994, WB Saunders.

260. Winter P: *Top 10 ways to monitor kids' computer health*, Sept, 2001, APTA press release.

261. Wirth MA, Rockwood CA: Acute and chronic traumatic injuries of the sternoclavicular joint, *J AAOS* 4:268-278, 1996.

262. Wysowski DK, Swann J, Vega A: Use of isotretinoin (Accutane) in the United States: rapid increase from 1992 through 2000, *J Am Acad Dermatol* 46:505-509, 2002.

263. Yawn BP, Amadio P, Harmsen WS: Isolated acute knee injuries in the general population, *J Trauma* 48:716-723, 2000.

264. Yawn BP, Yawn RA, Hodge D, et al: A population-based study of school scoliosis screening, *JAMA* 282:1472-1474, 1999.

265. Zachazewski JE, Magee DJ, Quillen WS: *Athletic injuries and rehabilitation*, Philadelphia, 1996, WB Saunders.

266. Zemper ED: A two-year prospective study of prophylactic knee braces in a national sample of college football players, *Sports Train Med Rehabil* 1:287-296, 1990.

Appendix **12-1** Pediatric Health Care Organizations, References, and Resources

- American Academy of Child and Adolescent Psychiatry: www.aacap.org
- AACAP resource links: www.aacap.org/resource
- American Academy of Family Physicians: www.familydoctor.org
- American Academy of Orthopaedic Surgery: www.aaos.org
- American Academy of Pediatrics: www.aap.org
- American Cancer Association: http://cancer.org
- American College of Allergy, Asthma & Immunology: www.allergy.mcg.edu
- American Dental Association: http://ada.org
- American Red Cross: www.redcross.org
- Best Start: Community Action for Healthy Babies: http://beststart@beststart.org
- Bicycle Helmet Safety Institute: www.bhsi.org
- Centers for Disease Control: www.cdc.gov
- Clinical Growth Charts: www.cdc.gov/growthcharts
- Drug Abuse Resistance Education (DARE): http://dare.com/
- Gay and Lesbian Medical Association: http://glma.org
- Healthy People 2010: www.health.gov/healthypeople
- Kaiser Family Foundation: www.talkingwithkids.org/
- Monitoring the Future: http://www.monitoringthefuture.org
- National Asthma Education and Prevention Program: www.nhlbi.nih.gov/about/naepp
- National Interscholastic Athletic Administrators Association: http://niaaa.org
- National Institute on Drug Abuse:http://drugabuse.gov
- National Institute on Mental Health: http://nimh.nih.gov
- National Sleep Foundation: http://sleepfoundation.org
- National Youth Sports Safety Foundation: www.nyssf.org
- Talking with Kids About Tough Issues: http://talkingwithkids.org
- United States Department of Agriculture: www.usda.gov

The Obstetric Patient   13

Jill Schiff Boissonnault, PT, PhD
Rebecca Gourley Stephenson, PT

Objectives

After reading the chapter, the reader will be able to:

1. Describe the roles of the caregivers for the obstetric patient.
2. Define terms unique to pregnancy and the postpartum period.
3. Describe the anatomic and physiological changes in pregnancy and the postpartum period.
4. Describe the common medical conditions and symptoms of pregnancy and the postpartum period, including those that warrant referral.
5. Describe the common symptoms and diseases that occur in pregnancy that imitate musculoskeletal conditions.
6. Describe examination modifications necessary for this population.
7. Describe the special issues of pregnant women with disabilities or chronic illness.
8. Describe medial diagnostic and pharmacologic challenges in the childbearing year.

Prenatal and Postpartum Issues

Interest in obstetric physical therapy has expanded concomitantly with increased attention directed toward research and advocacy for a broad range of women's health issues. As movement specialists, physical therapists (PTs) are ideally suited to adapt and expand their knowledge base to include evaluation and treatment of the pregnant and postpartum patient. This chapter highlights the anatomic and physiological changes in pregnancy and the postpartum period, common medical conditions, and screenings that warrant referral. Special conditions in pregnancy, examination modifications, medication concerns, and diagnostic challenges are also covered.

The design of this chapter is to assist the orthopedic PT in understanding the nomenclature necessary for interdisciplinary communication, the changes that occur during pregnancy and the postpartum period, the systems changes that affect the childbearing year, coverage of selected disease response to pregnancy, and information that might directly affect intervention or examination.

Armed with the information presented in this chapter, any PT should be able to confidently examine and then refer on an obstetric patient whose symptoms demand medical attention or specialty women's health physical therapy. Additionally, this chapter was written to enable PTs to treat pregnant and postpartum women without worry of unsafe positioning or intervention modalities and to familiarize the PT with the many complications and disease exacerbations that their patients may experience. This information should allow for more holistic care of this population and increased PT comfort in providing services for these women.

Defining Obstetric Terms

Many terms are used to describe number of pregnancies and deliveries and the stages of pregnancy, labor, and postpartum period (Table 13-1). These definitions are relevant to understanding the prenatal medical record and aid in communication with other health care practitioners.

Para, from the French word *parere*, meaning "to give birth," is the base word for the number of times a woman has given birth, regardless of the number of infants born (e.g., twins, triplets). *Gravida*, from the French word *gravis*, meaning "heavy," describes a woman who is or has been pregnant, regardless of the pregnancy outcome.

Past obstetric history can be documented in two different written forms. The *gravida para* method notes the number of pregnancies and births; for example, "gravida 3 para 2" means that a woman has been pregnant three times and has delivered two infants. The second, more complete method indicates reproductive history and is indicated by a series of numbers separated by dashes. The first number refers to the number of term infants, the second the number of preterm infants, the third the number of abortions, and the fourth the number of children currently alive. For example, an obstetric history in a chart with a number sequence of 3-1-2-3 indicates that the woman had 3 term deliveries, one preterm delivery, two abortions, and 3 children currently living.[41]

The Caregivers: Who They Are and Their Differences in Philosophy and Practice

Many health care professions are involved in the care of the pregnant woman. Overlap occurs in some of the roles.

Registered nurses can train to work in obstetrics by becoming additionally trained as a family, gynecologic, or women's health *nurse practitioner*. These programs consist of a formal curriculum leading to either a certificate or master's degree in nursing. Nurse practitioners typically work under the supervision of a physician and can order diagnostic procedures.

A *direct-entry midwife* has a certificate of midwifery studies without any other prerequisite. They have a limited scope of practice that is particular to home births, but they may also practice in birth centers. Direct-entry midwives learn by apprenticeship. Their birth philosophy is generally holistic and noninterventionist.

TABLE 13-1

Classification of Maternal Circumstance by Number of Pregnancies, Live Births, and Period During the Childbearing Year

Term	Definition
Nullipara	A woman who has not been pregnant or has never completed a pregnancy beyond 20 weeks of gestation.
Primipara	A woman who has had one delivery beyond 20 weeks of gestation.
Multipara	A woman who has delivered two or more pregnancies beyond 20 weeks of gestation regardless of whether the fetuses were born live or stillborn (not the number of fetuses delivered).
Nulligravida	A woman who is not now or who never has been pregnant.
Primigravida	A woman who has been pregnant once, regardless of outcome.
Multigravida	A woman who has had more than one pregnancy, regardless of the outcome. The number represents the number of pregnancies.
Postpartum	The period after childbirth, usually noted as the first 3-6 months after birth.
Puerperal	The period from the end of labor until the uterus returns to prepregnancy size, generally from 3-6 weeks postpartum. Puerpera refers to a woman who has just delivered.
Gestation	Duration of the pregnancy, usually 280 days, or 40 weeks, marked from the first day of the last menstrual period.
Trimesters	Division of weeks of pregnancy: first, 1-13 weeks; second, 14-17 weeks; third, 28-40 weeks.
EDC/EDD	"Expected date of confinement" (EDC) is an old-fashioned term indicating the date a woman was expected to deliver and be confined. A more modern term, estimated date of delivery (EDD), is now commonly used.
Parturient	A woman in labor.
Preterm labor	Labor that starts after the twentieth but before the thirty-seventh week.
Term labor	Labor initiated after the thirty-seventh week of pregnancy but before the forty-second week.
Postterm/postdates	Labor initiated after the thirty-seventh week of pregnancy but before the forty-second week.

A *nurse-midwife* is trained in both nursing and midwifery and attends to births in the hospital, the birthing center, and the home. The majority of these births (94%) are in the hospital.[74] Nurse-midwives practice in collaboration with physicians and are skilled at risk screening to make referrals to a physician when needed. They provide prenatal care, labor and delivery assistance, postpartum care, well-woman gynecology, normal newborn care, and family planning. They practice within the medical model but are less interventionist and more aligned with conservative care models than are allopathic physicians.

An *obstetrician* is a physician who has specialized in the management of pregnancy, labor, and postpartum care. They can manage all types of pregnancies; some may have subspecialty training in high-risk pregnancies. *Perinatologists* are obstetricians specializing in high-risk care.

Family practice physicians also attend deliveries and provide prenatal care. They do not manage high-risk pregnancies.

REFERRALS TO THE PHYSICIAN OR MIDWIFE. Table 13-2 lists some common prenatal and postnatal conditions and their corresponding symptoms and signs. The signs may not be available to the PT, as in the case of medically ordered diagnostic test results. The table lists some of the more likely conditions a PT working in an orthopedic setting might encounter in the prenatal and postnatal population that necessitate communication with the obstetric caregiver.

Examination and Treatment Precautionary Notes

Restrictions guide the PT when planning and administering an examination of obstetric patients. These constraints may impede standard physical therapy procedures, and accommodations

TABLE 13-2

Screening for Common Conditions of Pregnancy and the Postpartum Period that Warrant Communication with Midwife or Physician

Condition	Symptom	Sign/Positive Test Results
Preeclampsia	Headache, blurred vision	Edema (sudden onset, may be global), high blood pressure, proteinuria
Pregnancy-induced hypertension	Headache, blurred vision*	High blood pressure
Ectopic pregnancy	Severe lower abdominal pain,* dizziness or lightheadedness, nausea	Blood tests for progesterone and human chorionic gonadotropin levels; ultrasonography
Abruptio placentae	Severe lower abdominal pain,* vaginal bleeding	Positive ultrasonography
Fetal distress or demise	Decreased fetal movement*	Positive nonstress test or ultrasonography
Osteoporosis of pregnancy	Pain in hip or low back, pain with weight bearing	Empty or spasm end-feel in hip flexion; loss of height
Placenta previa	Vaginal bleeding*	Positive ultrasonography
Retained placenta	Increased postpartum bleeding,* uterine cramping, pelvic pain	Uterine tenderness to palpation
Mastitis	Localized breast tenderness	Localized breast redness, edema; fever may be present

*An urgent referral back to the care provider is warranted.

must be made accordingly. Pregnant women should avoid the following:

- Positions that involve abdominal compression in mid to late pregnancy (e.g., flat prone lying)
- Positions that maintain the supine position for longer than a few minutes after the fourth month of pregnancy
- Activities that strain the pelvic floor and abdominal muscles
- Positions that involve rapid uncontrolled bouncing or swinging movements
- Positions that encourage vigorous stretching of hip adductors
- Overheating
- Deep heat modalities or electrical stimulation over the trunk[70,148,160]

These restrictions are lifted once the mother has delivered. Consequently, most exercise positions and physical agents can be used for treatment in the postpartum period.

Modifications to the History and Physical Examination

HISTORY. A few additions to a standard subjective examination for musculoskeletal symptoms will ensure patient and fetal safety and assist the PT in making a physical therapy diagnosis. Special questions for the pregnant patient are listed in Table 13-3. Special questions for the postpartum patient are listed in Table 13-4.

PHYSICAL EXAMINATION. In addition to an awareness of the normal anatomic and physiological changes occurring in the pregnant and postpartum woman, PTs must also consider alterations in positioning for examination and treatment of this population. *Supine hypotension syndrome*, which occurs in approximately 10% of the pregnant population, can occur when women in the second half of pregnancy lie supine, compressing

---

TABLE 13-3	
Special Questions for History Taking of the Pregnant Patient	
Special Questions	**Ramifications**
Any complications with this pregnancy? (e.g., uterine bleeding, premature contractions, incompetent cervix, pregnancy-induced hypertension, preeclampsia, or other need for special tests or bed rest)	A positive response may alter the rigor of the physical exam and any exercise prescription given by the PT and may necessitate monitoring of vital signs and other signs and symptoms with each visit.
Any complications with a previous pregnancy or delivery that is placing you at high risk now?	For example, preterm labor in one pregnancy places a woman at risk for a similar outcome in subsequent pregnancies. Monitoring a woman for signs of preterm labor should occur with each visit.
Did you have any of your current musculoskeletal symptoms during a previous pregnancy, and, if so, what was done for them and was the treatment successful?	This information can aid the PT in treatment planning.
What medications are currently being taken and what medications did you stop because of the pregnancy?	Medications such as nonsteroidal anti-inflammatories, antidepressants, and migraine prescriptions that are contraindicated in pregnancy can affect symptoms of the musculoskeletal system and a patient's pain perception and affect.
Are you currently having any urinary stress incontinence?	Recognition of this condition will aid the PT and patient in treatment before and after delivery.

From Boissonnault JS, Bookhout MM: Course notes for physical therapy management of musculoskeletal dysfunction in the pregnant client, 2002; and Bookhout MM, Boissonnault WG: Physical therapy management of musculoskeletal disorders during pregnancy. In Wilder E: *Obstetric and gynecological physical therapy: clinics in physical therapy*, New York, 1988, Churchill Livingstone.

TABLE 13-4	
Special Questions for History Taking of the Postpartum Patient	
Special Questions	**Ramifications**
Was patient on bed rest during pregnancy? If so, for how long?	Debilitation may have resulted from prolonged bed rest and may necessitate treatment or modifications.
Did any of the following occur during delivery: regional anesthetic injection; forceps or vacuum extraction; episiotomy or tears of the perineum; cesarean?	Specific tissues may be affected by these procedures or occurrences and may necessitate treatment or referral to a PT with training in women's health.
Do you now have symptoms of urinary or fecal incontinence or organ prolapse?	Referral to a PT with training in rehabilitation of the pelvic floor would be appropriate.
Did you have your current symptoms during your pregnancy or after a previous pregnancy, and, if so, was there any treatment that was successful in ameliorating these symptoms?	A positive response may assist in determining cause, interventions, and prognosis.

From Boissonnault JS, Bookhout MM: Course notes for physical therapy management of musculoskeletal dysfunction in the pregnant client, 2002; and Bookhout MM, Boissonnault WG: Physical therapy management of musculoskeletal disorders during pregnancy. In Wilder E: *Obstetric and gynecological physical therapy: clinics in physical therapy*, New York, 1988, Churchill Livingstone.

returning blood flow by the inferior vena cava.[41,103] These women do not have adequate collateral circulation to the brain to avoid symptoms of shock.[103]

It is important for PTs to follow accepted medical guidelines regarding positioning of pregnant women during the second half of pregnancy. Although only a small percentage of women have overt signs of distress during supine lying, some research has shown that pregnant women have decreased cardiac output as a result of caval occlusion, with a subsequent decrease in uterine blood flow.[5,6] Although changes in fetal heart rate have not been routinely demonstrated,[11] the American College of Obstetricians and Gynecologists discourages exercise in the supine position in the second and third trimesters of pregnancy.[5,6] Extrapolation of these guidelines to PT practice infers avoidance of prolonged supine lying during examination and treatment as well as in exercise classes and home exercise sessions. Use of the supine position for brief palpation and treatment is sometimes necessary, but practices that require longer supine positioning should be done with the women turned 30 degrees to the left, supported with pillows or cushions under the right side.[152] This positioning is sufficient to shift the uterus to the left and relieve caval occlusion.

Modifications to examination and treatment in prone lying become necessary once the gravid uterus rises above the brim of the pelvis (12 to 16 weeks' gestation). Placing a pillow above or below the baby to create a nest for the belly or using an adaptive cushion system both work well for some women until late pregnancy. Women may become nauseated in prone lying, even with these modifications. Mobilization tables with a cutout for the gravid uterus are available in some locations. If prone lying is not possible, almost all examination and treatment techniques can be adapted to a sitting, side-lying, or four-point position.

Medications and Pregnancy

Many prescription and some over-the-counter (OTC) medications are contraindicated in pregnancy because of the risk to the fetus or the mother. Many texts are available to assist health professionals' decision making related to prescription drugs. Patients often take OTC medications or herbal remedies without physician knowledge. If the PT discovers such use, an awareness of any safety issues regarding these substances helps determine whether communication to the obstetric caregiver is warranted. Table 13-5 presents a list of the most common OTC medications and herbal remedies used during pregnancy and by the lactating woman after birth. In general, herbal remedies are not proven to be safe during pregnancy, so their use is discouraged.[41] PTs are also encouraged to visit the Food and Drug Administration (FDA) website (www.fda.gov) and to be cognizant of the FDA categories for medications and drugs in pregnancy. A brief explanation of the FDA categories follows:

- Category A: controlled studies in human beings have demonstrated no fetal risks.
- Category B: animal studies indicate no fetal risks (no human studies are available). It also can mean that adverse effects have occurred in some animal studies but not in well-controlled human studies.
- Category C: No adequate human or animal studies, or there are no human studies to substantiate negative animal studies.

- Category D: Some evidence to indicate fetal risk, but benefits are thought to outweigh these risks.
- Category X: Fetal risks outweigh any potential benefits.

Medical Diagnostic Challenges
Diagnostic Imaging

RADIOGRAPHY. Plain films should be avoided during the first trimester, and overall fetal x-ray exposure should be limited because of the risk of malformation with fetal exposure to more than 0.015 Gy (1.5 rad).[54] The total risk of fetal malformation is increased 1% with exposure to more than 0.1 Gy (10 rad). Abdominal lead shields will reduce the fetal radiation exposure to right-angle scatter by approximately 0.01 mGy (1 mrad), except in filming the lumbar spines and myelography, which should be especially avoided during the first trimester.[54] Standard x-ray films of the thoracic and lumbar spine will expose the fetus to 5 mGy (500 mrad) and 10 mGy (1000 mrad), respectively. Plain films are not an absolute contraindication after the first trimester and may be needed for diagnosis. A trauma series of an extremity, skull, or rib series delivers low doses to the fetus because of the distance from the screened area. A single-view pyelogram can locate a urolithiasis or other urinary obstruction that cannot be proved by ultrasound.[41]

COMPUTED TOMOGRAPHY SCAN. Computed tomography (CT) scans taken of the head and neck expose the fetus to the same minimal dose of radiation as a plain radiograph of the skull and cervical spine.[53] CT is commonly used when rapid diagnosis is needed to differentiate medical and surgical management. During a CT scan a pregnant woman should be positioned in left-lateral tilt with a wedge to avoid hypotension and aortic pulsations.[41]

MAGNETIC RESONANCE IMAGING. Magnetic resonance imaging (MRI) is believed to be safe in pregnancy and is considered low risk. However, MRI is not recommended for use in the first trimester.[41] MRI is used to diagnose arteriovenous malformations, nervous system abnormalities, spinal cord diseases, and demyelinating diseases. MRI is the preferred method of imaging the thoracic and lumbar regions because there is no effect on the fetus.[54] As in a CT scan, the pregnant woman must be in the left-lateral tilt position.

DIAGNOSTIC ULTRASOUND. Diagnostic ultrasound has been in existence since the late 1950s and is considered safe.[113] The sound waves are delivered at a high frequency, 3.5 to 5 MHz for transabdominal and 5 to 7.5 MHz for transvaginal transducers. Increased frequency will give a better resolution but less tissue penetration.[124] Diagnostic ultrasound is frequently used to determine fetal age and well-being, position, fetal cardiac activity, placenta placement, and amount of amniotic fluid. It is not currently recommended by the American College of Obstetricians and Gynecologists in routine low-risk pregnancies.[41]

In 1992, obstetric ultrasonography devices were outfitted with video displays that provided the diagnostician with indications of any ultrasound-induced bioeffects. The two effects of potential concern are (1) the thermal index, which indicates ultrasound-induced tissue heating, and (2) the mechanical index, which indicates inertial cavitation in body fluids and tissues. The concern with ultrasonography is in the third trimester, when the fetus

TABLE 13-5

Over-the-Counter Medications and Herbal Remedies in Pregnancy and for Lactating Women

Name of Drug	Recommendation in Pregnancy	Recommendation for Lactating Women	Negative Side Effects
Aspirin	Generally not recommended in pregnancy, especially in the third trimester.	Not recommended but may be taken in normal doses if breastfeeding is delayed for a few hours after ingestion. Ibuprofen is preferred to aspirin use in lactating women.	In third trimester more than 100 mg can lead to maternal and fetal platelet disorders and additional fetal and maternal complications. Postpartum concerns are similar.
Acetaminophen	Recommended pain reliever in pregnancy.	Recommended pain reliever during lactation.	None.
NSAIDs	Not recommended during pregnancy.	Ibuprofen is the recommended NSAID during lactation. Naproxen should be avoided (long acting).	Concerns about fetal complications in pregnancy as seen with aspirin, but not well studied. Naproxen may cause bleeding problems or gastrointestinal upset in the neonate from breast milk.
Antacids	General usage is OK, prolonged use should be checked with physician/midwife.	Safe to use in lactating women.	Potential toxicity if used long term in pregnancy.
Antihistamines	OTC versions found in cold medications are acceptable for use during pregnancy.	Those that are less sedating are preferred; recommended to avoid breastfeeding for a few hours after ingestion.	No large studies have shown ill effects on fetus or mother in pregnancy. In postpartum period sedating effects on infants with older, sedating antihistamines. Some concern about inhibition of lactation.
Decongestants	Discouraged in pregnancy.	Nasal spray recommended over oral route.	In pregnancy, may cause fetal tachycardia and increased fetal activity. In postpartum period, may cause infant irritability and suppress lactation.
Laxatives	Some are category B (lactulose and magnesium sulfate) and some category C (docusate, docusate sodium, and mineral oil the most common). Mineral oil may interfere with absorption of fat-soluble vitamins. Castor oil's irritant effects may induce premature labor.	Avoid those that contain aloe, cascara, anthraquinone, or phenolphthalein in lactating women. Bulking agents are safe, as are stool softeners such as docusate.	Laxative effect on the breastfed infant.
Antidiarrheals	Category C; caution is warranted.	Kaolin-pectin products are safe and preferred to other antidiarrheals.	Those with salicylates are contraindicated because of the aspirinlike effects.

NSAIDs, Nonsteroidal anti-inflammatory drugs.
Adapted from Anderson PO, Knoben JE, Troutman WG: *Handbook of clinical drug data*, ed 10, New York, 2002, McGraw-Hill; Cunningham FG, Gant NF, Leveno KJ, et al: *Williams obstetrics*, ed 21, New York, 2001, McGraw-Hill; Rebar RW: The breast and the physiology of lactation. In Creasy RK, Resnick RR, editors: *Maternal fetal medicine*, ed 5, Philadelphia, 1999, WB Saunders; and Riley MR, Burnham TH, Bastean JN, et al: *Drug facts and comparisons, 2001: pocket version*, ed 5, St Louis, 2001, Facts and Comparisons.

becomes somewhat warmer than the mother's core temperature. If the mother is febrile her core temperature will rise, and diagnostic ultrasound may be contraindicated.[113]

Chorionic Villus Sampling

Chorionic villus sampling (CVS) is an early detection test of genetic disorders that can be performed at 10 to 13 weeks of gestation and quickly provide results. This ultrasound-guided procedure removes some of the placental villi through the cervix, abdominal wall, or vagina. The chance of miscarriage is 1% to 2%.[124]

Amniocentesis

Amniocentesis tests for genetic disorders and abnormalities in growth patterns and is usually performed after 15 weeks of gestation. A physician inserts a hollow needle into the amniotic sac and withdraws fluid while being guided by simultaneous abdominal ultrasound. There is a 1 in 270 chance of a spontaneous miscarriage caused by the procedure. Consequently, amniocentesis is used for women older than 35 years and those with high-risk pregnancies.[41,124]

Laboratory Tests

In pregnancy, the intravascular volume in the blood results in dilutional anemia. Although there is an elevated erythropoietin level, which will lead to a compensatory increase in total red cell mass, some anemia is never fully corrected. There is a modest increase in white blood cell count during pregnancy and a marked elevation during labor and immediately after delivery. Pregnancy is a hypercoagulable state, and this increase protects the mother from too much blood loss at delivery but also enhances the risk of thromboembolism fivefold.[26,124]

A variety of blood tests are routinely performed in pregnancy. The most common are listed in Table 13-6.

TABLE 13-6
Commonly Performed Tests and Procedures in Pregnancy

Gestational Stage	Test	Indication
4-8 weeks	Transvaginal ultrasound	Screen for high-risk pregnancies, early diagnosis of multiple pregnancies
4 weeks; first prenatal visit	Blood screening	Blood screening for hematocrit, blood group, Rh, antibody screen, rubella status, syphilis screen, hepatitis B surface antigen, human immunodeficiency virus
Every prenatal visit	Urinalysis, urine culture	Test for protein and glucose
10-12 weeks	Chorionic villus sampling	Examine placental tissue for chromosomal and genetic information
16-18 weeks	Amniocentesis	Test amniotic fluid for chromosomal and genetic disorders
16-18 weeks	Alfa-fetoprotein	Test of blood to determine risk for neural tube disorder and Down syndrome
16-18 weeks	Multiple marker screening	Measure hormone and alfa-fetoprotein levels to screen for Down syndrome
18-20 weeks	Abdominal ultrasound	Measure fetal growth, check for placental position, congenital anomalies
24-28 weeks	Glucose screening	Blood test for gestational diabetes
Only when medically indicated	Radiograph	Determining fractures
35-37 weeks	Group B streptococcus bacteria screening	Screen for group B streptococcus cultures so that the mother does not pass it on to the baby during delivery

From Cunningham FG, Gant NF, Leveno KJ, et al: *Williams obstetrics*, ed 21, New York, 2001, McGraw-Hill; and Hayman B: A miracle in the making, Chicago, 2000, Budlong Press.

GLUCOSE TESTING. Screening and diagnosis of diabetes in pregnancy are done by using a glucose tolerance test. A 100-g dose of oral glucose is ingested and blood levels are measured every hour for 3 hours. A diagnosis of gestational diabetes is made when any two values in Table 13-7 are met or exceeded.

Common Medical Conditions and Symptoms of Pregnant and Postpartum Women

Table 13-8 presents an overview of common medical conditions and symptoms of pregnancy.

Differentiating Between High-Risk and Low-Risk Pregnancy

A high-risk pregnancy is distinguished by any fetal or maternal condition that can adversely affect the successful outcome of the pregnancy. By identifying pregnancies that are high risk, extra attention is given to those mothers who need the most medical care. Preexisting conditions such as heart and lung disease, diabetes, chronic illness, and disability can be identified before conception or within the first trimester and managed so that mortality and morbidity rates for the mother and child are decreased. Other women may start with a low-risk pregnancy but have complications develop—such as preeclampsia, premature labor, or multiple fetuses—that can threaten the completion of the pregnancy.

TABLE 13-7
Gestational Diabetes Diagnostic Values

Diagnostic 100-g Oral Glucose Tolerance Test	National Diabetes Data Group Conversion Plasma Glucose Level (mg/dL)
Fasting	105
1 hour	190
2 hours	165
3 hours	145

Adapted from Lucas MJ: Diabetes complicating pregnancy, *Obstet Gynecol Clin North Am* 28:513-536, 2001.

PTs who work with pregnant women must assess the woman within the physical restrictions set by her primary practitioner. Bed rest is prescribed for 18.2% of high-risk pregnant women.[108] Bed rest can be prescribed for preterm labor, premature rupture of membranes, amniotic fluid volume disorders, placental abnormalities, pregnancy-induced hypertension, pulmonary edema, hyperemesis gravidarum, cardiomyopathy, and a multifetal pregnancy.[160]

Classifications of bed rest are listed in Table 13-9.[61]

Overview of Physiologic and Anatomic Changes Associated with Pregnancy

The dynamic process of pregnancy changes the woman's anatomy and physiology, with changes occurring in every system. The pregnant woman's body changes internally and externally as she adjusts to fetal growth. Table 13-10 presents an overview of these anatomic and physiological changes by gestational month. Most of these changes listed in the table are covered in more detail throughout this chapter. Table 13-11 presents an overview of changes during gestation categorized by body system. Most of the changes listed in these tables are covered in more detail throughout the chapter.

Psychosocial Issues in Pregnancy and the Postpartum Period

The periods before and after childbirth are ones of great transition and adjustment for the pregnant woman and her family. PTs who commonly work with women during this life event are familiar with the signs of the emotional *work* women do during this time in their lives. Coombes and Darken[37] suggest that "Each trimester of pregnancy can generally be related to one of three psychological states: acknowledgment, consolidation and preparation" and that "A woman's mechanisms of coping throughout each stage are dependent upon such variables as her physical condition, social and family support networks, the reaction evoked in the woman by her pregnancy, and the significance she attaches to it." Anxiety, insecurity, joy and elation, stress, and

TABLE 13-8

Common Medical Conditions and Symptoms of Pregnancy

Condition	Symptom and Cause
Backache	Reported by 50% to 90% of pregnant women. Can be related to muscles, joints, or ligaments.
Breast tenderness	Tingling and tenderness are experienced in the early weeks of pregnancy. Breast size can increase by 500-800 g; veins become visible and nipples enlarge.
Carpal tunnel syndrome	Increased fluid volume in the wrist causes compression of the median nerve, resulting in wrist and hand pain and sensation change.
Constipation	Decreased elimination from decreased motility of the small bowel and increased ingestion of iron. Muscular relaxation of the colon with increased absorption of water.
Edema	Increased weight, gravity, and progesterone cause venous engorgement and swelling.
Fainting	Vasodilatation in early pregnancy and uterine pressure on the inferior vena cava in late pregnancy.
Fatigue	Increase in fatigue and excessive sleep in early pregnancy may be caused by progesterone. Usually subsides by the fourth month of pregnancy.
Headache	Frequent symptom in early pregnancy that decreases by midpregnancy; cause is usually not demonstrated. Severe headaches in later pregnancy may be related to hypertensive disorders.
Heartburn	Common symptom caused by gastric reflux into the lower esophagus, relaxation of the lower esophageal sphincter, and upward displacement and compression of the stomach by the uterus.
Hemorrhoids	Varicosities of the rectal veins related to increased pressure by obstruction of venous return of the expanding uterus with tendency toward constipation.
Insomnia	Increase in physical discomfort with increasing pregnancy. Anxiety and vivid dreams may decrease sleep.
Muscle cramps	Increased pressure of the expanding uterus on lower extremity nerves may cause ischemia.
Nausea/vomiting	Morning sickness often starts after the first 6 weeks of pregnancy. Multiple theories abound as to cause.
Urinary frequency	Pressure of the uterus on the bladder as pregnancy progresses.
Varicosities of the lower extremities, vulva, or rectum	Increased blood volume, pressure of the uterus on the pelvic veins, and swelling of veins causing regurgitation.

Adapted from references 41, 127, 130, 135, 141, and 144.

TABLE 13-9

Activity Restrictions for Patients on Bed Rest

Limitations of Activity	Toileting	Positions for Eating
Ad lib activity	No restrictions	No restrictions
Bed rest with bathroom privileges	May use toilet; shower in a shower chair	Limited sitting
Strict bed rest; no upright activity	Bedpan for all toileting; bed bath	May prop self up on elbow or elevate head of bed 30 to 45 degrees for eating
Strict bed rest in the Trendelenburg position, head of bed is 15 degrees lower than foot of the bed; no upright activity	Bedpan for toileting; bed bath	May roll side to side; may prop on elbow for eating

From Frahm J, Welsh RA: Physical therapy management of the high-risk antepartum patient, *Clinical Management* 9:15, 1999.

irritability are all emotions or experiences likely to surface in pregnant and postpartum women. Any PT treating or examining women during the childbearing year needs to be aware of the tremendous emotional challenges these women face.

The emotional status and childbirth practices of women are also influenced by culture and ethnicity. Multiple resources exist in today's literature that introduce the health care provider to cultural beliefs and practices common during pregnancy, childbirth, and the postpartum period.* Gaining perspective on a particular woman's emotional health necessitates an awareness of her cultural belief system. See Chapter 3 for additional information on diversity and multiculturalism.

Although a certain amount of emotional uncertainty and stress is normal during pregnancy, undue stress and high job strain (high demand, low control) have been shown to correlate with preterm delivery, pregnancy-induced hypertension, and preeclampsia.[109] These situations should therefore warrant referral to the medical care provider by the PT. It is certainly difficult for any health care provider to ascertain how much stress is normal and how much is "undue"; however, patients who overtly admit to being under a great deal of stress or whose conversations indicate very high-stress lives should signal a red flag for the PT involved in their care.

The following sections outline two additional issues facing pregnant and postpartum women in the psychosocial realm; domestic violence in pregnancy and prenatal and postnatal depression.

Domestic Violence in Pregnancy

Domestic violence, or battering, may be defined as "A pattern of physical, psychological, or sexual abuse between intimate partners."[31] The abuse is often episodic and chronic and can cause both physical and psychological injury.[31] The incidence of domestic violence in pregnancy is estimated to be approximately

*References 66, 93, 94, 96, 99, 133, 159.

TABLE 13-10

Overview of Anatomy and Physiology of the Childbearing Year

Month	Maternal and Physiological Changes	Anatomic Changes
1	Rise in temperature, vomiting, fatigue, breast discomfort, end of menses	Ovulation, fertilization, implantation of ovum, thickening of uterine lining from increased estrogen and progesterone
2	Positive pregnancy test; nausea subsiding; profuse, thick vaginal discharge; breast enlargement	Mucus plug forming in cervix; pressure on bladder with frequency of urination
3	Colostrum leaking from breasts; nausea subsiding; bladder pressure less	Placenta completely formed and secreting estrogen; uterine cavity filled; uterus rising from pelvic cavity into abdomen
4	Abdominal appearance of pregnancy; backache	Blood volume increasing; fundus half way between symphysis and umbilicus
5	Fetal movement called *quickening*	Placenta covers half of uterine wall
6	Stretch marks; linea nigra appears; possible chloasma (around eyes); period of greatest weight gain starts	Height of fundus at umbilicus; period of lowest hemoglobin level
7	Braxton Hicks contractions palpable; intermittent uterine contractions	Blood volume highest
8	Braxton Hicks contractions stronger; stretch marks more pronounced; backache possible	Longitudinal stretching of uterus
9	Umbilicus protrudes; shortness of breath, varicosities, swelling; descent of fetal head; *lightening* (baby "drops"); easier breathing; urinary frequency	Fundus just under diaphragm (before lightening); lightening more common in primiparas but can occur in multiparas; may drop just before birth

From Stephenson RG, O'Connor LJ: *Obstetric and gynecologic care in physical therapy*, ed 2, Thorofare, NJ, 2000, Slack.

10%, with a range of 4% to 20% reported in the literature, thus making it one of the most common complications of pregnancy.[31,46,69,110] Battering may begin during pregnancy; estimates are that as many as 25% to 45% of women who are victims of domestic violence before pregnancy will continue to experience it during pregnancy.[31,46,112] Adolescent pregnancies carry an even greater risk of abuse than do pregnancies begun in adulthood.[69,112] The abuse in pregnancy escalates after delivery of the child; Mezey and Bewley[112] report that the risk of moderate to severe violence appears to be highest in the postpartum period.

In general, abusers tend to target a woman's head, neck, breasts, abdomen, pelvis, and buttocks. Pregnant women often experience physical abuse directly to the abdomen.[31,112] Outcome studies on women who have suffered abuse during

TABLE 13-11

Overview of Pregnancy Changes by System

System	Change
Gastrointestinal	Nausea and vomiting may occur in early pregnancy, intestinal motility slows, constipation can develop.
Urogenital	Glomerular filtration rate increases by 50%, renal function increases with increased urinary output, reproductive organs hypertrophy from edema and increased vascularity.
Cardiovascular	Blood volume increases 40%-50%; stroke volume increases 20%-40% in mid pregnancy, then decreases after 28-32 weeks until term; resting heart rate increases an average of 20 beats/min throughout pregnancy; cardiac output increases at twelfth week and peaks at 28-32 weeks
Endocrine	Adrenal, thyroid, parathyroid, and pituitary glands enlarge. Hormones increase to support the pregnancy, and placenta, and to prepare the mothers body for labor. Hormones cause generalized increase in joint laxity and return to prepregnant values by 3-6 months postpartum.
Respiratory	Oxygen consumption increases by 18%, carbon dioxide output increases, tidal volume increases 40%, vital capacity increases 5%, residual volume decreases 20%, ventilation increases up to 40%, diaphragm elevates and central part flattens. Breathing is more costal than abdominal.
Metabolic	Increased demand for tissue growth; insulin is elevated from plasma expansion, and blood glucose is reduced for a given insulin load. Renal threshold for glucose drops because of increased glomerular filtration rate; fats and minerals are stored for maternal use; increase in sodium and water retention.
Musculoskeletal	Rib cage circumference increases 4 cm, increasing the subcostal angle and the transverse diameter. Rectus muscles may separate and form a diastasis. Posture changes caused by change in center of gravity, weight gain, and decrease in spinal curves.
Neurologic	Swelling and increased fluid volume can cause nerve compression at the thoracic outlet, wrists, or groin (brachial plexus, median nerve, and lateral femoral cutaneous nerves, respectively).
Integumentary	Pigmentation may increase around eyes, face, linea alba, areolas; spider nevi, telangiectasia, and palmar erythema appear due to increase in estrogen and capillary dilations. Striae gravidarum (stretch marks) appear. Increases in sweating, hirsutism, and varices may appear but resolve postpartum.
Psychiatric	Pregnancy-related depression and postpartum depression may occur.

From Crapo RO: Normal cardiopulmonary physiology during pregnancy, *Clin Obstet Gynecol* 39:3-16, 1996; and Cunningham FG, Gant NF, Leveno KJ, et al: *Williams obstetrics*, ed 21, New York, 2001, McGraw-Hill.

pregnancy have shown negative outcomes, though not across the board.[31] These negative outcomes may include preterm labor and low-birth-weight babies[31,93] and can include a host of other maternal and fetal complications. Some of these complications are a direct result of violent encounters (e.g., fetal injury or death, maternal fractures) and some are from indirect effects of violence such as emotional stress or decreased access to health care.[36,46] Table 13-12 lists potential adverse effects of domestic violence perpetrated during pregnancy.

Clinical presentation is likely to be extremely variable. Patients who are victims of domestic violence may have symptoms directly related to the injury that they have sustained from the violent encounter but will more likely have vague physical and psychological symptoms such as headache, chronic pelvic pain, sleep disorders, and depression or anxiety.[31] Particularly telling for physical therapy patients is the common denominator of patients seeking care for relatively minor symptoms and those who do not comply with prescribed treatment regimens (although the latter is a scenario PTs find in the general physical therapy population as well).

A partner who does not allow a patient to speak for herself, refuses to let the PT interview the patient alone or leave the area during examination or treatment, or in some other way seems overly protective should raise the suspicion of domestic abuse. Every PT should have training in spotting domestic violence and should have a plan of how to question patients regarding abuse and how to offer assistance if such violence is disclosed. Because battering is so common during pregnancy, the primary care PT should consider it a possibility with every pregnant patient seen and should routinely screen for it. Suggestions for specific, direct questions related to abuse detection in pregnancy can be found in many hospital policies and in multiple texts and articles. Examples of such questions include the following:

- Since you have been pregnant, have you been hit, slapped, kicked, or otherwise physically hurt by someone?[31]
- Because domestic abuse is common during pregnancy, I routinely ask my patients if this is a problem for them. Are you in a relationship with someone who threatens or physically hurts you?[46]

TABLE 13-12
Adverse Perinatal Effects from Domestic Abuse

Direct	Indirect
Abruptio placentae	Elevated maternal stress
Fetal fracture	Isolation of mother
Uterine rupture	Inadequate health care
Rupture of maternal liver	Inadequate nutrition
Rupture of maternal spleen	Substance abuse
Pelvic fracture	Late entry into prenatal care
Antepartum hemorrhage	Unintended pregnancy
Preterm labor/delivery	Lack of breastfeeding
Preterm premature rupture of the membranes	Sexually transmitted disease

From Dattel BJ: Domestic violence. In Sanfilippo JS, Smith RP, editors: *Primary care in obstetrics and gynecology: a handbook for clinicians*, New York, 1998, Springer-Verlag, p 216.

Additional information on domestic violence as it applies to the primary care PT, as well as general questions related to abuse detection, are found in Chapter 5.

Depression in the Prenatal and Postnatal Periods

Postnatal depression has been documented to occur in 5% to 20%[30,79,122,144] of all postpartum women. Josefsson et al[79] found the prevalence of depressive symptoms during late pregnancy (35 to 36 weeks' gestation) to be 17%, higher than their postpartum prevalence of 13%. Depressive postpartum disorders range from "postpartum blues," which occurs from 1 to 5 days after birth and lasts for only a few days,[51] to postpartum depression and postpartum psychosis. The latter two are more serious conditions and require medical or social intervention to avoid serious ramifications to the family unit. The "baby blues" are said to be related to the dramatic shift in maternal hormones that occurs immediately after delivery.[51,76] The etiology of the more serious postpartum depression is still unclear, but recent studies have shown that depression during pregnancy is often predictive of postpartum depression.[30,79,122] Other factors such as maternal age, parity, prepregnancy history of affective disorders, low socioeconomic status, non-European race, social isolation, and thoughts of death and symptoms of insomnia in the first postpartum month have all been demonstrated in the literature to be predictive of postpartum depression.[30,79,122,144]

Abnormalities of postpartum thyroid function are said to occur in 4% to 7% of the population[149] and may account for some postpartum depression. Postpartum thyroiditis is a condition marked by a transient swing between a thyrotoxic phase with symptoms of fatigue, weight loss, palpitations, and dizziness followed by a hypothyroid phase with symptoms of fatigue and weight gain. The thyrotoxic phase is most common at 2 to 3 months postpartum, whereas the hypothyroid phase usually occurs between 4 and 8 months postpartum.[149] Depression is a common symptom associated with hypothyroidism and has been successfully treated with thyroid hormone therapy.[149] Seely and Burrow[149] state that "although suggestive, the relationship between postnatal depression and thyroid dysfunction remains speculative."

Postpartum depression commonly begins at 6 weeks to 4 months postpartum with a duration ranging from 2 weeks to 12 months.[122,144] It has been shown that postpartum depression can affect the cognitive development of the infant[34,151] and is theorized to have an impact on a woman's marital relationship, mother-infant relationship, and even survival of the infant.[79,122,144]

A commonly used validated, screening tool for postpartum depression, the Edinburgh Postnatal Depression Scale,[40] is one tool the PT can use to assess for possible postpartum depression. The tool is easily administered in 5 minutes[79] and has demonstrated good specificity and sensitivity.[40,79] A validation study showed that mothers who scored above threshold (92.3%) were likely to have a depressive illness of varying severity.[40] The authors warn that the score should not override clinical judgment. Once the screen has been used and a score of greater than 10 has been achieved, a referral to medical care is warranted. The tool is simply a screen and does not diagnose depression. The scale indicates how the mother has felt during the previous week; in doubtful cases it may be repeated after 2 weeks. The scale does not detect mothers with anxiety, neuroses, phobias, or personality disorder.[40] The Edinburgh Postnatal Depression Scale is presented in Appendix 13-1.

Postpartum psychosis is a much more serious disorder occurring in approximately 1 to 2 women per 1000 and should be treated as a medical emergency.[144] Signs of postpartum psychosis include symptoms of both mania and depression. The woman may experience hallucinations and delusions, especially concerning her child, with the disorder placing the woman at risk for suicide and infanticide.[144] This condition usually occurs within the first 2 weeks postpartum and may be related to the hormonal changes mentioned in relation to the postpartum blues.[144] Early recognition and proper treatment are imperative for the safety of the mother and baby.

Additional information on depression related to the primary care PT can be found in Chapters 5 and 7.

Gastrointestinal System

Common gastrointestinal symptoms during pregnancy include nausea and vomiting, esophageal reflux, intestinal motility, and an increase in incidence and symptoms of gallbladder disease. Of these, only the gallbladder problems present a diagnostic challenge to the primary care PT; gallbladder symptoms can mimic musculoskeletal dysfunction and pain, and accurate differential diagnosis is helpful in preserving the health of the mother. The other issues interfere with the woman's quality of life, but only in rare cases do they present significant morbidity concerns.

NAUSEA, VOMITING, AND HYPEREMESIS. Nausea is reported to occur in approximately 50% to 80% of pregnancies,[12,41,59,146] with vomiting complicating approximately 40% of pregnancies.[146] These symptoms are generally confined to the first 16 weeks of pregnancy but occasionally remain throughout the entire 10 lunar months. Women carrying multiple fetuses may have more intense or prolonged symptoms than women carrying one fetus. Velacott, Cooke, and James[167] reported that one quarter of the pregnant women reporting nausea and vomiting require time off from work because of these symptoms, and that nearly half of employed women cite job inefficiency as a result of this early complication.

Hyperemesis gravidarum, a condition resulting from continued and prolonged vomiting in pregnancy, occurs in 5% or fewer of pregnant women[12] but may require hospitalization and nutritional and fluid support as well as electrolyte balancing. Hyperemesis gravidarum can result in weight loss, dehydration, acidosis from starvation, alkalosis from loss of hydrochloric acid in vomitus, and hypokalemia.[41] Patients reporting severe vomiting and weight loss should be encouraged to contact their obstetric caregiver or their primary care provider if they have not yet seen a midwife, obstetrician, or obstetric family practitioner.

ESOPHAGEAL REFLUX AND HEARTBURN. Fifty percent to 80% of women report heartburn (pyrosis) during pregnancy, with its incidence peaking in the third trimester.[41,59,146] Pregnant women are generally not thought to be at risk for esophagitis or occult esophagitis and stricture and are therefore not candidates

for invasive diagnostic studies or aggressive treatment. They are treated for the nuisance and discomfort with advice on posture (assuming an upright posture and avoiding forward bending activities after meals), reduction in volume but increase in frequency of meals, diet modification (decrease fatty and spicy foods), smoking cessation, and medications such as antacids or acid-suppressing drugs when necessary.

MOTILITY ISSUES AND CONSTIPATION. Whether the gastrointestinal system in pregnancy slows down or not is a matter of controversy. Minimal, as well as conflicting, scientific investigation exists on the matter. It has been a commonly held dictum by those in the obstetric field that constipation is a common symptom of pregnancy because of decreased intestinal motility, but the few studies that have surveyed women on the incidence of this problem demonstrate equivocal results.[146] Nonetheless, when present, symptoms of constipation may be quite distressing for the pregnant woman and may include abdominal bloating, straining to pass stool with potential pelvic floor dysfunction exacerbation (prolapse of organs), and hemorrhoids. To ensure that women with this problem obtain symptomatic relief, the PT should encourage the woman to report her symptoms to her obstetric caregiver.

GALLBLADDER DISORDERS. Pregnancy increases a woman's risk of cholelithiasis (gallstones),[41,59,136,146,156] most likely from (1) increased bile production with a concomitant increase in the percentage of cholesterol in the bile; and (2) decreased gallbladder emptying time or incomplete emptying.[41,146,156] Smith[156] reports a symptomatic incidence of 3% to 4% in pregnant women, with increased parity a significant risk factor.

Symptoms of gallstones include intermittent right upper abdominal quadrant pain referred to the back and scapular areas. Additionally, fatty food intolerance and nausea and vomiting may be present. Because these latter symptoms are common symptoms of pregnancy, gallstones may be overlooked as the source of these symptoms. Differential diagnosis to rule out musculoskeletal dysfunction as a source of the upper quadrant symptoms may be necessary.

Ultrasonography is the preferred diagnostic tool for this condition. Confirmed diagnosis may require surgical intervention, especially when acute cholecystitis results.[41] Safe outcomes for mother and fetus have been reported, especially in the second trimester.[146] Laparoscopic cholecystectomy is the procedure now commonly performed.[41]

Urogenital System

Anatomic and hormonal changes during pregnancy place the pregnant woman at risk for both lower and upper urinary tract infections and for urinary incontinence. Events of labor and delivery (the puerperium) place a woman at risk for de novo development of urinary and fecal incontinence and pelvic organ prolapse. Although PTs are not responsible for treatment of urogenital infection during pregnancy, they need to recognize the symptoms of such infections (see Chapter 7) and refer the patient to the primary physician or obstetric caregiver. Differentiating signs and symptoms of upper and lower urinary tract infections from symptoms of back or pelvic pain of musculoskeletal origin is a primary function of any PT treating pregnant women.

Pregnant and postpartum women with incontinence symptoms (fecal and urinary) and urogenital supportive dysfunction, such as prolapsed uterus, prolapsed bladder (cystocele), or prolapsed rectum (rectocele), should be referred to PTs specializing in this area of practice. The Section on Women's Health, American Physical Therapy Association, can assist in locating such specialized practitioners. The primary care PT is in a unique position to screen for these common disorders in postpartum women and should take advantage of the opportunity to improve the quality of life for the women they treat and perhaps prevent additional or continued urogenital dysfunction in later years.

URINARY TRACT INFECTIONS. The frequency of both upper (kidney: acute pyelonephritis) and lower (bladder: acute cystitis) urinary tract infections is increased during pregnancy. The anatomic and physiological changes of pregnancy place the pregnant woman at greater risk for these infections. These changes include dilation of ureters and kidneys, compression of the ureters at the pelvic rim by mid-pregnancy, and softening of the angle of insertion at the ureterovesical junction. All contribute to vesicoureteral reflux and increased risk of kidney infection.[41,47,117,144] Increased glomerular filtration rate, decreased bladder capacity and emptying, decreased drainage of blood and lymph of the bladder, and urinary stasis because of collagenous changes in the urinary tract contribute to increased risk of acute cystitis.[41,47,117,172]

Pyelonephritis is said to be the most common serious medical complication of pregnancy and remains the leading cause of septic shock during this period.[41] In perhaps as many as 40% of untreated cases of acute cystitis, the infection ascends to the kidneys and results in acute pyelonephritis.[41] Thus identification and subsequent treatment of both of these entities are imperative for maternal-fetal well-being.

ACUTE CYSTITIS. Acute cystitis occurs in approximately 1% of pregnancies.[47] Symptoms of acute cystitis may include urinary frequency, urinary urgency, suprapubic discomfort or pain, and pain and burning with voiding.[41,47,156] Referred pain may be experienced over the sacral spine.[15] Some of these symptoms are hard to distinguish from the normal symptoms of pregnancy (frequency and urgency, abdominal discomfort) or from musculoskeletal dysfunction (sacroiliac joint problems), further complicating differential diagnosis. Medical treatment should be sought and most commonly includes antibiotics, sulfonamides, and cephalosporins.[95]

ACUTE PYELONEPHRITIS. Acute pyelonephritis occurs in approximately 2% of pregnancies.[47] Symptoms include flank pain; fever; nausea and vomiting; and, though not in all cases, symptoms of lower urinary tract involvement such as urgency, frequency, and dysuria.[41,47] Percussion over the costovertebral angle usually elicits flank tenderness, but this may also be present with musculoskeletal dysfunction of the lower ribcage in pregnancy and therefore may be diagnostically less than helpful. Pyelonephritis during pregnancy usually requires hospitalization, and suspicions of this condition should be immediately reported to the patient's medical care provider. Women with acute pyelonephritis in pregnancy are at risk for relapse and recurrence,[59] thus warranting continued vigilance of those women who have had such an occurrence.

An interesting aside to urinary tract infections in pregnancy is the apparently rare incidence of sacroiliitis associated with pyelonephritis. Egerman et al[58] describe such a case and review the literature on this infection and "unusual cause[s] of back pain." Recent history of peripartal infection with failure to reduce symptoms of sacroiliac dysfunction should lead the PT to consider referral to the primary care provider for further investigation of the pain symptoms.

URINARY INCONTINENCE. Current literature supports the long-held belief that women have increased incidence of urinary incontinence during pregnancy.[25,111,118,144,167,173] Prevalence rates of stress urinary incontinence (incontinence resulting from increased intra-abdominal pressure, such as a cough or sneeze) range from 20% to 67%,[111] with most researchers noting rates between 30% and 55%.[111,118,168] Comparing this to estimates of the incidence of stress incontinence in women who had never been pregnant (6% to 28%[111,118,144]) shows an increased incidence during pregnancy. Viktrup et al reported a 7% incidence of stress incontinence that began immediately or shortly after delivery.[168] Estimates of the prevalence of urinary incontinence (urge and stress incontinence) after birth range from 6% to 38%[111,118] and include statistics of the numbers of women who have urinary incontinence develop de novo and those whose incontinence began during pregnancy and did not resolve in the postpartum period.

Clearly, urinary incontinence is an issue affecting many women during and after pregnancy and could easily be screened for by the primary care PT who sees these women incidentally.

Fecal Incontinence

Urinary incontinence has "come out of the closet," so to speak, over the past decade, with patients consulting medical practitioners about this problem more readily than in the past. This has not occurred in the case of fecal incontinence. There has been a significant increase in research dollars spent on the investigation of fecal incontinence resulting from labor and delivery, but this has not affected public awareness. Patients rarely volunteer information on involuntary loss of stool or gas even though they often demonstrate profound changes in quality of life. Screening and obtaining treatment for these issues can become part of a primary care PT's common practice with a little background knowledge and the right set of questions to ask the patient. These questions, like those that screen for urinary incontinence, can be incorporated into the health history questionnaire (see Chapters 5 and 7).

The incidence of fecal incontinence (often referring to both inadvertent stool and gas loss) is much lower than urinary incontinence. Postpartum estimates of fecal incontinence range from 2.7% to 13%.[144] Regarding obstetrically related fecal incontinence, etiology points to either pudendal nerve damage or anal sphincter disruption and damage, both occurring during delivery.[48,144,163] Symptoms may include rectal urgency or urge incontinence of stool or passive or insensitive loss of rectal contents, including stool or gas.[144]

Organ Prolapse Related to Obstetrics

Compared with incontinence, there is very little written or researched in medical literature about postpartum urogenital prolapse. Sapsford and Markwell[144] briefly discuss postpartum uterine, bladder (cystocele), rectal (rectocele), and intestinal prolapse (enterocele) and the need for pelvic floor rehabilitation to provide support for these entities. Surgical repair is commonly performed for cystoceles or rectoceles that compromise normal voiding or defecation functions, and hysterectomy is commonly performed for a uterine prolapse that protrudes beyond the introitus (opening of the vaginal vault). Theoretically, the combination of endocrine changes of pregnancy with resultant connective tissue laxity and trauma occurring within the maternal pelvis during fetal descent can result in any one or a combination of these supportive disorders. Mild prolapse of organs often spontaneously resolves by 3 to 6 months postpartum. Moderate prolapse may be given a trial of pelvic floor rehabilitation before surgical options are explored. The pessary, a supportive device, may be another nonsurgical option for women with cystocele or uterine prolapse.

Symptoms of prolapse may include a feeling of incomplete emptying of the bladder or rectum, depending on the organ involved,[144] and rubbing or irritation at the introitus. Patients with uterine prolapse sometimes report aching in the area of the sacrum, possibly because of increased torsion placed on the uterosacral ligament.

Endocrine System

Endocrine system changes during pregnancy occur as a result of physiological alterations in the secretions of the endocrine glands. This system is extremely sensitive and is vital to the support of a thriving pregnancy. The endocrine system regulates how the body responds to thermal changes. As the pregnant woman's metabolism increases, surplus heat is dissipated by peripheral vasodilation and acceleration of sweating occurs. Consequently, she may frequently experience heat intolerance and exhaustion after minimal activity.[162] The functions of many hormones change during pregnancy, including the action of hormones on the musculoskeletal system. (See Table 13-11 for information on effects of the endocrine system and hormones on the musculoskeletal system.) Certain diseases within the endocrine system are common to pregnancy and, with close medical supervision, can coexist with a successful outcome.

GESTATIONAL DIABETES. Gestational diabetes mellitus (GDM) is defined as carbohydrate intolerance diagnosed during pregnancy, regardless of whether insulin is required for treatment. The development of this disease during pregnancy may be caused by exaggerated physiological changes in carbohydrate metabolism, which affect 1% to 14% of the population.[4] GDM may also be a maturity onset of type 2 diabetes that is uncovered during pregnancy.[41] There is a 33% to 50% probability of gestational diabetes in subsequent pregnancies and a 50% increased lifetime risk of developing non-insulin-dependent diabetes mellitus.[4,115] Women with GDM and all types of diabetes are at an increased risk of developing hypertensive disorders and preeclampsia and requiring a cesarean deliv-

ery.[4,104] There is additional evidence for long-term obesity and diabetes in offspring of diabetic mothers.[41]

GDM is associated with an increased risk of congenital malformations, macrosomia (infants large or heavy for gestational age), and perinatal morbidity and death.[115] Large infants can be difficult to deliver and have a greater chance of developing shoulder dystocia with resulting brachial plexus neuropathy from prolonged compression during delivery.

There is controversy regarding the optimal approach to screening for GDM because of the lack of data from well-designed studies.[7,41] Typical protocols call for all pregnant women to be screened for GDM between the twenty-fourth and twenty-sixth week of pregnancy with a 50-g oral glucose load. If the blood glucose result is greater than 130 to 140 mg/dl, then a full 3-hour glucose tolerance test with a 100-g oral glucose load follows the initial screening.[104,115]

Women with GDM must strictly monitor and control their blood glucose level through dietary changes during pregnancy, monitor and decrease strenuous work and lifestyle, and have other medications checked with a primary care physician.[4] At the 6-week postpartum checkup women should have their blood glucose level rechecked.

TYPE 1 DIABETES MELLITUS. The risk of malformations in infants of mothers with type 1 diabetes mellitus is two to three times that of the general population.[104] An increased rate of stillborn and macrosomic newborns is also attributed to pregestational diabetes.[104] Management of pregnant women with type 1 diabetes includes treatment with insulin, frequent monitoring of blood levels, diet control, and repeat sonograms to measure for infant size. There is usually a decrease in insulin needed in the third trimester, and hypoglycemia needs to be monitored because fetal loss is associated with low blood sugar.[104]

Cesarean sections are performed in 50% to 75% of insulin-treated diabetic mothers.[104] Prophylactic cesarean deliveries are sometimes performed if the fetal weight is estimated to exceed 4500 g. The PT working with this population may be involved with exercise regulation and abdominal rehabilitation after delivery.

TYPE 2 DIABETES MELLITUS. Type 2 diabetes occurs when there is abnormal insulin secretion and insulin resistance in the target tissues.[41] Type 2 diabetes is more common in women, especially in those with a history of gestational diabetes.[165] Most patients have inherited the disease and are obese. It is speculated that peripheral insulin resistance, which is induced by obesity, leads to β-cell exhaustion.[41] During the postpartum period, the newborn should be monitored for low glucose levels, low blood calcium and magnesium levels, excess of red blood cells, neonatal jaundice, and breathing problems. The mother will likely have a change in her insulin levels after delivery and should be routinely monitored.

EXERCISE FOR PREGNANT WOMEN WITH DIABETES. Control of all forms of diabetes during pregnancy requires home monitoring, diet change, exercise, insulin or other medications, and prenatal care. Pregnant women with diabetes should regularly exercise to enhance insulin sensitivity, decrease cardiovascular risk factors, and increase muscular strength and sense of well-being.[165] Because exercise reduces the amount of insulin necessary for normal blood glucose levels and the effect of exercise on metabolism is complex, the woman with diabetes and her health care practitioner should decide what type of exercise is best.[4,115]

For women with GDM, a program involving cardiovascular conditioning improves glycemic control better than diet control alone.[80] Exercise levels can be safely increased without fear of fetal distress if, during exercise, the lower body is kept from an excessive weight-bearing load.[41] Jovanovic-Peterson and Peterson[81] reported that with upper body cardiovascular training, a decrease in glucose levels became apparent after 4 weeks of exercise.

Cardiovascular System

Cardiovascular problems can arise in pregnancy and in the postpartum period as a result of preexisting diseases, disorders, or physiological changes that take place in pregnancy. The cardiovascular system normally undergoes rapid and broad changes as the blood volume increases by 40%.[124] The combined effect of underlying cardiovascular disease and physiological changes in pregnancy puts the mother and fetus at risk for serious complications.

Advances in cardiac surgery and medical therapy have increased the number of women with congenital heart disease living to reproductive age. Pulmonary hypertension and cyanotic disease present a 50% risk of maternal death, so antenatal counseling should be tailored to their specific condition.[105]

The PT involved in the care of pregnant women with cardiovascular disease needs to obtain guidelines from the cardiologist, obstetrician, or midwife who is managing the mother's overall care before planning a physical therapy program. PTs working with pregnant patients should be aware of the clinical indicators of heart disease during pregnancy (Box 13-1).

BOX 13-1

Clinical Indicators of Heart Disease During Pregnancy

SYMPTOMS
Progressive dyspnea or orthopnea
Nocturnal cough
Hemoptysis
Syncope
Chest pain

CLINICAL FINDINGS
Cyanosis
Clubbing of fingers
Persistent neck vein distention
Systolic murmur grade 3/6 or greater
Diastolic murmur
Cardiomegaly
Persistent arrhythmia
Persistent split-second sound
Criteria for pulmonary hypertension

From Cunningham FG, Gant NF, Leveno KJ, et al: *Williams obstetrics*, ed 21, New York, 2001, McGraw-Hill, p 1183.

The prognosis for pregnant women with heart disease depends on functional cardiac capacity, clinical conditions, medications, and the specific nature of the condition. Cardiac function has been classified by the New York Heart Association (Table 13-13).

Sickle Cell Disease

Sickle cell anemia decreases the blood cells' ability to transport oxygen throughout the body and complicates 1 in every 500 pregnancies among African Americans.[116,120] In this condition blood cells clump together and can cause clogging in capillaries. The blockages cause a decrease in blood flow and can bring on a painful crisis in the pregnant woman.[116] Oxygen flow can be compromised to the uterus as blood is shunted to vital organs, resulting in decreased oxygenation to the fetus, who may become severely compromised.

Pregnant women with sickle cell disease are at increased risk for preterm labor, abruptio placentae, placenta previa, and toxemia of pregnancy.[85] All tissues and organs are at risk for an ischemic injury because of decreased blood flow. Symptoms of the hypoxic injury are often acute and are delineated by painful episodes. PTs working with this population should be aware of the patient's preexisting condition because a painful crisis may mimic musculoskeletal conditions. The PT needs to differentiate quickly so that the woman can obtain appropriate care (see Table 13-16).

Patients with sickle cell disease have the increased likelihood of seizure activity, thrombosis, and hemorrhage. Headaches can often be the first sign of an acute central nervous system event.[85] Patients with sickle cell disease also have the potential for acute pleuritic-type chest pain, urinary tract infections, and acute cholecystitis.

Supine Hypotension Syndrome

Supine hypotension syndrome is defined as a hypotensive state brought on by compression of the inferior vena cava (and sometimes the aorta) by the gravid uterus when the women assumes a supine position or during prolonged standing or semirecumbent sitting.[5] Symptoms may include nausea, bradycardia, and syncope. Only 8% to 10% of women seem to demonstrate any signs or symptoms of hypotension; these women are said to have inadequate collateral paravertebral circulation.[103] It appears that all women in the latter half of pregnancy have decreased cardiac

---

TABLE 13-13

New York Heart Association Classification of Maternal Heart Disease

Class I	Uncompromised	No limitation of Normal Physical Activity
Class II	Slightly compromised	Slight limitation of normal physical activity
Class III	Markedly compromised	Symptoms with normal activity
Class IV	Severely compromised	Symptoms at rest

From Norwitz E, Schorge J: *Obstetrics and gynecology at a glance*, Oxford, 2001, Blackwell Science.

output in a fully supine position, but the effect on the fetus is not fully understood. There is disagreement concerning at what point in pregnancy the gravid uterus is large enough to cause the occlusion, but the American College of Obstetricians and Gynecologists suggests that women in the second trimester of pregnancy and beyond follow the recommendation to avoid exercise in the supine position.[5] Consensus opinion considers right or left side-lying or a 30-degree turn to the left from supine to relieve the caval occlusion.

Hypertensive Disorders in Pregnancy

Hypertensive disorders complicating pregnancy are the most common medical risk factor (3.7% to 7% of all pregnancies) responsible for maternal morbidity and death related to pregnancy.[41,44,101] Twenty percent to 40% of pregnant women with chronic renal disease, essential hypertension, diabetes mellitus, or lupus erythematosus will have hypertensive complications.[44] Hypertensive disorders complicating pregnancy have been divided into five types: gestational hypertension (pregnancy-induced hypertension), preeclampsia, eclampsia, preeclampsia superimposed on chronic hypertension, and chronic hypertension.

Despite decades of research, the relation between pregnancy and aggravation of hypertension remains unknown.[41]

Hypertension is diagnosed when blood pressure is 140/90 mm Hg or greater.[41] Edema is no longer a diagnostic criterion for hypertension because too many normal pregnant women also have edema.[3] Table 13-14 summarizes the types of hypertension.

PTs should check the pregnant woman's blood pressure if she has not had it taken within the last week and look for sudden onset of edema. Signs of hypertension such as visual changes, headaches, blood pressure change above baseline, and sudden onset of edema should be reported to the primary caregiver. Abruption of the placenta is a possible sequela to hypertension, preeclampsia, or eclampsia in pregnancy (see Table 13-14). Abruptio placentae may mimic groin pain but will be long lasting and not mechanical in origin.

Venous Thromboembolism

Venous thromboembolism (VTE) is a complicating factor in 0.5 to 3.0 of every 1000 pregnancies, a rate five times higher than in nonpregnant women of similar age.[9,98] Pulmonary embolism, a complication of VTE, is the primary cause of maternal death in the United States[52,97] and the United Kingdom.[152] In untreated cases of deep vein thrombosis, pulmonary embolism will develop in 24% of pregnant women, resulting in a mortality rate of 15%.[9] However, patients who

---

TABLE 13-14

Summary of Types of Hypertension During Pregnancy

Disorder/Incidence	Definition	Diagnostic Criteria	Signs/Symptoms
Gestational hypertension: affects nulliparous women most often	Diagnosis made retrospectively when preeclampsia does not develop and blood pressure returns to normal by the twelfth week postpartum	Blood pressure 140/99 mm Hg or greater for the first time during pregnancy; no proteinuria; blood pressure returns to normal by 12 weeks' postpartum	Epigastric pain, thrombocytopenia, headache
Preeclampsia: 5% incidence influenced by parity, race, ethnicity, and environmental factors	Pregnancy-specific syndrome of reduced organ perfusion from vasospasm and endothelial activation	Blood pressure 140/90 mm Hg or greater after 20 weeks' gestation; proteinuria: 300 mg or more of urinary protein in a 24-hour period or persistent 30 mg/dL in random urine samples	The more severe the hypertension or proteinuria, the more certain is the severity of preeclampsia; symptoms of eclampsia, such as headache, cerebral or visual disturbance, and epigastric pain can occur
Eclampsia: 1 in 3250 in United States (in 1998)	Seizures in a pregnant woman with preeclampsia not assigned to other causes	Grand mal seizures appearing before, during, or after labor; in nulliparas, seizures may develop 48 hours to 10 days after delivery	Mother may develop abruptio placentae, neurological deficits, aspiration pneumonia, pulmonary edema, cardiopulmonary arrest, acute renal failure; maternal death
Superimposed preeclampsia on chronic hypertension	Chronic hypertensive disorders predispose to development of superimposed preeclampsia or eclampsia	New onset proteinuria of 300 mg or more in 24 hours in hypertensive women; no proteinuria before 20 weeks' gestation	Risk of abruptio placentae; fetus at risk for growth restriction and death
Chronic hypertension: strong familial history of essential hypertension and or multiparous women with hypertension complicated by a previous pregnancy beyond the first one	Hypertension that persists longer than 12 weeks after delivery	Hypertension 140/90 mm Hg or greater before pregnancy; hypertension 140/90 mm Hg or greater detected before 20 weeks, gestation; persistent hypertension long after delivery	Risk of abruptio placentae; fetus at risk for growth restriction and death; pulmonary edema; hypertensive encephalopathy; renal failure

Adapted from American College of Obstetrics and Gynecology: Chronic hypertension in pregnancy. Practice Bulletin 29, *Obstet Gynecol* 98:177-185, 2001; Cunningham FG, Gant NF, Leveno KJ, et al: *Williams obstetrics*, ed 21, pp. 1210-1220, New York, 2001, McGraw-Hill; and Livingston JC, Baha MS: Chronic hypertension in pregnancy, *Obstet Gynecol Clin North Am* 28:447-463, 2001.

are managed will have less risk (4.5%) of pulmonary embolism and a less than 1% mortality rate.[9]

All the risk factors for VTE (all potentially present in pregnancy)—hypercoagulability, venous stasis, vascular damage, and changes in the coagulation system—contribute to increased risk for venous thromboembolism.[9] Additional risk factors for pregnancy-associated deep vein thrombosis and pulmonary embolism are tobacco smoking, prior superficial vein thrombosis, and varicose veins. Women who smoke or have varicose veins also have a risk for overall primary pulmonary embolism during the postpartum period.[45]

Risk factors for VTE in the postpartum period include age greater than 40 years, smoking, obesity, blood group other than type O, congenital or acquired thrombophilia, immobility, congestive heart failure, malignancy, hypertension, delivery by cesarean section, preeclampsia, and eclampsia.[153] Simpson et al[153] estimated that 38% of puerperal deep vein thrombosis and 22% of puerperal pulmonary emboli manifest after discharge from the hospital. Consequently, twice as many postnatal as antenatal events are identified.[153]

PTs working with pregnant and postpartum women should be aware of the acute symptoms of deep vein thrombosis because patients may report these symptoms during classes or therapy. Symptoms include pain in the proximal thigh, inguinal region, or calf. Often these symptoms are nonspecific, with the patient reporting diffuse tenderness and leg pain. Signs of deep vein thrombosis include skin discoloration, edema, prominent superficial veins, and a positive Homans' sign.[150] Homans' sign is positive if the ankle is passively dorsiflexed and the patient reports any sudden increase of pain in the calf or popliteal space.[140]

Pulmonary embolism is uncommon during pregnancy and the puerperium but is responsible for approximately 10% of maternal deaths.[41] This incidence averages approximately 1 in 64,000 pregnancies, divided equally in the antepartum and postpartum periods.[41] The common symptoms of pulmonary embolism disease are dyspnea, chest pain, cough, tachycardia, syncope, and hemoptysis. Sometimes there is an increased pulmonic closure sound, rales, or a friction rub on auscultation.

Respiratory System

Disorders of the respiratory system severe enough to cause respiratory distress are rare in pregnancy. Comfort and oxygen exchange issues influence physical therapy treatment of the pregnant patient.

Dyspnea, often one of the first signs of pregnancy, occurs as the level of progesterone increases. The mother initiates "overbreathing" in response to increased sensitivity of the respiratory center in the brain to carbon dioxide.[33] Sixty percent of pregnant women report dyspnea. The elevation of the diaphragm by approximately 4 cm and the flaring of the lower ribs during pregnancy[114] improve the mother's capacity to breathe deeply, ensuring oxygen supply to the fetus.[33] Implications for the PT include consideration of dyspnea during maternal exercise.

Asthma

Asthma in pregnancy occurs in 4% to 5% of the population, which is the same for the general population.[78] During the course of pregnancy one third will get better, one third will get worse, and one third will have no change in their asthma.[78,172] Effects of asthma on pregnancy include increased incidence of preterm low-birth-weight infants, preeclampsia, and perinatal morbidity.[172] There is also an association of pregnancy-induced hypertension in women with asthma.[172] The fetus is susceptible to maternal respiratory changes; the placenta consequently functions as a concurrent oxygen exchange organ. The fetus may develop hypoxemia before maternal perception of any respiratory compromise.

Exercise-induced asthma is brought on by smooth muscle constriction in the walls of the airways that respond to changes in airway temperature and hydration. The constriction increases the resistance to air flow, making it difficult to breathe deeply fast enough to keep up with oxygen needs for exercise. Hormonal changes in pregnancy decrease the smooth muscle constriction, thereby improving symptoms. Adequate hydration and use of respiratory inhalers before exercise can prevent exercise-induced asthma.[33]

Cystic Fibrosis

Cystic fibrosis (CF) is a genetic disease marked by exocrine gland dysfunction with production of thick, viscous secretions. The eccrine sweat gland is the foundation for the sweat test, characterized by elevated chloride, potassium, and sodium levels.

The frequency of CF is estimated to be 1 per 1500 white births and 1 per 17,000 African American births. The median survival rate has increased from 14 years in 1969 to 30 years in 1995.[137] Because of improved diagnostics and treatment, 80% of women with CF will likely survive to adulthood, and the North American Cystic Fibrosis Foundation estimates that 4% of women with CF become pregnant each year.

The concern for a pregnant patient with CF relates to her ability to support her own pulmonary and nutritional needs as well as those of a fetus. Chronic lung disease, hypoxia, and frequent lung infections can be dangerous to the fetus. Cor pulmonale and pancreatic dysfunction frequently develop. Pulmonary involvement, hypoxia, and repeated lung infections can be harmful to pregnancy. The patient with CF who chooses to become pregnant is best managed with serial pulmonary function testing for infection, development of diabetes, and heart failure. Heart failure is reported in 13% of pregnant women with CF, and pancreatic dysfunction can also contribute significantly to inferior maternal nutrition.[41]

Pregnant women with CF can have a successful pregnancy. The Shwachman-Kulczycki, or Taussig, score (0 to 100) is used to rate the severity of CF symptoms based on radiologic and clinical criteria. Women who have a Shwachman-Kulczycki score greater than 75, good nutrition, and a forced expiratory volume in 1 second of 70% usually tolerate pregnancy well.[41] Physical therapy may be indicated for postural drainage and respiratory therapy for bronchodilation.

The PT working with mothers with CF should know that preterm labor and delivery are a significant risk to fetal well-being. Perinatal death rates are higher in infants of women with CF because of preterm deliveries.[41] Patients with any signs of preterm labor such as increased vaginal discharge, vaginal bleeding, onset of regular contractions, and an increased pressure sensation should be referred to their primary obstetric caregiver as an emergency. For operative delivery an epidural analgesia is recommended. Postpartum, breastfeeding is not contraindicated as long as the mother can provide adequate caloric intake for herself and for the production of breast milk.

Musculoskeletal System

Pregnancy and the postpartum period present a unique challenge to the musculoskeletal system of a woman. At no other time in a woman's life does she experience the need for such a relatively quick adjustment in posture, such a profound alteration in the distensibility and load requirements of the abdominal wall or pelvic floor, or such an increase in the amount of joint play available in and around the bony pelvis. A number of pathologic conditions of the musculoskeletal system are more prevalent during the childbearing year, such as transient osteoporosis of the hip, spine, and wrist, and diastasis recti abdominis, a separation at the tendinous aponeurosis that lays between the two bellies of the rectus abdominis. Low back pain, said to occur in approximately 50% to 90% of pregnant women,[23,62,127] pelvic ring pain (pain in the joints of the sacroiliac or pubic symphysis), patellofemoral dysfunction and pain, rib and thoracic spine pain, coccydynia, and headaches are some of the commonly occurring musculoskeletal dysfunctions seen in the pregnant population.

The primary care PT needs to be aware of the relative ligamentous laxity, both capsular and extracapsular, exhibited by many pregnant women, especially at the sacroiliac joints and pubis. Increased extensibility of many of the soft tissues of the body occurs in most pregnant women,[27,145] and when combined with increased weight gain and fluid retention, may lead to conditions otherwise normally seen only as a result of trauma or repetitive stress. In pregnancy, it may take very little force or torque to result in significant dysfunction. Soft tissue injury or dysfunction may also occur without concomitant joint dysfunction, as in diastasis recti abdominis or urinary stress incontinence. It is also important to recognize, however, that even though there is generalized increased soft tissue mobility, localized soft tissue or joint restriction may also occur. Joint or soft tissue mobilization is appropriate in these cases. PTs must respect soft tissue laxity by avoiding positioning that places joints in closed-packed, end-range positions and by using treatment techniques that impart the least amount of force needed to accomplish the treatment goal. Awareness of these issues and of the more common musculoskeletal conditions in pregnancy may assist the PT in appropriate treatment strategies and in developing the prognosis.

Any PT working with this population should recognize the potential for significant postural changes in the pregnant woman and the need for relatively quick adaptation to postural change in the postpartum period. In general, the curves of the cervical, thoracic, and lumbar spine all increase in the pregnant woman, as does the inclination of the sacrum.[123,151] Although the center of gravity shifts anteriorly in response to weight gain and the growing uterus, research has shown that the change in curvature is not correlated with the onset of low back pain.[24,62]

Low Back Pain in Pregnancy

As mentioned before, the incidence of low back pain in pregnancy is quite high. Alexander and McCormick[2] report a 24% incidence of severe or moderate low back pain in pregnancy. PTs usually get involved in management of low back pain in pregnancy when it affects a woman's ability to function at work (at home or outside the home) or in her leisure time. Ostgaard[129] reports a ratio of low back pain to sacroiliac joint pain in pregnancy of 1:4.

True first incidence of disc herniation in pregnancy is reported to be 1 in 10,000,[90] and exacerbation of existing disc disease has not been reported. Because the annulus is considered a ligamentous structure and ligaments soften during pregnancy, it could be speculated that disc herniation would be higher during this period than in the nonpregnant state. Statistics do not, however, bear this out. Disc herniation does occur in pregnancy and the presentation in pregnancy is unlikely to be significantly different than in the nonpregnant state, although changes in bowel and bladder habits may be harder to discern because of changes commonly seen in these functions during pregnancy. MRI can be safely used in pregnancy to make a definitive diagnosis but is generally reserved for surgical candidates.[65,90] A pregnant woman will occasionally have a very flattened lumbar spine unrelated to disc disease and a lumbar lateral trunk shift. One explanation for this may be that in some women, tight dorsolumbar fascia exerts an overwhelming pull on the spine in the frontal plane, disallowing significant sagittal plane mobility. PTs should not be fooled into thinking that all flat backs represent signs of disc lesions.

Mechanical low back pain is much more common than disc herniation or disc degeneration in this population and can be assessed in pregnancy just as in the nonpregnant state. The pregnant woman in the first trimester may have increased range of active trunk motion compared with her nonpregnant state. In later pregnancy, active movements of the spine may be limited because of the bulk of the fetus and the stretch on dorsolumbar fascia. PTs may note what would normally be considered increased mobility to posteroanterior pressures of the spine during this period. This hypermobility should be considered normal in the pregnant woman when it is generalized to the whole spine.

PTs should always consider the possibility of kidney infection as a source of back pain in pregnancy. As mentioned, pregnant women are at greater risk for kidney infections than the nonpregnant population, and PTs should therefore screen all patients with symptoms of thoracolumbar or posterior rib pain for this condition.

Sacroiliac Joint Dysfunction

The incidence of pelvic ring dysfunction (also commonly called pelvic girdle relaxation, pelvic insufficiency, or symptom-giving pelvic girdle relaxation) in pregnancy ranges from 0.8% to 50%.[43,72,73,126,128] This variation may result from differences in inclusion criteria, type of study (retrospective vs. prospective), and possibly ethnicity. This syndrome includes posterior pelvic pain, which is discussed here as sacroiliac (SI) joint pain, and pain around the pubic symphysis. Aggravation of SI pain occurs during weight shifting activities such as sit-to-stand, rolling in bed, donning shoes or socks, getting up from a chair, and in gait or stair climbing.[73,91] Women with SI joint pain commonly report sharp pain in and around the sacrum and buttock with referral around the entire pelvic region and often down one or both lower extremities to the knee. The literature notes that referral is possible down the lower extremities, occasionally to the foot.[13] This pain pattern may make differentiation between nerve root compression with radicular pain and SI dysfunction a challenge.

There is much debate in the literature concerning the role of the hormone relaxin in the cause of SI joint dysfunction in pregnancy,[72,87,106,131] but authors do agree that increased SI joint mobility, whatever the mechanism, allows the condition to occur. Damen et al[43] noted that the increased SI joint laxity found in pregnant women is not associated with posterior pelvic pain but demonstrated that asymmetric laxity of the SI joints is implicated in this dysfunction. Figure 13-1 demonstrates the significant increase in SI joint mobility during pregnancy compared with men and nonpregnant women throughout the lifespan.

Albert et al[1] have developed a scheme to determine prognosis for pelvic ring dysfunction that begins in pregnancy. According to their classification, women who exhibit symptoms unilater-

ally or bilaterally at the sacrum or the pubis are much more likely to have their symptoms resolve within 6 months after delivery. It took up to 2 years in women who had pain in all three joints for their symptoms to resolve. The women with three-joint involvement fare the worst regarding disablement.

In addition to joint and soft tissue mobility, examination of the pelvic ring should include assessment of intrinsic support about the pelvis, body mechanics and posture, environmental factors such as chairs and bed cushioning (softer is often better in this population), and job and family demands.

Observation of unusual presentation should suggest conditions that warrant referral back to the obstetric caregiver or primary care physician. Sacroiliitis, a condition of inflammation and erosion of the bone at the margins of the SI joints caused by infection, can present with signs and symptoms similar to the more typical SI joint dysfunction encountered in pregnancy. However, the condition will not respond to joint or soft tissue mobilization but may improve with external stabilization (a belt or support). Sacroiliitis has been reported as a complication of peripartal infection, including with urinary tract infection or after surgery of the urogenital system.[58] Postpartum medical imaging or perinatal MRI will demonstrate changes representative of this condition. Intensity of symptoms with difficulty in resolution should raise suspicion for this condition. Similarly, transient osteoporosis of the spine or hip may be confused with mechanical dysfunction at the lumbar spine or pelvic ring; PTs should consider it as a possible cause of pain around the hips and pelvis.

Pubic Symphysis Dysfunction

Groin or pubic pain, with possible referral to the medial thigh(s) or along the pubic rami, is also a relatively common musculoskeletal symptom during the childbearing year. There is potential for increased incidence of pubic symphysis dysfunction in pregnancy and the postpartum period because of increased joint mobility around the pelvis before and after delivery and because of significant force on the joint during parturition. Dysfunction may include a relatively simple shifting of the rami cephalad or caudad (*pubic shears*) or a more complex and painful condition called *pubic symphysis separation*. In later postpartum months, the condition of *osteitis pubis* may occur, perhaps as a result of periosteal trauma that has occurred during pregnancy or the puerperium. Lentz,[97] in a review article on osteitis pubis, states that "although the pathogenesis of osteitis pubis is not clear, periosteal trauma seems to be an important initiating event."

All three types of pubic dysfunction may share common symptoms of painful gait and weight-shifting activities, especially in bed mobility activities, as well as painful abduction of the lower extremities. A separated symphysis generally results in greater intensity of symptoms. Pubic shears will yield positive palpatory findings of asymmetry at the pubic tubercles. Pubic symphysis separation and osteitis pubis can be confirmed with medical imaging techniques. Plain radiograph findings may lag behind the symptoms of osteitis pubis by as much as 4 weeks, but the results of bone scans will be positive much sooner.[97] Scriven et al[147] recommend ultrasound as the medical imaging

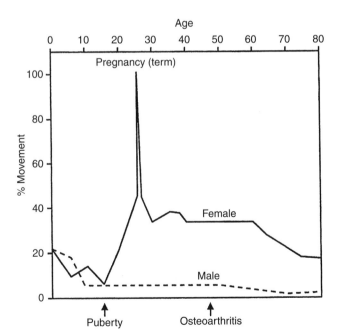

FIGURE 13-1 Sacroiliac joint mobility related to age in the man and woman. (From Bookhout MM, Boissonnault JS: Musculoskeletal dysfunction in the female pelvis, *Orthop Phys Ther Clin North Am* 5:23-45, 1996. Adapted from Vleeming A, Mooney V, Snijders C, et al, editors: First interdisciplinary world congress on low back pain and its relation to the sacroiliac joint, San Diego, 1992, with permission of the authors.)

modality of choice for separated symphyses because of its ability to detect trauma to organs and other soft tissues associated with the separation and because of its relatively low cost. However, plain radiographs do provide an adequate picture of the bony separation (Figure 13-2).

There are few estimates of the incidence of pubic symphysis separation during pregnancy, but postpartum incidence ranges from 1 in 300 to 1 in 30,000 births, with a general consensus of 1 in 600 births.[20,28,157] Separation is generally defined as a widening at the pubis of greater than 10 mm.[50,61,100] The woman who has this separation is generally aware of the inability to get out of bed and walk immediately after birth and will require significant family support to get through the first 3 to 6 weeks postpartum. Physical therapy is appropriate for these patients and includes provision of external support (a trochanteric belt), education in appropriate body mechanics and bed mobility techniques, limited weight bearing, and eventually (6 to 12 weeks postpartum) joint mobilization and stabilization exercises.[10,17,102] The PT should consider the diagnosis of separated symphysis under the following conditions: significant pain at the pubis and surrounding tissues, with onset immediately postpartum or occasionally prenatally; a lack of positive palpatory findings; and occasional bladder dysfunction (inability to void or hematuria).

Osteitis pubis is more of a chronic condition and, as mentioned, is more likely to occur later in the postpartum period but has been reported as early as 3 weeks postpartum after a woman participated in a household move.[68] This condition is also seen after bladder repair[82,169] and in athletes. This latter population is often treated aggressively with joint injections and short-term immobilization with a strong trochanteric belt.[77] Postpartum women who demonstrate radiographic signs of loss of smooth cortical periphery at the pubic symphysis, superficial bone destruction and sclerosis, and occasional heterotopic ossification coupled with symptoms of pain at the joint or in surrounding tissues, aggravated with weight shift or abduction, and in whom joint infection and separation have been ruled out, earn this same diagnosis.[97] The treatment offered to athletes with osteitis pubis can be effective in the postpartum population. Because the condition is often more chronic in postpartum women, external support may be necessary for many months compared with the few weeks common with an acute athletic injury.

Thoracic Spine and Rib Dysfunction

The ribcage undergoes significant anatomic change during pregnancy (Figure 13-3, Table 13-11) and does not fully revert to the nonpregnant state once childbirth has occurred. These profound changes likely account for the joint dysfunction that may occur at the sternocostal joints anteriorly or at the costotransverse joints and costovertebral joints posteriorly. Women who demonstrate this type of dysfunction often report pain, stiffness, or pressure in the vicinity of the mechanical problem but may also demonstrate referred pain with or without concomitant soft tissue restrictions and trigger points. In the third trimester, when the fundus of the uterus is elevated nearly to the xiphoid process, decreased trunk mobility coupled with an elevated diaphragm and thoracocostal or sternocostal dysfunction can produce significant impediment to daily function. The woman may not be able to sit or work in a seated position (especially during keyboarding or desk tasks) or assume recumbent positions without disabling pain or discomfort. Understanding the anatomic changes and propensity for dysfunction in this body region may assist the primary care PT in

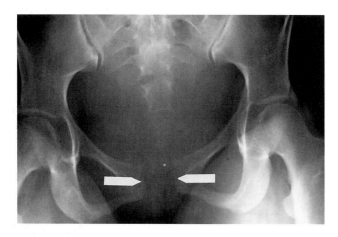

FIGURE 13-2 Plain radiograph, anteroposterior view, illustrating postpartum separated pubis.

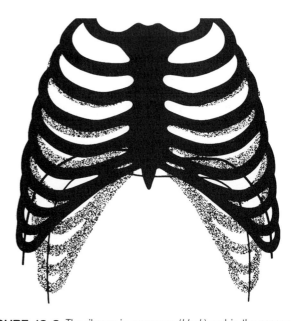

FIGURE 13-3 The ribcage in pregnancy (*black*) and in the nonpregnant state (*stippled*) showing the increased subcostal angle, increased transverse diameter, and raised diaphragm in pregnancy. (From deSwiet M: The respiratory system. In Hyten FE, Chamberlain G, editors: *Clinical physiology in obstetrics*, ed 2, Oxford, 1991, Blackwell, p 88.)

recognizing these issues and result in prompt therapeutic intervention. As mentioned, screening for kidney infection is an important step in examination of the pregnant woman with symptoms in the posterior thoracolumbar region.

Headaches and Cervical Spine Dysfunction

Headaches in pregnancy are usually either migraines or tension headaches.[60,71] A certain proportion of prepregnancy headaches get better during pregnancy, supposedly because of the increase in estrogen during this period. Reports of as high as a 70% remission in migraine have been noted in the literature.[71] Headache in pregnancy may be the result of endocrine system–mediated effects on the neurotransmitters or on the vascular system of the brain.[60] However, upper cervical mechanical dysfunction and stress/tension increased with associated soft tissue changes have also been implicated in headaches in the general population.[60]

Migraines are seldom said to begin in pregnancy.[71] A summary of symptoms and treatments for these types of headaches during pregnancy can be found in Table 13-15.[60] Headaches may also be caused by various pathologic processes such as pregnancy-induced hypertension and preeclampsia. These conditions are discussed in the cardiovascular section of this chapter, and the differential diagnosis of these conditions should be part of the screening process with any pregnant patient with headaches.

Physical therapy treatment of existing soft tissue and joint dysfunction along with any positive neural tension signs is one intervention used to reduce headaches in this population. In pregnancy, with the increase of curvature throughout the spine,[23,71] there exists a potential for aggravation of facet joint problems where the normal lordosis is increased, as in the lumbar and cervical regions.[71] The same anatomic changes predispose women to adaptive shortening of the posterior musculature and soft tissues in the suboccipital area that can lead to increased soft tissue tension and potentially to pressure on the suboccipital nerve. The soft tissue tension and nerve compression can both result in headaches. Reducing forward head posture and addressing needed workstation adaptations may reduce the need for additional acute, hands-on intervention. Because stress plays such a large role in all headaches, screening for undue stress and assisting women in obtaining appropriate stress-reduction strategies or therapies should be part of an overall prenatal PT headache treatment plan.

Postpartum headache may be a result of the spinal anesthesia used[102] or from dural puncture as a complication of epidural anesthesia.[161] Resolution generally occurs (unless the dural puncture has resulted in a subdural hematoma, which is quite rare), but a blood patch may be required.[166] Postpartum migraine headaches are said to be common in women with a history of prepregnancy headaches and are theorized to result from the precipitous drop in estrogen that accompanies delivery.[71]

Extremity Dysfunction

Nerve entrapment syndromes of the extremities are detailed in Table 13-16. Patellofemoral dysfunction in the form of chondromalacia patellae is said to occur with greater frequency in pregnancy because of ligamentous laxity,[160] increased load on the knees, and increased fluid retention.[88] Symptoms of pain at the patella during prolonged or end-range flexion of the joint and patellar tracking problems are likely with this diagnosis.[88] Treatment can be similar to that offered during nonpregnant periods, but, because of the transient mechanical changes, should not involve purchase of expensive orthotics.

The same advice holds true for changes to the foot during pregnancy. Because the changes may not be permanent or may continue into the postpartum period and not stabilize for many months, expensive foot orthotics should be avoided during this time period. Off-the-shelf or temporary orthotics that support the arch of the foot and provide some cushioning are preferred in pregnancy. The foot may undergo anatomic change during pregnancy because of ligamentous laxity, including softening of

---

TABLE 13-15

Summary of Symptoms and Treatment for Tension-Type and Migraine Headache During Pregnancy

Type of Headache	Symptoms	Treatment
Tension-type	Bilateral, dull, steady pain that worsens throughout the day	Identify stress- and tension-producing situations
	Pressure that feels like a tight rubber band around the head	Develop new ways of coping
	Last 4 to 24 hours	Rest, use of ice packs
	Areas of tenderness on head and neck	Biofeedback, relaxation techniques, physical therapy
	Onset gradual and sometimes slight; anxiety, nausea, or dizziness present	Analgesics, sedatives, and others that have no or few effects on fetus
Migraine	Severe, throbbing, one-sided pain	Avoid triggering factors such as foods high in tyramine, nitrites and nitrates, MSG, alcohol, weather changes, activity changes, stress, hunger, changes in sleep patterns
	Last 4 to 72 hours	Develop lifestyle changes
	May be accompanied by nausea, vomiting, dizziness, tremors, and increased sensitivity to sound and light	Biofeedback
	Classic migraine (with aura) warning symptoms include visual disturbance, numbness in extremities, strange olfactory sensations, and possible hallucinations	Analgesics, β-blockers, sedatives, and others that have no or few adverse effects on fetus

From Feller CM, Franko-Filipasis KJ: Headaches during pregnancy, *J Perinatal Neonatal Nurs* 7:1-10, 1993.

TABLE 13-16

Nerve Entrapments and Palsies Found in Pregnancy and the Postpartum Period

Nerve Injury	Mechanism and Structure	Result
Bell's palsy (cranial nerve VII)	Compression on facial nerve	Facial paralysis, pain, and numbness
Thoracic outlet syndrome (C5, 6, 7, 8; T1)	Caused by posture changes of head and neck forward, causing compression of the brachial plexus nerve fibers, subclavian artery, and vein at the cervicothoracic dorsal outlet	Pain and paresthesia in neck, shoulder, or hand; vascular/autonomic changes in the hand
Carpal tunnel syndrome (C6, 7, 8; T1)	Compression of the median nerve by the flexor retinaculum and increased fluid volumes of pregnancy	Numbness, tingling, and pain in the thumb, index and middle fingers, and lateral aspect of the ring finger; positive Tinel's sign
Radial nerve palsy (C5, 6, 7, 8)	Squatting, resting forearms over the birthing bar	Weakness of forearm and wrist extensors
Lumbosacral plexus injury (T12-L4)	Compression on the lumbosacral plexus by the fetal head and forceps or retractor against the pelvic wall	Lumbosacral plexopathy; unilateral foot drop
Ilioinguinal neuropathy (L1)	Entrapment after low and wide abdominal incision	Paresthesia of mons pubis, labium, medial thigh
Iliohypogastric neuropathy (T12-L1)	Entrapment after low and wide abdominal incision	Paresthesia in the hypogastric region
Genitofemoral neuropathy (L1-L2)	Injury under the inguinal ligament	Paresthesia in lateral thigh and labium
Meralgia paresthetica or lateral femoral cutaneous neuropathy (L2-L3)	Painful dysesthesia in the third trimester results from entrapment of the sensory lateral femoral cutaneous nerve between inguinal ligament and the enlarging abdomen and iliacus fascia	Unilateral or bilateral paresthesias, numbness and tingling over the lateral aspect of the thigh; spontaneously resolves after delivery
Femoral neuropathy (L2-L4)	Compression on femoral nerve with retractor or dorsolithotomy position	Paresthesia in anterior thigh, weak quadriceps
Obturator neuropathy (L2-L4)	Compression through labor or postpartum hematoma	Paresthesia in medial thigh, weakness in thigh muscles
Pudendal neuropathy (S2-S4)	Pudendal block, forceps, prolonged labor, or fetal head pressure during delivery	Perineal neuralgia Levator ani weakness
Common peroneal neuropathy (L4, L5-S1, S2)	In labor pressure on the common peroneal nerve between leg holders and fibular head	Foot drop; dorsiflexors and evertors affected

Data from references 35, 41, 53, 64, 84, and 154.

the supportive ligaments with resultant loss of arches and increased size. These changes may or may not produce symptoms. Cognizance of the possibility of this type of anatomic change in the feet will improve holistic therapeutic management of a whole host of musculoskeletal symptoms during pregnancy.

Osteoporosis in Pregnancy

Osteoporosis in pregnancy is said to be transient and to affect the lumbar spine, hip, and wrist.[63,143] The condition is not always associated with any symptoms and rarely causes a hip or wrist fracture, although compression fractures of the spine have been reported.[155] The decreased bone density can, and does, result in significant pain and disability in some women, probably because of joint effusion and irritation.[19] Suspected diagnosis is made by ruling out other mechanical causes of pain coupled with pain that does not change with physical therapy interventions such as joint mobilization, soft tissue work, or physical agents (although some relief may be achieved by ameliorating secondary symptoms of edema and muscle spasm). Empty or spasm end-feels at the hip, spine, and wrist are also possible signs. Generally, there will be no history of trauma as a precipitating factor to the patient's pain. Onset of pain in tran-

sient osteoporosis of the hip has been cited as most commonly occurring in the third trimester and with an antalgic gait or inability to weight bear on the affected side.[155] Pregnancy-related osteoporosis of the spine will also present most commonly in the third trimester and may be associated with back pain and change in height from compression fracture of the vertebral column.[155] A confirmed diagnosis is made postpartum, when medical imaging techniques can demonstrate the decreased bone density necessary for a diagnosis of osteoporosis.

Every PT who cares for pregnant women must keep the possibility of this diagnosis in mind when examining patients. The incidence of osteoporosis in pregnancy is unknown. There are numerous cases of transient osteoporosis of the hip in pregnancy found in the literature,[19,55,63,155] but there are no large epidemiologic studies that attempt to estimate the incidence, prevalence, or true longevity of this condition during the childbearing year. There are many theories regarding the cause of osteoporosis in pregnancy,[29,32,56] but none of them have been substantiated through clinical investigation. Preexisting osteopenia has been shown, however, to predispose a pregnant woman to this condition.[83] Prolonged use of corticosteroids, heparin, cigarettes, and alcohol are risk factors for osteopenia and should raise suspicion of this condition in women with this type of history. In addition, numerous other diseases place a woman at risk of osteopenia and osteoporosis. These include rheumatoid arthritis; hyperthyroidism and hyperparathyroidism; eating disorders; and cancers such as multiple myeloma, lymphoma, and leukemia.[92]

Treatment of osteoporosis in pregnancy, when symptomatic, is largely aimed at preserving joint integrity and minimizing disability. During pregnancy, for the spine and hip, minimizing weight bearing with lifestyle changes and gait aids, education in positioning for rest and sleep, and general body-mechanics instruction are the main intervention strategies used. Osteoporosis at the wrist may benefit from adaptive activities of daily living strategies, with likely referral to occupational therapy. Postpartum, after definitive diagnosis is made, the patient can gradually progress through a gentle mobility and strengthening program. Aquatic therapy is a safe way to begin.[19] Eventually, weight-bearing exercise should be implemented as pain resolves and the danger of joint collapse or damage diminishes.

Abdominal Musculature and Diastasis Recti Abdominis

Diastasis recti abdominis (DR) is defined as a separation of greater than two fingertip widths of the two bellies of the rectus abdominis muscle at the linea alba (or linea nigra, in pregnancy).[19,123] This painless condition occurs most frequently in relation to pregnancy but can be found in patients with chronic pulmonary conditions, in children younger than 2 years, and in men with "beer bellies."[16] Because the condition changes the integrity of the abdominal wall and trunk, it has theoretically been linked to low back pain and urinary incontinence; dysfunction may correlate with altered intra-abdominal pressure gradients or abdominal muscle function. However, the repercussions of DR are not well researched.

DR is commonly noted in primiparas in the third trimester and seems to resolve spontaneously in most women as they progress through the postpartum period.[18] However, DR will not resolve spontaneously in all women and exercise aimed at strengthening the recti without increasing intra-abdominal pressure will reduce the gap.[16,18,123,160] The separation may be noted anywhere along the linea alba (or nigra) and may or may not appear as a distinct bulge noted during movements that involve abdominal contraction with increased intra-abdominal pressure (e.g., a curl-up). The most common assessment technique for this condition is to have the woman perform a curl-up while the PT palpates horizontally between the two sides of the contracted recti. The PT notes the number of fingertips she/he is able to place within the potential separation of the two bellies of the muscle. Greater than two fingertips is considered a diastasis (Figure 13-4).[18,123]

It is suggested that women work to eliminate DR after birth and before resuming more stressful abdominal muscle strengthening, such as curl-ups.[123] Transversus abdominis work or other exercises for the abdominals that do not result in increased intra-abdominal pressure should be safe even in the presence of DR. During pregnancy, because of the changes in hormones and the advancing weight and size of the fetus, resolution of this condition is not possible. The abdominal wall changes considerably during pregnancy as the fetus exerts force against it, and increased maternal hormones soften its structures. The rectus abdominis elongates during pregnancy and seems to curve around the gravid uterus rather than maintain its nonpregnant linear orientation.[67]

After delivery, the rectus suffers from stretch weakness. The linea alba, which has darkened and become the linea nigra, also stretches to accommodate the fetal growth; in some women it tears, but in most it becomes elongated and flaccid (moved beyond its elastic limit).[86] Because the linea alba is a tendinous aponeurosis and not composed of contractile tissue, it cannot resume its prepregnancy condition and will therefore remain loose even as the rectus regains its size and tensile force. As the two sides of the rectus regain their pre-pregnancy position, the line alba will continue to lay between them as an overstretched, sagging structure. This makes the likelihood of DR in subsequent pregnancies quite high, although this has not been established in the literature.

The abdominal wall, with or without DR, exhibits diminished functional capacity as pregnancy progresses. Gilliard and Brown[67] examined the ability of pregnant women to stabilize the pelvis against resistance. They found that pregnant women, when compared with nonpregnant control subjects, could not accomplish this task in the later stages of pregnancy. Pregnancy and the early postpartum period are times of great stress on the abdominal wall and times of relative weakness of these structures. Proper rehabilitation may have a significant impact on a woman's urogenital and musculoskeletal health as she moves through the remainder of her life. Referral to a women's health PT specialist is appropriate to accomplish this rehabilitation when DR is noted by the primary care PT.

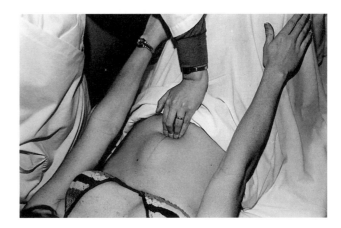

FIGURE 13-4 Diastasis recti abdominis assessment with patient supine. This patient had a diastasis recti of four finger widths. (From Boissonnault JS, Kotarinas RK: Diastasis recti. In Wilder E, editor: *Obstetric and gynecologic physical therapy*, New York, 1988, Churchill Livingstone, p 75.)

Coccydynia

Coccydynia is defined as pain in and around the region of the coccyx.[175] Perinatal coccydynia is most likely to result from parturition-related trauma such as sacral-coccygeal subluxation or fracture or to a stretch injury to the sacral-coccygeal ligaments or sacrococcygeal or intercoccygeal discs.[107,132,142] Patients will have pain in the region of the coccyx or perineum, with sitting as the most common aggravating factor. In addition to the localized trauma to the joint and bone itself, there may be associated soft tissue dysfunction (often classified as "levator ani syndrome"), particularly in the coccygeus and levator ani musculature that makes up part of the pelvic floor.[119,164]

Providing the patient with seating adaptation to lessen the weight on the coccyx (this can be done simply by placing toweling under each thigh or by purchasing an appropriate cushion) and to support the lumbar spine to maintain lordosis and disallow lumbar flexion with posterior pelvic tilt will aid in healing of tissues and should provide some pain relief. If the patient is still symptomatic after following this postural adaptation for a few weeks postpartum, then manual therapy to treat any joint subluxation or concomitant soft tissue dysfunction should be initiated. Some PTs have advocated the use of iontophoresis with dexamethasone for this condition, especially if there is significant pain provoked on the dorsal surface of the sacrococcygeal surface (personal communication between authors). Others have advocated high-volt galvanic stimulation to the area by a rectal probe[125,158] or internal soft-tissue mobilization.[164] Wray et al[175] reported on outcomes of a series of patients with coccydynia (some were postpartum women) and found that combining joint manipulation under general anesthesia and injection around the coccyx provided the best results.

Primary coccydynia (i.e., pain in the coccyx region that emanates directly from these tissues) that begins during pregnancy is uncommon. Because coccydynia is such a difficult condition to overcome, some women will continue to have symptoms from this dysfunction into their subsequent pregnancies. Legitimate fear of delivery trauma may bring them to a PT during a subsequent pregnancy. Instruction in sitting and body mechanics along with suggestions for positions in labor and delivery that allow for full mobility of the coccyx are welcome therapeutic interventions for this population.

Symptoms that Can Mimic Musculoskeletal Conditions in Pregnancy

Table 13-17 contains a partial list of symptoms during pregnancy that may result from musculoskeletal dysfunction or from medical conditions. The table lists common presenting symptoms, the pregnancy-related condition, the musculoskeletal dysfunction that might be responsible, and differential tests.

TABLE 13-17

Symptoms that Can Mimic Musculoskeletal Conditions in Pregnancy

Symptoms	Possible Medical Condition	Possible Musculoskeletal Dysfunction	Differentiating Tests or Measures
Calf, proximal thigh, or inguinal pain	Deep vein thrombosis	Gastrosoleus sprain; radicular symptoms from nerve root impingement; compartment syndrome; pubic symphysis dysfunction	Duplex ultrasonography; positive Homans' sign; assessment of response to treatment and provocation of pain by musculoskeletal examination of the pelvis and lower quadrant
Urinary incontinence	Urinary tract infection	Pelvic floor muscle dysfunction; cauda equina syndrome	Urinalysis; assessment of onset (acute or gradual) and aggravating factors
Lower abdominal pain	Abruption of the placenta; ectopic pregnancy	Pubic symphysis dysfunction (shears or separation)	Assessment of nature of pain (constant or intermittent) and aggravating factors; provocation of pain by musculoskeletal assessment of the pelvis; diagnostic ultrasound
Low back pain or hip pain	Osteoporosis of pregnancy with or without fracture	Mechanical dysfunction of the low back or pelvic ring; disc disease; spondylolisthesis	Height assessment; pain pattern assessment; objective findings (provocation tests, palpatory findings, neurologic findings, end-feels)
Flank pain	Upper urinary tract infection (kidney)	Rib or thoracic spine dysfunction	Percussion over the ribs; assessment of response to Rx and provocation of pain by musculoskeletal examination of the thorax; fever assessment; urinalysis
Right upper quadrant/ scapular pain	Gallstones	Shoulder girdle or thoracic spine/ rib dysfunction	Diagnostic ultrasound; assessment of response to treatment and nature of symptoms (whether pain is constant or provoked by activity)
Headache	Pregnancy-induced hypertension or preeclampsia	Upper cervical dysfunction or tension-type headache	Blood pressure assessment for hypertension; signs of recent onset of edema; provocation of headache by musculoskeletal assessment of the upper cervical spine

Neurologic System

Neurodiagnostic procedures are not contraindicated during pregnancy. Electromyography and electroencephalography can be undertaken without risk. Pregnancy does not alter the cerebrospinal fluid or the indications for examination of cerebrospinal fluid.[53] It is wise to limit fetal x-ray exposure, although there is no absolute contraindication for any neuroradiologic study. During the first trimester, x-ray exposure should be limited because there is an increased risk of malformation with fetal exposure to more than 0.015 Gy (1.5 rad).

Neurologic disorders of the central nervous system are rare in pregnancy. Brain tumor incidence in pregnancy is 1 in 1000,[41] and epilepsy is said to complicate 1 in 200 pregnancies.[124] Peripheral nervous system disorders are more common and are summarized in Table 13-16 by structures, mechanism of injury, and results of commonly found peripheral nerve entrapments and palsies in pregnancy and the postpartum period.

Peripheral Nervous System Disorders

Peripheral nervous system disorders can result from compression injuries and surgical neuropathies. Increases in extracellular fluid and weight gain, along with hormonal changes, are largely responsible for the neuropathic conditions seen during pregnancy. Most postpartum peripheral nervous system damage is caused by trauma incurred during labor and delivery, such as radial nerve palsies from holding on to the squat bar incorrectly or femoral nerve damage from lithotomy position. Additionally, pelvic floor dysfunction may develop as a result of sacral plexus or pudendal nerve damage from vaginal delivery or the use of forceps and vacuum extractors.

Epilepsy

Pregnancy can change the pattern of seizures and how a woman's body reacts to her antiepileptic drugs (AEDs). Seizures need to be avoided because they can affect the growing fetus. There is cause for concern because as many as one third of epileptic women will have an increase in the number of seizures during pregnancy despite taking AEDs.[41] Additionally, these women will have an increase in high blood pressure. Seizures can also increase the risk of falls that can result in serious injury.

There is a 2% to 3% increase in fetal anomalies found in pregnant women who take anticonvulsant drugs. Children born to mothers with epilepsy have a four-fold increase of developing a seizure disorder.[124] During labor and delivery women are monitored, and the experience is usually uneventful. AEDs will need to be readjusted after delivery, and these mothers will need counseling because all anticonvulsant medications will cross into breast milk to some degree, although this is not a contraindication to breastfeeding.[124,134] Studies of seizure frequency show that 35% of pregnant women will have an increase in seizures, 15% report a decrease, and 50% find no change in seizure activity.[41] In women with an increased rate of seizures there is a return to prepregnancy seizure rates after delivery.[134]

Multiple Sclerosis

During pregnancy, there is a trend toward lower relapse rates followed by an increase in relapse during the 6-month postpartum period. Initial onset of multiple sclerosis (MS) during pregnancy is uncommon and occurs in fewer than 10% of patients with MS.[42] Women with MS who have a singleton infant are no more likely to have complications in pregnancy or during delivery than women without MS. However, they are more likely to have a hospitalization during the first 3 postpartum months.[121] Damek[42] has also shown that women who have had children either before or after their diagnosis of MS may have positively altered the course of the disease over the long term.

Physical therapy management of pregnant women with MS is the same as for nonaffected women. Evaluation should include careful attention to the effects of potential balance and gait disturbances and spasticity on activities of daily living and functional activities. The enlarging uterus can affect the function of an already neurogenic bladder and increase the episodes of cystitis. Labor itself remains unchanged, but extensor or flexor spasms can be triggered by labor pain.[54]

In the postpartum period the PT can assist the new mother by encouraging her to obtain adequate rest, arrange for adequate child care, and obtain community support if she has an exacerbation.

Restless Legs Syndrome

Restless legs syndrome affects approximately 10% of pregnant women and should not be confused with leg cramps, which affect the gastrocnemius muscles only. Symptoms develop within 10 to 20 minutes after getting into bed. Patients report a feeling of "a wormy, burning ache developing" in their legs.[53] The syndrome is idiopathic in pregnancy but may improve with iron for women with anemia.

Spinal Cord Injury

In the United States, more than 30,000 women have spinal cord injuries (SCIs).[171] SCIs with cervical or thoracic lesions caused by trauma or tumor are not a contraindication to conception, pregnancy, or delivery. Women with SCIs have lower-birth-weight infants and have more complications in pregnancy. These complications include bacteriuria, urinary tract infections, pyelonephritis, pressure sores of the insensate skin, bowel dysfunction, respiratory problems, preterm contractions, and autonomic dysreflexia.[41,171] The perinatal mortality rate is 3.9%, and the preterm delivery rate is 20%.[41]

In lesions above T10, respiratory function and cough reflex will be compromised, which can affect pulmonary function in pregnancy. Women with these level lesions may need ventilatory support in late pregnancy or during labor. In lesions above T5-T6, autonomic hyperreflexia can occur, which is a potentially life-threatening situation. The splanchnic nerves are excited and are not dampened because of the lack of central inhibition.

Concomitantly, sudden sympathetic stimulation of nerves below the cord lesion can cause throbbing headaches, facial flushing, sweating, bradycardia, and paroxysmal hypertension. Culpable stimuli could include examination of pelvic structures; uterine contractions; cervical dilation; and urethral bladder, rectal, or cervical distention and catheterization. This can precipitate dangerous hypertension and require immediate attention. Support during labor often includes spinal or epidural anesthesia; these measures can prevent dysreflexia and are begun at the start of labor.

The level of the lesion does not affect uterine contractions for all spinal cord lesions. In lesions below T12, contractions are felt normally. Women with lesions above T12 are instructed in how to palpate uterine contractions or monitor with home tocodynamometry. The American College of Obstetricians and Gynecologists recommends continuous cardiac and intraarterial pressure monitoring.

During the postpartum period the mother with an SCI may have poor episiotomy healing and deep vein thrombosis. Blood loss during delivery may complicate the common anemia seen in pregnancy. This can lead to decreased energy levels and difficulty in the extra demands that parenting can have.[171] PTs can teach safe transfer techniques to avoid injury when the mother is fatigued.

Neural Tube Defects

Spina bifida (SB) is diagnosed in 2000 infants every year in the United States.[171] Through corrective surgery and adaptive technology, many of the women with spina bifida have full lives, including pregnancy. The incidence of women with SB giving birth to infants with SB is 2% to 4% higher than the general population.[171] Folic acid intake needs to be increased if a woman has already had one child with SB.

Poorly developed pelvic floor structures of these women can influence labor. Complications can result from previous bladder and bowel surgeries resulting in renal function deterioration, pain with intraperitoneal adhesions, increased incontinence, urinary tract infections, pyelonephritis, and obstruction with shifting of the intra-abdominal contents as the uterus expands.[171]

MRI pelvimetry may be necessary for pregnant women who have SB and a contracted pelvis. The deformity can result in an obstructed birth with cephalopelvic disproportion. Labor and delivery can be protracted, resulting in permanent loss in perineal muscle strength. Women with SB are at higher risk for pelvic organ prolapse without any effect of vaginal delivery. Spinal anesthesia for these women can be complex because of the level of their spinal lesion.

Guillain-Barré Syndrome

There is no increased incidence of Guillain-Barré syndrome in pregnancy, but there is a threefold increase in the first 30 days after delivery.[41]

Migraine

See the musculoskeletal section of this chapter for discussion on migraine headaches.

Integumentary System

Changes to the integumentary system during pregnancy usually occur for one of three reasons: physiological skin changes, dermatologic conditions that are unique to pregnancy, and preexisting skin diseases that complicate pregnancy. These conditions are rarely harmful to the pregnant patient but can be inconvenient and bothersome. PTs have a responsibility and opportunity to report any unusual skin changes because they see large areas of the patient's skin when examining and treating. It is helpful for clinicians to know what these skin changes are so that they can act as a resource for the patient and refer the patient for further consultation.

Physiological Changes

Hormonal changes during pregnancy have an extensive impact on the skin. These changes include hyperpigmentation, connective tissue and collagen changes, hair growth, vascular modifications, and glandular activity.

Increased skin darkening is observed in 90% of all pregnant women and is one of the most recognized changes of pregnancy.[14] This hyperpigmentation can occur in the nipples, areolae, linea alba, perineum, recent scars, moles, freckles, vulva, and perianal region. These areas of pigmentation usually increase in the first trimester, especially in dark-complexion and dark-haired women, and fade in the postpartum period. However, the pigmentation seldom returns to the prepregnancy level.[14]

Chloasma or melasma, also called the "mask of pregnancy," consists of irregular brownish patches of pigmentation that occur in 70% of women during the second half of pregnancy. The pattern of increased pigmentation can cover the forehead, cheeks, upper lip, nose, and chin. Other separated patterns are limited to the cheeks, nose, and mandible. Melasma occurs as well in 30% of women taking oral contraceptives. All these pigmentation changes are thought to be mediated by hormonal responses. No medical treatment is needed for chloasma.[41]

Vascular changes can affect the skin, causing edema in the face and hands in approximately 50% of all pregnant women. Edema of the legs, not associated with preeclampsia, develops in 80% of all pregnancies.[14] The swelling is worse in the morning, is nonpitting, and is caused by increases in fluid retention, vascular permeability, blood flow, and decreased colloid osmotic plasma pressure. PTs can assist in management of the edema by patient education in appropriate use of gradient pressure stockings and body positioning for optimal return of blood and lymph.

Spider nevi (dilated arteriole, or angioma, in the skin with radiating capillary branches)[57] and palmar erythema (redness in the palms) are thought to appear because of an increase in estrogen production.[160] Spider nevi appear between the second and fifth months of pregnancy in approximately 57% of white and 10% of black women.[14] They usually occur in the areas that are drained by the superior vena cava on the upper trunk and face and disappear by the seventh postpartum week. Palmar erythema develops in the first trimester in 70% of white and 35% of black women, resolving quickly after delivery.[14]

Varices most often involve the saphenous veins in the legs, vulva, and hemorrhoidal tissue. These dilated vessels result from increased venous pressure from compression of the pelvic and femoral veins by the enlarging uterus, increased blood volume, increased collagen fragility, and a hereditary tendency to varicose veins. As the vein swells, the valve inside the vein does not completely close, and retrograde flow forms varices. These subside after birth, but often not fully. Rest with the legs elevated and support stockings to increase the pressure on the leg, decreasing the swelling within the vein, are treatments and possible preventions of varices.

There is a familial tendency for connective tissue changes affecting the skin that occur most often in the second half of pregnancy.[14] These striae gravidarum, or stretch marks, are most frequently clustered on the abdomen, breasts, and thighs. The collagen and elastic fibers rupture with the increased stretching of the abdominal wall. Estrogen and relaxin are thought to increase the separation of the collagen fibers.[14] During the second half of pregnancy skin tags may develop on the pregnant woman's face, neck, axillae, and under the breasts. These usually recede postpartum.

Dermatoses

There are five types of dermatoses that are unique to pregnancy: herpes gestationis, polymorphic eruption of pregnancy, prurigo of pregnancy, pruritic folliculitis of pregnancy, and cholestasis of pregnancy. PTs need to be alert to skin changes because they may be seeing a woman during a skin eruption, necessitating a referral to a dermatologist.

Herpes gestationis, or pemphigoid gestationis, is a rare condition characterized by intensely pruritic papules with blistering skin eruptions in the second or third trimester of pregnancy. It occurs in 1 in 10,000 multiparous women.[41] In subsequent pregnancies, herpes gestationis is likely to appear earlier and with increased severity. It can sometimes appear in early pregnancy and up to 1 week after birth. These lesions vary in form from erythematous and edematous papules to large, tense bullae and vesicles.[41] These eruptions appear on the abdomen and extremities. Babies born to mothers with herpes gestationis may have a tendency for premature delivery, which may put the infant at risk for increased morbidity.[14] The cause of herpes gestationis is thought to be an immunopathologic, autoimmune, organ-specific blistering skin disease.[41] Treatment includes antipruritics, topical corticosteroids, and oral corticosteroids if the symptoms are severe.

Pruritic urticarial papules and plaques of pregnancy (PUPP), also referred to as polymorphic eruption of pregnancy, is the most common of the pruritic dermatoses of pregnancy, occurring in 0.25% to 1% of pregnancies.[41] These intensely pruritic cutaneous eruptions appear in late pregnancy, developing on the abdomen around the striae and spreading to the buttocks, thighs, and extremities. This disease is common in nulliparas and rarely occurs in later pregnancies. The pathogenetic pathology is unknown. Treatment with topical corticosteroid ointments and oral corticosteroids helps if itching is severe. The rash most often disappears within several days of delivery, and there is no evidence of perinatal morbidity.

Prurigo of pregnancy, also known as prurigo gestationis or papular dermatitis, is uncommon, with a rate of 1 in 300 to 1 in 2400 pregnancies. This type of dermatosis is characterized by small skin eruptions on the forearms and trunk. The lesions appear at 25 to 30 weeks of gestation with no adverse outcome to mother or fetus. The itching is controlled by antihistamines and topical corticosteroid creams.

Impetigo herpetiformis is a rare skin eruption seen in late pregnancy consisting of pustules that form themselves around the margin of erythematous patches. Itching is not severe but there are signs of nausea, vomiting, diarrhea, chills, and fever. The pustules may become infected after rupture, and sepsis can be a major concern. Treatment consists of systemic corticosteroids and antimicrobials to treat secondary infection. This disease can persist for several months after delivery, and fetal morbidity and mortality rates can be affected by the severity of the maternal infection.[41]

Cholestasis (inflammation of the gallbladder) in pregnancy involves intense pruritus without lesions and is common in 1% to 2% of pregnancies, resolving after birth. This skin disease is a mild form of cholestatic jaundice with onset in the third trimester generalized throughout the body. There is an increase in the rate of perinatal morbidity.[41]

Preexisting Skin Diseases

The hormones of pregnancy can have an effect on existing skin diseases. An improvement of psoriasis during pregnancy occurs in 65% of women, but 90% report a flare of the psoriasis in the postpartum period.[41] Psoriasis may remain unchanged, clear, worsen, or appear for the first time during pregnancy.[14] The effect of pregnancy on acne is unpredictable. Acne can improve or worsen in pregnancy. It can also appear for the first time, along with hirsutism. Retinoids and tetracyclines are highly teratogenic during pregnancy and are contraindicated. As a result, the withdrawal of these drugs may cause a flare of the acne. Candidiasis is 10 to 20 times more common in pregnancy because the lowered vaginal pH and increased sweating create a favorable environment. Treatment is topical with nystatin or miconazole.[14]

Special Considerations During Pregnancy and the Postpartum Period

Systemic Lupus Erythematosus

Systemic lupus erythematosus (SLE) is an autoimmune disorder that can be affected by the hormonal changes of pregnancy. SLE in pregnancy has three main outcomes: it increases late pregnancy miscarriage from hypertension and renal failure, it can cause heart block and other cardiac defects in the newborn, and it can increase the risk of abortion.

SLE is a fluctuating illness and pregnancy does not affect the long-term prognosis of the disease, but it may cause more flare-ups, particularly in the postpartum period. If the fetus lives to full gestation, there is an increased risk of fetal distress.[49] Women with SLE can have many complications of hypertension and renal failure, or may have no medical complications.

Rheumatoid Arthritis

Pregnancy usually improves the inflammatory component of rheumatoid arthritis. Symptoms and complications occurring during pregnancy are rare.[41,49] The pregnant woman with RA may feel a relief of her pain and stiffness. However, in the postpartum period there is a six-fold likelihood of exacerbation within the first 3 months. There is a small risk of congenital heart block in the newborn. The PT working with these pregnant women can caution against potential problems resulting from adduction of the mother's legs during delivery and hyperextension of her neck for intubation in general anesthesia.[49]

Women who have juvenile rheumatoid arthritis report similar results of decreased disease activity during pregnancy, with flare-ups in the postpartum period. Additionally, joint deformities are common and cesarean deliveries are performed for contracted pelves or joint prostheses.

Teen Pregnancy

The rate of teen and adolescent pregnancies fluctuates with the success rate of pregnancy prevention programs. Adolescents are at increased risk for preterm labor and psychological problems.[41] By 1996 the teenage birth rate was 54.7 live births per 1000 population. Ninety percent of these teens described their pregnancies as unintended.[38]

Teen pregnancies are complicated by incomplete pelvic growth, lack of psychological maturity, lack of prenatal care, and inadequate weight gain. As the teen continues to grow herself, she must gain enough for her own nutritional needs as well as for the growing fetus. Pregnant teens grow at a slower rate than their nonpregnant peers. Consequently pregnant adolescents have more than twice the mortality rate of adult pregnant women.[170]

The PT involved with this population can support the teenager in understanding the nutritional, physical, emotional, and nurturing changes that she will be confronted with. The PT can serve as a resource outside the family unit.

Cesarean Deliveries

Cesarean, or abdominal birth, is the delivery of the infant through the abdominal wall. In 1985 the cesarean delivery rate in the United States reached an all-time high of 24.4% of all births. Each year, 1 of every 10 pregnant American women has had a previous cesarean delivery.[41] Because of this large increase, in 1991 the United States Public Health Service set a goal of an overall 15% cesarean rate.

There are many reasons for cesarean deliveries. More than 85% are performed because of prior cesareans, labor dystocia, fetal distress, and breech presentation.[41] In subsequent pregnancies, women who have had a cesarean delivery may be given a chance to try a vaginal delivery as long as the risk factors are low. Vaginal birth after cesarean can be associated with a small but significant risk of uterine rupture, with poor outcomes for the mother and infant.[41]

Most often the surgical approach is made transversely through the lower uterine segment above the pubic bone. The classic cesarean incision vertically from umbilicus to pubis is now used in emergency situations. For a planned procedure, the patient may have options for anesthesia.

Early postpartum management by the PT is similar to any surgical patient: active movement of the extremities to prevent venous stasis and peripheral edema. Some women may have labored for an extensive period before requiring a cesarean section. Consequently, these women may need assistance in recovery from the major abdominal surgery as well as from the labor. In the later postpartum period, the PT can assist the patient in the full recovery of body mechanics, activities of daily living, abdominal wall strength, and return to an endurance and exercise program.

Summary

Pregnancy and the 3 months after delivery present unique challenges to examination and intervention of the obstetric patient. The primary care PT needs to be able to make an accurate physical therapy diagnosis and adapt the examination and treatment interventions to meet the obstetric patient's anatomic and physiological needs. As the health care field encourages that more obstetric patients be seen by PTs, a broader base of knowledge is required to examine, diagnosis and treat this population effectively.

The interaction of all body systems is taken into account because the pregnant patient goes through profound changes during the childbearing year. The primary care PT must weave together all the standard physical therapy information while accounting for the biomechanical forces that change.

Suggested readings are included for further study of obstetric physical therapy, and a list of related organizations can be found in Appendix 13-2, *Obstetric Resources*.

REFERENCES

1. Albert H, Godskesen M, Westergaard J: Prognosis in four syndromes of pregnancy-related pelvic pain, *Acta Obstet Gynecol Scand* 80:510, 2001.
2. Alexander JT, McCormick PC: Pregnancy and discogenic disease of the spine, *Neurosurg Clin North Am* 4:153-159, 1993.
3. American College of Obstetrics and Gynecology: Chronic hypertension in pregnancy. Practice Bulletin 29, *Obstet Gynecol* 98:177-185, 2001.
4. American College of Obstetrics and Gynecology: *Diabetes during pregnancy*, Patient Education Bulletin AP051. Washington, DC, 1996, American College of Obstetrics and Gynecology.
5. American College of Obstetrics and Gynecology: *Exercise during pregnancy and the postpartum period*, Technical Bulletin 189. Washington, DC, 1994, American College of Obstetrics and Gynecology.
6. American College of Obstetricians and Gynecologists: Committee opinion: exercise during pregnancy and the postpartum period, *Obstet Gynecol* 99:171-173, 2002.
7. American College of Obstetricians and Gynecologists: *Gestational diabetes*, ACOG Practice Bulletin 30, *Obstet Gynecol* 98: 525-538, 2001.
8. Anderson PO, Knoben JE, Troutman WG: *Handbook of clinical drug data*, ed 10, New York, 2002, McGraw-Hill.
9. Andres RL, Miles A: Venous thromboembolism and pregnancy, *Obstet Gynecol Clin North Am* 28:613, 2001.
10. Association of the Chartered Society of Physiotherapists in Women's Health: *Pubic symphysis dysfunction*, London, 1997, Association of Chartered Physiotherapists in Women's Health.
11. Backe B, Brodtkorb CJ, Giltvedt J, et al: Fetal and maternal aortic flow in two different maternal positions, *Ultrasound in Medicine and Biology* 9:587-593, 1983.
12. Belluomini J, Litt RC, Lee KA, et al: Acupressure for nausea and vomiting of pregnancy: a randomized blinded study, *Obstet Gynecol* 84:245-248, 1994.
13. Berg G, Hammar M, Moller-Nielsen J, et al: Low back pain during pregnancy, *Obstet Gynecol* 71:71-75, 1988.
14. Black MM, Mayou SC: Skin diseases in pregnancy. In de Swiet M, editor: *Medical disorders in obstetric practice*, ed 3, Oxford, 1995, Blackwell Science, pp 610-624.
15. Boissonnault WG: Male urogenital system. In Boissonnault WG, editor: *Examination in physical therapy practice: screening for medical disease*, ed 2, Philadelphia, 1995, Churchill Livingstone.
16. Boissonnault JS, Kotarinos RK: Diastasis recti. In Wilder E, editor: *Obstetric and gynecologic physical therapy: clinics in physical therapy*, New York, 1988, Churchill Livingstone.
17. Boissonnault JS, Bookhout MM: Course notes for physical therapy management of musculoskeletal dysfunction in the pregnant patient. 2002.

18. Boissonnault JS, Blaschak MJ: Incidence of diastasis recti abdominis during the childbearing year, *Phys Ther* 68:1082-1086, 1998.
19. Boissonnault WG, Boissonnault JS: Transient osteoporosis of the hip associated with pregnancy, *J Ortho Sports Phys Ther* 31:359-367, 2001.
20. Boland BF: Separation of symphysis pubis: report of ten cases occurring during delivery, *N Engl J Med* 208:431-438, 1933.
21. Bookhout MM, Boissonnault JS: Musculoskeletal dysfunction in the female pelvis, *Ortho Phys Ther Clin North Am* 5:23-45, 1996.
22. Bookhout MM, Boissonnault WG: Physical therapy management of musculoskeletal disorders during pregnancy. In Wilder E, editor: *Obstetric and gynecological physical therapy: clinics in physical therapy*, New York, 1988, Churchill Livingstone.
23. Bullock-Saxton J: Musculoskeletal changes associated with the perinatal period. In Sapsford R, Bullock-Saxton J, Markwell S, editors: *Women's health: a textbook for physiotherapists*, Philadelphia, 1998, WB Saunders.
24. Bullock JE, Jull GA, Bullock MI: The relationship of low back pain to postural changes during pregnancy, *Aust J Physiother* 33:10-17, 1987.
25. Burgio KL, Lovher JL, Zyczynski H, et al: Urinary incontinence during pregnancy in a racially mixed sample: characteristics and predisposing factors, *Int Urogynecol J* 7:69-73, 1996.
26. Burtis CA, Ashwood ER: *Tietz textbook of clinical chemistry*, ed 2, Philadelphia, 1994, WB Saunders, pp 2107-2148.
27. Calguneri M, Bird H, Wright V: Changes in joint laxity occurring during pregnancy, *Ann Rheumatic Dis* 41:126-128, 1982.
28. Cappiello GA, Oliver BC: Rupture of symphysis pubis caused by forceful and excessive abduction of the thighs with labor epidural anesthesia, *J Florida Med Assoc* 82:438-443, 1995.
29. Carbonne LD, Palmieri GMH, Graves SC, et al: Osteoporosis of pregnancy: long term follow-up of patients and their offspring, *Obstet Gynecol* 86:664-666, 1995.
30. Chaudron LH, Klein MH, Remington P, et al: Predictors, prodromes and incidence of postpartum depression, *J Psychosomatic Obstet Gynecol* 22:103-112, 2001.
31. Chez RA: Women battering in pregnancy. In Sapsford R, Bullock-Saxton J, Markwell S, editors: *Women's health: a textbook for physiotherapists*, Philadelphia, 1998, WB Saunders.
32. Chigara M, Watanabe H, Udogowa E: Transient osteoporosis of the hip in the first trimester of pregnancy, *Arch Orthop Trauma Surg* 107:178-180, 1998.
33. Clapp JF III: *Exercising through your pregnancy*, Omaha, Neb, 2002, Addicus Books.
34. Cogill SR, Caplan HL, Anexandra H, et al: Impact of maternal postnatal depression on cognitive development of young children, *BMJ* 292:1165-1167, 2002.
35. Cohen Y, Lavie O, Granovsky-Grisaru S, et al: Bell palsy complicating pregnancy: a review. *Obstet Gynecol Survey* 55:184-188, 2002.
36. Cokkinides VE, Coker AL, Sanderson M, et al: Physical violence during pregnancy: maternal complications and birth outcomes, *Obstet Gynecol* 93:661-666, 1999.
37. Coombes K, Darken R: Psychological and emotional aspects of child bearing. In Sapsford R, Bullock-Saxton J, Markwell S, editors: *Women's health: a textbook for physiotherapists*, Philadelphia, 1998, WB Saunders.
38. Committee on Adolescence: Adolescent pregnancy-current trends and issues: 1998, *Pediatrics* 103:516-520, 1999.
39. Crapo RO: Normal cardiopulmonary physiology during pregnancy, *Clin Obstet Gynecol* 39:3-16, 1996.
40. Cox JL, Hoden JM, Sagovsky R: Edinburgh Postnatal Depression Scale (EPDS), *Br J Psych* 150:782-786, 1987.
41. Cunningham FG, Gant NF, Leveno KJ, et al: *Williams obstetrics*, ed 21, New York, 2001, McGraw-Hill.
42. Damek DE, Shuster EA: Pregnancy and multiple sclerosis, *Mayo Clin Proc* 72:977-989, 1997.
43. Damen L, Buyrak HM, Stam CJ, et al: Pelvic pain during pregnancy is associated with asymmetric laxity of the sacroiliac joints, *Acta Obstet Gynecol Scand* 80:1019-1024, 2001.
44. Danforth DN, Scott JR, editors: *Obstetrics and gynecology*, ed 5, Philadelphia, 1986, JB Lippincott.
45. Danilenko-Dixon DR, Heit JA, Silverstein MD, et al: Risk factors for deep vein thrombosis and pulmonary embolism during pregnancy or post partum: a population-based, case-control study, *Am J Obstet Gynecol* 184:104-110, 2001.
46. Dattel BJ: Domestic violence. In Sanfilippo JS, Smith RP, editors *Primary care in obstetrics and gynecology: a handbook for clinicians*, New York, 1998, Springer-Verlag.
47. Davison JM, Lindheimer MD: Renal disorders. In Creasy RK, Resnik R, editors: *Maternal-fetal medicine*, ed 4, Philadelphia, 1999, WB Saunders.
48. DeLeeuw JW, Vierhout ME, Struijk PC, et al: Anal sphincter damage after vaginal delivery: functional outcome and risk factors for fecal incontinence, *Acta Obstet Gynecol Scand* 80:830-834, 2001.
49. de Swiet M: Systemic lupus erythematosus and other connective tissue diseases. In de Swiet M, editor: *Medical disorders in obstetric practice*, ed 3, Oxford, 1995, Blackwell Science.
50. Dhar S, Anderton JM: Rupture of the symphysis pubis during labor, *Clin Orthop Rel Res* 283:252-257, 1992.
51. Division of Maternal Fetal Medicine Dartmouth-Hitchcock Medical Center: *Depression in pregnancy*, 2002, accessed at www.dartmouth.edu/~obygn/mfm/patiented/depression.html.
52. Dixon-Townson D: Pregnancy-related venous thromboembolism, *Clin Obstet Gynecol* 45:363-368, 2002.
53. Donaldson JO: Neurologic complications. In Burrow GN, Duffy TP, editors: *Medical complications during pregnancy*, ed 5, Philadelphia, 1999, WB Saunders, pp 401-414.
54. Donaldson JO: Neurological disorders. In de Swiet M, editor: *Medical disorders in obstetric practice*, ed 3, Oxford, 1995, Blackwell Science, pp 535-551.
55. Drinkwater BL, Chestnut CH III: Bone density changes during pregnancy and lactation in active women: a longitudinal study, *Bone Mineral* 14:153-160, 1991.
56. Dunne F, Walters B, Marshall T: Pregnancy associated osteoporosis, *Clin Endocrinol* 39:487-490, 1993.
57. Dox I, Melloni JB, Eisner GM: *Melloni's illustrated medical dictionary*, Baltimore, 1979, William & Wilkins.
58. Egerman RS, Mabie WC, Eifrid M, et al: Sacralilitis associated with pyelonephritis in pregnancy, *Obstet Gynecol* 85:834-835, 1995.
59. Enkin E, Keirse MJNC, Neilson J, et al: *A guide to effective care in pregnancy & childbirth*, Oxford, 2000, Oxford University Press.
60. Feller CM, Franko-Filipasis KJ: Headaches during pregnancy, *J Perinatal Neonatal Nurs* 7:1-10, 1993.
61. Frahm J, Welsh RA: Physical therapy management of the high-risk antepartum patient, *Clin Management* 9:15, 1989.
62. Franklin ME, Conner-Kerr T: An analysis of posture and back pain in the first and third trimesters of pregnancy, *J Orthop Sports Phys Ther* 28:133-138, 1998.
63. Funk JL, Shovack DM, Grnant HK: Transient osteoporosis of the hip in pregnancy: natural history of changes in bone mineral density, *Clin Endocrinol* 43:373-382, 1995.
64. Furman GJ: *Anatomy in outline* Oxford, 2001, Blackwell Science.
65. Garmel SH, Guzelian GA, D'alton JG, et al: Lumbar disk disease in pregnancy, *Obstet Gynecol* 89:821-822, 1997.
66. Giger JN, Davidhizar R: *Transcultural nursing assessment and intervention*, St. Louis, 1995, Mosby Year-Book.
67. Gilliard WL, Brown JM: Structure and function of the abdominal muscles in primigravid subjects during pregnancy and the immediate postbirth period, *Phys Ther* 76:750-762, 1996.
68. Gonik B, Stringer CA: Postpartum osteitis pubis, *Southern Med J* 78:213-214, 1985.
69. Goodwin MM, et al, for the PRAMS Workgroup: Pregnancy intendedness and physical abuse around the time of pregnancy: findings from the Pregnancy Risk Assessment Monitoring System, *Maternal Child Health* 4:85-92, 2000.
70. Griffin JE, Karselis TC: *Physical agents for physical therapists*, Springfield, Ill, 1982, Charles C. Thomas.
71. Hainline B: Headache in neurologic complications of pregnancy, *Neurologic Clin* 12:443-460, 1994.
72. Hansen A, Jensen DV, Larson E, et al: Relaxin is not related to symptom giving pelvic girdle relaxation in pregnant women, *Acta Obstet Gynecol Scand* 75:245-249, 1996.
73. Hansen A, Jensen DV, Wromslev M, et al: Symptom-giving pelvic girdle relaxation in pregnancy II: symptoms and clinical signs, *Acta Obstet Gynecol Scand* 78:111-115, 1999.
74. Hayman B: A miracle in the making, Chicago, 2000, Budlong Press.
75. Hedegaard M: Life style, work and stress, and pregnancy outcome, *Curr Opin Obstet Gynecol* 11:553-556, 1999.
76. Hoffman CM. Depression in pregnancy: a frequent problem that is frequently missed, *North Carolina Med J* 56:212-213, 1995.
77. Holt MA, Keene JS, Graf BK, et al: Treatment of osteitis pubis in athletes, *Am J Sports Med* 23:601-606, 1995.
78. James AW: Asthma. In Vogt V, Elmore TD, Ling FW, editors: *Obstetrics and gynecology clinics of North America*, Philadelphia, 2001, WB Saunders.
79. Josefsson A, Berg G, Nordin C, et al: Prevalence of depressive symptoms in late pregnancy and postpartum, *Acta Obstet Gynecol Scand* 80:251-255, 2001.

80. Jovanovic-Peterson L, Durak EP, Peters CM: Randomized trial of diet versus diet plus cardiovascular conditioning on glucose levels in gestational diabetes, *Am J Obstet Gynecol* 161:415, 1989.

81. Jovanovic-Peterson L, Peterson CM: Dietary manipulation as a primary treatment strategy for pregnancies complicated by diabetes, *J Am Coll Nutr* 9:320, 1990.

82. Kammerer-Doak DN, Cornella JL, Magrina JF, et al: Osteitis pubis after Marshall-Marchetti-Krantz urethropexy: a pubic osteomyelitis, *Am J Obstet Gynecol* 179:586-590, 1998.

83. Khastigir G, Studd JW, King H, et al: Changes in bone density and biochemical markers of bone turnover in pregnancy-associated osteoporosis, *Br J Obstet Gynaecol* 103:716-718, 1996.

84. Kopell HP, Thompson WAL: *Peripheral entrapment neuropathies*, Huntington, NY, 1976, Robert E. Krieger, p 86.

85. Koshy M, Burd L: Management of pregnancy in sickle cell syndromes, *Hematology/Oncology Clin North Am* 5:585-596, 1991.

86. Kotarinos RK: Diastasis recti: clinical assessment versus surgical observation, *J Obstet Gynecol Phys Ther* 15:9-12, 1991.

87. Kristiansson P, Svardsudd K, Von Schoultz B: Serum relaxin, symphyseal pain, and back pain during pregnancy, *Am J Obstet Gynecol* 175:1342-1347, 1996.

88. Kurzel RP. Friedman MJ: Orthopedic injuries in pregnancy. In Mittlemark RA, Wiswell RA, Frinkwater BL, editors: *Exercise in pregnancy*, ed 2, Baltimore, 1991, Williams & Wilkins.

89. LaBan MM, Perrin JCS, Latimer FR: Pregnancy and the herniated disc, *Arch Phys Med Rehab* 64:319-321, 1983.

90. LaBan MM, Viola S, Williams DA, et al: Magnetic resonance imaging of the lumbar herniated disc in pregnancy, *Phys Med Rehab* 74:59-61, 1995.

91. Larsen EC, Wilken-Jensen C, Hansen A, et al: Symptom-giving pelvic girdle relaxation in pregnancy. I: prevalence and risk factors, *Acta Obstet Gynecol Scand* 78:105-110, 1999.

92. Larson J: Osteoporosis. In Sapsford R, Bullock-Saxton J, Markwell S, editors: *Women's health: a textbook for physiotherapists*, Philadelphia, 1998, WB Saunders.

93. Lauderdale J: Childbearing and transcultural nursing care issues. In Andrews MM, Boyle JS, editors: *Transcultural concepts in nursing care*, Philadelphia, 1999, JB Lippincott.

94. Leavitt R, editor: *Cross-cultural rehabilitation: an international perspective*, Philadelphia, 1999, WB Saunders.

95. Lederer E: Urinary tract infections. In Sanfilippo JS, Smith RP. editors: *Primary care in obstetrics and gynecology*, New York, 1998, Springer-Verlag.

96. Leininger M, editor: *Transcultural nursing: concepts, theories, research, and practices*, New York, 1995, McGraw-Hill.

97. Lentz SS: Osteitis pubis: a review, *Obstet Gynecol Survey* 50:310-315, 1995.

98. Lepercq J, Conard J, Borel-Derlon A, et al: Venous thromboembolism during pregnancy: a retrospective study of enoxaparin safety in 624 pregnancies, *Br J Obstet Gynaecol* 108:1134-1140, 2001.

99. Lipson JP, Dibble SL, Minarik PA: *Culture & nursing care: a pocket guide*, San Francisco, Calif, 1996, UCSF Nursing Press.

100. Lindsey RW, Leggon RE, Wright DW, et al: Separation of the symphysis pubis in association with childbearing: a case report, *J Bone Joint Surg* 70:289-292, 1988.

101. Livingston JC, Baha MS: Chronic hypertension in pregnancy, *Obstet Gynecol Clin North Am* 28:447-463, 2001.

102. Livingstone L: Postnatal management, In Sapsford R, Bullock-Saxton J, Markwell S, editors: *Women's health: a textbook for physiotherapists*, Philadelphia, 1998, WB Saunders.

103. Livingstone L: Physiology of labour. In Sapsford R, Bullock-Saxton J, Markwell S, editors: *Women's health: a textbook for physiotherapists*, Philadelphia, 1998, WB Saunders.

104. Lucas MJ: Diabetes complicating pregnancy. In *Obstet Gynecol Clin North Am*, Philadelphia, 2001, WB Saunders, pp 513-536.

105. Lupton M, Oteng-Ntim E, Ayida G, et al: Cardiac disease in pregnancy, *Curr Opin Obstet Gynecol* 14:137-143, 2002.

106. MacLennan AH: The role of the hormone relaxin in human reproduction and pelvic girdle relaxation, *Scand J Rheumatol* 88:7-15, 1991.

107. Maigne J, Guedj S, Straus C: Idiopathic coccygodynia, *Spine* 19:930-934, 1994.

108. Maloni JA: Bed rest and high-risk pregnancy, *Nurs Clin North Am* 31:313-325, 1996.

109. Marcoux S, Berube S, Brisson C, et al: Job strain and pregnancy induced hypertension, *Epidemiology* 10:376-382, 1999.

110. Martin SL, Mackie L, Kupper LL, et al: Physical abuse of women before, during and after pregnancy, *JAMA* 285:1581-1584, 2001.

111. Mason L, Glenn S, Walton I, et al: The prevalence of stress incontinence during pregnancy and following delivery, *Midwifery* 15:120-128, 1999.

112. Mezey GC, Bewley S: Domestic violence and pregnancy, *Br J Obstet Gynaecol* 104:528-531, 1997.

113. Miller MW, Brayman AA, Abromowicz JS: Obstetric ultrasonography: a biophysical consideration of patient safety. The "rules" have changed, *Am J Obstet Gynecol* 179:241-254, 1998.

114. Mittelmark RA, Wiswell RA, Drinkwater BL, editors: *Exercise in pregnancy*, ed 2, Baltimore, 1986, Williams & Wilkins.

115. Mokshagundam SPL: Diabetes mellitus. In Sanfilippo JS, Smith RP, editors: *Primary care in obstetrics and gynecology*, New York, 1998, Springer-Verlag, pp 194-206.

116. Montgomery KS: Caring for the pregnant woman with sickle cell disease, *MCN J Am J Matern Child Nurs* 21:224-228, 1996.

117. Morin KH: Urologic consequences of childbirth: a review of the literature, *Urol Nurs* 14:41-45, 1994.

118. Morkved S, Bo K: Prevalence of urinary incontinence during pregnancy and postpartum, *Int Urogynecol* J 10:394-398, 1999.

119. Morris L, Newton RA: Use of high voltage galvanic stimulation for patients with levator ani syndrome, *Phys Ther* 67:1522-1525, 1986.

120. Mou Sun P, Wilburn W, Raynor BD, et al: Sickle cell disease in pregnancy: twenty years of experience at Grady Memorial Hospital, Atlanta, Georgia, *Am J Obstet Gynecol* 184:1127-1130, 2001.

121. Mueller BA, Ahang J, Critchlow CW: Birth outcomes and need for hospitalization after delivery among women with multiple sclerosis, *Am J Obstet Gynecol* 186:446-452, 2002.

122. Nielsen Forman D, Videbech P, Hedegaard M, et al: Postpartum depression: identification of women at risk, *Br J Obstet Gynaecol* 107:1210-1217, 2000.

123. Noble E: *Essential exercises for the childbearing year*, ed 2, Boston, 1982, Houghton Mifflin.

124. Norwitz E, Schorge J: *Obstetrics and gynecology at a glance*, Oxford, 2001, Blackwell Science.

125. Ostergaard GC, Rubin RJ, Salvati EP, et al: Electrogalvanic stimulation in the treatment of levator ani syndrome, *Dis Colon Rectum* 28:662-663, 1988.

126. Ostgaard M, Bonde B, Thomsen BS: *Pelvic insufficiency during pregnancy*. Summary in English, Ugeskr Laeger 154:3568-3572, 1992.

127. Ostgaard HC, Andersson GBJ, Karlsson K: Prevalence of back pain in pregnancy, *Spine* 16:549-552, 1991.

128. Ostgaard HC, Andersson GBJ, Schultz AB, et al: Influence of some biomechanical factors on low back pain in pregnancy, *Spine* 18:61-65, 1993.

129. Ostgaard HC, Zetherstrom G, Roos-Hansson E, et al: Reduction of back and posterior pelvic pain in pregnancy, *Spine* 19:894-900, 1994.

130. Perkins J, Hammer RL, Louber P: Identification and management of pregnancy-related low back pain, *J Nurse Mid* 43:331-340, 1998.

131. Petersen LK, Hvidman L, Uldbjerg N: Normal serum relaxin in women with disabling pelvic pain during pregnancy, *Gynecol Obstet Invest* 38:21-23, 1994.

132. Peyton FW: Coccygodynia in women, *Indiana Medicine* 81:697-698, 1988.

133. Purnell LD, Paulanka BJ, editors: *Transcultural healthcare: a culturally competent approach*, Philadelphia, 1998, FA Davis.

134. Pschirrer ER, Maonga M: Seizure disorders in pregnancy, *Obstet Gynecol Clin North Am* 28:601-611, 2001.

135. Rath JD, Rath R, Mielcarski E, et al: Low back pain during pregnancy: helping patients take control, *J Musculoskel Med* 17:223-232, 2000.

136. Ramin KD, Ramsey PS: Disease of the gallbladder and pancreas in pregnancy, *Obstet Gynecol Clin North Am* 28:571-580, 2001.

137. Ramsey BW: Management of pulmonary disease in patients with cystic fibrosis, *N Engl J Med* 335:179, 1996.

138. Rebar RW: The breast and the physiology of lactation. In Creasy RK, Resnick RR, editors: *Maternal fetal medicine*, ed 5, Philadelphia, 1999, WB Saunders.

139. Riley MR, Burnham TH, Bastean JN, et al: *Drug facts and comparisons, 2001*, pocket version, ed 5, St Louis, 2001, Facts and Comparisons.

140. Rothstein JM, Roy SH, Wolf SL: *The rehabilitation specialist's handbook*, Philadelphia, 1991, FA Davis.

141. Rungee MAJ: Low back pain during pregnancy, *J Orthop* 16:1339-1343, 1993.

142. Saluja PG: The incidence of ossification of the sacralcoccygeal joint, *J Anat* 156:11-15, 1988.

143. Samdani A, Lachman E, Nogler W: Transient osteoporosis of the hip during pregnancy: a case report, *Am J Phys Med Rehab* 77:153-156, 1998.

144. Sapsford R, Markwell, S: Pelvic floor dysfunction in the perinatal period. In Sapsford R, Bullock-Saxton J, Markwell S, editors: *Women's health: a textbook for physiotherapists*, Philadelphia, 1998, WB Saunders.

145. Schauberger CW, Rooney BL, Goldsmith L, et al: Peripheral joint laxity increases in pregnancy but does not correlate with serum relaxin levels, *Am J Obstet Gynecol* 174:664-671, 1996.

146. Scott LD: Gastrointestinal disease in pregnancy. In Creasy RK, Resnik R, editors: *Maternal-fetal medicine*, Philadelphia, 1999, WB Saunders, pp 1038-1053.

147. Scriven MW, Jones DS, McKnight L: The importance of pubic pain following childbirth: a clinical and ultrasonographic study of the pubic symphysis, *J Royal Soc Med* 88:28-30, 1995.

148. Section on Obstetrics and Gynecology, APTA, Perinatal exercise guideline, Alexandria, Va., 1986.

149. Seely BL, Burrow GN: Thyroid disease and pregnancy. In Creasy RK, Resnik R, editors: *Maternal-fetal medicine*, Philadelphia, 1999, WB Saunders, pp 996-1014.

150. Shankman G: Thromboembolic disease anticoagulation therapy, *Ortho Prac* 13;3:14-15, 2001.

151. Sharp D, Paulby FH, Dale S, et al: The impact of postnatal depression on boys intellectual development, *J Child Psychol Psychiatry* 36:1315-1316, 1995.

152. Sharpe R: Pregnancy and the puerperium: physiological changes. In Sapsford R, Bullock-Saxton J, Markwell S, editors: *Women's health: a textbook for physiotherapists*, Philadelphia, 1998, WB Saunders.

153. Simpson EL, Lawrenson RA, Nightingale AI, et al: Venous thromboembolism in pregnancy and the puerperium: incidence and additional risk factors from a London perinatal database, *Br J Obstet Gynaecol* 108:56-60, 2001.

154. Silva M, Mallinson C, Reynolds F: Sciatic nerve palsy following childbirth, *Anaesthesia* 51:1144-1148, 1996.

155. *Smith R, Athanasou NA, Ostlere SJ, et al: Pregnancy-associated osteoporosis, Q J Med* 88:865-878, 1995.

156. Smith RP: Gastrointestinal disorders. In Sanfilippo JS, Smith RP, editors: *Primary care in obstetrics and gynecology: a handbook for clinicians*, New York, 1998, Springer-Verlag, pp 231-243.

157. Snow RE, Neubert AG: Peripartum pubic symphysis separation: a case series and review of the literature, *Obstet Gynecol Survey* 52:438-433, 1997.

158. Sohn N, Weinstein MA, Robbins RD: The levator syndrome and its treatment with high voltage electrogalvanic stimulation, *Am J Surg* 144:58-62, 1982.

159. Spector RE, editor: *Cultural diversity in health and illness*, Stamford, Conn, 1996, Appleton & Lange.

160. Stephenson RG, O'Connor LJ: *Obstetric and gynecologic care in physical therapy*, ed 2, Thorofare, NJ, 2000, Slack Inc.

161. Stocks GM, Wooller DJA, Young JM, et al: Postpartum headache after epidural bloodpatch: investigation and diagnosis, *Br J Anaesthesiol* 84:407-410, 2000.

162. Strauhal MJ: Therapeutic exercise in obstetrics. In Hall CM, Brody LT, editors: *Therapeutic exercise: moving toward function*, Philadelphia, 1999, Lippincott Williams & Wilkins, pp 213-232.

163. Sultan AH, Kamin MA, Hudson CN: Pudendal nerve damage during labour: a prospective study before and after childbirth, *Br J Obstet Gynaecol* 101:22-28, 1994.

164. Thiele GH: Coccygeus and piriformis muscles: its relationship to coccygodynia and pain in the region of the hip and down the leg, Transcript of the American Proctology Society 37:145-155, 1936.

165. Umpierrez GE, Kitabchi AE: Management of type 2 diabetes: evolving strategies for treatment. In *Obstetrics and gynecology clinics of North America*, Philadelphia, 2001, WB Saunders, pp 401-421.

166. Vaughan DJA, Stirrup CA, Robinson PN: Cranial subdural haematoma associated with dural puncture in labour, *Br J Anaesthesiol* 84:518-520, 2000.

167. Vellacott ID, Cook E, James CE: Nausea and vomiting in early pregnancy, *Int J Gynecol Obstet* 27:57-62, 1998.

168. Viktrup L, Lose G, Rolff M, et al: The symptom of stress incontinence caused by pregnancy or delivery in primiparas, *Obstet Gynecol* 79:945-949, 1992.

169. Vincent C: Osteitis pubis, *J Am Board Fam Pract* 6:492-496, 1993.

170. Wahl R: Nutrition in the adolescent, *Pediatr Ann* 2:107-111, 1999.

171. Welner S: Pregnancy in women with disabilities. In Cohen WR, editor: *Cherry and Merkatz's complications of pregnancy*, ed 5, Philadelphia, 2000, Lippincott Williams & Wilkins, pp 829-838.

172. Wendel PJ: Asthma in pregnancy, *Obstet Gynecol Clin North Am*, Philadelphia, 2001, WB Saunders, pp 537-551.

173. Wijma J, Potters AEW, deWolf B, et al: Anatomical and functional changes in the lower urinary tract during pregnancy, *Br J Obstet Gynaecol* 108:678-683, 2001.

174. Wing DA: Pyelonephritis, *Clin Obstet Gynecol* 41:515-526, 1998.

175. Wray CC, Eason S, Hoskinson J: Coccydynia, *J Bone Joint Surg* 73-B:335-338, 1991.

SUGGESTED READINGS

Exercise in Pregnancy

Clapp J: *Exercising through your pregnancy*, Omaha, Neb, 2002, Addicus Books.

Mittlemark RA, Wiswell RA, Drinkwater BL: *Exercise in pregnancy*, ed 2, Baltimore, 1990, Williams and Wilkins.

Section on Obstetrics and Gynecology, APTA: *Perinatal exercise guidelines*. Alexandria, Va, 1986, Section on Obstetrics and Gynecology of the APTA.

Musculoskeletal

Vleeming A, Mooney V, Dorman T, et al: *Movement, stability and low back pain: the essential role of the pelvis*, New York, 1999, Churchill Livingstone.

Obstetrics and Gynecology

Creasy RK, Resnik R: Maternal-fetal medicine, ed 4, Philadelphia, 1999, WB Saunders.

Cunningham FG, Gant NF, Leveno KJ, et al: *Williams obstetrics*, ed 21, New York, 2001, McGraw-Hill.

Danforth DN, Scott JR. editors: *Obstetrics and gynecology*, ed 5, Philadelphia, 1986, JB Lippincott.

Niswander KR. editor: *Manual of obstetrics*, ed 3, Boston, 1987, Little, Brown.

Obstetrics/Gynecology Books by Physical Therapists

Noble E: *Essential exercises for the childbearing year: a guide to health before and after your baby is born*, ed 4, Boston, 1987, Houghton-Mifflin.

Pauls JA: *Therapeutic approaches to women's health: a program of exercise and education*, Frederick, Md, 1996, Aspen.

Polden M, Mantle J: *Physiotherapy in obstetrics and gynecology*, London, 1990, Butterworth-Heinemann.

Sapsford R, Bullock-Saxton J, Markwell S: *Women's health: a textbook for physiotherapists*, London, 1998, WB Saunders.

Stephenson RG, O'Connor LJ: *Obstetric and gynecologic care in physical therapy*, ed 2, Thorofare, NJ, 2000, Slack.

Wilder E, editor: *Clinics in physical therapy*. Vol 20: *Obstetric and gynecologic physical therapy*, New York, 1988, Churchill-Livingstone.

Appendix **13-1** Edinburgh Postnatal Depression Scale (EPDS)

Instructions for Administrators

The mother is asked to underline the response that comes closest to how she has been feeling in the previous 7 days. All 10 items must be completed.

Care should be taken to avoid the possibility of the mother discussing her answers with others. The mother should complete the scale herself unless she has limited English or has difficulty with reading.

The EPDS may be used at 6 to 8 weeks after delivery to screen postnatal women. The child health clinic, postnatal checkup, or a home visit may provide suitable opportunities for its completion.

Instructions for Users

Because you have recently had a baby, we would like to know how you are feeling. Please UNDERLINE the answer that comes closest to how you have felt IN THE PAST 7 DAYS, not just how you feel today.

1. **I have been able to laugh and see the funny side of things.**
   As much as I always could
   Not quite so much now
   Definitely not so much now
   Not at all

2. **I have looked forward with enjoyment to things.**
   As much as I ever did
   Rather less than I used to
   Definitely less than I used to
   Hardly at all

3. **I have blamed myself unnecessarily when things went wrong.***
   Yes, most of the time
   Yes, some of the time
   Not very often
   No, never

4. **I have been anxious or worried for no good reason.**
   No, not at all
   Hardly ever

Yes, sometimes
Yes, very often

5. **I have felt scared or panicky for no very good reason.***
   Yes, quite a lot
   Yes, sometimes
   No, not much
   No, not at all

6. ***Things have been getting on top of me.***
   Yes, most of the time I haven't been able to cope at all
   Yes, sometimes I haven't been coping as well as usual
   No, most of the time I have coped quite well
   No, I have been coping as well as ever

7. **I have been so unhappy that I have had difficulty sleeping.***
   Yes, most of the time
   Yes, sometimes
   Not very often
   No, not at all

8. **I have felt sad or miserable.***
   Yes, most of the time
   Yes, quite often
   Not very often
   No, not at all

9. ***I have been so unhappy that I have been crying.***
   Yes, most of the time
   Yes, quite often
   Only occasionally
   No, never

10. ***The thought of harming myself has occurred to me.***
    Yes, quite often
    Sometimes
    Hardly ever
    Never

Response categories are scored 0, 1, 2, and 3 according to increased severity of the symptoms. Items marked with an asterisk are reverse coded (3, 2, 1, and 0). The total score is calculated by adding together the scores for each of the 10 items.[40]

Appendix **13-2 Obstetric Resources**

Maternal-Child Health Organizations

American Academy of Husband-Coached Childbirth (AAHCC)
The Bradley Method
PO Box 5224
Sherman Oaks, CA 91413
(818) 788-6662
(800) 423-2397
www.bradleybirth.com

American College of Nurse-Midwives (ACNM)
1522 K Street NW, Suite 1120
Washington, DC 20005
(202) 347-5445
www.acnm.org
Gives listing of nurse-midwives and nurse-midwifery training programs.

American College of Obstetricians and Gynecologists (ACOG)
409 12th Street, SW
Washington, DC 20024
(202) 638-5577
www.acog.org
Brochure: "Exercise and Fitness: A Guide for Women and Women and Exercise." Technical Bulletins: *Women and Exercise, Exercise During Pregnancy and the Postpartum Period.*

Birth Works, Inc.
PO Box 2045
Medford, NJ 08055
888-862-4784
www.birthworks.org
Offers a holistic approach to childbirth and provides information from a holistic standpoint.

Council of Childbirth Education Specialists, Inc.
PO Box 2000
Williamsburg, VA 23187-2000
757-258-5282
www.councilces.org
Childbirth organization offering certification to nurses and PTs; offers introductory and advanced seminars.

International Childbirth Education Association (ICEA)
PO Box 20048
Minneapolis, MN 55420
(612) 854-8660
www.icea.org
Certifies childbirth educators, has mail-order bookstore, and offers information about pregnancy and childbirth education.

International Organization of Physical Therapists in Women's Health (IOPTWH)
Subgroup of the World Confederation for Physical Therapy (WCPT)
335 Main Street
Medfield, MA 02052
(508) 359-2427
www.ioptwh.org

La Leche League International
9616 Minneapolis Avenue
PO Box 1209
Franklin Park, IL 60131
(212) 455-7730
www.lalecheleague.org
Headquarters for the 3000 groups throughout the world offering support for breastfeeding through individual counseling and education.

Lamaze International (formerly known as the American Society for Psychoprophylaxis in Obstetrics)
1840 Wilson Boulevard, Suite 204
Arlington, VA 22201
(703) 524-7802
(800) 368-4404
www.lamaze.org

Offers certification in Lamaze method of childbirth preparation, publishes the *Lamaze Parents* magazine, and provides information about pregnancy and childbirth-related topics.

National Domestic Violence Hotline
(800) 799-SAFE

National Family Violence HelpLine
(800) 222-2000

National Institutes of Health (NIH)
U.S. Department of Health and Human Services
Building 31, Room 7A-32
Bethesda, MD 20205
(301) 496-4000
www.nih.gov
Offers all NIH publications and information on antenatal diagnosis, cesarean birth, toxoplasmosis, and ultrasound imaging.

Association of Women's Health, Obstetric and Neonatal Nurses (AWHONN)
2000 L Street, NW, Suite 740
Washington, DC 20036
(202) 261-2400
(800) 673-8499
Organization for nurses specializing in obstetric, gynecologic, and neonatal nursing, with many publications related to pregnancy and childbirth, continuing education programs, and current maternal and child health information.

Sidelines National Support Network
2805 Park Place
Laguna Beach, CA 92651
(714) 497-2265
(602) 941-0176
www.sidelines.org
Support for women with high-risk pregnancies.

U.S. Department of Agriculture
WIC Supplemental Food Section
1103 North B Street, Suite E
Sacramento, CA 95814
(916) 322-5277
www.usda.gov
Offers information on nutrition for pregnant and nursing women.

Audiovisual Aids for Patient Education

American Physical Therapy Association
Section on Women's Health
1111 North Fairfax St.
Alexandria, VA 22314
(703) 684-2782
(800) 999-2782
www.apta.org

Lamaze International
1840 Wilson Boulevard, Suite 204
Arlington, VA 22201
(703) 524-7802
(800) 368-4404
www.lamaze.org

Childbirth Graphics
PO Box 17025
Rochester, NY 14617
(716) 266-6769
www.childbirthgraphics.com
Perinatal education materials company providing more than 1100 products, including models, posters, slides, and brochures.

International Childbirth Education Association (ICEA)
PO Box 20048
Minneapolis, MN 55420
(612) 854-8660
www.icea.org
Materials include patient education booklets, community education programs in slide format, pelvic floor evaluation forms, courses, and PT referral forms.

The Work-Injured Population

Deborah Lechner, PT, MS

Joe Daly, PT, MA, MHS

Kathryn Maltchev, OTR/L

Barbara McKelvy, PT

Sherry Fadel, PT, MS

Objectives

After reading this chapter, the reader will be able to:

1. Describe the impact that state and federal regulations have on the delivery of care to the workers' compensation population.
2. Provide an overview of commonly used assessments, including functional capacity evaluation, job demand analysis, work risk analysis, and post-offer screening.
3. Describe roles that physical therapists can play in the prevention of work-related injuries.

Primary care for injured workers requires a treatment model that involves much more than direct access to services and the delivery of acute care interventions. Certainly physical examination skills are important and have been addressed by other authors in this text. But physical examination skills are only the beginning. Treating the injured worker requires that the physical therapist (PT) must be knowledgeable regarding (1) the nature of the patient's work, (2) the psychosocial issues and culture of the workplace, and (3) the most appropriate avenues for minimizing work loss while maximizing recovery for a specific patient and workplace. For many injured workers this approach includes patient management strategies long after the acute phase of clinical care is complete.

Communication with multiple parties is often required and is a time-consuming part of patient care for patients with work-related injuries. The physician, case manager, employer, insurer, and sometimes attorneys are all stakeholders in the return to work process. It is often a challenge for physicians and case managers to make appropriate return to work decisions. Returning to work prematurely may result in reinjury or a new injury for the patient. Delayed return to work or providing unnecessary care costs the employer and insurer time, productivity, and money. Our entire society ultimately pays the bill in higher insurance premiums. If a lawsuit has been filed, then at least two attorneys with opposing viewpoints will be involved with the case. The plaintiff attorney will want the patient to appear as disabled as possible so as to achieve a maximum settlement. The defense attorney will want to prove that the patient's injuries are minimal so as to minimize the liability for the insurance company and employer.

Regardless of the type of work performed by the patient, one fact remains constant: to effectively treat the injured worker, the PT must have an understanding of all aspects of the patient's work. This understanding begins with the patient and employer interview, but optimal treatment generally requires that the PT go to the worksite and see, firsthand, the demands of the job. The importance of information on work demands cannot be overemphasized in terms of facilitating a successful outcome. The skills necessary for the PT to practice effectively in the area of occupational health are outlined in Box 14-1. Many of these skills are not taught in entry-level physical therapy programs and must be acquired through continuing education courses or on-the-job training.

This chapter reviews the areas of examination, plan of care, and treatment specifically required for the appropriate management of patients with work-related injuries. The impact of the state workers' compensation systems and the federal regulatory bodies on occupational health physical therapy practice is discussed. Patient assessments are reviewed, including functional capacity evaluation, job demands analysis, work risk analysis, and post-offer screening. Effective post-acute treatment interventions unique to the injured worker population will also be described and compared. The role of the PT in prevention is explored throughout the chapter.

Regulatory Influences on the Practice of Occupational Health Physical Therapy

Workers' Compensation

The rules and regulations of individual state's workers' compensation systems are the primary factors influencing the provision of physical therapy services for patients with work-related injuries. Workers' compensation systems arose in the early 1900s. Before their establishment, workers who were disabled because of injury or work-related disease were essentially destitute, and few could afford the legal expenses to sue their employers. By the same token, small employers could be wiped out by one successful lawsuit. The workers' compensation systems therefore evolved as a no-fault system that pays all medical benefits and replaces salary (usually at 66%) until recovery occurs. In turn, employees forfeit the right to sue their employers for damages.

BOX 14-1

Skills and Knowledge Necessary for the Occupational Health PT

- Management of acute musculoskeletal dysfunctions
- Management approaches for cumulative trauma disorders
- Functional capacity evaluation
- Job demands analysis
- Post-offer screening
- Work risk analysis
- Worksite modification
- Work conditioning
- Work simulation
- Job coaching
- Occupational Safety and Health Administration regulations
- Equal Employment Opportunity Commission regulations
- Americans With Disabilities Act provisions
- State workers' compensation regulations
- Social Security Administration regulations

BOX 14-2

ADA Major Life Activities

- Caring for self
- Performing manual tasks
- Walking
- Seeing
- Hearing
- Speaking
- Breathing
- Learning
- Working
- Participating in community affairs

To obtain these benefits the employee must prove that he or she has sustained a traumatic injury or has an illness related to prolonged exposure to work. The laws vary from state to state, but most states identify four types of disability[8]:

- Temporary partial
- Temporary total
- Permanent partial
- Permanent total

If the patient is capable of employment, but return to the former job is not possible, the disability is considered partial. Permanent partial disability benefits are usually paid according to a prescribed schedule for a specific number of weeks. Permanent total disability means that the employee cannot return to any gainful employment, and lifetime benefits are provided to the employee. In some states the employee can choose the health care provider seen, whereas in other states the employers choose the health care provider. Many states have a prior approval process for medical expenses, and some states have implemented a utilization review process that allows the necessity of certain medical services to be challenged.

Americans With Disabilities Act

The federal Americans With Disabilities Act (ADA) was designed to eliminate employment discrimination as well as architectural and communication barriers for persons with disabilities who otherwise qualify for employment (i.e., having the education, training, skills, experience, and other job-related credentials). To qualify as a person with disability, the individual must have a physical or mental impairment that substantially limits the performance of one or more major life activities. A list of major life activities can be found in Box 14-2. The job applicant must be able to perform the *essential functions* of the job with or without accommodations on the part of the employer. A function is defined as essential if: (1) it is the reason the position exists, (2) there are a limited number of employees who can perform that function, or (3) the function is highly specialized so that the person is hired specifically for the ability to perform that function. According to the ADA, the employer must make reasonable accommodations to allow a qualified person with a disability the opportunity for employment unless doing so would create *undue hardship* for the employer. The criteria for undue hardship have not been specifically defined by the ADA and vary from employer to employer. Therefore what is an undue hardship for a small company may not be so for a large one. The ADA has specific criteria for the hiring practices of most employers, including the post-offer screening process.

Occupational Safety and Health Administration

The goal of the Occupational Safety and Health Administration (OSHA) is to create a safe and healthy working environment for Americans. Employers must provide employment that is free from recognized hazards, and employees must adhere to safety and health standards. OSHA rules and regulations cover record keeping regarding injuries, citations for OSHA violations, and information regarding employee and employer rights under the act. An employer may receive a citation under OSHA for violating the act. OSHA had attempted to release an "ergonomic standard" for the past several years but has met with much political resistance. Instead of enforceable standards, they are currently targeting specific industries where injury rates are high and are issuing general guidelines for appropriate ergonomic modifications in those industries. The National Institute for Safety and Health (NIOSH) is the research arm of OSHA. This institute is responsible for carrying out research that underpins the regulations established by OSHA.

Social Security Act

The act creating the Social Security Administration established an entitlement program that provides income to disabled Americans who are incapable of gainful employment because of a "medically determined physical or mental impairment. To receive Social Security benefits, the worker must be unable to perform *any* 'substantial gainful' employment (considering age, education, and work experience) that exists in the national economy," not just be unable to return to a former job. To qualify as "existing in the national economy" means that jobs for which the worker is qualified must exist in significant numbers in the geographic region where the worker resides or in several regions of the country. A sequential five-step evaluation process is used to determine disability.

1. Determine if the claimant is engaged in substantial gainful employment. If yes, then disability is denied. If no, proceed to step 2.
2. Determine if the claimant has a severe impairment. If yes, proceed to step 3. If no, disability is denied.
3. Determine if the claimant's impairment meets the "listings" (a list of impairments that by definition are considered so severe as to automatically classify the claimant as disabled). If yes, then disability is awarded. If no, proceed to step 4.
4. Determine if the claimant's impairment prevents return to past relevant work. If yes, proceed to step 5. If no, the claimant is denied.
5. Determine if the claimant's impairment prevents return to any work that exists in the national economy, considering age, education, and past relevant work. If yes, then disability is awarded. If no, then the claimant is denied.

Dictionary of Occupational Titles

The Dictionary of Occupational Titles (DOT)[7] is a reference manual published by the U.S. Department of Labor (DOL) that describes and defines the nature of work in more than 12,000 jobs in the U.S. economy. The DOT was initially published in 1939 and has undergone multiple revisions with the last release (fourth edition) occurring in 1991. The DOT reports job requirements and demands according to a federally sanctioned classification system. Field job analysts, who analyzed representative jobs from each occupation, collected the data for the DOT. Another reference that provides additional data on the physical and dexterity demands of the jobs listed in the DOT is the *Classification of Jobs*. This reference provides information about the duration of the day spent performing various non–materials handling tasks of the job. Boxes 14-3 and 14-4 provide examples of the terminology used to classify work according to the DOT. This terminology is important to the PT working in occupational health physical therapy because it is used to classify the physical abilities of injured and noninjured workers as well as the demands of work.

Use of Functional Capacity Evaluations in Primary Care for Work-Related Injuries

Without functional capacity evaluations (FCEs), return-to-work decisions would be based on patient self-report, physician intuition, medical diagnosis, and impairment measures. Self-report and physician intuition can be clouded by patient motivation or clinician bias. In addition, many of the "traditional" medical diagnoses and impairment measures are often unrelated to function. Alternatively, well-designed FCEs offer performance-based measures and can provide objective information essential for the necessary clinical decision-making.

Purpose

An FCE is a test of work-related physical function that provides performance-based measures. FCEs are typically composed of a battery of tasks that involve testing of manual materials handling abilities (lifting, carrying, pushing, and pulling) and non–materials handling abilities (activities or positions required for work that do not involve handling significant weights). Boxes 14-3 and 14-4 list the physical demands and classifications of work defined by the DOT that are typically tested during an FCE. Patients are asked to perform functional work tasks while an evaluator observes and rates their performance. At the conclusion of the test, a report is generated that defines the intensity and duration of work that the patient is capable of performing.

Methods

Some FCE protocols can vary according to a number of factors. Controversy abounds regarding the most effective and valid approach to FCEs. Randomized controlled studies comparing the different approaches are not currently available. Some clinics use their own approach, whereas others purchase a commercially available FCE system. The test length can range from 1 hour to multiple weeks. The clinician's goal should be to perform no more testing than is necessary to provide accurate results and recommendations. There is literature that reports

---

BOX 14-3

Physical Demands of Work Defined by the DOT

- Strength demands
  - Lifting: Raising or lowering an object from one level to another
  - Carrying: Transporting an object, usually holding it in the hands or arms
  - Pushing: Exerting force on an object so that it moves away from the force
- Pulling: Exerting force on an object so that it moves toward the force
- Standing: Remaining on one's feet in an upright position without moving about
- Walking: Moving about on foot
- Sitting: Remaining in a seated position
- Climbing: Ascending or descending ladders, stairs, scaffolding, ramps, poles, etc.
- Balancing: Maintaining body equilibrium to prevent falling
- Stooping: Bending the body downward and forward by bending the spine at the waist

- Kneeling: Bending the legs at the knees to come to rest on knee or knees
- Crouching: Bending the body downward and forward by bending the legs and spine
- Crawling: Moving about on hands and knees or hands and feet
- Reaching: Extending arms and hands in any direction
- Handling: Seizing, holding, grasping, turning, or working with hands
- Fingering: Picking, pinching, or otherwise working primarily with the fingers
- Feeling: Perceiving attributes of items as size, shape, temperature
- Talking: Expressing or exchanging ideas by means of the spoken word
- Hearing: Perceiving the nature of sounds by the ear
- Tasting/Smelling: Distinguishing flavors or odors with the tongue and/or nose
- Near Acuity: Clarity of vision at 20 inches or less
- Far Acuity: Clarity of vision at 20 feet or more

Adapted from Field JE, Field TF: *Classification of jobs*, Athens, Ga, 1992, Elliott and Fitzpatrick.

Definitions of Work Intensity and Frequency

Strength Demands

Sedentary: Exerting up to 10 lb of force occasionally and/or a negligible amount of force frequently to lift, carry, push, pull, or otherwise move objects, including the human body. Involves sitting most of the time but may involve walking or standing for brief periods of time.

Light: Exerting up to 20 lb of force occasionally and/or up to 10 lb force frequently and/or a negligible amount of force constantly. Even when weight lifted is negligible, a job is rated light when (1) it involves walking or standing to a significant degree; (2) it requires sitting most of the time but involves pushing and/or pulling of arm or leg controls; (3) it involves working at a production rate that requires constant pushing or pulling of materials.

Medium: Exerting 20 to 50 lb of force occasionally and/or 10 to 25 lb force frequently and/or up to 10 lb of force constantly. Physical demand requirements are greater than those required for light work.

Heavy: Exerting 50 to 100 lb of force occasionally and/or 25 to 50 lb force frequently and/or 10 to 20 lb of force constantly. Physical demand requirements are greater than those required for light work.

Very heavy: Exerting greater than 100 lb of force occasionally and/or greater than 50 lb force frequently and/or greater than 20 lb of force constantly. Physical demand requirements are greater than those required for light work.

Frequency Demands

Never: Activity or condition does not exist.
Occasionally: Activity or condition exists up to one third of the time.
Frequently: Activity or condition exists from one to two thirds of the time.
Constantly: Activity or condition exists two thirds or more of the time.

Adapted from Field JE, Field TF: *Classification of jobs*, Athens, Ga, 1992, Elliott and Fitzpatrick.

---

the reliability and validity of an FCE performed with PT observation, minimal equipment, and a scoring system in a 1-day, 3- to 4-hour format.[18,19] Whether reliability and validity would be enhanced with different test lengths or high-tech equipment has not yet been addressed in the peer-reviewed literature.

Reporting Process and Format

The primary elements of the report should include:

1. The patient's overall level of work, ranging from sedentary to very heavy
2. Abilities on specific tasks within that overall level
3. Tolerance for an 8-hour day
4. Level of cooperation with the testing or sincerity of effort
5. Comparison of the patient's abilities with the job demands or former occupation
6. Conclusion/summary/recommendations (This portion of the report may not be desired by all referral sources and should be discussed before report preparation.)

FCEs also vary in terms of the time required to score and write the report. Some require hours, whereas others provide scoring and report-generating software that allow the examiners to complete the report in minutes.

Professional Qualifications for Administration

Occupational therapists were the first professionals to perform FCEs, followed soon after by PTs. Individuals from other disciplines, such as exercise physiologists, kinesiologists, athletic trainers, and physicians have also become involved in FCEs. Insurance plans in many states often restrict who can be reimbursed for performing FCEs. Perhaps this controversy is best addressed by establishing the competencies necessary to safely, reliably, and accurately perform an FCE. Training courses could then require clinicians to demonstrate those competencies through written and practical testing to achieve certification.

Equipment and Space Requirements

Space requirements for an FCE also vary according to the FCE protocol used. In general, a dedicated private area for the evaluation is optimal but not required. Lifting and position-tolerance testing generally require at least a 10×10 ft area to allow for adequate visualization of the entire body. In some cases it will be important to view the patient from a specific perspective; therefore having an uncluttered evaluation area is helpful. For carrying, pushing, pulling, walking, and crawling activities, a 25×30 ft walkway, with the ability to view the patient in either the sagittal or frontal planes, is optimal. Short or narrow walkways make visual observation difficult and may adversely affect reliability and validity. Access to stairs and adequate ceiling height for ladder climbing are also important when assessing potential space for an FCE.

Projecting Performance for an 8-Hour Day

During an FCE, each physical demand of work is typically assessed for a brief period, usually no more than 5 to 10 minutes. The examiner must then decide, based on this brief assessment, the duration of day that this level of demand could be performed by the worker. For example, if the examiner watches a patient perform the "stooping" task of an FCE, it must be determined whether the patient can perform stooping either "constantly, frequently, occasionally, or never," as defined by the DOL. These projections are often made based on the PT's experience and judgment. In unpublished pilot studies the primary author (D.L.) has found this intuitive approach to be unreliable from PT to PT. A scoring system of systematic data collection and rating performance according to operational definitions and algorithms helps minimize much of this variability.

Patient Sincerity of Effort

One of the most challenging and controversial aspects of the FCE involves determining the patient's sincerity of effort. Patients who perceive secondary financial gain through the workers' compensation system may exaggerate their symptoms and limitations. As a result, many methods for detecting these patients have evolved (Box 14-5). A thorough discussion of these approaches and the literature supporting them is beyond the scope of this text and is the subject of a critical review.[28] New approaches, such as the X-RTS upper extremity and lever

BOX 14-5
Methods of Determining Sincerity of Effort

- Waddell's nonorganic signs
- Coefficient of variation
- Bell-shaped curve
- Rapid exchange grip
- Correlation between musculoskeletal evaluation and FCE
- Documentation of pain behavior
- Documentation of symptom magnification
- Ratio of heart rate and pain intensity

arm protocols, have been developed that show great promise and are supported through research. The clinician who is performing the FCE is advised to be keenly aware of the literature or lack of literature supporting these various approaches and to select the approach carefully.

Safety Precautions

Injury during an FCE can occur as a result of exceeding the patient's musculoskeletal, cardiovascular, or neurologic system tolerances. Safety is enhanced by having clear, well-defined end points for halting the tasks. Specific decision-making criteria help to standardize the process and protect the patient from overexertion. Teaching proper lifting techniques before testing will also minimize the risk of reinjury during testing. If the patient requires instruction in body mechanics before the evaluation, the need for further instruction should be documented in the summary report so that additional assistance can be provided before return to work.

Controversy exists surrounding the safety of isometric lift testing. Some examiners insist that isometric lifting is safe, whereas others report that injuries have occurred from isometric lifting. One possible explanation for the reported injuries with isometric lifting is that the patient can build up a significant amount of force with little accompanying observable biomechanical evidence of effort. This lack of visual feedback limits the examiner's ability to stop the patient before a safe maximum is exceeded.

If the patient reports symptoms related to radiculopathy or vertebral artery compromise, special precautions should be taken during an FCE. Blood pressure should be monitored before initiating an FCE. If the blood pressure significantly exceeds the predetermined cutoff (the authors use 150 to 160/100 mm Hg), the FCE should be deferred until this problem is resolved. If the patient's blood pressure only slightly exceeds the cutoff point, the PT may try to proceed carefully with the testing, rechecking blood pressure after or during every task. If the blood pressure stays the same or decreases with physical activity, the examiner should proceed while frequently rechecking the pressure throughout the evaluation. If the patient's blood pressure increases with activity, the examiner should terminate the FCE and refer the patient for medical management. See Chapter 9 for a detailed description of blood pressure assessment and interpretation.

Monitoring the patient's heart rate with a device that has an upper-limit alarm helps prevent patients from performing tasks that exceed their cardiovascular capabilities. When patients are taking heart rate–suppressing drugs such as β-blockers or calcium channel blockers, however, heart rate can no longer be used as an indicator of overexertion. Instead, the clinician must rely on the patient's perceived exertion level and clinical signs of overexertion, such as respiratory rate and color, to determine safe exertion levels.

Training Requirements

The training requirements for those administering an FCE vary, ranging from 0 to 5 days in length. Certain FCE systems require that participants pass a competency requirement to be certified, whereas others have no training or competency testing. Some PTs simply learn on the job. This lack of formal training is of concern because few, if any, physical or occupational therapy programs include FCE training as part of the curriculum. However, there is no peer-reviewed, published evidence regarding the extent of training necessary to achieve a reliable, valid FCE. Unpublished pilot studies conducted by the primary author (D.L.) suggested that for one FCE protocol, the Physical Work Performance Evaluation, 3 days of training were needed.

Comparison with Normative Databases

Since passage of the ADA in 1992, return-to-work and pre-employment/post-offer decisions must be made by comparing the patient's abilities to the job demands. Regardless of whether the individual's abilities are in the fifth or ninety-fifth percentile of a normative database, if abilities meet the job demands then the patient can return to work or the job applicant can be hired. Therefore, in the authors' opinion, normative databases are of relatively little value in FCEs. The exception is manual dexterity testing, the results of which must first be translated into a percentile score and then into an aptitude score for comparison to DOL classifications of the dexterity demands of jobs.

Comprehensive Versus Job-Specific Functional Capacity Evaluations

FCEs can be subclassified into two broad categories: comprehensive and job specific. When administering the comprehensive FCE, most evaluators use a complete battery of tasks that cover all physical demands listed in the DOT. In job-specific testing, the evaluator tests only those tasks that are related to the person's job. The disability insurance industry typically differentiates among three different types of FCEs: own job, own occupation, and any occupation. For an own-job FCE, patient abilities are compared with demands of a former or current job. For an own-occupation FCE, patient abilities are compared with a generic type of work. For an any-occupation FCE, a comprehensive test is administered and no comparisons to job or occupations are made.

Use in Acute Care

FCEs are grossly underused in general practice. They are typically reserved for those cases in which intervention has failed, poor motivation is suspected, return to work attempts have not been successful, or the patient is in the chronic phases of impairment. These are all appropriate times to perform a comprehensive FCE; however, if FCE components were used at the conclusion of the acute care when the initial return-to-work decision is being made, fewer cases would become chronic, and efficient and effective return to work could be facilitated. Consider the following example. A patient with a diagnosis of patellofemoral joint dysfunction is completing 4 to 6 weeks of acute care physical therapy. Three of the most demanding aspects of the patient's job require him to lift 56 lb from floor to waist, walk constantly, and kneel occasionally. During the final acute care physical therapy visit, the PT administers these three functional tasks from a comprehensive FCE as part of the discharge evaluation. The patient was able to successfully complete the walking and lifting but had difficulty tolerating the kneeling. The patient was returned to work with the restriction of avoiding kneeling for 2 weeks and to continue physical therapy to improve kneeling tolerance. After 2 weeks of continued treatment and modified work, the kneeling task was readministered and the patient demonstrated improved tolerance to kneeling at the occasional level. The patient was released to work full duty and therapy was discontinued. The FCE tasks helped set realistic return-to-work parameters and gradually return the patient to full duties.

Directing Work Conditioning/Work Hardening

If patients are to begin a program of work simulation and conditioning after acute care treatment, FCEs (combined with job demands information) can be used to help establish the focus and goals of the program. There are many work-related functions that the patient could perform as part of an industrial rehabilitation program. FCEs result in the patient's program being more focused, efficient, and cost effective. Weekly progress on functional activities can then be monitored by two or three specific tasks of the FCE that relate to the tasks and goals of the work simulation program. Suppose the patient needs to be able to lift 42 lb from the floor to a waist-height table for her job. On the initial FCE she was only able to lift 26 lb. In the work simulation program, she would likely be working on improving her floor-to-waist lifting and could be retested weekly on this task until she meets the work-related goal of 42 lb.

Use of Job Demands Analysis in Primary Care for the Work-Injured Patient

An objective, well-executed job demands analysis (JDA) can provide the same information about job demands that the FCE provides about patient abilities, allowing the patient's abilities to be matched to job demands. The purpose of the JDA is to define the physical demands of work by using the DOL classification system described in Boxes 14-3 and 14-4. The JDA is not to be confused with hazard identification or work risk analysis (WRA). In the WRA, the purpose is to identify elements of the job that might create excessive stress for the worker. In JDA, the purpose is to define or classify the demands of work regardless of the hazard. Some employers may expect the PT to combine JDA and WRA. However, such a directive should be clarified with the employer before the analysis.

Methods

Information regarding job demands can be acquired from a variety of sources, but the most frequently used method is the patient or employer self-report. The accuracy of this self-report process is questionable because employees and employers often overestimate or underestimate the demands of work. In the authors' opinions, worksite assessment of the job demands is the optimal method. Performing a worksite assessment of the job demands provides additional opportunity to develop the relationship between the employer and the clinician. At the worksite, the clinician can observe job tasks being performed, talk to workers performing the job, measure the forces required to perform the work, and in some cases videotape the jobs for further analysis or patient education.

Test Length and Equipment

The time required for self-report job analysis is approximately 10 to 30 minutes per interview. The time required for observation-based JDA varies greatly with the job. For assembly line work, a position on the line could be analyzed in approximately 15 to 30 minutes. For a construction or maintenance position, where job duties vary from day to day, the analysis could take the better part of a day or require an analysis that stretches over a several-day period to accurately capture all job tasks. The equipment needed for the self-report approach is minimal, usually a questioning process and forms for recording data. The observation-based approach requires a force gauge to measure forces and a video camera if videotaping is desired.

Reporting Process and Format

The JDA report should define the tasks of the job and the physical demands required to perform those tasks. For example, a hospital housekeeper might have to mop floors as one of the essential tasks of the job. The physical demands to perform the task might include standing, walking, lifting, and pushing. The environmental conditions to which the worker is exposed and the protective equipment the worker must wear are also important aspects of the report. If the JDA is being done to develop post-offer screening, the employer may expect to see the screening tasks and cut points for the screening process as part of the report. Similarly, if the employer wants a transitional duty program established for an injured worker, those recommendations may be part of the report as well.

Professional Qualifications

The professional qualifications for JDA differ from those of FCE or post-offer screening because patient involvement is not a part of the process. In the authors' opinion physical and occupational therapists are not the only discipline that can effectively perform JDAs. Case managers, vocational evaluators, safety officers, and human resource professionals can be effectively trained to perform JDAs.

Objectivity

There is a paucity of data regarding the reliability of the JDA. A recent reliability study of JDAs involving case managers, vocational evaluators, and physical and occupational therapists indicated that all these disciplines are capable of performing highly reliable JDAs, provided they use a standardized, objective process.[17]

Safety Precautions

Safety precautions related to JDA primarily involve the safety of the analyst. Many industrial environments are full of hazards, particularly to the person unfamiliar with the environment. For this reason, most companies require the job analyst to have an official company escort and to wear safety equipment, such as a hard hat, metal-toed shoes, earplugs, safety glasses, hairnets, or protective clothing. Therefore the job analyst must clarify any safety equipment requirements before making the worksite visit.

Clinical Use of JDAs

JDA data can be effectively used throughout the course of patient management. At any point in the delivery of care in which a return-to-work decision is being made, information regarding job demands can provide objective information for comparison with the patient's abilities. If a work conditioning or work simulation treatment program is required, JDA data can be used to make the program more job specific. If a transitional duty program is needed, job demands information may be needed on a variety of jobs that are involved in the patient's transition back to full duty. The clinician cannot just report the physical demands of the work but must help the employer understand the link between physical demands and the job tasks with which they are associated. Transitional duty plans must be written in terms of job tasks rather than physical demands to be meaningful to the employer. For example, the hospital housekeeper's return-to-work restrictions may be written to avoid lifting more than 50 lb and standing more than occasionally. However, the employer needs to know which tasks this employee with these restrictions can perform, such as mopping, dusting, cleaning the bathroom, and changing the linen.

Use of Work Risk Analysis in Primary Care for the Work-Injured Patient

A WRA is a systematic assessment of the work environment and the fit of the worker to the environment with the objective of identifying risk factors for injury. In addition, the assessment could provide cost-effective solutions to decrease the noted risks. The WRA is designed to decrease the risk of injury and trauma by appropriately adapting the worker to the demands of the workstation and the job tasks. Recommendations are determined through the analysis of the biomechanical and postural risks observed while the worker is performing the job.

WRAs may be completed for an individual patient before returning to work or on a larger scale for a number of jobs for an employer. In either case, the goal is to identify risks and provide realistic solutions to decrease those risks. It is important for the clinician to keep this tool in mind while working with patients to assist them in preventing recurrence of the musculoskeletal condition for which they required therapy. If the biomechanical stresses are not reduced when the worker returns to the job, the symptoms will likely return. It is not realistic to eliminate every risk factor for a job, but the emphasis is placed on decreasing repetitive biomechanical stress to tissues. WRAs should be performed in the presence of the supervisor to collaborate on potential solutions, which may help create a positive rapport. Management must be a part of the process for long-term successful changes in the environment.

Differences from a Job Demands Analysis

A WRA should not be confused with a JDA. A JDA is completed to evaluate and measure the physical demands required to complete the essential functions of a job by using the DOT classification system. Potential risk factors may be identified while performing a JDA but are typically not a component of the final report. The clinician may bring the concerns regarding the potential risk factors to the employer's attention and suggest further assessment in the form of a WRA. The WRA is a narrative description of the job with emphasis on identification of observed risk factors in the demands of the job, the job environment, and the behaviors of the worker. This process combines the qualitative and quantitative information obtained from the JDA and the observed risk factors and corrective solutions of the WRA for a complete assessment of the job with the interaction of the worker.

Performing a Work Risk Analysis

The WRA contains the following elements[11]:
- A qualitative description of the workstation design, job demands, and worker habits
- A narrative description of observed risks for musculoskeletal injury and cumulative trauma
- A list of practical, low-cost solutions to lower risk factors
- The foundation of an injury prevention plan

If a WRA is requested by an employer as a component of an ergonomic assessment of the company, evaluation of the OSHA 300 logs should be the first step. The 300 log compiles all the recorded injuries and resultant restricted duty or lost work days for each job. Understanding the information provided in the 300 logs will point to those jobs that carry the highest risk and for which a WRA should be performed first. If the employer is not willing to share OSHA 300 logs, interviews with management and supervisors can provide the necessary information.

Office Environment

A WRA assesses three primary areas in an office environment: the workstation layout, mechanical forces and repetitive motion, and environmental factors. Proper workstation layout is critical to decreasing the biomechanical stress on tissues. The positions of the computer monitor and keyboard, chair, mouse, and accessories such as document holders are analyzed. The worker's posture and position in relation to workstation layout are documented. The worker is observed for use of excessive force while operating the computer, using the stapler, or performing any job task. The impact of environmental factors, including lighting and temperature, is also noted.

Industrial Environment

In the industrial environment, a WRA assesses the workstation design, worker behaviors, and environmental factors. The workstation design is analyzed for efficiency of required tasks and promotion of a variety of postures. Tools are assessed for condition, performance, and appropriate fit to the worker. Worker behaviors are observed for unnecessary repetitive motions, reaching, improper lifting, choice of poor postures, and improper tool use, such as excessive grip force. As in the office environment, the environmental factors of lighting and temperature are noted.

In any environment, the WRA is the framework for determining an effective corrective action plan and prevention program. Prevention strategies are discussed in the following section and may be used to provide recommendations for reducing observed risks during the WRA assessment.

Effective Post-Acute Intervention

Many injured workers are able to return to full duty work after the acute or subacute phase of rehabilitation. For injured workers who have not attained the physical abilities to return to the demands of the job, *work conditioning/general occupational rehabilitation programs* or *work hardening/comprehensive occupational rehabilitation programs* can be used to optimize work capacity. The PT is the ideal clinician to help oversee management of the injured worker and should take the initiative to recommend and defend the medical necessity of these programs when appropriate.

History

In the 1980s, rehabilitation professionals from many disciplines were entering the field of post-acute rehabilitation for injured workers. A large variety of programs with varying philosophies, goals, and interventions were developed. In an attempt to standardize post-acute injury intervention, the Commission on Accreditation of Rehabilitation Facilities (CARF) defined standards for general occupational rehabilitation programs (work conditioning) and comprehensive occupational rehabilitation programs (work hardening).[27] In 1991, the American Physical Therapy Association (APTA) formed the Industrial Rehabilitation Advisory Council (IRAC) to classify the levels of occupational rehabilitation.[11]

Work Conditioning/General Occupational Rehabilitation Program

The work conditioning program is a work-related, outcomes-focused conditioning program designed to restore physical capacity and function so the patient can return to work. Specific goals may be improvement of cardiopulmonary function, including aerobic capacity and endurance, and improvement of neuromusculoskeletal abilities such as strength, flexibility, stability, and motor control. Work conditioning is a program designed for the post-acute injured worker with continuing physical impairments. The appropriate candidate for this program is beyond the initial healing phase—typically 4 to 6 weeks after injury, with remaining physical and functional needs that can be addressed by one discipline, such as physical therapy.

Components of a work conditioning program include strengthening, flexibility, aerobic exercises, work-related activities, and education. Strengthening exercise programs are designed according to the specific needs of the injured worker and the demands of the job. Flexibility exercises are used both to restore tissue length and to teach the injured worker to decrease stresses brought on by job postures and activities. Aerobic conditioning is designed to improve the patient's cardiovascular status to meet the job demands. Work-related activities are used to improve functional performance of the activity, instruct in appropriate body mechanics specific to the job task, and develop problem-solving skills to improve work performance and safety. Injured worker independence in performing the prescribed program is emphasized and progressed as skills are developed, decreasing dependence on the PT, improving self-esteem, and decreasing return-to-work anxiety.

Some examples of work-related activities include the following:

- Sorting bolts in a work-related position, such as standing
- Climbing ladders
- Moving clothespins on a curtain in a work-related position, such as overhead
- Lifting and carrying boxes
- Pushing/pulling activities with a pulley system

Work-related activities are performed at established workstations in the clinic. The activities are customized to meet the specific needs of each injured worker by adjusting the duration of the activity, heights of the activity, and the number of repetitions. The PT prescribes the most appropriate work methods for the injured worker as determined by the worker's current physical capabilities and the demands of the job. For example, a worker who is required to sit several hours a day will spend more time at the sitting workstation, whereas a worker who is required to lift floor to waist throughout the day will spend more time at the lifting workstation. The PT also sets goals for the injured worker on the basis of job demands. Goals should include attaining the abilities to perform the physical requirements necessary to complete job tasks. For example, increasing sitting tolerance may be an appropriate goal for a worker required to sit for several hours a day, and increasing lifting ability to complete a necessary job task may be an appropriate goal for an injured worker required to lift throughout the day. Education of the injured worker within the work-conditioning program focuses on injury prevention and safe work practices. Lastly, throughout the program, emphasis is placed on reestablishing worker traits such as punctuality, time management, teamwork, and responding to direction.

Work Hardening/Comprehensive Occupational Rehabilitation Program

The work hardening program is an interdisciplinary, highly structured, goal-oriented program designed to restore the physical, functional, and behavioral status of the injured worker to promote a return to work. Specific goals may include improvement of cardiopulmonary and neuromusculoskeletal function, physical tolerance, worker behavior, and productivity. A work hardening program is designed for the injured worker to address any behavioral and vocational impairment along with the physical impairments. The appropriate candidate for this program is beyond the subacute phase of rehabilitation—typically 10 to 12 weeks after injury—and requires intervention from professionals from multiple disciplines such as PTs, occupational therapists, psychological services, and vocational services.

The primary component of a work hardening program is work simulation. Total body conditioning, education, and psychological support are secondary components. Total body conditioning involves worker-specific strengthening, flexibility, and cardiovascular conditioning. Education programs are multifaceted, with injured workers participating in groups, and individual education sessions on body mechanics, injury prevention, nutrition, and fitness. Psychological support is customized to address any issues that may be inhibiting return to work and may include stress relief, employee interpersonal issues, and substance abuse.

Work simulation involves specifically practicing job tasks with actual worksite equipment whenever possible. The injured worker learns optimal postures and body mechanics, improves technique, and becomes conditioned to perform the task for the appropriate length of time required on the job. An additional goal of work simulation is for the injured worker to learn self-management techniques for symptom control and postural stress relief while performing job tasks.

Some examples of work simulation include the following:
- A shovel pit filled with soil and a specific shovel to simulate digging for an underground utilities worker
- A ladder, paint, paintbrushes, rollers, and cardboard attached to the ceiling to simulate overhead painting for a house painter
- A pipe tree station and hand tools to simulate pipe work for a plumber

Throughout the work hardening program, the injured worker is taught responsibility for self-management while gaining confidence and competence in performing job tasks.

Evidence of Effectiveness

Several studies in the literature have attempted to document the efficacy of work conditioning and work hardening. Most studies report positive results, but there are relatively few randomized, controlled studies that demonstrate a higher percentage of return to work and earlier return to work for injured workers in work conditioning/hardening programs compared with control groups.[4,5] The few work hardening studies that were randomized and controlled did show a favorable outcome. The studies indicate that the worksite interventions of worksite evaluations and modifications were key elements of successful outcomes.[16] Most studies that evaluate return-to-work percentages among injured workers 3 months after completion of a work hardening program report a range of 60% to 82% return to work in some capacity.[3,36] More research is needed to demonstrate the effectiveness of work conditioning and work hardening interventions.

Importance of Injury Prevention Education

The challenge of occupational injury prevention is to balance the demands of the work with the worker's capacity. Prevention of occupational injuries can include services that are primary, secondary, and tertiary in nature:
- *Primary prevention*: Measures that prevent the primary or first occurrence of injury.
- *Secondary prevention*: Measures that decrease the duration of recovery from injury through early detection and intervention.
- *Tertiary prevention*: Measures that limit the degree of disability for injured workers.

Strategies to prevent injuries focus on the worksite environment to decrease unsafe conditions and improve worker behaviors to minimize unsafe actions. Prevention approaches can be used for any phase, but the majority of interventions are targeted to affect primary prevention.

Worksite Environment

The goal of prevention in the worksite environment approach is to minimize the worker's exposure to risk factors for injury through adaptation of the physical environment of the workplace. Adaptations or interventions are further categorized as engineering controls and administrative controls. Engineering controls focus on decreasing the physical demands of a job. Common engineering controls include workstation design, work method design, and tool design.

The workstation layout can be adapted to decrease the need for extreme and sustained postures and to minimize repetitive motion activities. For example, adjustment of the height and angle of a work surface can promote proper posture, and the improved placement of necessary work tools can decrease repetitive motion stresses. Work method design involves changing processes to also decrease mechanical stresses on the body. Incorporating the use of a mechanical lift aide such as a lift table is an example. Tool design can be adapted to decrease the mechanical load necessary for worker force production. For example, tool handles may be ergonomically adjusted to decrease the muscle contraction force necessary to operate the tool.

Administrative controls focus on decreasing worker exposure to risk factors by changing the way that work is assigned through management policy and procedure. Administrative controls may include altering job tasks, job pace, or production requirements. Interventions that reduce the number of task repetitions per employee include job rotation, job enlargement, and work/rest schedules. Job rotation is the practice of workers rotating among more than one job. Job enlargement involves changing a job description to include a greater variety of tasks. Work/rest schedules include regular breaks from a job task. Administrative controls that ensure safe and proper functioning of equipment include preventive maintenance, tool inspection, and housekeeping.

Worker Behaviors

The goal of prevention in the worker behavior approach is to equip the worker to prevent injury through safe job performance. It is estimated that up to 80% of occupational injuries are caused in some part by worker behaviors. The primary components of this approach are safety training, exercise, and use of safety equipment. The background of a PT is ideal to promote and institute these safety interventions.

Safety training is designed to educate the worker on proper posture and technique for job task performance. Training program content typically includes basic anatomy, specific risk factors for injury, proper work posture, lifting technique, and body mechanics. Effective training presentations combine lecture, body mechanics practice, and proper work technique simulation with worksite equipment. For safety training to be successful, management must be engaged in the process. Company supervisors should receive training on the systems to be put in place to support and reinforce the education. This creates a culture supportive of safety and the worker, which is the foundation of an effective safety program.

The exercise component may focus on stretching to relieve work-induced stresses or on wellness by incorporating strengthening and aerobic conditioning to improve worker capacity. On-the-job stretch breaks may be mandatory or optional and should be designed to relieve stress on body tissues and promote proper tissue flexibility. Strengthening and aerobic conditioning programs are typically designed to be performed outside work hours at a company-owned fitness area or facility.

Safety equipment is intended to protect the worker while performing a high-risk activity such as heavy lifting or repetitive wrist motion. Common forms of safety equipment include back belts, wrist supports, hard hats, and steel-toed shoes.

Post-Offer Screening

Another strategy to prevent injury is to attempt to match the physical demands of a job with the abilities of the prospective worker through a post-offer screening process. Some employers have used pre-offer screens; however, post-offer screens are preferred to pre-offer screens for the following reasons:
1. They are viewed more favorably by the Equal Employment Opportunity Commission
2. In a pre-offer screen, monitoring of heart rate and blood pressure is not permitted
3. A medical screen by a physician is not permitted in a pre-offer screen
4. A post-offer screen is more cost effective because only viable candidates are tested

Post-offer functional screening should occur after a conditional offer of employment and before the applicant begins work. The post-offer screen may contain several components, including a medical examination by a physician, a drug screen, and the physical abilities test. The physical abilities should primarily focus on the applicant's ability to perform the specific demands of the job such as lifting, carrying, pushing, and pulling. All test items must be related to the job and necessary to the performance of the job. If the applicant is unable to perform a test item and does not have a qualified disability, the employer can choose to withdraw the offer of employment. The employer, however, may choose to offer a less physically demanding job or offer remediation to the applicant. This often depends on the job market and the availability of applicants. It is important that the employer's policies are consistent and in writing.

Evidence of Effectiveness of Injury Prevention Programs

The primary measure of the effectiveness of an injury prevention program is demonstration of a decrease in the rate of injury. Relatively few studies in the literature cite injury rate as an outcome. Many studies that analyze injury rates do not show injury rate reduction. However, many current studies look at an individual prevention intervention, such as one specific engineering control. Research that investigates application of multiple injury prevention strategies may best demonstrate potential effect on injury rates.

Overall, more support in the literature exists for worksite environment interventions than for worker behavior interventions. For example, several studies in an office environment show improved posture and/or decreased muscle activation with computer monitor positioning at or slightly above eye level.[14,30] In contrast, multiple studies do not show any changes in back pain or back injuries with the use of a back belt.[6]

To summarize, although the literature does not currently contain overwhelming evidence of the effectiveness of injury prevention strategies, there are many examples of anecdotal evidence supporting a decrease in injury rate and severity from focused injury prevention. Research is needed to demonstrate

---

PATIENT CASE

The following example incorporates components of the *worksite environment* and *worker behavior* approaches to injury prevention.

Job: Palletizer

Description: The worker stands at the end of a shoulder-height conveyor belt. Boxes of computer components ranging in weight from 10 lb to 75 lb come down the conveyor belt in random order. The worker picks up the box, walks 25 feet to a pallet on the floor, and stacks the boxes to a height of 7 feet. Another worker removes the loaded pallet with a forklift and replaces it with an empty pallet.

Worksite Environment

Engineering controls: Workstation design recommendations
• Adapt the height of the terminus of the conveyor belt to waist high
• Place the empty pallet closer to the terminus of the conveyor belt

Engineering controls: Work method design recommendations
• Design product flow so that the heavier boxes arrive first to become the lower layers of the pallet, followed by lighter boxes for the higher layers of the pallet

Administrative controls: Job rotation recommendations
• Assign the palletizer and the fork lift driver to rotate positions at the completion of each pallet

Worker Behavior

Safety Training
• Educate the worker on safe lifting technique at multiple heights

Exercise Training
• Implement 3-minute hourly stretching routine for trunk and extremity muscle groups

the effectiveness of both the worksite environment and the worker behavior approaches to injury prevention.

Worksite Physical Therapy

Worksite therapy offers another opportunity for PTs to become involved in primary care for injured workers. In addition, recent changes in the insurance industry have influenced PTs in developing new methods of delivery. Worker compensation costs have influenced companies to find more effective methods for medical cost containment. Thus physical therapy and industry have found a symbiotic relationship in worksite therapy services.

Worksite therapy, also known as on-site therapy, is the treatment of patients with musculoskeletal injuries or disorders in their work setting. Although the majority of PTs who work on-site typically work in industrial or manufacturing settings, they may also provide services in offices, to the transportation industry, and in off-shore rigging operations. The options are limitless. Depending on the specific company needs, worksite therapy treatment facilities range from being a small 10 × 12-foot treatment space to a fully functioning gym with private treatment rooms. The equipment used is also as varied. Many PTs function on-site with few to no modalities or exercise equipment. Others use a full complement of modalities, exercise, and high-tech work simulation devices. In addition to the standard rehabilitation equipment, worksite PTs also benefit from access to the workstations and equipment used by employees on a daily basis. The use of the actual work equipment offers PTs significant advantages when developing work-related treatment protocols and goals.

A variety of opportunities are available to worksite PTs. PTs can offer many types of on-site care: triage, acute care physical therapy, JDAs, post-offer screening, FCEs, hazard identification, and abatement recommendations. In addition, worksite PTs can become involved with employee injury prevention education through "back schools" and ergonomic training. PTs can also assist in developing, supervising, and participating in ergonomic teams, hazard identification and abatement projects, and injury investigations. Options for physical therapy involvement are limited only by company needs, time, and the PT's skill and confidence.

PTs can provide the services mentioned above as the sole worksite medical provider, or they may work with occupational health physicians, nurses, occupational therapists, and case managers. When a worksite PT works independently, worksite triage becomes a significant asset for the company and deserves special mention. The PT is uniquely positioned to provide this service because of the in-depth training related to examination and treatment of musculoskeletal disorders and medical screening they receive both initially and throughout their careers. The cost savings for the company is also significant. Not only are they able to provide a musculoskeletal evaluation the day the injury occurs, but the company can also save the cost of a physician evaluation on many of the less complicated cases.

For example, a worker with moderate low back pain after lifting an object can be evaluated and treated the day the injury occurs. The next day, the worker can begin a modified job and continue with therapy as needed. The company saves the cost

of lost production, salary for time off, and a physician referral, thus resulting in a total cost savings of several hundred dollars. PTs who work in direct access states and perform primary care will typically see workers with repetitive strain injuries or injuries that develop over a period of time. If the worker does not improve within 2 to 3 weeks of therapy and a physician referral is needed, the PT can play a valuable role in directing the worker to an appropriate specialist, thus avoiding costly evaluations for additional referrals.

Some companies refer workers with sudden-onset, traumatic injuries to a physician whereas PTs see the workers with repetitive trauma. For example, one large manufacturing corporation uses on-site therapy and off-site physician services. This company has instituted a policy that the PTs may evaluate and treat workers who report repetitive motion symptoms (symptoms that have a gradual onset with no specific injury). The company further states that any worker sustaining an injury with a specific time, date, and location of incidence will be automatically sent to a physician. Although this represents a pattern of practice noted by the authors, other practice patterns in which the PT is the primary care practitioner for soft tissue trauma may emerge in the future.

Currently more than 35 states allow some form of direct access. However even in some of the states that do not currently allow direct access, PTs can still perform triage services to a limited extent. This restricted therapy access allows the PT to perform a musculoskeletal and pain screen to determine whether a physician referral is warranted or if additional evaluation and treatment would be beneficial.

Once confidence and trust are established, employees will occasionally seek advice for minor discomforts. Such early reporting can identify and prevent more significant injuries, and a brief musculoskeletal examination to identify any impairment combined with a simple ergonomic evaluation and adjustment of worker technique is often enough to relieve any discomfort. Continued follow-up will determine if the situation is relieved, continues, or worsens and whether further assessment or treatment is needed. When working independently, it remains extremely important that the PT understands and does not exceed the scope of practice established by the individual state licensing boards and the APTA.

Clinic-Based Practice Versus Worksite Intervention

The comparison of clinic-based practice with on-site therapy is best understood if we follow two workers (Ted and Bill) with low back injuries. Ted works for ABC Manufacturing and is sent to an off-site clinic for his medical care. Ted is seen by a physician outside the company the day the injury occurs and is taken off work. Because of insurance verification, limited openings for new evaluations, and transportation problems, an additional 3 days pass before Ted is able to see a clinic-based PT. During the initial evaluation, Ted's PT learns that Ted's physician encouraged him to remain off work, rest, and restrict his daily activities. The doctor also wrote a prescription for therapy to consist primarily of a series of passive modalities. Ted's PT knows that Ted should begin a more active program and would like for him to begin modified duty if available. Ted attends three therapy appointments before the PT can speak with the physician to modify the orders. However, the physician does not feel that Ted is ready for modified duty, so this is put on hold. Ted, still having some discomfort, assures his physician and employer that he is not ready to return to work.

A few more weeks pass, and because Ted is still off work, the PT attempts to integrate some work simulation and education into Ted's treatment. The PT covers some very general ergonomic principles. Ted thinks the suggestions make sense and are beneficial, but he has difficulty imagining putting them into practice in his own job. ABC Manufacturing provides the PT with a very general job description, and Ted attempts to fill in missing information. Ted's job involves loading large metal bathtubs onto a cart, coating the inside surfaces with a special paint, and pushing the cart into large furnaces for firing.

The PT has never seen Ted's job, and the case manager would not reimburse for an on-site evaluation. The company also refused when she asked for temporary use of a cart, bathtub, and paint sprayer to use in Ted's therapy sessions. The PT works very hard to simulate the tasks, and it takes several attempts before Ted says that the simulation "somewhat" resembles his actual job. The PT knows that the more information she gathers about Ted's ability to perform the job, the more realistic she can make the simulation. Ted is asked to wear his uniform, which is specially made to endure the heat of the furnace and keep the paint spray off his skin. However, after wearing the uniform the first day, Ted feels uncomfortable and embarrassed in front of all the other patients, and he does not wear it again.

Finally, it is time for Ted to return to work. He is very nervous about becoming reinjured and does not feel confident that he will be able to do his job safely. The PT writes several recommendations for modifying his job, but his supervisor and the plant engineer tell Ted that the suggestions are not feasible for the company to implement. Unfortunately, the PT does not receive this information. On his first day back, the other employees tease Ted about taking an extended vacation, and he has a lot of difficulty reacclimating to the cumbersome uniform and the excruciating heat. Ted resumes his previous poor mechanics because "that is the way everyone does it" and continues to have difficulty performing his job tasks. Ted is subsequently reinjured within the first few months of his return.

In comparison, Bill works for XYZ Manufacturing and is referred directly to a worksite PT the same day his injury occurred. Bill reports persistent pain but is able to complete a variety of stabilization, strengthening, and mobility exercises. The PT applies manual therapy to promote pain reduction and proper alignment. The PT also emphasizes the importance of remaining active and maintaining function. Although Bill requires a few days off after his injury, the PT is able to find a suitable modified position for Bill to start the next week.

Bill's primary job is similar to Ted's, but the PT had previously performed a JDA for Bill's position and is familiar with the work. Bill cannot tolerate the pushing and pulling of the carts or the trunk rotation required to spray the bathtubs. However, a polishing position (cleaning and "finishing" pieces before they are crated for shipping) is available and a perfect match for Bill's current physical abilities. The PT discusses this option with Bill's supervisor, and Bill is able to take the temporary position as a polisher with a few added stretch breaks and time off for 3 hours per week for therapy.

Bill's goal remains to return to his previous position, so the PT takes Bill out to the furnaces. Bill dons the uniform the other employees wear to spray the bathtubs and push the carts into the furnace. The PT slowly guides Bill through the different tasks this job requires. She notices several biomechanical changes Bill can make to minimize the risk for reinjury and make his job less physically demanding. The PT also notices that the wheels on several carts do not turn properly, which significantly increases the force required to push and pull the carts. Maintenance is able to fix the wheels the next day.

After a few weeks, Bill continues to report some pain but says he is feeling stronger and more comfortable with the work simulation. He is able to safely perform all the physical demands except pushing and pulling the heaviest (200-lb) bathtubs. Again, the PT discusses the options with the supervisor and discovers that Bill can return to his primary job 2 days per week when they are not scheduled to produce the 200-lb bathtubs. After 2 more weeks of modified duty, Bill is able to return to his primary position full time at the same work level he was performing before the injury.

This example illustrates four primary factors that help differentiate on-site therapy from off-site clinic-based practice. First, the worksite PT has direct access to the worker's actual job and equipment. This availability allows the PT to perform job analysis and worker observation as needed, use actual job equipment for assessment and treatment purposes, and directly consult with supervisors, managers, and other personnel to determine modified duty options. The PT in a community- or clinic-based setting is often able to provide general patient education and ergonomic suggestions, but because a formal job analysis may be denied by insurance or the company, the PT is unable to determine if these suggestions are feasible. Worksite PTs know the specific modifications the worker can make and whether engineering or administrative controls can be feasibly implemented. Thus the worksite PT has a better understanding of the physical demands of the job, the equipment used, and worksite "culture," which can all play important roles in successfully returning the employee back to work.

The second advantage of the worksite PT is the ability to provide early intervention for acute injuries and apply corrective treatments before muscle imbalances and soft tissue asymmetries become a problem. Typically, the sooner the injured employee is seen by the PT, the faster he is able to return to work. Often, if seen on the same day, no time off may be necessary. Research suggests that early evaluation and treatment within 2 days of an injury can significantly reduce the number of treatment visits and lost work days.[22,32] Additional studies conclude that the longer injured workers remain off work, the less likely they are to return.[37]

The third factor is the communication that further enhances the team approach. Worksite PTs can more easily have face-to-face relationships with everyone involved in returning the injured employee back to work. The PT is perceived as and becomes part of the team. This communication allows the PT to understand what modifications, alternate methods, or equipment can be feasibly implemented to keep an employee working. By understanding the PT's concerns and issues with safely returning the employee to the job, supervisors can be encouraged to find or create available accommodations. Studies addressing worksite "politics" emphasize the importance of understanding and addressing potential problems that may hinder the injured worker's ability or willingness to return to work.[12,20,26] All parties working together can significantly decrease lost time and costs associated with occupational injuries.

The fourth factor that separates on-site therapy from clinic-based therapy is cost containment. Research suggests that aggressive therapy initiated within the first 2 days after injury significantly reduces lost time.[20,37] Even a few days of lost time can potentially result in hundreds of dollars in lost productivity, salary, and additional medical costs. For example, if an employee earning $15 per hour remains off work for 3 days after an injury, the employer must pay $360 in nonproductive salary. The company also saves money by directly contracting or employing a PT. Conservatively speaking, if the injured employee attends 5 to 6 therapy sessions and a community-based practice charges approximately $75 for each session, the employer will pay $450 in therapy services offered off-site. The total payment equals $810 for an injury that could have cost the employer less than $300 in contracted time if the employee had been seen by a worksite PT. The following illustration outlines this example:

Employee hourly wage ($15) $\times$ hours/day (8) $\times$ days off work (3)
= $360 in total nonproductive wages

Cost per therapy session ($75) $\times$ number of sessions (6) = total cost of therapy sessions ($450)

Total cost of therapy sessions ($450) + total nonproductive wages ($360) = total cost of wages and therapy ($810)

The following studies further detail the cost-benefit analysis and offer examples of managing injury costs with on-site therapy services.

Evidence of Effectiveness for Worksite Programs

Few studies have attempted to address the effects of offering worksite therapy, and those available are case examples with no comparison group. However, these studies help demonstrate the significant contribution worksite therapy can make to successful cost management programs in industry. For example, Dumont and Vance[9] reported a cost-saving analysis of an on-site physical therapy clinic in a Maine shipyard. The physically demanding work, often in confined spaces and with awkward positioning, was difficult to modify or correct through ergonomics. A worksite PT provided evaluations and traditional services emphasizing early mobility, patient education, and function. Within the first year of implementation, the company reported a reduction of approximately $3 million in travel and time-off costs. In addition, total lost work days decreased by more than 10,000 days, and both costs and lost work days continued to drop over the next year.

Another study conducted by Hochanadel and Conrad[13] reported the effects of an on-site physical therapy program in a research and manufacturing plant for the U.S. Department of Energy. PTs stressed the importance of early intervention, aggressive care, and patient education. When an employee was referred for treatment, clinicians performed worksite and work practice analyses to determine possible causes or aggravators of the injury. A retrospective analysis of cost savings for worksite therapy was calculated over a 10-year period. During the years analyzed, the authors calculated a total savings of $3.2 million in treatment costs, $2.4 million in travel time saved by offering services on-site, and $3.2 million in reduced time off. After gross operational expenditures for the on-site clinic were deducted, the company's annual savings averaged $830,000.

In a more recent study reported as a letter to the editor, Scruby, Denham, and Larkin[29] compared associated costs between on-site therapy services in a pharmaceutical company and local community clinics. They found that the on-site clinical costs averaged approximately $40 less per visit than similar community-based clinic visits. This seemingly small amount per visit resulted in savings of almost $400,000 during the 4-year study period. In addition, the on-site clinic reported fewer total therapy visits on average and improved productivity for workers attending therapy appointments. The total annual savings were calculated at more than $240,000 for offering therapy services on-site.

Investigators attempting to evaluate on-site services admit difficulties in reporting clear and accurate information. Problems include difficulty separating the effects of multiple interventions applied simultaneously,[9,13] database issues such as lack of financial data in therapy records and time required to cross-compare lost time data with payroll records,[13] and difficulty calculating the effect on worksite programs. Despite this, the above studies suggest that worksite therapy is beneficial and results in considerable cost savings for companies. Nevertheless, additional studies conducted with comparison groups addressing single interventions and using a comprehensive database could significantly enhance the acceptance and implementation of on-site therapy services by industry.

Physical Therapy Skills Needed for Worksite Therapy

PTs working in industry must be highly skilled and confident in identifying, diagnosing, and treating musculoskeletal disorders as well as screening workers for situations that require the expertise of other health care practitioners. Because the PT often works independently of other PTs and occasionally independently of other medical professionals (e.g., occupational health physicians and nurses), limited opportunity exists to discuss challenging cases or learn new techniques from others. This autonomy can be isolating and may be difficult for PTs new to industrial rehabilitation.

In addition, working for industry instead of the medical community requires a balance of sometimes conflicting interests. Although PTs certainly maintain a role as patient advocate, they must also consider company goals and concerns. This delicate balance of maintaining the confidence of the workers and management influences how recommendations to accommodate an injured worker are made. The PT must be aware of all consequences other employees may experience from any job modification. For example, if the PT recommends that an injured worker take 5-minute stretch breaks every hour, the effect the break has on the rate of productivity the company must maintain, the additional workload other workers have to pick up, and maintenance issues if the line must be stopped or slowed must be considered. The needs of the injured worker may exceed the scope of what the company is capable or willing to accommodate. Thus pressure may be placed on the PT to generate a solution acceptable to both parties. This process requires creativity and is time consuming, but the contribution to both the workers and employers is enormous.

Worksite therapy services require the PT to have good communication skills. These skills include active communication among everyone involved with the injured worker, an understanding of roles and priorities, and an understanding of what information can and should be given to whom. Most clinicians are familiar with and have experience working with physicians, nurses, and case managers. However, worksite PTs often develop very close working relationships with these individuals. For example, an on-site physician may recruit the assistance of a PT to assist in diagnosing orthopedic injuries and consult with the PT on a regular basis to determine treatment options. When a physician is not available on-site, an occupational health nurse can serve as a liaison between PTs working on-site and community-based physicians or specialty providers. Communication among all medical providers is imperative for proper injury management.

Managers/supervisors, safety personnel, noninjured workers, team leaders (e.g., safety, ergonomics), engineers, ergonomists, and maintenance personnel are just a few of the other members that play important roles in returning injured workers and keeping them on the job. The PT must understand the goals and concerns of these individuals to maintain that balance between the injured worker and the company. Managers and supervisors play an important role in keeping employees on the job or returning them to work. A proactive manager can contribute significantly to the treatment of the injured worker by implementing administrative controls (e.g., modified duty, transitional duty, task rotations, reduced work days, and reduced productivity standards). However, it is important for the PT to remember that the primary concern of the manager and supervisor is productivity. When making suggestions for modification, transitional duty, or other return-to-work strategies, PTs should always consider whether the recommendations could potentially reduce the overall productivity or hinder another employee's productivity.

Safety personnel and ergonomists, whose concerns are often similar to those of the PT, are often the largest supporters of on-site therapy. Safety personnel focus primarily on the overall reduction of injuries and illnesses, lost work days, and all related costs. Ergonomists primarily focus on reducing injury rates and prevention of musculoskeletal occurrences. Both of these team members can be valuable resources for identifying jobs, determining appropriate modifications, and integrating

the worker back into the job. They often have more experience in working directly with management and workers and can facilitate communication between these groups and the PT. Maintenance personnel and engineers ensure proper machine functioning at the rates and productivity standards outlined by management. However, they can often be recruited to identify possible engineering controls such as physically modifying existing equipment or even creating new pieces to accommodate physical limitations.

Finally, the PT must interact with noninjured workers. Not only does this build the trust and confidence mentioned earlier, but it also allows the PT to become part of the organization. In fact, the more the PT can interact with noninjured workers, the better the relationships. PTs who have attempted the jobs the workers perform daily and who interact with employees on all levels develop a higher level of respect within the organization.

Despite the above, worksite therapy does contain some disadvantages. For example, an injured employee working for the company may view the PT as an agent for the company. A company that requires the PT to compromise quality of care may fuel this employee concern. When pursuing a position on-site, PTs must ask related questions about the type of care the company is willing and wanting to give. Speaking to several of the people mentioned earlier (worksite physicians, occupational health nurses, safety officers, and ergonomists) will assist in defining the work culture and expectations. This initial communication may also help determine the willingness of the company to implement prevention strategies. If a company is not supportive of prevention, the PT may have difficulty working with management in other areas. For this reason, the PT should always work with the company to outline goals, expectations, and measures of success to avoid future problems. For example, the PT may have difficulty justifying services if the company does not wish to support and finance prevention strategies yet bases therapy reviews on decreasing injury rates.

Worksite therapy offers both the PT and the company numerous advantages and few significant disadvantages. Although often challenging, worksite therapy is a unique opportunity for PTs to significantly improve their skills, independence, and confidence.

Transitional Work Programs

A transitional work program (TWP) uses a continuum of proactive and reactive interventions to identify the targeted return to work (RTW) job and productive alternative jobs that can be used to maximize the safe work capacities of an injured worker. A TWP transitions the worker to full duty through the implementation of timely progressions based on TWP performance.[31] The employer and the clinician must have a clear understanding of the TWP process. All team members must establish ownership in the process and must respect each other's contributions. Team member interaction should be nonadversarial, using negotiation as an integral part of TWP. The continuum of long-term TWP services is ensured through partnerships. Resources, information, education, and a clear definition of the decision-making process are needed to accomplish return to full duty goals. The TWP is organized to emphasize the needs of the worker and to maximize their participation. Therefore TWP services provided at the worksite are designed to improve continuity of care, quality of care, and operational efficiency. Cross-training to produce multi-skilled TWP providers and a decentralization/redeployment of TWP provider services is inherent.

Co-workers must accept a TWP worker in production, supervisors must be comfortable with the job assignment, and employers must establish eligibility criteria, often within the framework of a union contract. Production is paramount to the employer. TWP providers need to factor productivity into account when assessing worker fit into the production schedule. The short- and the long-term impact on quotas, quality, and production processes as well as the effect on the clinical status of the worker must be considered.

Transitional Work Program Objective

A comprehensive TWP is well planned and may involve significant resources from the employer and the provider. The program provides organization, structure, and accountability to the RTW process. The TWP conveys the corporate philosophy regarding RTW issues and provides a clear vision and expectations of the RTW process. The TWP reorganizes the employer's and the worker's responsibilities so that the worker can work at his or her maximum safe capacity, contributing to productivity and competitiveness. The TWP provides case resolution within the medicolegal system with the multidisciplinary team approach. Closure is important and all goals should be met or redirected in a defined time frame. The emphasis of the TWP is on a safe and long-term productive RTW and should not be seen as a "quick fix" for RTW issues. The TWP can prevent an impairment (a medical condition that results in a quantifiable loss) from becoming a disability (loss of capacity to engage in gainful employment).

Clinical Perspective

PTs implementing a TWP need to have the appropriate clinical background. Clinical expertise in orthopedics, chronic pain management, and in the sports medicine approach to RTW is fundamental. Because the TWP is provided in an industrial environment, certification in CPR and universal first-aid is advised. The *Guide to PT Practice* describes the elements of generally accepted PT practice, defines standardized terminology, and delineates preferred practice patterns.[2] Familiarity with the APTA's Occupational Health Special Interest Group Guidelines for Legal and Risk Management and Injury Prevention is advised. Best practices can be researched through the APTA's Hooked on Evidence project, which allows members to post summaries of clinical studies with outcome data from peer-reviewed articles to an online database. The use of scientific basis methods, critical pathways, and treatment algorithms facilitates the collection of functional outcomes that will establish evidence-based TWP protocols.[24]

Industrial Perspective

The out-of-clinic experience mandates exposure to production processes; personal protective equipment; tools and machines; work shifts; and federal, state, and union workplace regulations and policies. Journals that can be reviewed for specific industrial information include *Ergonomics, Human Factors, Work Study,* and the *International Journal of Ergonomics.*

Documentation

TWP-specific information must be added to physical therapy documentation: initial and discharge reports, progress reports, and exercise programs. The TWP requires documentation regarding the worker's abilities, productivity, attitude, and behavior.[33,35] TWPs must assess psychosocial factors such as satisfaction, depression, hysterical personality, aging, dependent or immature personality, substance abuse, secondary gains, sociopathy, learned helplessness, fear avoidance, motivation, locus of control, life stressors, and self-deprecation for successful RTW closure. This can be accomplished by a variety of psychosocial assessment tools such as the Modified Work Apgar, RTW Forcefield Analysis, WRI, Behavioral Health Inventory, North American Spine Society's Outcome Questionnaire, or Oswestry/Modified Oswestry Questionnaire.[10,15]

The work log collects information regarding pain levels and location, work performance and tolerance, safe work practices, and job assignments. It is completed daily by the worker throughout the TWP. The information obtained through the work log is used for progress reports to the various TWP team members and to direct TWP progression.

A successful TWP incorporates goals and action plans identified by the RTW Forcefield Analysis (or similar tool) so that a realistic direction for TWP resolution can be achieved. The TWP team assigns a program manager to facilitate TWP action plans. The program manager oversees the implementation, modification, and monitoring of the action plans throughout the TWP.

Program Evaluation

To establish the effectiveness of TWPs, outcome-based objective data are collected. Sources for the collection of data include goal sheets (before and after ratings), work logs (tolerances, pain levels, performance levels), satisfaction questionnaires (employer, physician, worker, case manager, supervisor), program management reports (action plans), OSHA 300 logs, workers' compensation billing records, medical/health records, and discharge summaries (case resolution, case velocity, RTW Forcefield Analysis).

Outcome-based objective data to be collected include lost time days, restricted days, productivity levels, RTW rate, number of claims, incident rates, total recordable injuries, severity rates, medical costs, reinjury rates, legal costs, and nonphysical psychosocial test scores. These multivariate data can then be analyzed to determine such factors as cost effectiveness, worker retention, case velocity, programmatic content, and TWP critical pathways and algorithms.

Transitional Work Program Benefits

The benefits of a TWP are program specific, but all TWPs should realize most of the following benefits if the program is implemented appropriately. A TWP facilitates the employer management of the work environment by maximizing internal policy and procedures, thus meeting ownership and partnership obligations. Corporate competitiveness is enhanced because of the improvement to the bottom line and the availability of productive workers. A TWP promotes early and proactive interventions emphasizing the determination of a specific diagnosis with concurrent specific treatment within 4 to 6 weeks of date of injury. This results in appropriate care by the appropriate health care provider at the appropriate time. A TWP improves the management of external resources by providing a common ground for addressing RTW issues and an awareness of availability of these resources (networking). A TWP improves workforce morale and protects worker employability through ADA and OSHA Ergonomic Guidelines compliance. It promotes the labor-management collaboration in the RTW process, thereby reducing the adversarial nature of the work injury. Finally, a TWP promotes worker locus of control in the RTW process by identifying the strengths and weaknesses for RTW and incorporating the worker as an active TWP team member to resolve them.

Transitional Work Program Outcomes

The outcomes-based data in Table 14-1 were collected from two central Ohio–based companies that have an evidence-based TWP. Each program has specific TWP policies and procedures, a long-standing worksite PT who is present one to three times per week, a relationship with an occupational medicine facility, a network of consultant/treatment health care providers, an external case manager, and the support of management to implement proactive intervention.

Future Changes

The workforce of the new millennium will continue to change. The Bureau of Labor Statistics describes a workforce that is currently 55% female (a large proportion being single mothers), multiethnic, and poorly educated. The current business environment responds to a service-oriented economy that continually expands and contracts. The result is a decreasing number of skilled trade workers and an increasing use of temporary or leased workers. In many sectors of business (e.g., the steel industry, car manufacturing) the workforce is aging and unionized. The union seniority system has its advantages, but the workforce experiences normal physiological changes associated with the aging process and the subsequent comorbidities associated with working lifestyles. In other business sectors (e.g., technology) there is evidence of a new work ethic: one that values a balance and synergy between work and family, considers work as a noble cause, strives for personal growth and development, builds a partnership and trusting relationship with the employer, and fosters a community spirit at work.

The challenge for TWP is to devise a new work strategies paradigm that will benefit the future workforce. Many data sources are available to construct and validate a new paradigm. The federal government has specific initiatives to address the work environment. *Healthy People 2010* has been pursued over the past 2 decades.[34] *Healthy People 2010* is grounded in science, built through public consensus, and designed to measure progress. Its goals are to increase the quality and years of healthy life and to eliminate health disparities. These goals are supported by specific objectives in 28 Focus Areas. Focus Area 20 is occupational safety and health, which has the goal of promoting the health and safety of people at work through prevention and early intervention objectives. There are 11 specific objectives in Focus Area 20, which include reducing work-related injuries resulting in medical treatment, lost time from work or injury, and illness cases involving days away from work because of overexertion or repetitive motion. The OSHA ergonomic guidelines will continue to be formulated through consensus of labor, government, business, health, and litigation. 0*NET is being developed as a replacement for the DOT. 0*NET classifies physical demands by subjective assessment and may be unsuitable for the purposes of rehabilitation and disability determination (e.g., FCEs, JDAs). Legal issues such as the recent ADA rulings and the use of genetic testing (e.g., sickle cell anemia, carpal tunnel) will influence TWP as well as the administration of post-offer/essential functional testing.

Evidence-based disability guidelines are increasingly being used to facilitate and validate the RTW process.[25] The four major guidelines are the Official Disability Guidelines (Work Loss Data Institute), the Medical Disability Advisor (Reed Group), the Health Management Guidelines (Milliman and Robertson), and the Occupational Medicine Practice Guideline (American College of Occupational and Environmental Medicine). The new TWP work strategies paradigm dictates that disability guidelines are to be based on objective data and take into account all the factors affecting RTW (e.g., type of intervention, severity, type of job).

Research for Occupational Safety and Health is being pursued by NIOSH and by the APTA research program, Foundation for Physical Therapy. NIOSH established the National Occupational Research Agenda in 1996 and targeted 21 areas (e.g., low back disorders; musculoskeletal disorders of the upper extremity; intervention effectiveness research; and

---

TABLE 14-1

Outcomes-Based Data from Two Evidence-Based Transitional Work Programs

	Steel Foundry, Columbus, Ohio		
	1999	**2000**	**% Change**
Incident rates	24	21	−11
Total recordable injuries	340	246	−28
Severity rates	970	682	−29
Total lost and restricted days	13,730	7864	−43
Total lost work days	11,706	5948	−49
Medical costs	Proprietary information	Proprietary information	−38

	Automotive Supplier, Canal Winchester, Ohio		
	1991	**1992**	**1993**
Carpal tunnel disability costs	$87,605	$59,570	$44,678

illness and injury surveillance research methods) for specific research priority. Research in physical therapy has established evidence-based treatment protocols for modalities such as ultrasound and electrical stimulation. TWP will need to incorporate as much information as possible from research to effectively resolve RTW issues.

Education and certification requirements will affect the TWP. The emergence of doctorate of physical therapy programs and the physical therapy certifications in areas such as orthopedics and neurology ensure that a more qualified TWP provider will be available. Other professional certifications that enhance TWP provider expertise include ergonomics (Board of Certification in Professional Ergonomics), FCEs (various systems), and OSHA (course work).

The behavior-based safety coaching process uses a systematic approach to develop and sustain safe work practices.[1] The TWP process can implement this model by identifying at-risk behaviors, writing observable behavior definitions, installing interventions, monitoring performance, and providing immediate feedback. The benefits of utilizing a behavior-based approach to TWP include increasing the worker's involvement, allowing the worker locus of control, promoting team work and partnering, improving communication, reinforcing desired behavior, changing undesirable behavior, and maximizing TWP efficiency.

The goal of the TWP is to conserve workforce productivity and health to promote corporate competitiveness. To accomplish this, implementing evidence-based interventions and protocols, with research and professional resources and a grounding in medicolegal business issues, will ensure the delivery of validated and effective work strategies.

Summary

The scope of practice in primary care for the injured worker is extremely broad, ranging from appropriate management and triage of acutely injured workers to facilitation of disability decisions. The injured worker arena requires a thorough understanding of state and federal regulations and of the roles filled by other professionals. Working effectively with all the players can make or break the resolution of the case and the ultimate outcome of the treatment. Facilitating effective teamwork may be an inportant role of the PT.

REFERENCES

1. AON: Safety coaching process. In *Training manual 2000*, Dallas, 2000, AON Risk Services of Texas.
2. APTA: Guide to physical therapist practice, ed 2, *Phys Ther* 81:9-744, 2001.
3. APTA: Effective prevention and management of work-related injuries. In *Home Study Course 12.3*, Alexandria, Va, 2002, Orthopedic Section APTA.
4. APTA: *Industrial Rehabilitation Advisory Committee guidelines*, Alexandria, Va, 1992, APTA.
5. CARF: *Medical rehabilitation standards manual*, Tucson, Az, 2002, Commission on Accreditation of Rehabilitation Facilities.
6. De Wall M, Van Riel M, Aghina J, et al: Improving the sitting posture of CAD/CAM workers by increasing VDU monitor working height, *Ergonomics* 35:427-436, 1992.
7. *Dictionary of occupational titles*, ed 4, vol I and II, 1991, Washington, D.C. U.S. Department of Commerce, Bureau of Census.
8. Dommer TM: Regulatory agencies and legislation. In King PM, editor: *Sourcebook of occupational rehabilitation*, 1998, New York, Picnum Press, p 62.
9. Dumont D, Vance S: Industrial physical therapy: a model of on-site intervention, *Work Injury Management* 3:1-4, 1992.
10. Frymoyer JW: Predicting disability from low back pain, *Clin Orthop Rel Res* 279:101-109, 1992.
11. Hebert L: Cumulative trauma prevention, *Clin Management* 10:5, 1990.
12. Hebert L: The politics of work injury prevention, *Industrial Safety and Hygiene News* May, 1992.
13. Hochanadel C, Conrad D: Evolution of an on-site physical therapy program, *J Occup Med* 35:1011-1016, 1993.
14. Johnson L, Archer-Heese G: Work hardening: Outdated fad or effective intervention? *Work* 16:235-243, 2001.
15. Kielhofner G, Brauman B, Baron K, et al: The model of human occupation: understanding the worker who is injured or disabled. *Work* 12:3-11, 1999.
16. Lechner D: Work hardening and work conditioning interventions: do they affect disability? *Phys Ther* 74:471-493, 1994.
17. Lechner D, Bradbury S, Bradley L: Detecting sincerity of effort a summary of methods and approaches. *Phys Ther* 78:867-888, 1998.
18. Lechner D, Jackson J, Rosh D, et al: Reliability and validity of newly developed test of physical work performance, *J Occup Med* 36:997-1004, 1994.
19. Lechner DE, Sheffield G: Predictive validity of the physical work performance evaluation. *Phys Ther* 76:881, 1996.
20. Linton SJ, Hellsing AL, Anderson D: A controlled study of the effects of an early intervention on acute musculoskeletal pain problems, *Pain* 54:353-359, 1993.
21. Melnik M: Enlisting participation in an injury prevention and management program, *Work* Fall, 1990.
22. NIOSH: *Workplace use of back belts: review and recommendations*, Cincinnati, Ohio, 1994, National Institute for Occupational Safety and Health.
23. Nordin M, Weiser S, Halpern N: Prevention and treatment of low back disorders. In Frymoyer J, editor: *The adult spine*, vol I, Philadelphia, 1991, Lippincott-Raven.
24. Philadelphia panel evidence-based clinical practice guidelines on selected rehabilitation interventions for low back pain, *Phys Ther* 81:1641-1674, 2001.
25. Prezzia C, Donniston P: Evidence-based duration guidelines, *J Workers Comp* 10:43-53, 2001.
26. Rosta P: Industrial workers excel with work hardening, *Rehab Management* April-May, 1991.
27. Rothstein JM, Echternach JL: *Primer on measurement: an introductory guide to measurement issues*, Alexandria, Va, American Physical Therapy Association, pp 78-80, 1993.
28. Scalzitti DA: Screening for psychological factors in patients with low back problems: Waddell's nonorganic signs, *Phys Ther* 77:306-312, 1997.
29. Scruby D, Denham S, Larkin G: Economic impact of on-site physical therapy, *J Occup Environ Med* 43:670-671, 2001.
30. Scully-Palmer C: Outcome study: an industrial rehab program, *Work* 15:21-23, 2000.
31. Shrey DE, Lacerte M: *Principles and practices of disability management in industry*, Winter Park, Fla, 1995, GR Press.
32. Sommerich C, Joines S, Psihogios J: Effects of computer monitor viewing angle and related factors on strain, performance, and preference outcomes, *Hum Factors* 43:39-55, 2001.
33. Toeppen-Sprigg B: Importance of job analysis with functional capacity matching in medical case management: a physician's perspective, *Work* 15:133-137, 2000.
34. US Department of Health and Human Services: *Healthy People 2010: understanding and improving health*, ed 2, Washington, DC, 2000, US Government Printing Office.
35. Waddell G: A new clinical model for the treatment of low back pain, *Spine* 12:632-644, 1987.
36. Weir R, Nelson W: Interventions for disability management, *Clin J Pain* 17(suppl 4):128-132, 2001.
37. Zigenfus G, Yin J, Giang G, et al: Effectiveness of early physical therapy in the treatment of acute low back musculoskeletal disorders, *J Occup Environ Med* 42:35-39, 2000.

The Geriatric Population 15

Jennifer M. Bottomley, PT, MS, PhD

Objectives

After reading this chapter, the reader will be able to:

1. Explain the distinctions between normal and pathologic aging.
2. Describe the working definitions of frailty and wellness as they apply to the geriatric population.
3. Describe the medical diagnostic challenges associated with the geriatric population, including polypharmacy, nutritional deficits, dehydration, poor levels of fitness, and sudden changes in cognition.
4. Explain the clinical considerations specific to the geriatric population associated with diseases common to this group.

Today there are 78 million American baby boomers—persons between ages 35 and 53—making up one third of the U.S. population. All of these people will soon be considered the elderly of our nation.[27] From a rehabilitative, physical-therapy perspective, observers predict that this new cohort of elders, the aging boomers, will crave vigor, vitality, and extended life. In addition to this evolving demographic phenomenon, the portion of the American population currently 65 and older is growing rapidly, and the group 85 years and older is the largest growing segment of our population.[5]

The irony of past medical successes is that they have produced many long-lived elders who struggle with the very problems of long-term disability that the American health-care system is ill-prepared to handle, such as heart disease, cancer, arthritis, osteoporosis, and Alzheimer's.[15] This results in many elders needing rehabilitative services in primary-care outpatient clinics.

The good news is that through proper preventive interventions, which can be incorporated in the primary-care setting, we have the potential to produce a healthier version of aging at a lower cost than the current health care delivery system. Physical therapy, as a profession, is poised to help meet the primary-care needs of the aging population. Through direct access, PTs often will be the practitioner of choice for many of these patients/clients. In addition to our traditional roles in rehabilitation, we will shift our clinical interventions toward prevention of disease, injury, and disability.

PTs in primary-care outpatient settings encounter geriatric patients each day. In fact, in many clinics, elderly patients make up the largest proportion of the non–hospital-based ambulatory-care patient population. It is important, therefore, for PTs to develop expertise in the management of geriatric patients in a primary-care environment. PTs in the primary-care venue need to be an integral part of the interdisciplinary approach inherent in a family or general-medicine practice or non–hospital-based outpatient physical-therapy clinic. The goal of this chapter is to provide the clinician working in a primary-care setting an understanding of the principles and practices needed to adequately address the outpatient physical-therapy needs of an aging patient population.

Primary Care in Geriatric Physical Therapy

The *Guide to Physical Therapist Practice* describes primary care as "the provision of integrated, accessible health care services by clinicians who are accountable for addressing a large majority of personal health care needs, developing a sustained partnership with patients, and practicing within the context of family and community."[3] These components are crucial to the holistic and comprehensive care of aged individuals.

The PT is often a part of a primary-care team, and in many cases the entry point into the health care system for elderly patients. The concept of *multi*disciplinary care has long been a cornerstone of geriatric care.[91] The newer models of primary care in geriatrics support the concept of *inter*disciplinary care, whereby the PT working in a primary-care setting in outpatient medical clinics is working in concert with physicians, nurse practitioners, nutritionists, pharmacologists, behavior medicine specialists, health-education specialists, and a variety of other clinicians. Each team member contributes his or her expertise to the comprehensive care of an elderly individual and has the responsibility of referring patients to the appropriate disciplines within the team, as well as outside of the primary-care team, as the patient's condition and status warrant.

Often the patient is screened over the telephone when she or he calls to consult with the clinic, and is scheduled to see a PT because of musculoskeletal symptoms without seeing any other team members. Or, patients are referred to physical therapy after a quick screen by a physician or nurse practitioner upon their first visit. Therefore the PT becomes the key primary-care provider and coordinator of care for this patient. The PT then is considered central to the successful implementation of geriatric assessment, treatment, and appropriate referral in primary care.

As the potential entry point into a primary-care clinic the PT must have a sound educational background in differential diagnosis and acute management of musculoskeletal conditions and other pathologies specific to the elderly population, and a working knowledge of radiology, pharmacology, nutrition, laboratory technology, team building, and communication skills. It is recommended that an outpatient physical-therapy clinic have a geriatric certified specialist (GCS) on staff who is knowledgeable and capable of providing high-quality care for the more complex elderly patients. If this is not the case, however, the clinic must develop an academic and consultative specialty that would integrate geriatrics *into* the primary-care and specialty-care physical-therapy setting and act as a potential referral source for the PTs at the clinic.

The field of geriatrics requires a strong clinical team leader to bring together a variety of disciplines in a coordinated way.[20] As a subspecialty, geriatrics physical therapy must go beyond classic physical-therapy models of care and work closely with other health fields, such as social work, nursing, nutrition, occupational therapy, and pharmacy, in providing clinical services and education in a primary-care setting. Geriatrics should be seen as a *perspective* concerned with a stage of life that calls for an interdisciplinary approach with collaboration among specialties. This is the core premise of primary care in physical-therapy management of the geriatric client.

Geriatric Assessment and Managed Care

With the reorganization of the financing of health care and the creation of systems of care, it is possible to design and implement organizational interventions to improve the care of older persons beyond the services that can be provided by an individual provider.[86] Changing the structure of delivery to an interdisciplinary, primary-care model is a potentially powerful method of influencing health-care and maintaining the health of older persons.

Managed care for older people is growing very rapidly.[85] Risk and value of services are central concepts that affect managed care of this population. The Balanced Budget Act of 1997 brought several changes in Medicare Managed Care. However, managed care offers the potential for improved models of care delivery to older adults. It not only offers coordinated, patient-centered assessment and intervention, but if properly implemented, the managed-care model offers the greatest continuity of care across the care-giving spectrum for older people.[79]

The concept of interdisciplinary primary care is an integral part of managed care in the elderly.[51,71] Comprehensive geriatric assessment is considered an important and effective element of secondary and tertiary preventive care for the frail elderly.[37] Appropriate screening and appraisal for health and functional risks can identify those elderly individuals who have the greatest risk of developing morbidity and disability. Cohen and associates,[18] in a controlled trial, found that primary care in inpatient geriatric units and outpatient geriatric clinics had no significant effects on survival. However, there were significant reductions in functional decline with inpatient geriatric evaluation and management and improvements in mental health and functional status with outpatient primary-care evaluation and management, with no increase in costs.[18]

Effective new strategies that complement primary care are needed to reduce disability risks and improve self-management of chronic illness in frail older people living in the community. Leveille et al[65] evaluated the effect of a 1-year, senior-center–based chronic illness self-management and disability-prevention program on health, functioning, and health care utilization in frail older adults. This project produced evidence that a community-based collaboration with primary-care providers can improve function and reduce inpatient utilization in chronically ill older adults. Linking organized medical care with complementary community-based interventions may be a promising direction for research and practice.[65] Survey findings also point to the potential importance of primary-care programs for long-term nursing home residents.[5,33]

In traditional fee-for-service primary-care practices, comprehensive assessment of older patients is provided at the site of care by an interdisciplinary team. Targeting this complex, costly, and time-consuming process to individuals who have the potential to benefit the most from subsequent interventions (i.e., the highest-risk elderly population) is vital to the success of primary care within a managed-care environment.

It is often difficult for most Medicare providers to conduct all-inclusive examinations because of the time and personnel required for interdisciplinary geriatric care. However, the economic and clinical forces of managed care promote creativity and innovation in the development of targeted programs that provide the most efficient and effective interventions for geriatric patients. For example, disease-management programs generally include the identification of high-risk members and the targeting of coordinated care to those individuals.[88] A model in physical therapy would be screening for risk of falls, identifying those elderly who are most likely to experience a fall, and intervening by strengthening weak muscles, promoting erect posture, and facilitating sensory-organization strategies to accommodate for instabilities around the center of gravity. In the long run, treating before the fall is intuitively much less costly than intervening after the fall. Targeting allows the available resources of the interdisciplinary geriatric team to be directed to individuals with the greatest potential to benefit. High-risk screening or health-risk appraisals often are used to identify elders requiring primary, secondary, or tertiary preventive health interventions. High-risk individuals then can be triaged to interventions such as physical therapy.

Unique Clinical Characteristics of the Aging Population

One primary concept associated with the geriatric population is that of *variability*. More than any other age group, the aged vary in their level of functional capabilities. In the clinic, we often see 65-year-old individuals who are severely physically disabled, sitting right alongside individuals who are 65 years old and still building houses and felling trees. Even in the "old-old" category, variability in physical and cognitive functioning is remarkable.[8]

Another important element in geriatric physical therapy is the concept of *activity versus inactivity*. The most common reason for losses in functional capabilities in the aged is inactivity or immobility. The aged become immobilized for many reasons. Acute immobilization often is considered to be accidental immobilization and can be associated with acute catastrophic illnesses, including severe blood loss, trauma, head injury, cerebral vascular accidents, burns, and hip fractures. The patient's activity level often is severely curtailed until the acute illnesses become medically stable.

Chronic immobilization may result from long-standing problems that are undertreated or left untreated and include cerebral vascular accidents (strokes), amputations, arthritis, Parkinson's disease, cardiac disease, pulmonary disease, and low back pain. Environmental barriers are a major cause of accidental immobilization in both the acute and chronic-care settings. These include bedrails, the height of the bed, physical restraints, an inappropriate chair, lack of physical assistance, fall precautions imposed by medical staff, lack of orders in the chart for mobilization, social isolation, and environmental obstacles (e.g., stairs or doorway thresholds). Cognitive impairments, central nervous system (CNS) disorders (such as cerebral vascular accidents, Parkinson's disease, and multiple sclerosis), peripheral neuropathies resulting from diabetes, and pain with movement also can severely reduce mobility. Affective disorders such as depression, anxiety, or fear of falling also may lead to accidental immobilization. In addition, sensory changes, terminal illnesses (such as cancer or cirrhosis of the liver), acute episodes of illness like pneumonia or cellulitis, or an attitude of "I'm too sick to get up" can reduce mobility.[8]

Another key clinical principle in geriatric rehabilitation is the principle of *optimal health*. The great English statesman Benjamin Disraeli said, "The health of people is really the foundation upon which all their happiness and their powers as a state depend." The World Health Organization defines health as a state of complete physical, mental, and social well-being, not merely the absence of disease or infirmity.[111] The presence of complete physical health refers to the absence of pathology, impairment, or disability and is quite achievable. Mental and social well-being are closely related, and possibly less easy to obtain in this age. Mental health as defined by the World Health Organization includes cognitive and intellectual intactness as well as emotional well-being. The social components of health include living situation, social roles (e.g., mother, daughter, vocation), and economic status.

The clinician must consider these unique clinical characteristics of aging as part of a comprehensive screen and examination of an elderly individual entering the primary-care environment.

Normal-Version Pathologic Aging

Aging is considered a normal physiological process because of its universality. As much as the aging process may affect the predisposition to disease, aging in and of itself is not considered to be pathologic. This distinction seems conceptually clear, but the fine line between aging and disease often is blurred when applied to specific cases, and some degree of decrease in biological, physiological, anatomical, and functional capabilities occurs as one ages. Some degree of atrophy

is evident in all tissues of the body. A variety of degenerative processes are called "normal aging" until they proceed far enough to cause clinically significant disability.

Although aging may not be considered a disease process, the time-dependent loss of structure and function in all organ systems leads to pathologic end states. Age brings a general decline in structure, function, and number of many cell types. Consider these examples: Cellular aging is accompanied by denaturation of extracellular proteins, and the collagen and elastin of the skin become irreversibly crystalline and broken. The hyaline cartilage on articular surfaces of joints becomes fibrillar and fragmented, and the beautifully ordered structure of the eye lens becomes brittle and chaotic as lens protein is gradually denatured. The most important aging changes occur at the molecular level. Small injuries occurring within the cell result in the loss of genetic memory and progressive crosslinking of collagen, the chief structural protein in the body.

Disease is defined as the reaction to injury.[58] If aging is a gradual accumulation of incompletely repaired injuries caused by microtrauma through the life course, aging may not be normal, despite its universality. Perhaps "aging" is a pathologic process resulting from tissue reactions to imperceptible injuries that could have been avoided.

In the primary-care model, PTs play a major role in preventing the disabilities that result from these insidious microtraumas. Screening and subsequent evaluation and interventions for the limitations and disabilities identified could preserve health and function. For example, preventive strengthening and conditioning exercises, positioning, joint and tissue mobilization, and the many other treatments that could be employed all affect functional capabilities, especially in an aged population. Preventing disabilities that can result from pathologic processes greatly improves the level of function and the quality of life. Certainly some changes that occur in aging need not be inevitable.[9]

Anatomical and Physiological Features of the Aging Process

Many changes are associated with aging throughout adulthood and into old age. Table 15-1 summarizes these system changes. One must remember that individuals age at different rates. Therefore, while it is useful to summarize age-related changes in a table, the PT must remember that any one individual may vary remarkably from her or his peers.

Defining Frailty

Defining the term *frailty* is difficult, but the *image* of frailty is well understood in geriatric rehabilitation. The concept of frailty invokes a clear mental image for most clinicians; the components of frailty include compromises in cognition, reductions in sensorimotor input and integration,[67] polypharmacy, dehydration, and malnutrition. The decline in muscle strength and mass,[36] respiratory reserve, and cardiovascular functioning; kyphotic postural changes; compromised eyesight; poor hydration and marginal nutritional intake; and many other physiological and physical changes associated with inactivity and aging lead to

TABLE 15-1

Summary of Multisystem Changes in the Elderly

MUSCULOSKELETAL SYSTEM

- Muscle mass and strength decrease at a rate of about 30% between the ages of 60 and 90.
- Change in muscle fiber type, white and red. Type II fibers (fast twitch) decrease by about 50%.
- Change in clear differentiation of fiber type, with the red increasing in speed of contraction and the white fibers decreasing in the speed of contraction
- Decrease in recruitment of motor units
- Decrease in the speed of movement
- Decreased tensile strength of bone (more than 30% of women over age 65 have osteoporosis)
- Females lose about 30% of bone mass by age of 70; males lose about 15% by age of 70.
- Joint flexibility reduced by 25% to 30% over the age of 70
- Decrease in enzymatic activity, cell count, and metabolic substrates in cartilage (collagen fibers increase their cross-linking, resulting in increase in soft-tissue density)

NEUROMUSCULAR SYSTEM

- Atrophy of neurons; nerve fibers decrease and change in structure
- Myoneural junction decreases in transmission speed.
- Mitochondrial activity decreases.
- Dopamine level depletion
- Decrease in nerve conduction velocity by about 0.4% per year after age 70
- Slowing of motor-neuron conduction, which contributes to alterations in the autonomic system
- Decrease in reflexes result from decrease in nerve conduction. In a population of those 70-80 years old: ankle jerk is absent in about 70%, and knee and biceps jerk are absent in about 15%.
- Overall slowed and decreased responsiveness in reaction time (simple reflexes less than complex)
- Increased postural sway (less in women than in men with linear increase with age)
- Changes in sleep patterns that affect neuromuscular functioning

NEUROSENSORY SYSTEM

- Decrease in sweating (implications for modalities and exercise)
- 10% to 20% decrease in brain weight by age 90
- Decrease in mechanoreceptors
- Decrease in efficiency of the neuroendocrine system (i.e., decrease in calcium control, affecting heart contraction and causing osteoporosis; thymus function decreases 90% between ages 20 and 80)
- Decrease in visual acuity and ability to accommodate to lighting changes resulting from increased density of lens
- Decrease in hearing capabilities
- Decrease in the senses of smell and taste

CARDIOVASCULAR AND PULMONARY SYSTEMS

- Decrease in cardiac output by about 0.7% per year after 20 years of age (5 L/min CO at age 20 versus 3.5 L/min by age 75)
- Increased vascular resistance
- Decreased arterial elasticity
- Decreased cardiac reserve, decreased physical and psychological response to stress
- Decrease in lipid catabolism, which may increase risk for heart disease; about 50% of adults between ages 65 and 74 have evidence of heart disease, and about 30% in this age range have sustained myocardial infarction even in the absence of symptoms of ischemia (in CHF, MIs exceed 50%).
- Increased irritation of myocardium contributes to increased risk of atrial fibrillation and arrhythmias.

- Decrease in lung function (from age 25 to age 85 as much as 50% decrease in maximal voluntary ventilation due to an increase in air resistance; get about 40% decrease in vital capacity)
- Respiratory gas exchange surface decreases at a rate of about 0.27 square meters a year (maximum oxygen consumption for sedentary individuals of any age is 0.6 to 0.7 mL/min).
- Decrease in elastin in the lungs (increased rigidity) and chest wall soft tissues results in decrease in chest wall compliance.
- Decrease in vital capacity and decrease in pulmonary blood flow contribute to lower oxygen saturation levels
- Residual volume doubles.
- Decreased cough reflex
- Decreased ciliary response
- Work capacity declines about 30% between the ages of 40 and 70.

UROGENITAL/RENAL SYSTEMS

- Gradual overall structure change in all renal components
- Decreased glomerular filtration rate and creatinine clearance
- Change in response to sodium intake
- Muscle hypertrophy in the urethra and bladder
- Decreased ability to concentrate urine

GASTROINTESTINAL SYSTEM

- Decrease in number of taste buds and ability to taste
- Decreased peristalsis
- Diminished secretions of pepsin and acid in the stomach
- Decrease in hepatic and pancreatic enzymes

IMMUNOLOGIC SYSTEM

- Decrease in overall function with respect to infection
- Decreased temperature regulation
- Decrease in T cells
- Decrease in neuroendocrine system efficiency, diminishing responsiveness

GENERAL FACTS ABOUT AGING

- About 50% of decreased function is attributed to pathology rather than "normal" aging changes. Organ systems decline at a rate of about 0.75% to 1% per year starting at the age of 30.
- One in three individuals have sustained a fall by 80 years of age. Hip surgery is the third-most-common surgery for those over the age of 65, and this risk doubles every 5 years after the age of 60.
- The overall efficiency of body systems decreases.
- Many responses that are normal in younger individuals are blunted or slowed in the geriatric population.
- The presence of chronic illnesses also may affect response.

EFFECTS OF BEDREST

- Maximum oxygen uptake decreases by 20% to 40% within 3 days.
- Ventilatory volume at rest and during functional activity declines by as much as 50% within the first week of bedrest.
- Stroke volume decreases by about 10% within the first week and decreases at about 10%/week each week thereafter.
- Work capacity declines as much as 25% after 3 weeks of bedrest, declining at a rate of about 1%/day.
- Blood volume decreases by 700 to 800 mL, resulting in hypovolemic manifestations of tachycardia and orthostatic hypotension as well as increasing thromboembolic risk within first 3 days.
- Nitrogen spilling into urine increases, indicative of protein wasting within 3 days.
- Bone mass is lost at a rate of about 1.4%/day without weight bearing (starting day 1). About 40% of bone mass can be lost after 6 weeks of bedrest.
- Decrease in the skeletal muscle mass and contractile strength and efficiency by about 10% to 15% within first week of bedrest.

Continued

TABLE 15-1

Summary of Multisystem Changes in the Elderly—cont'd

EFFECTS OF EXERCISE

- Ten weeks of aerobic training results in a 10% to 15% increase in maximum oxygen consumption, stroke volume, and cardiac output.
- Maximal oxygen consumption in elderly over the age of 80 increases by 0% to 38% with endurance training of as little as 6 weeks.
- One hour of exercise class (seated exercises) four times a week has shown a favorable effect on aerobic parameters.
- Exercise for 70-year-olds, three times a week for 12 weeks (45 minute sessions), increased static and dynamic strength at all velocities, increased type-II muscle fibers, and showed improved enzymatic responses.

- Muscle activation (neural factors) increase with little hypertrophy in the elderly related to strength training.
- Less stretch is required to produce maximum twitch tension after resistance training in individuals 70 to 95.
- Balance exercises improve postural control, trunk strength, and speed of reaction time in elderly over the age of 70.
- There are significant improvements in muscle strength and muscle cross-sectional area, improved mobility (including increased walking speed, improved stair-climbing ability, and higher functional capabilities), improved dietary intake, and increased spontaneous physical activity in "frail" elderly with high-intensity, progressive resistance exercise training.

From Bottomley JM: Summary of system changes. Comparing and contrasting age-related changes. In Bottomley JM, Lewis CB: *Geriatric rehabilitation: a clinical approach*, ed 2, Upper Saddleback, NJ, 2003, Prentice Hall Publishers, pp 50-75.

frailty. Any of these conditions, in isolation or in combination, can create frailty. Concomitant diseases such as congestive heart failure, renal disease, osteoporosis, diabetes, chronic lung disease, and arthritis all add to the level of frailty.

Medical Complexity/Multisystem Involvement

Impaired physical functioning has been documented in one third of older hospitalized patients.[56] Any older person who is admitted for acute illnesses or injury faces significant short-term deterioration in mobility and other functional domains.[107] Decline in physical function, while a negative outcome in itself, also has been associated with many adverse consequences such as falls, disability, and mortality.[39,40,107]

Functional dependence develops in about 10% of nondisabled community-dwelling persons over the age of 75 each year.[39] Increasing levels of disability are associated with substantial morbidity leading to the adverse outcomes of hospitalization, nursing home placement, and greater use of home-care services.[40] Functional dependence leads to increasing levels of frailty, especially in the medically complex, multisystem-involved elder. With each medical insult and hospitalization, the patient faces a decreasing level of physiological capacity, which is associated with greater difficulty in recovering his or her premorbid functional abilities.[13,81]

The movement of frail older people through the health care system is important to clinicians. Cost-containment strategies that encourage providers to substitute less-costly care in the community for the more-expensive care in hospitals and nursing homes may have implications for the patient's functioning, ability to remain at home, or other treatment outcomes.[1,40] An understanding of this issue is essential to ensure that frail older patients receive the services they need and are treated appropriately. The primary-care model works well in the frail elderly population.

Polypharmacy

The presence of multiple diagnoses in the elderly leads to multiple drug and nutrient interactions and complex medical management, with the resulting side effects of progressive loss of functional reserve and physiological homeostasis.

Many medications are absorbed, distributed, metabolized, and excreted (pharmacokinetics) differently in the elderly, and the action of drugs (pharmacodynamics) may be exaggerated or reduced (see Chapter 16).[38] Of special significance in the geriatric population, different drugs interact with each other either by pharmacokinetic inhibition or induction of drug metabolism or by pharmacodynamic potentiation or antagonism. Knowledge of these pharmacologic pathways has a profound effect on the quality of care. The problem of polypharmacy, defined here as the long-term use of two or more medications, is significant in the older patient.[47,52]

Medication mishaps in the elderly occur for many reasons. Multiple providers often are unaware of one another's new prescriptions or medication changes, especially after hospitalization. Older patients often have visual or cognitive impairments (or both) that lead to errors in self-administration. Patients may be unable to afford their medicines, so they take only some of what is prescribed based on how they are feeling, or they cut doses down to save money and extend the life of their prescription. Functional illiteracy, which is not uncommon among the elderly, makes adherence to a medical regimen difficult. Cultural diversity also affects some older people's perspective about the value of taking a certain medication when some natural alternative has been used for centuries in their culture to treat the same condition.[10]

PTs in a primary-care setting, where they may be the sole clinician working with an elderly individual, must understand the actions and interactions of drugs for several reasons.[10] First, with direct access, PTs may be the entry point of care, making it important for the therapist to have a working knowledge of the drugs that elderly individuals are taking and the potential interactions and side effects of the multipharmacy regimen. Second, PTs design and monitor exercise programs that can adversely affect the pharmacokinetics of many drugs. Fat-soluble drugs, for example, may be affected by a person's decrease in fat after participation in an exercise program, and, therefore dosages will need to be adjusted accordingly. Finally, therapists often see patients regularly and can easily note adverse reactions, such as dizziness, confusion, and slurred speech.

If adequately educated in pharmacology, therapists can suggest modifications of drug regimens to the physician or nurse practitioner in the primary-care team based on patient symptoms. Appropriate medication management is an interdisciplinary concern. Other health care team members, not just the physician or nurse practitioner, must take responsibility for the supervision and coordination of drug interventions, especially in a primary-care setting.

Nutritional/Hydration Considerations

Aging processes and lifelong eating patterns are often associated with diseases and disorders such as atherosclerosis, hypertension, osteoporosis, diabetes, cancer, Alzheimer's disease, renal disease, dental disease, obesity, and impaired immunity that affect the life span.[72] The prevalence of many chronic degenerative diseases increases with advancing age. These disease states may have synergistic negative effects on individuals whose physiological function is already compromised by the aging process. Many chronic conditions have dietary implications that alter the need for nutrients, the physical and metabolic form in which nutrients are delivered, and the activities of daily living related to food and eating. Modifications in the type or amount of energy or the energy-providing nutrients, vitamins, and minerals may be required to provide nutritional support or to control the progression of chronic degenerative diseases. Unfortunately, manifestations of malnutrition, such as cracks in the mouth or a bright-red tongue, are overt signs of a problem that is far advanced. Physical signs of dehydration usually are not apparent until it is in the advanced stages. It is important for the primary-care PT to be familiar with the subtle signs of malnutrition and dehydration.

Clinical Features of Malnutrition

There are several physical findings related to a client's nutritional status, and many of the normal changes of aging mimic clinical findings described as pathognomic of malnutritive states in the elderly.[99] Clinically overt malnutrition rarely is caused by a primary deficit in nutritional intake, rather it is more likely associated with gastrointestinal tract disorders or with one of the chronic debilitating illnesses common to the elderly.

In contrast, subclinical malnutrition,[32] which is by definition undetectable by physical findings on clinical evaluation, is probably common in certain at-risk elderly populations. These subgroups might include those who are institutionalized, those with mental disturbances or gross CNS disease, or those at or below the poverty level. In subclinical malnutritive states, an elderly individual may manifest depleted nutritional reserves as a failure to thrive. Reduced nutritional reserves may contribute to postoperative confusion, delayed recovery times of homeostatic function, delayed wound healing, and increased susceptibility to infection.[42]

The clinical examination, including the history and physical examination, may reveal findings associated with nutritional deficiencies.[26,104] This clinical assessment should include weight history (current, usual, and ideal); assessment of changes in oral intake (type and duration); symptoms affecting nutrition (including anorexia, nausea and vomiting, diarrhea, constipation, stomatitis/mucositis, dry mouth, taste/olfactory abnormalities, and pain); medications that may affect intake or metabolic requirements; other medical conditions that may affect nutritional intake or nutrition intervention options; and evaluation of performance status. Physical examination entails a general assessment of physical condition, including evidence of weight loss, loss of subcutaneous fat, muscle wasting, presence of sacral or tibial edema, or ascites.

Table 15-2 presents possible clinical manifestations of nutritional deficiencies that can occur in the aged. The PT should remember that before ascribing any physical findings elicited during physical examination to nutritional problems, he or she should consider whether the findings are consistent with normal aging or with an underlying disease state.

Clinical Features of Dehydration

Dehydration, a decrease in total body water, is the most common fluid and electrolyte disturbance in the elderly.[82] In many cases in the elderly, cognitive or physical disabilities reduce the ability to recognize thirst, express thirst, or obtain access to water.[74] In addition, healthy elderly individuals seem to have reduced thirst in response to fluid deprivation.[82] Elderly individuals also produce less concentrated urine after fluid deprivation. Because elderly subjects have higher vasopressin levels in response to dehydration, the reduced capacity to concentrate the urine is most likely at the renal level.[82]

An increase in serum sodium concentration results from a loss of body water in excess of salt loss. Among elderly patients, hypernatremia (dehydration with elevated sodium levels in the serum) is most common in those who are not given sufficient water to satisfy their thirst or in those whose thirst sensation is reduced by impaired CNS functioning. A net deficit of water is associated with vomiting, diarrhea, diabetes insipidus, and hyperpyrexia (excessive sweating). In general, older patients appear to be predisposed to the development of hypernatremia. Surgery, febrile illnesses, infirmity, and diabetes mellitus account for most of these incidences.[63] Finally, diuretic-acting fluids, such as coffee and soft drinks, should be avoided.

Many pharmacologic agents can lead to dehydration. Older people have an increased sensitivity to dehydration as a result of physiological changes, including an increase in fat and a decrease in lean body mass, which corresponds with reduced total body water in the elderly. Other drug-related changes with age include the kidneys' reduced ability to conserve water and concentrate urine, increased secretion of antidiuretic hormone, and impaired renal sodium conservation. Dehydration often is iatrogenic, resulting from low-salt diets and volume-depleting drugs, which include most cardiovascular medications (particularly the diuretics), many of the psychotropic and gastrointestinal medications, and many of the commonly used pain-relieving drugs prescribed or purchased over the counter. Many of the drugs prescribed, such as those in the cardiovascular class, are accompanied by recommendations to reduce fluid

TABLE 15-2

Physical Manifestations of Malnutrition

Nutrient Deficiency	Physical Manifestation
Protein	Edema, hypoalbuminemia, enlarged liver, diarrhea
Protein/energy	Muscle wasting; sparse, thin, dry, brittle hair; dry, inelastic skin; muscle weakness
Vitamin A	Poor visual accommodation to dark, Bitot's spots (eyes), dryness of the eyes, hair loss, impaired taste, gooseflesh
Vitamin D	Bowed legs, beading of ribs, and other skeletal deformities (rickets)
Vitamin K	Bleeding (poor coagulation of blood)
Thiamin (B_1)	Cardiac enlargement; mental confusion; irritability; calf-muscle tenderness and foot drop; hypoflexia; hyperesthesia; paresthesia
Riboflavin (B_2)	Fissures around mouth; reddened, scaly, greasy skin around the nose and mouth; magenta-colored tongue
Niacin (B_3)	Bright red, swollen, painful tongue; pellagrous dermatitis; depression; insomnia; headaches; dizziness; dementia; diarrhea
Pyridoxine (B_6)	Neuropathies; glossitis, nasolabial seborrhea
Folic acid	Red, painful, shiny, smooth tongue; skin hyperpigmentation
Vitamin B_{12}	Mild dementia; sensory losses in hands and feet; red, smooth, shiny, painful tongue; mild jaundice; optic neuritis; anorexia; diarrhea
Vitamin C	Joint tenderness and swelling; hemorrhages under the skin; spongy gums that bleed easily; poor wound healing; petechiae
Essential fatty acids	Sparse hair growth; dry, flaky skin; depression and psychosis; dementia
Calcium	Poor reflexes; poor cardiovascular accommodation to activity; slow mental processing; depression; dementia
Magnesium	Lethargy and weakness; anorexia and vomiting; tremor; convulsions
Iodine	Goiter
Iron	Pallor; pale, atrophic tongue; spoon-shaped nails; pale conjunctivae
Zinc	Sluggish muscle contraction; poor wound healing; diminished taste and appetite; dermatitis; hair loss; diarrhea

From Bottomley JM: Exploring nutritional needs in the elderly. In Bottomley JM, Lewis CB: *Geriatric rehabilitation: a clinical approach*, ed 2, Upper Saddleback, NJ, 2003, Prentice Hall Publishers, p 212.

consumption, further increasing the risk of complications from dehydration.

Examination findings common to dehydration should alert the primary-care therapist to further assess an older person for this condition:

- Weight loss
- Altered mental status
- Agitation or lethargy
- Lightheadedness
- Confusion
- Syncope
- Orthostatic hypotension[73]
- Weakness
- Lethargy

The therapist must consider dehydration as part of the medical-screening process when examining an elderly individual and should encourage hydration when appropriate. About 1.5 quarts of water or other water-based fluids per day is a reasonable goal to seek in the aged.

Screening the Geriatric Population

Older individuals at high risk for negative health outcomes often can be identified effectively by self-reported health screenings or assessments that take into account the unique health problems of this population.[19,80] Such instruments have demonstrated a positive effect on health and utilization outcomes when they have been integrated into a comprehensive geriatric assessment program.[105]

Some assessment instruments for health-risk appraisals attempt to gather large amounts of data on the patient's health

status. Other high-risk screening instruments are brief and attempt only to identify members at high risk for adverse health outcomes and increased use of services. A limited number of specific variables have been shown to predict increased medical utilization and adverse health outcomes.[78,80] Such variables as prior hospitalization, advanced age, number of medications, and self-reported health status therefore have been incorporated into scoring algorithms.

Most Medicare HMOs gather patient information from such sources as insurance claims, pharmacy records, and encounters with primary-care providers. These administrative data have been employed for health-risk assessment of geriatric populations.[19,78,105] They also can be used for assessing quality of care.[55,89] Administrative data are readily available in most Medicare HMOs and are relatively inexpensive. The Center for Medicaid and Medicare Services (CMS) (formerly HCFA) has implemented a system of health-risk-adjusted payment rates for Medicare + Choice Coordinated Care Plans that uses administrative data on patient diagnosis.

Screening in the outpatient physical-therapy clinic should be a part of routine protocol as the entry point into the primary-care setting. Many diseases can be prevented or forestalled by identifying and avoiding high-risk history and behaviors. Others can be treated in the early stages, reducing the risk of disability or death. Yearly physical assessments are the preferred means of identifying problems, but most people 65 years of age and over do not seek medical attention on an annual basis. As a result of initiatives implemented by the Surgeon General in the early 1980s, many agencies now offer preventive health programs, including screening for high-risk behaviors and the presence of disease.[11] The costs associated with the treatment of chronic disease are clearly not desirable in today's malnourished economy. Health screening and early detection of disease processes can reduce the costs substantially.

Screening programs for the elderly need to address behavior patterns such as smoking, level of activity, dietary habits, living environment, and health care needs such as dental and foot care, and immunization history. Screening programs are aimed at identifying any problems and addressing these problems from an educational perspective. Ideally, screening programs should have a follow-up mechanism or referral sources for evaluating and treating physical or medical problems identified during the screen. Screening programs for the elderly can be holistic, screening all systems of the body, or system/disease–specific (e.g., blood pressure screening, diabetes screening, cholesterol screening, dental screening).

Primary prevention screening programs should include such areas as immunizations, screening for falls and accident prevention, posture and flexibility assessment, nutritional considerations, screening for environmental modifications, and assessment of health-risk behaviors such as smoking, poor nutrition, inactivity, isolation, and other psychosocial factors. Secondary preventive screening focuses on early detection and treatment of disease and is particularly applicable in disorders such as hypertension, vision and hearing impairments, musculoskeletal problems, neuromuscular conditions, depression, and iatrogenic adverse drug effects. Tertiary preventive screening focuses on functional assessment and maximizing physical potential and environmental efficiency to prevent the progression of functional decline.

The U.S. Preventive Services Task Force[109,110] has identified screening interventions that successfully alter the outcomes of various diseases. Its recommendations emphasize the importance of educating the elderly population in modification of high-risk behaviors. For example, the task force advised that elderly individuals be given educational material about the benefits of physical activity in disease prevention and that guidance in selecting appropriate exercise levels and modes of exercise be provided individually to each person screened. Other components in the task force's recommendations include smoking cessation programs; dietary modification to prevent diseases associated with dietary excesses or imbalances (e.g., osteoporosis, heart disease, some cancers, cerebral vascular accidents, dental diseases); alcohol cessation programs when abuse is identified; home modification screening to reduce the potential for accidental injuries; vaccination programs for pneumococcal, influenza, and tetanus immunization; and screening for preventive "chemo-prophylaxis" programs such as low-dose aspirin therapy (e.g., 325 mg every other day) for those at risk for cardiovascular diseases and estrogen replacement therapy for women who are at increased risk for the development of osteoporosis.

Examination and Evaluation of the Elderly Patient

The long-term efficacy of interdisciplinary outpatient primary-care evaluation and management depends greatly on the screening information for high-risk elders that is gathered, subsequent referrals and interventions, and follow-up to determine the effectiveness of care provided.[14] Comprehensive and efficient primary geriatric care is provided through the process of geriatric assessment combined with traditional medical care. Comprehensive geriatric assessment is a structured approach to measuring physical, mental, and social functioning of older people to identify needs and to plan care.[83] It employs the team approach to the evaluation and management of the elderly patient with complex interdisciplinary health care needs and is accomplished through the use of an organized set of instruments to ensure that the assessment process is structured and quantitative, and expedites care.[41]

The four essential components of a comprehensive geriatric assessment are physical health, functional health, mental health, and social health. Assessment of a geriatric patient's physical health typically includes a geriatric medical history, a physical examination, and such tests as gait/falls/mobility and incontinence assessments. Assessments of functional health include the patient's ability to perform the activities of daily living, such as feeding himself or herself, dressing, and bathing, as well as the instrumental activities of daily living, which include such areas as light housework, yard work, money management, and transportation.

A comprehensive geriatric assessment also addresses an elderly patient's mental health, including a cognitive assessment to determine whether dementia or deliriums are present and an affect assessment to determine whether such mental disorders as depression are involved. Finally, the comprehensive assessment examines the patient's social health, including economic condition, the presence or absence of caregivers and their ability to give care, whether the patient has a health care proxy, and whether the patient has done needed estate planning.

Frail elderly patients may benefit from admission to an acute setting for inpatient comprehensive geriatric assessment when an outpatient assessment would require many clinic or office visits over the course of several weeks or months, during which time the patient might progressively deteriorate as a result of unresolved problems and be at great risk for further morbidity or even mortality. Thus the concept regarding admissions for "geriatric assessment" under Medicare is that of multiple diagnoses in frail elderly patients for whom the diagnostic sum is greater than its parts. That is, although no single diagnosis might justify the admission of an individual patient, a multitude of diagnoses might equal an "acute" admission because the sum of the complex problems results in a geometric increase in morbidity. Although hospitalization carries obvious risks, these might be outweighed by the benefits of a relatively quick and comprehensive evaluation of complex problems.

Medicare does not provide a diagnosis-related group (DRG) for geriatric assessment. Therefore the performance of geriatric assessment for Medicare beneficiaries must be an efficient and comprehensive process that does not prolong hospital length of stay. Some DRGs of the Medicare Prospective Payment system also can be employed for admitting these frail patients. DRG diagnoses such as change in mental status, Alzheimer's disease or senile dementia, dementia, urinary incontinence, sleep disorders, cachexia, malnutrition, or weight loss are applicable. If the PT performing the initial screening and assessment refers to other disciplines to address these diagnostic categories, admission for a more comprehensive assessment is a realistic goal. The most important aspect is documentation that clearly explains the acuity of the patient's condition, particularly from an expert geriatric rehabilitative perspective.

The major differences in evaluation of older individuals arise in the way one collects data, attention to detail in physical examination, and the high suspicion for disease required when nonspecific symptoms are encountered. Assessing in such detail undoubtedly takes more time, but the clinician who is familiar with evaluation of the elderly watches every interaction for subtle clues that might point toward a diagnosis. The possibility of successful therapeutic interventions in the geriatric population, especially when disease and dysfunction are detected early, should be adequate incentive to take the extra steps necessary for proper and comprehensive evaluation of the elderly individual.

Medical Diagnostic Challenges

For all disease states and in every older adult, the atypical presentation of illness cannot be overemphasized. In the aged, diseases may have unusual presentations with clinical symptoms and signs that can be confusing. Congestive heart failure, for example, often has the presenting problem of urinary incontinence. Elders rarely experience angina; rather, chest pain presents itself as shortness of breath. Hyperthyroidism may present as lethargy and intellectual blunting in what is termed the *apathetic hyperthyroid* state. At other times, disease may present nonspecifically as merely failure to thrive, anorexia, change in alertness, or, to the caregiver, as simply "a change."[60]

The classic signs and symptoms of disease may be absent in the elderly. It is not uncommon to find clinically important congestive heart failure without the presence of rales. The clinical signs of pulmonary consolidation occur much later in the aged in the presence of pneumonia as proven by fever, sputum production, and radiographic changes. An elderly individual's core temperature often runs lower than normal because of inactivity, a decrease in metabolic rate, and reduced neuroendocrine activity (see Chapter 7). The result is that *fevers* go undetected and elders are in the advanced stages of infection when the pathology is finally detected. Hypothyroidism may lack change in voice, skin findings, and constipation; and may produce confusion alone.[66,97]

Because of the often complex and atypical presentation of medical conditions in the elderly, the PT must be an astute observer. The old axiom *"when you hear hoof beats under your window, you should think of horses before you think of zebras,"*[95] does not hold true in elderly patients. Uncommon presentations of common medical conditions are a frequent occurrence in this population.[60,97] As PTs move toward establishing functional and physical-therapy diagnoses, it is imperative that they look beyond the obvious when assessing and diagnosing symptoms in this population.

Although most physical health problems seen in the elderly are not rare, the symptoms of illness often do not adhere to typical differential diagnostic algorithms. The PT especially

must consider the unusual when working with older adults with a history of reduced cognitive functioning or lack of ability to communicate verbally. One of the most common symptoms in an outpatient setting is a loss in cognitive ability or confusion. Patients or family members will often say, "I can't seem to think clearly," or "Dad hasn't been himself lately," or "Mom used to do this every day and now can't." These symptoms usually result from an alteration in mental status—a sentinel event for many underlying medical problems in the elderly. Although the most common fear is that the elder has suffered a stroke, other conditions are more often the underlying cause of a change in cognition or behavior. A sudden increase in restlessness, confusion, apathy, agitation, or lethargy can indicate an adverse change in physical status. Changes in sleeping patterns or decreased appetite also can signal underlying acute medical problems.

Because a change in mental status may be the presenting symptom of an underlying physical problem, the change should not automatically be considered neurologic in origin. Pre-existing impairments in speech, vision, or hearing can complicate the therapist's assessment of cognitive changes.

When a change in mental status occurs, one must differentiate dementia from delirium or depression. Delirium has an acute onset, most often related to a physical cause. Acute illness, medication toxicity, or other adverse drug interactions are often contributors to sudden confusion. If the accompanying physical condition is adequately treated, symptoms of delirium will disappear.

In contrast, dementia has a slower, progressively worsening onset. However, nutritional or neuroendocrine disorders such as a vitamin B_{12} deficiency or hypothyroidism can cause symptoms that mimic dementia; these should be ruled out in a differential diagnosis. Conversely, Alzheimer's disease, the most common type of dementia, has been linked to physical symptoms such as urinary incontinence and gait apraxia.[94]

Many cognitive, behavioral, and psychological tests are used in primary-care settings to screen for dementia.[66] Such instruments also may help to rule out depression as a cause for a change in mental status. In acute situations, using a few questions from the Mini Mental State Evaluation, such as asking the patient to identify the place and date and the current and immediate past president of the United States, can provide a brief assessment of cognition. A baseline evaluation and subsequent use of the entire scale are necessary to determine progression of dementia. Other tests, such as the 7-Minute Screen, have been shown to differentiate between normal cognition and the presence of dementia secondary to Alzheimer's disease.[98]

These are only a few examples of a long list of nonspecific and atypical presentations in the older adult.

Many drugs have paradoxical or bizarre side effects when given to the older adult. One should be suspicious of every drug the patient is taking, including over-the-counter medications, especially when CNS abnormalities are the problem. The interactions between drugs increase as the number of drugs increases, and the elderly are often taking multiple medicines (see Chapter 16).[10]

Psychosocial Issues of Aging

Depression

Depression has been termed the common cold of the elderly.[7,102] It is important for the primary-care PT to recognize depressive symptoms (see Chapters 5 and 7) because many elders see this as a character flaw and will not admit to feeling blue. Diagnosed depressive illness can be found in 5% to 65% of the older population, depending on the source cited.[30,48,102] Nevertheless, studies show that it is not aging per se that causes depression, but the added variables of cognitive impairment, incontinence, chronic conditions, and disabilities, as well as significant personal and emotional losses.[34]

Depression is usually associated with cognitive symptoms such as poor concentration, low self-esteem, indecisiveness, feelings of guilt, hopelessness, and, at its extreme, suicidal ideations.[102] Somatic symptoms often accompany depression in the elderly, and an atypical description of symptoms (see Chapter 6) should alert the therapist to explore for the presence of depression. Patients often report a combination of the following symptoms:

- Fatigue
- Altered sleep patterns
- Weight gain or loss
- Tearfulness
- Agitation
- Heart palpitations
- Nonspecific generalized weakness
- Sadness
- Anxiety
- Irritability
- Fear
- Anger
- Depersonalization
- Feelings of isolation

The primary-care therapist should understand some of the themes that emerge when working with the depressed older patient. Depression often will be concomitant with the elder's adjustment to new family roles, new body image, or increased dependency. Physical and functional losses have a significant effect on emotional well-being. Elderly patients often are grieving the many losses they experience throughout a lifetime of living. In screening an elderly patient population, determining the presence of depression will greatly affect subsequent treatment outcomes. The depressed older person often will be unmotivated and noncompliant with treatment recommendations because he or she fails to find value in *being*, and consequently sees little need for exercise, activity, or even attending physical-therapy sessions. See Chapter 4 for a description of communication strategies when working with a patient who is depressed and Chapter 5 for information about recognizing patients who may be considering suicide.

Dementia

Recognition and documentation of dementia in the primary-care setting have been found to be inconsistent, and such cognitive deficits often go undiagnosed in the early stages.[103]

Diagnosis of dementia in primary care is difficult but important.[24] Cognitive impairment in older primary-care patients has been found to have a tremendous effect on morbidity and mortality after controlling for the confounding effects of demographic and comorbid chronic conditions.[100] The mortality rate increases steeply with the degree of severity of dementia. In fact, the remaining life expectancy of the demented elder depends primarily on the severity of the dementia, the patient's age, and his or her general physical health.[24,100]

Dementias are characterized by a slow onset of increasing intellectual impairment, including disorientation, memory loss, reduced ability to reason and make sound judgments, loss of social skills, and development of regressed or antisocial behavior.[7] Depression often is superimposed on dementia as a reaction to the perceived loss of intellectual skills and leads to further cognitive impairment.[2]

Alzheimer's disease and multi-infarct dementia are the two most common forms of irreversible dementia. Each has a fairly characteristic pattern of onset and findings. Alzheimer's disease, involving multiple areas of cognition and function, usually begins gradually and is slowly progressive.[69] It is not associated with focal neurologic deficits or abrupt changes in severity. Patients typically begin with short-term memory deficits and progress to severely regressed behavior, an inability to learn or remember new tasks, and loss of ability to perform ADLs.[54] Early diagnosis is key because it can initiate the process of patients and family adapting to and managing disease symptoms.[69] Moreover, certain pharmacologic interventions can impede symptom progression and significantly improve quality of life. A spectrum of basic tests and instruments make clinical diagnosis of Alzheimer's possible in the primary-care setting.[69]

Multi-infarct dementia is usually of more rapid onset, occurs in younger individuals, and progresses in a step-wise fashion with abrupt worsening and subsequent plateaus of function. The patient often has focal neurologic deficits, such as paresis and paresthesias.[23] The individual often is hypertensive, has diabetes, or both, and also may show evidence of generalized atherosclerosis.[49]

It is important to distinguish between Alzheimer's and multi-infarct dementias. The prevention of recurrent cerebral infarction may arrest the progression of multi-infarct dementia, which has as its pathophysiological basis irreversible brain damage resulting from repetitive ischemic injury caused by emboli or bleeding. Normalization of blood pressure is the most effective intervention known. Other types of reversible dementia, such as those resulting from hypothyroidism, vitamin B_{12} deficiency, and normal pressure hydrocephalus, can become "fixed" and unresponsive to treatment unless identified and treated at an early stage. Early identification of these correctable dementias is essential, although no curative intervention currently is available for Alzheimer's disease.

Regardless of the etiology of dementia, when reversible causes have been ruled out, the main tasks of the clinical team are to minister to the patient's emotional needs, assist in the act of grieving for lost function, alter the environment so that the patient's remaining skills can be used, augment the patient's capacity to successfully undertake ADLs, educate the family, provide emotional and physical support to the family and caretakers, and give the patient and family a realistic prognosis. Any superimposed illness can cause a rapid and prolonged decline in mental status, which may totally resolve as the underlying illness is treated.

Elder Abuse

For many elders, the entry point into a primary-care setting unfortunately is the identification and the subsequent reporting of elder abuse. As the practice of rehabilitation typically involves development of an ongoing relationship with the patient and may also include frequent contact with the patient's families, PTs must know how to identify and effectively intervene in situations of suspected abuse.

The common types of elder maltreatment include caregiver neglect and self-neglect, emotional and psychological abuse, fiduciary exploitation, and physical abuse.[21] Elder abuse occurs most often in the home rather than institutional settings. Victims of elder abuse most likely know their perpetrator.[59,70] Potential risk factors for mistreatment of older people include age, race, low income, functional or cognitive impairment, a history of violence, and recent stressful events.[21,70] Both depression and dementia have been identified as particularly strong risk factors associated with abuse of the elderly.[4,28] The literature offers little information about the clinical profile of mistreated older people.

Assessment consists of a comprehensive history and physical examination, including scrutiny of the musculoskeletal system, neurologic and cognitive testing, and detailed social and sexual histories.[46] See Chapters 5 and 7 for additional information about screening for abuse. Clinical findings that cannot be explained medically may signal elder abuse. To properly intervene, clinicians should be familiar with state laws governing reporting procedures and patient privacy; in some states reporting is mandatory, whereas in others it may be voluntary.[17,108]

Common Medical Conditions in the Elderly

Although this chapter is not the place for an extensive review of pathologies associated with the aging process, the most common medical conditions are mentioned in the next section. For a more comprehensive review of pathologic manifestations of aging, see reference number 9 of this chapter.

As age advances there is a marked increase in many diseases, including hypertension, atherosclerosis, myocardial degeneration, arthritis, osteoporosis, cerebral vascular accidents, and cancers of all types. Rates of change in physiological function with age directly affect risk of age-related morbidities, such as changes in cognitive function, bone density, vital capacity, visual capacity, and blood pressure. Suppression in homeostatic functions, such as glucose tolerance, blood pressure stability, and balance also can result in significant pathologic consequences.[9]

This section will cover some of the more common conditions that affect functional activities of daily living.

Musculoskeletal Pathologies
Sarcopenia

Sarcopenia is an age-associated loss in lean muscle mass and results in a significant decrease in muscle power. This process starts earlier in the life cycle and is accelerated with inactivity. Although the condition itself is not considered pathologic, it can progress to the point that it affects functional capabilities such as standing, transfers, and ambulation, and increases the likelihood of falls.[9] Clinically, the surface muscle appear atrophied, and manual muscle tests reveal a decrease in maximal force produced. Patients often complain of poor endurance in activities such as walking or tasks that require repeated muscle activity.

Myopathy and Myositis

Myopathy, myositis, and other related muscle disorders in the elderly usually are the result of toxic or metabolic factors acting on the muscle rather than any intrinsic etiologies.[22] Hip-girdle weakness with difficulty rising from a chair and a waddling gait are symptoms suggesting myopathy. The weakness also may involve the shoulder girdle, with the individual complaining about an inability to lift items, especially above shoulder height. Myopathy typically does not present with muscle soreness, so the report of muscle pain indicates the possibility of the muscle inflammation associated with myositis. Polymyositis is not uncommon, and although the cause is usually idiopathic, it may result from underlying carcinoma, so one should refer the elder to the physician for further work-up. Fibromyalgia is another common form of non-articular rheumatism that can cause diffuse musculoskeletal aching and tender muscular trigger points, and would be part of the differential diagnostic consideration.[45]

Osteoporosis

With advancing age, increasing levels of bone loss can lead to osteoporosis. The presenting features of this disease are a decrease in height; postural changes including a forward head, kyphosis in the thoracic spine, a decrease in lordosis of the lumbar spine, and accommodative hip and knee flexion; the presence of a fracture with symptoms of pain and muscle splinting often is noted immediately over the site of fracture. The most common sites of fracture include the vertebral column (thoracic and lumbar), femur, and radius. Osteoporosis often is asymptomatic until the fracture occurs and a seemingly benign activity, such as leaning over to tie one's shoe, may be the precipitating event.[101]

Osteoporosis may not be a presenting diagnosis for the patient, but any patient with a history of chronic renal or gastrointestinal disease, rheumatoid arthritis, long-term corticosteroid use, or chronic alcohol abuse should be suspect for reduced bone density.

Osteomalacia

Other bone-related pathologies also affect the elderly more than other age groups. Osteomalacia is a softening of bone owing to poor mineralization generally associated with vitamin D and calcium deficiencies. Diagnosis often is delayed because of the initial presentation of fatigue and general, diffuse aching. In contrast to osteoporosis, other symptoms include weakness (proximal myopathy) and sensory polyneuropathies. Concomitant weight loss also is a presenting symptom, and osteomalacia often accompanies chronic gastrointestinal conditions such as irritable bowel syndrome or Crohn's disease.

Paget's Disease

Paget's disease is a disorder that results in the remodeling of bone characterized by increased bone resorption and bone formation. Although often asymptomatic and identified only by abnormal findings on plain films, symptomatic patients present with bone pain (often noted at night; see Chapter 6), pathologic fractures, and deformities in the long bones, clavicles, and skull. The long bones, such as the tibia or femur, may be bowed. Bony impingement on soft-tissue structures at the base of the skull may result in slurred speech, double vision, swallowing problems, and incontinence. In addition, these patients often complain of dizziness, vertigo, tinnitus, and hearing loss. Spinal-nerve entrapment syndromes may surface when the thoracic or lumbar vertebrae are involved. Another classic sign is hypervascularity of the skin covering the involved bones. Cardiac involvement ultimately resulting in heart failure also is associated with Paget's disease.

Osteoarthritis

Degenerative arthritis or osteoarthritis (OA) is characterized by an inflammation within the joint space that causes pain, loss of mobility, and deformity of the joint.[62] The joints most often affected by degenerative joint disease are the hands, knees, hips, lumbar spine, and cervical spine. It is manifested clinically by stiffness and pain that increase with use. Impaired mobility causes difficulty in performing routine activities of daily living (ADLs).[25]

The symptoms of osteoarthritis can occur insidiously or suddenly. Generally, joint destruction occurs gradually and progresses slowly. Pain is described as a deep ache, can occur at rest, and often awakens the individual at night. Stiffness of the involved joint(s) occurs after periods of inactivity and usually is resolved after a relatively short period of movement. Loss of flexibility is associated with soft-tissue contractures, intra-articular loose bodies, ostephytes, and loss of joint-surface congruity.[92] This condition is important to differentiate from joint rheumatic disorders that can cause rapid joint destruction.

Rheumatoid Arthritis

The initial manifestations of rheumatoid arthritis (RA) typically occur at younger ages, but as one ages the potential multisystem complications associated with this systemic illness can affect one's quality of life. RA typically is characterized by the abrupt onset of symmetric joint swelling, erythema, and pain. Inflammation of the synovial membrane results in the release of proteolytic enzymes that perpetuate inflammation and joint damage.[92] Symptoms usually are insidious and progress slowly as the disease progresses. Symptoms of joint pain, muscle

fatigue and weakness, weight loss, and general loss of stamina are common. Inflammation and musculoskeletal symptoms are localized to the specific joint, although multiple joints usually are involved. Morning stiffness is more pronounced and of longer duration than in osteoarthritis. Intense pain can occur after periods of rest. The involved joints tend to be the small joints of the hands and feet, the wrists, shoulders, elbows, hips, knees, and ankles. Essentially every joint is involved in this autoimmune, systemic condition. Eventually deformities occur, affecting mobility and basic ADLs. Rheumatoid arthritis is a systemic disease; therefore other signs and symptoms often are present, including: fever, fatigue, malaise, poor appetite, weight loss, nutritional deficiencies, weakness, anemia, enlarged spleen, and lymphadenopathy (disease of the lymph nodes), symptoms not typically associated with OA.[62]

Gout

Gout is a form of arthritis that usually affects only a few joints. Needle-like crystals of uric acid (monosodium urate crystals) are deposited in joints, tendons, and bursae; they incite a rapidly progressive inflammatory reaction. The result is the abrupt onset of severe pain and development of an acutely tender and inflamed joint (most often the first metatarsophalangeal, knee, wrist, and elbow) that can rapidly incapacitate the individual. In middle age, gout is episodic, but in later years it tends to occur with greater frequency and in more joints.[9] Gout tends to affect men more than women and occurs spontaneously or as a result of other illnesses or treatments. Some diuretics used to treat congestive heart failure or hypertension may cause gout because they interfere with the secretion of uric acid from the kidney, thereby causing an elevated level of uric acid. Other causes of gout include rapid tissue turnover, such as seen in lymphoma, leukemia, thalassemia, psoriasis, and pernicious anemia. Acidosis of any cause, such as in diabetes, alcohol abuse, or renal failure, also can precipitate gout. When crystals other than monosodium urate crystals are found, such as calcium pyrophosphate dihydrate crystals, the condition is called *pseudogout*.

Temporal Arteritis/Polymyalgia Rheumatica

Temporal arteritis and polymyalgia rheumatica are seen more often in older adult populations. Inflammation of small and medium-size arteries that are derived from the aortic arch give rise to a condition called giant cell arteritis or temporal arteritis (TA). This condition is part of a spectrum of conditions that include the entity of polymyalgia rheumatica (PMR), which is only seen in individuals over the age of 50.[9] Neck/shoulder and pelvic-girdle stiffness and pain, an elevated erythrocyte sedimentation rate, low-grade anemia, fever, weight loss, elevated globulins, and rapid response to steroids are the characteristics of polymyalgia rheumatica. Of the greatest clinical significance is the high incidence of sudden monocular blindness, which can result from the obliteration of the ophthalmic artery by the TA.[12] This potential outcome necessitates early and aggressive evaluation and treatment of anyone suspected of having PMR/TA. The diagnosis is established by biopsy of the temporal artery, looking for evidence of arteritis. Early diagnosis is important, because this is one of the most common preventable causes of blindness in the aged. Warning signs of this dangerous situation (TA) include sudden onset of a throbbing temporal headache, scalp sensitivity, and jaw claudication.

Spondyloarthropathies

Spondyloarthropathies are a group of disorders that include ankylosing spondylitis, Reiter's syndrome, and psoriatic arthritis. These conditions often begin at earlier ages, but all are more common in older adults.[92] Ankylosing spondylitis is an inflammatory arthropathy that involves the sacroiliac joints, apophyseal joints, intervertebral disc articulations, and the costovertebral joints. This pathology also can affect the large peripheral joints, including the hip, knee, and shoulder.[92] Ultimately, this disorder leads to fibrosis, calcification, and ossification of the involved joints and is associated with a marked loss of functional mobility. The onset is insidious back pain and stiffness with pain described as an ache. These patients experience considerable morning stiffness that is reduced with activity and increased with rest. The recumbent position is not tolerated well. As the disease progresses, the cervical and thoracic spines and the chest cage become involved. Radiating pain generally is reported in the lower and upper extremities as spinal mobility is compromised. Symptoms of pain usually are accompanied by symptoms of weight loss, fever, and fatigue. As the spine fuses, the patient is at risk for developing osteoporosis and fracture, especially of the lower cervical spine.

Reiter's syndrome is a reactive arthritis in which an inflammatory arthropathy follows an infective process, such as bacillary dysentery or venereal disease. A triad of symptoms is associated with this syndrome, including urethritis and conjunctivitis, which occur early in the disease, and arthritis, which is typically asymmetric and involves the joints of the lower extremities.[53] The digits, especially the toes, can become swollen and distended (dactylitis). The arthritis can progress and spread to the spine and the upper extremities. Other potential manifestations include mouth ulcers, skin rashes, and inflammation of the glans penis or clitoris. Low back pain is a common symptom.[53]

Psoriatic arthritis is an inflammatory joint disorder affecting individuals with psoriasis. It leads to erosion of the periarticular bone and significant joint destruction. There is a lymphocyte infiltration into the synovium and the appearance of edematous granulation tissue that leads to thickening of the synovium. As the disease progresses, the joint space often is lost to the build-up of dense fibrous tissue. The distal interphalangeal joints of the hands and feet are involved most often, with concomitant joint deformities (e.g., claw deformity) and flexor tenosynovitis. Pitting of the nail beds also is commonly associated with psoriatic arthritis and may be noted during the history-taking process (see Chapter 8). The sacroiliac joint also can be involved and typically is involved unilaterally. Other problems associated with psoriasis include inflammatory eye disease, including conjunctivitis and iritis; renal disease; mitral valve prolapse; and aortic regurgitation.

Cardiovascular Pathologies

Ischemic Heart Disease

Ischemic heart disease, commonly called *coronary artery disease* (CAD), results from blockage of blood flow to cardiac muscle. Gross obstruction of the major coronary vessels results in anginal pain typically brought on by vigorous exercise.[29] In the elderly, however, anginal pain is not a consistent symptomatic indicator of ischemia of the cardiac tissue. The elderly more often report dyspnea (shortness of breath). Clinically, shortness of breath is a much more reliable indicator of ischemia than anginal pain in the elderly individual.[31] ST-segment depression on the ECG generally correlates with the onset of anginal symptoms, although in the elderly, marked ST-segment depression occurs with dyspnea without the development of the characteristic anginal pain.[31]

Cardiomyopathies

Cardiomyopathies are conditions in which the heart muscle hypertrophies and cardiac function is impaired, often resulting in congestive heart failure.[84] The weakening results in dilation of the heart and can lead to congestive heart failure because the heart cannot contract strongly enough to empty a sufficient amount of blood into the peripheral vasculature to meet the body's needs. The hypertrophied heart is stiff and does not easily fill with blood. As a result, the heart contracts vigorously, but there is little forward circulation to show for the effort, and the body's energy and oxygen needs are not met.

In hypertrophic cardiomyopathy, the muscle abnormally contracts, actually creating an obstruction to the outflow of blood from the heart. The more strongly the heart contracts, the greater is the obstruction. In dilated cardiomyopathies, the heart is not strong enough to move blood against the pressure in the blood vessels.[61] As a result, fluid builds up in the pulmonary circulation, causing pulmonary edema, difficult breathing, low blood oxygen, and further difficulty in meeting the metabolic needs of the contracting cardiac muscle. Manifestations of cardiomyopathy generally are similar to those of heart failure: dyspnea, orthopnea, tachycardia, palpitations, peripheral edema, and distended jugular vein.

Conduction System Diseases

Conduction system diseases are those that affect the rate and rhythm of the heart's contractions.[84] The electrical wave that results in the coordinated contraction of the heart muscle is propagated in the two pacemaker sites in the heart and carried along specialized pathways that spread the wave throughout the heart, also known as the conduction system. The pacemakers and pathways can be damaged by many different agents, including those that result in cardiomyopathies and myocardial infarction. The most common consequences of pacemaker dysfunction are extremely rapid (tachycardic) contractions, poorly coordinated (dysrhythmic) contractions, or extremely slow (bradycardic) contractions that are less effective in moving blood and result in reduced cardiac output.[84] Low cardiac output can result in confusion, fatigue, poor exercise tolerance, and congestive heart failure. Rapid reductions in cardiac output can cause syncope.

Valvular disease of the heart involves the heart valves, which function to keep the blood flowing in one direction. Defects of the heart valves are of two types: stenosis or narrowing of the valve, restricting blood flow,[84] and insufficiency or regurgitation, resulting in the backward flow of blood. Both conditions increase the workload on the heart and greatly reduce its efficiency.[96]

Two valves, the mitral and aortic valves, are affected most often. Of the two, the aortic valve is involved more often in the elderly, with aortic stenosis usually being asymptomatic until middle or old age. Aortic-valve disease is common in the aged and results from rheumatic valve disease, which increases damage to a congenitally malformed valve, or the progression of age-related injury to an otherwise normal valve.[93] The latter results from the gradual build-up of scar tissue and calcium on the valve leaflets as part of the normal aging of the valve. The most clinically significant lesion is stenosis of the aortic valve. This results in a progressive increase in resistance to the flow of blood out of the heart, and, as a result, the heart pumps blood against increasingly greater afterload.[84] Patients can experience angina even without coronary artery disease, because even normal coronary arteries are unable to deliver sufficient blood to meet the metabolic demands of the overtaxed heart muscle. As the stenosis increases, transient decreases in cardiac output caused by arrhythmias or ischemia result in syncope.[96] Finally, when the heart is no longer able to compensate by hypertrophy for the increasing resistance to flow, congestive heart failure supervenes. See Chapter 9 for a description of auscultation as a clinical tool that may detect the abnormality before any symptoms are noted.

Rheumatic Valve Disease

Rheumatic valve disease, caused by earlier episodes of rheumatic fever, is the most common cause of mitral stenosis and insufficiency in the aged.[93] Congestive heart failure, arrhythmias, and embolization of blood clots from the heart to the brain and other organs are the most common complications associated with mitral valve disease. These patients require attentive medical management, including the use of anticoagulants to prevent emboli, diuretics to control congestive heart failure, and digitalis or other medications to control the heart rate.[84] Nutritional support often is required to ensure compliance with a low-sodium diet. Protective intervention should focus on skin protection and maintenance of maximal functional capabilities, with close monitoring of the older person's vital signs (see Chapter 9) and subjective responses of perceived tolerance to increasing activity levels.

Endocarditis

Infection of the heart valve, or endocarditis, is a rare but significant illness in the aged.[84] This is due not only to its potential for causing death or severe disability but also to its subtle presentation. Lethargy, fatigue, anorexia, failure to thrive, anemia, worsening congestive heart failure, progressive renal failure, low-grade fever, embolic stroke or transient ischemic attack,

worsening control of diabetes, and development of a new heart murmur all are potentially caused by bacterial endocarditis.[93]

Hypertension

Hypertension is another common condition affecting the cardiovascular system. The aged with systolic blood pressures above 160 mm Hg and diastolic pressures above 95 mm Hg clearly are at increased risk for stroke, congestive heart failure (hypertensive cardiomyopathy), and renal failure. Isolated systolic hypertension carries a similar risk,[84] because much of the cardiovascular morbidity and mortality in the elderly is related to hypertension. See Chapter 9 for a detailed discussion of hypertension and the assessment of blood pressure and other related vascular measures.

Myocardial Degeneration

Myocardial degeneration is the general decline of cardiac performance with age and with inactivity; it affects elderly individuals' ability to function at their maximum. The recognized changes in cardiac function include a decrease in right ventricular work rate and a variable change of left ventricular work rate, depending on the relative magnitudes of the reduction in maximum cardiac output and the increase of systemic blood pressure.[96] Symptoms of shortness of breath in the elderly often reflect problems with getting enough oxygen to the working muscle through a failing circulatory system.

Individuals with a seriously reduced cardiac reserve report a marked need for rest after even mild physical activity.[9] In addition to persistent and undue fatigue, an inadequate cardiac response to exercise usually causes acute shortness of breath (dyspnea), while a restriction of blood flow to the heart itself may produce anginal pain. Inadequate blood flow to the peripheral tissues may give the skin a bluish hue (peripheral cyanosis). The pulse rate typically rises over the day, with a slow and incomplete recovery during rest pauses.[96] Activities of daily living are notably difficult for these elderly individuals. Lying down can induce a sharp recurrence or increase of dyspnea and create a "fear of sleeping" that further aggravates the severe fatigue experienced on minimal activity by an individual with myocardial degeneration.

Respiratory Pathologies
Pneumonia

Pneumonia is the most common infectious cause of death in the elderly[44] and the most common infection requiring hospitalization. The increased incidence of pneumonia with aging is due in part to the weakening of the local pulmonary defenses; however, the high mortality of pneumonia is largely due to its more subtle and atypical presentation in the elderly. Typical symptoms such as a productive cough, fever, and pleuritic chest pain often are absent, but subtler symptoms, such as confusion, alteration of sleep-wake cycles, increased congestive heart failure, anorexia, and failure to thrive, are more common. Noting any of the above manifestations in the elderly should prompt the therapist to auscultate the chest wall (see Chapter 9).

Obstructive Airway Disease

Conditions that cause obstruction to air flow within the lungs are called obstructive airway diseases, while conditions that cause resistance to air flow are called resistive airway diseases. They share the common characteristic of increased resistance to air flow within the airways.[61] Chronic obstructive pulmonary disease (COPD) includes conditions of increased airway resistance that are irreversible because of permanent structural damage and obstruction resulting from cigarette smoking, infections, toxic exposures, or any combination of these. *Emphysema* is a term used to describe the permanent destruction of alveoli with the resulting expansion of the remaining alveoli. A consequence of emphysema is a reduction in the area in which gas exchange can occur. This causes a perfusion/ventilation mismatch and hypoxia. Emphysema is associated with increased airway resistance resulting from collapse of small airways.

Chronic bronchitis is a different disease process in which there is chronic inflammation of the small airways, with resulting increased mucus, airway plugging, and destruction of small airways.[44] As a consequence, air flow is reduced because of permanent narrowing of the small airways. There is often a reversible component of the airway obstruction superimposed on the chronic changes. Cigarette smoking is the leading cause of chronic bronchitis and multiplies the deleterious effects of other environmental agents, such as asbestos, silica, coal dust, and fibers. Emphysema and chronic bronchitis often coexist.

Patients with obstructive airway diseases usually manifest disabilities that result from hypoxia, hypercapnia, or dyspnea. Both hypoxia and hypercapnia can cause confusion, fatigue, and worsening heart failure. Breathlessness, or dyspnea, is usually the most limiting symptom of COPD. Functional impairment caused by COPD can be severe, and COPD often is fatal. See Chapter 7 for detailed discussion of symptoms associated with pulmonary disorders and Chapter 9 for a discussion of auscultation for pulmonary disorders.

Neurologic and Neurosensory Pathologies

Parkinson's Disease

Parkinson's disease (PD) is the most common type of parkinsonism, a clinical syndrome caused by lesions in the basal ganglia, predominantly in the substantia nigra, that produce deficits in motor behavior.[106] Parkinsonism is a clinical rather than an etiologic entity because it is associated with several pathologic processes that damage the extrapyramidal system.[106] This syndrome results in a reduction in muscle power, rigidity, and slowness of movement (akinesia). There is a characteristic tetrad of symptoms, including resting tremor, cogwheel rigidity, bradykinesia or akinesia, and an impairment in postural reflexes. Of this tetrad, only resting tremor is truly suggestive of PD, an early sign that may remain prominent even late in the disorder.[1] The others occur in varying degrees in other forms of parkinsonism.

Because the onset of PD is typically in the fifth or sixth decade of life and is progressive, the complications of the aging process are superimposed on the progression of this disease. Lack of mobility, loss of balance, and weakness result in more falls. The complications of immobility such as osteoporosis, cardiovascular deconditioning, muscle weakness, and loss of flexibility are other considerations in the treatment of patients with PD. Despite the progressive nature of this illness, many patients can maintain full function for several decades with a combination of physical and occupational therapy and drug intervention.[106]

Cervical Spondylosis

Cervical spondylosis, another pathology often seen in an elderly population, is caused by impingement on the cervical spinal cord by bony spurs resulting from severe degenerative arthritis.[61] Because patients usually develop a clumsy, spastic, and stiff gait, incontinence, and reduced sensation in the lower extremities, this condition can be overlooked while other neurologic disorders are considered first in the diagnostic process. Causing confusion is that the patient may present with few if any cervical-spine symptoms other than a little stiffness. Cervical computed tomography scanning, myelograms, and magnetic resonance imaging (MRI) can establish the location and extent of spinal-cord impingement.

Peripheral Nervous System Disorders

Peripheral nervous system disorders often are diagnosed in an aged population. With aging, the number and size of peripheral nerve fibers diminish with a concomitant decrease in conduction velocity.[6] There is often a clinically insignificant decrease in touch and vibration sense. The peripheral nerves, however, are easily affected by nutritional deficiencies, toxins, and endocrine disorders.[93] The resulting neuropathies can cause marked loss of position sense, resulting in instability, falls, chronic pain,[64] and dysesthesia (painful and persistent sensation induced by a gentle touch of the skin).

A common example is diabetic neuropathy, which can take several forms. There is a distal sensory polyneuropathy that affects the hands and feet, with diminished sensation and burning pain; a proximal motor neuropathy resulting in proximal muscle wasting and weakness; and a diffuse autonomic neuropathy resulting in orthostatic hypotension, neurogenic bladder, obstipation (intractable constipation), and bowel immotility.[43] In addition to these diffuse forms of neuropathy, single nerves can be affected. The resulting mononeuropathies can cause loss of ocular muscle function and painful nerve root and branch dysfunction wherever an involved nerve travels.

Vestibular Disorders

Vestibular symptoms have been reported in more than 50% of elderly people.[16] The central mechanisms that are involved in the control of balance do not appear to change excessively with age but are more likely to be affected by degenerative neurologic diseases such as Alzheimer's or Parkinson's disease. However, age-related changes in the peripheral vestibular system do occur. Hair cell receptors decrease in number, and there is a loss of the vestibular receptor ganglion cells. The myelinated nerve cells of the vestibular system decrease by as much as 40%.

There is a reported increase in the incidence of *benign paroxysmal positioning vertigo* (BPPV) with symptoms of dizziness with head movements. This may be due to an increase in the deposits in the posterior semicircular canal. Partial loss of vestibular function in the elderly can lead to symptoms of dizziness, with less ability of the nervous system to accommodate to positional changes.[16] Coupled with the vestibular losses, there is concomitant loss in vision and somatosensation, which severely affects sensory input used in the maintenance of balance.

Various pathologic conditions can affect the peripheral vestibular system, producing vertigo or disequilibrium. Benign paroxysmal positional vertigo is the most common cause of vertigo with changes in head position in an older-adult population. BPPV generally is associated with the deposition of otoconial material in the cupula of the posterior semicircular canal. The otoliths adhere to the cupula in some cases and retard its return to a resting position after head rotation, or obstruct the flow of endolymph, producing symptoms from the affected posterior semicircular canal by impeding or stopping stimulation to the vestibular nerve. The condition can be unilateral or bilateral. Prolonged inactivity also can lead to symptoms of BPPV.

Acute vestibular neuritis, also known as *labyrinthitis*, is the second-most-common cause of vertigo in the elderly.[35] It is associated with a viral infection that causes inflammatory changes of branches of the vestibular nerve. In the elderly, the onset usually is preceded by upper-respiratory-tract or gastrointestinal-tract infections. The chief symptom is the acute onset of prolonged severe rotational vertigo that is exacerbated by movement of the head. Symptoms include spontaneous horizontal-rotatory nystagmus with beating toward the good ear, postural imbalance, and nausea.[35] Antiviral medications are used in this condition, and habituation exercises help to resolve this condition quickly after the infection clears.

Ménière's disease is a disorder of the inner-ear function that can cause hearing problems and vestibular symptoms in the elderly.[35] The patient complains of a sensation of fullness of the ear, a reduced ability to hear, and tinnitus. These symptoms are accompanied by rotational vertigo, postural imbalance, nystagmus, and nausea and vomiting, which can last for long periods of time. A phenomenon identified in Ménière's disease is *endolymphatic hydrops*, a condition in which malabsorption of endolymph results in an increase in endolymphatic fluid pressure in the endolymphatic duct and sac.

Bilateral vestibular disorders may occur secondary to other diseases or could be drug induced in the elderly. Conditions that may lead to vestibular problems include meningitis, labyrinthine infections, otosclerosis, Paget's disease, polyneuropathy, bilateral tumors (acoustic neuromas in neurofibromatosis), endolymphatic hydrops, bilateral vestibular neuritis, cerebral hemosiderosis, ototoxic drugs, inner-ear autoimmune disease, or congenital malformations of the inner ear.[35] Autoimmune conditions such as rheumatoid arthritis, psoriasis, ulcerative colitis, and Cogan's syndrome (iritis accompanied by vertigo and sensorineural hearing loss) can lead to a progressive, bilateral sensorineural hearing loss often accompanied by bilateral loss in vestibular function. In addition, the toxic effects of alcohol may cause an acute vertigo as the dehydration created by alcoholic substances may change the specific gravity of the endolymph. Other agents that may cause vertigo include organic compounds of heavy metals and aminoglycosides.[35]

PTs are well trained to assist in the differential diagnostic process when faced with symptoms of dizziness and then to provide the necessary rehabilitation for these patients.

Endrocrine Pathologies

Diabetes Mellitus

Diabetes mellitus is a chronic endocrine disease that affects a significant number of elderly people in the United States.[43] The complex nature of diabetes creates a broad spectrum of physical complications and reactions, which can make the condition extremely dangerous. Diabetes is the leading cause of blindness and can cause glaucoma and cataracts. People with diabetes are twice as likely to have heart attacks and strokes, five times more prone to foot ulceration with the development of gangrene, and 17 times more prone to kidney disease compared with the general population.[57] Complications of diabetes also affect the mouth, reproductive system, nervous system, vascular system, muscular system, and skin. They also reduce an individual's defense mechanisms against infection.

Symptoms of diabetes include increased urination, thirst, hunger, fatigue, and lethargy; weight loss; and numbness or tingling in the feet and hands. Although no clear understanding of the cause of diabetes has been found and there is no cure, the disease has been found to be controllable by achieving and maintaining normal levels of blood glucose.[43] This requires a careful balance of four critical components: diet, exercise, education for self monitoring, and drug therapy.

Signs of *hyperglycemia* may be caused by a missed insulin dose, overeating, failure to follow the diabetic diet, or a fever or infection. These signs include excessive thirst, urination, dry mouth, drowsiness, flushed, dry skin, fruitlike breath odor, stomach ache, nausea, vomiting, and difficulty in breathing.

Signs of *hypoglycemia* may be caused by excessive insulin, skipping of a snack or meal, sickness, excessive exercise, drinking of alcoholic beverages, or taking of medications that contain alcohol. Symptoms include anxiety, chills, cold sweats, cool, pale skin, confusion, drowsiness, excessive hunger, headache, nausea, nervousness, shakiness, vision changes, and unusual tiredness or fatigue. If these symptoms occur, the consumption of a sugar-containing food (e.g., orange juice or honey) should reverse the symptoms.

Thyroid Disease

Diseases of the thyroid gland, although more often diagnosed at younger ages, are more common in the elderly population. Significant morbidity and even death can result from both excessive and insufficient thyroid hormone. In both hyperthyroidism and hypothyroidism, the presentation of the syndrome can be very different in the aged from its presentation in younger patients. As is the rule in most illnesses in the aged, the presentation is usually more subtle, and the symptoms and signs are less specific.[76]

Hypothyroidism is common in the aged and results from failure of the thyroid gland to elaborate sufficient thyroid hormone despite maximum stimulation of the gland by TSH.[87] Vague symptoms, such as the following, abound:

- Dry skin
- Chronic muscle and joint pains
- Lethargy
- Confusion
- Weight gain
- Edema
- Depression
- Apathy
- Sensitivity to sedatives
- Cold intolerance

Patients with severe hypothyroidism develop hypothermia and have cognitive dysfunction resembling dementia. These hypofunctions are seen most often in the hospitalized elderly patient who experiences the stress of surgery or other acute illness. Subtler abnormalities, such as pseudo dementia, depression, and lethargy, are more common in ambulatory patients.

In the aged, *hyperthyroidism* results most often from an excess of thyroid hormone released from a multinodular goiter. Although many symptoms of hyperthyroidism in the aged are similar to those in the younger patient, they usually are subtler. Common manifestations include the development of glucose intolerance (diabetes mellitus), congestive heart failure, atrial fibrillation, muscle weakness, weight loss, diarrhea, and agitation. However, there is a small group of the aged with "apathetic hyperthyroidism," in which the presentation of disease is diametrically different from the usual.[77] These individuals show depression, apathy, failure to thrive, and constipation. Although their symptoms are similar to those of patients with hypothyroidism, correction of the elevated thyroid hormone level abolishes the symptoms.

Summary

If the unprecedented increase in life expectancy has a down side, it is the increased risk of chronic age-related disorders. As clinicians work to foster healthy aging, we must seek ways to prevent the disabling disorders that keep many older people from enjoying their longevity. The high prevalence of chronic illness and functional limitation among older individuals underscores the need for strategically directed health and social services.[15] Under a primary-care model of geriatric intervention, successful patient management must extend beyond diagnosis and disease treatment and include promotion of function and prevention of decline. Achieving this goal requires a seamless continuum of management and interdisciplinary care. We also must focus on improving the understanding of the science of aging so that preventive approaches can be employed to prevent the development of chronic illness and disability.

This chapter has addressed primary-care considerations important for the outpatient PT treating elderly patients. Emphasis has been placed on the need to develop clinical decision-making skills necessary for the provision of safe, effective, and efficient physical-therapy examination and intervention in a geriatric population. The distinctions between normal and pathologic aging have been explored, with emphasis on the need to improve clinical examination and treatment skills in working with this very diverse population. Working definitions of the concepts of frailty and wellness have been presented and will be important as the PT communicates with others involved in the care of this population. Common musculoskeletal, cardiovascular, respiratory, neurologic, neurosensory, and endocrine pathologies seen in elderly patients were presented. Screening and therapeutic interventions that address the prevention of ill health also have been addressed. Medical diagnostic challenges such as multisystem involvement, multipharmacy, sudden changes in cognition, poor nutrition, and poor fitness levels were explored to assist the reader in developing skills for accurately assessing an elderly population in a primary-care setting.

REFERENCES

1. Adams RD, Victor M, Ropper AH. *Principles of neurology.* Ed 6, New York, 1997, McGraw-Hill, pp 1067-1078.
2. Alexopoulos GS, Abrams RC, Young RC, et al: Cornell scale for depression in dementia, *Biol Psychiatr* 23:271-284, 1988.
3. American Physical Therapy Association: *The guide to physical therapist practice,* ed 2, Alexandria, Va, 2001, APTA.
4. Anetzberger GJ, Palmisano BR, Sanders M, et al: A model of intervention for elder abuse and dementia, *Gerontologist* 40:492-497, 2000.
5. Bailey ML: Care coordination in managed care. Creating a quality - continuum for high risk elderly patients, *Nurs Case Manag* 3:172-180, 1998.
6. Baloh RW: Neurology of aging: vestibular system. In Albert ML, ed: *Clinical neurology of aging.* New York, 1984, Oxford University Press.
7. Bettes S: Depression: the "common cold" of the elderly, *Generations* 3:15, 1979.
8. Bottomley JM: Principles and practice in geriatric rehabilitation. In Bottomley JM and Lewis CB: *Geriatric rehabilitation: a clinical approach,* ed 2, Upper Saddleback, NJ, 2003, Prentice Hall Publishers, pp 292-328.
9. Bottomley JM: Pathological manifestations of aging. In Bottomley JM, Lewis CB: *Geriatric rehabilitation: a clinical approach,* ed 2, Upper Saddleback, NJ, 2003, Prentice Hall Publishers, pp 76-100.
10. Bottomley JM, Lewis CB: Pharmacology. In Bottomley JM and Lewis CB: *Geriatric rehabilitation: a clinical approach,* ed 2, Upper Saddleback, NJ, 2003, Prentice Hall Publishers, pp 247-291.
11. Bottomley JM: Establishing community based screening programs. In Bottomley JM, Lewis CB: *Geriatric rehabilitation: a clinical approach,* ed 2, Upper Saddleback, NJ, 2003, Prentice Hall Publishers, pp 528-548.
12. Boyer GG: Vision problems. In Camevali E, Patrick C, eds: *Nursing management for the elderly,* Philadelphia, 1989, JB Lippincott.
13. Buchner DM, Wagner EH: Preventing frail health, *Clin Geriatr Med* 8:1-17, 1992.
14. Burns R, Nichols LO, Martindale-Adams J, et al: Interdisciplinary geriatric primary care evaluation and management: two-year outcomes, *J Am Geriatr Soc* 48:8-13, 2000.
15. Cassel CK: Successful aging. How increased life expectancy and medical advances are changing geriatric care, *Geriatrics* 56:35-39, 2001.
16. Chandler JM, Duncan PW: Balance and falls in the elderly: issues in evaluation and treatment. In Guccione AA, ed: *Geriatric physical therapy,* St Louis, 1993, Mosby-Year Book, pp 237-252.
17. Ciolek DE, Ciolek CH: *Guidelines for recognizing and providing care for victims of elder abuse and neglect,* Alexandria, VA, 1999, Section on Geriatrics—American Physical Therapy Association.
18. Cohen HJ, Feusser JR, Weinberger M, et al: A controlled trial of inpatient and outpatient geriatric evaluation and management, *N Engl J Med* 346:905-912, 2002.
19. Coleman EA, Wagner EH, Grothaus LC, et al: Predicting hospitalization and functional decline in older health plan enrollees: are administrative data as accurate as self-report? *J Am Geriatr Soc* 46:534-535, 1998.
20. Coleman EA, Grothaus LC, Sandhu N, et al: Chronic care clinics: a randomized controlled trial of a new model of primary care for frail older adults, *J Am Geriatr Soc* 47:775-783, 1999.

21. Collins KA, Bennett AT, Hanzlick R: Elder abuse and neglect. Autopsy Committee of the College of American Pathologists, *Arch Intern Med* 160:1567-1568, 2000.

22. Cress ME, Schultz E: Aging muscle: functional, morphologic, biochemical, and regenerative capacity, *Top Geriatric Rehabil* 11-19, 1985.

23. Cummings JL, Miller B, Hill MA, et al: Neuropsychiatric aspects of multi-infarct dementia and dementia of the Alzheimer type, *Arch Neurol* 44:389-393, 1987.

24. De Lepeleire J, Heyrman J: Diagnosis and management of dementia in primary care at an early stage: the need for a new concept and an adapted procedure, *Theor Med Bioeth* 20:215-228, 1999.

25. Donatelli R, Owens-Burkart H: Effects of immobilization on the extensibility of periarticular connective tissue, *J Orthop Sport Phys Ther* 3:67-71, 1981.

26. Duerksen DR, Yeo TA, Siemens JL, et al: The validity and reproducibility of clinical assessment of nutritional status in the elderly, *Nutrition* 16:740-744, 2000.

27. Dychtwald K: "Age power": how the new-old will transform medicine in the 21st century, *Geriatrics* 54:22-27, 1999.

28. Dyer CB, Pavlik VN, Murphy KP, et al: The high prevalence of depression and dementia in elder abuse or neglect, *J Am Geriatr Soc* 48:205-208, 2000.

29. Ellestad MH: *Stress testing-principles and practice*, ed 2, Philadelphia, 1985, Davis.

30. Epstein L: Symposium of age differentiation in depressive illness: depression in the elderly, *J Gerontol* 31:278, 1976.

31. Ewing DJ, Campbell IN, Clarke BF: Heart-rate response to standing as a test for automatic neuropathy, *Br Med J* 1(6128):1700, 1978.

32. Exton-Smith AN: The problem of subclinical malnutrition in the elderly. In Exton-Smith AN, Scott DL, eds: *Vitamins in the elderly*, Bristol, U.K., 1968, Wright and Sons, pp 12-18.

33. Farley DO, Zellman G, Ouslander JG, et al: Use of primary care teams by HMOs for care of long-stay nursing home residents, *J Am Geriatr Soc* 47:139-144, 1999.

34. Ferucci LI, Guralnik J, Marchionni N, et al: Aging and prevalence of depression, *Gerontologist* 30:314A, October, 1990.

35. Fetter M: Vestibular system disorders. In Herdman SJ, ed: *Vestibular rehabilitation*, Philadelphia, 1994, FA Davis, pp 80-89.

36. Fiatarone MA, O'Neill EF, Ryan ND, et al: Exercise training and nutritional supplementation for physical frailty in very elderly people, *N Engl J Med* 330:1769-1775, 1994.

37. Fillet HM, Picariello GP, Warburton SW: Health risk appraisals in the elderly: results from a survey of 70,000 Medicare HMO members, *J Clin Outcomes Meas* 4:23-29, 1997.

38. Fillet HM, Gutterman R, Orland BI, et al: Polypharmacy management in Medicare managed care: changes in prescribing by primary care physicians resulting from a program promoting medication reviews, *Am J Manag Care* 5:587-594, 1999.

39. Fried LP, Guralnik JM: Disability in older adults: evidence regarding significance, etiology, and risk, *J Am Geriatr Soc* 45:92-100, 1997.

40. Fried TR, Mor V: Frailty and hospitalization of long-term stay nursing home residents, *J Am Geriatr Soc* 45:265-269, 1997.

41. Fulmer T, Gallo JJ, Paveza GJ, et al: *Handbook of geriatric assessment*, ed 3, Gaithersburg, MD, 2000, Aspen Publishers.

42. Gambert SR, Guansing AR: Protein-calorie malnutrition in the elderly, *J Am Geriatr Soc* 28:272-275, 1980.

43. Gambert SR: *Diabetes mellitus in the elderly: a practical guide*, New York, 1990, Raven Press.

44. Gladman JRF, Barer D, Venkatesan P, et al: The outcome of pneumonia in the elderly: a hospital survey, *Clin Rehabil* 5:201-204, 1991.

45. Gowin KM: Diffuse pain syndromes in the elderly, *Rheum Dis Clin North Am* 26:673-682, 2000.

46. Gray-Vickery P: Recognizing elder abuse, *Nursing* 29:52-53, 1999.

47. Gupta S, Rappaport HM, Bennett LT: Polypharmacy among nursing home geriatric Medicaid recipients, *Ann Pharmacother* 30:946-950, 1996.

48. Gurland B: The comparative frequency of depression in various adult age groups, *J Gerontol* 31:283-292, 1976.

49. Hachinski VC, Illiff LD, Zilhka E, et al. Cerebral blood flow in dementia, *Arch Neurol* 32:632-637, 1975.

50. Ham RJ, Marcy ML, Holtzman JM: The aging process: biological and social aspects. In Wright J, ed: *Primary care geriatrics*, Boston, 1983, PSG.

51. Hamerman D: Geriatric practice revisited: toward collaboration with primary care medicine, *J Am Geriatr Soc* 50:971-972, 2002.

52. Hanlon JT, Schmader KE, Koronkowski MJ, et al: Adverse drug events in high risk older populations, *J Am Geriatr Soc* 45:945-958, 1997.

53. Hellman DB: Arthritis and musculoskeletal disorders. In Tierney LM, McPhee SJ, Papadakis MA, eds: *Current medical diagnosis and treatment*, ed 34, Norwalk, CT, 1995, Appleton & Lange, pp 726-732.

54. Hughes CP, Berg L, Danziger WL, et al: A new clinical scale for the staging of dementia, *Br J Psychiatr* 140:566-572, 1982.

55. Iezzoni LI: Assessing quality using administrative data, *Ann Intern Med* 127:666-674, 1997.

56. Inouye SK, Wagner DR, Acampora D: A predictive index for functional decline in hospitalized elderly medical patients, *J Intern Med* 8:645-652, 1993.

57. Jackson RA: Mechanisms of age-related glucose intolerance, *Diabetes Care* 13(suppl 2):9-19, 1990.

58. Johnson HA: Is aging physiological or pathological? In Johnson HA, ed: *Relations between normal aging and disease*, Aging Series vol 28, New York, 1985, Raven Press, pp 239-247.

59. Jogerst GJ, Dawson JD, Hartz AJ, et al: Community characteristics associated with elder abuse, *J Am Geriatr Soc* 48:513-518, 2000.

60. Keen P: Atypical presentation of medical conditions in the elderly, American Academy of Nurse Practitioners Sixteenth Annual National Conference, conference proceedings, programs, and abstracts, Austin, Tex., June 28-July 1, 2001, Medscape Portals.

61. Kenney RA: *Physiology of aging: a synopsis*, Chicago, 1982, Year Book Medical Publishers.

62. Klein FA, Rajan RK: Normal aging: effects on connective tissue metabolism and structure, *J Gerontol* 40:579-585, 1985.

63. Lavizzo-Mourey R, Johnson J, Stolley P: Risk factors for dehydration among elderly nursing home residents, *J Am Geriatr Soc* 36:213-218, 1988.

64. Leland JY: Chronic pain: primary care treatment of the older patient, *Geriatrics* 54:22-28, 33-37, 1999.

65. Leveille SG, Wagner EH, Davis C, et al: Preventing disability and managing chronic illness in frail older adults: a randomized trial of a community-based partnership with primary care, *J Am Geriatr Soc* 46:1191-1198, 1998.

66. Lewis CB: Assessment instruments. In Bottomley JM, Lewis CB: *Geriatric rehabilitation: a clinical approach*, ed 2, Upper Saddleback, NJ, 2003, Prentice Hall Publishers, pp 152-190.

67. Lundin-Olsson L, Nyberg L, Gustafson Y: Attention, frailty, and falls: the effect of a manual task on basic mobility, *J Am Geriatr Soc* 46:758-761, 1998.

68. Manton KG, Corder L, Stallard E: Chronic disability trends in elderly United States populations: 1982-1994, *Proc Natl Acad Sci USA* 94: 2593-2598, 1997.

69. Marin DB, Sewell MC, Schlechter A: Alzheimer's disease. Accurate and early diagnosis in the primary care setting, *Geriatrics* 57:36-40, 2002.

70. Marshall CE, Benton D, Brazier JM: Elder abuse. Using clinical tools to identify clues of mistreatment, *Geriatrics* 55:42-44, 47-50, 53, 2000.

71. McCormack B: Clinical effectiveness and clinical teams: effective practice with older people, *Nurs Older People* 13:14-17, 2001.

72. McGee M, Jensen GL: Nutrition in the elderly, *J Clin Gastroenterol* 30:372-380, 2000.

73. Mentes J, Adkins J, Culp K: *Hydration management research-based protocol*, Iowa City, IA, 1998, University of Iowa Gerontological Nursing Interventions Research Center.

74. Miller PD, Krebs RA, Neal BJ, et al: Hypodipsia in geriatric patients, *Am J Med* 73:354-356, 1982.

75. Molsa PK, Paljarvi L, Rinne JO, et al: Validity of clinical diagnosis in dementia: a prospective clinicopathologic study, *J Neurol Neurosurg Psychiatry* 48:1085-1090, 1985.

76. Morley JE: Geriatric endocrinology. In Mendelsohn G, ed: *Diagnosis and pathology of endocrine disease*, Philadelphia, 1988, JB Lippincott.

77. Morley JE: The aging endocrine system, *Postgrad Med* 73:107-120, 1983.

78. Mukamel DB, Chou C, Zimmer JG, et al: The effect of accurate patient screening on the cost-effectiveness of case management programs, *Gerontologist* 37:777-784, 1997.

79. Nazarko L: Continuity of care for older people, *Nurs Stand* 12:42-45, 1998.

80. Pacala JT, Boult C, Reed RL, et al: Predictive validity of the P_{ra} instrument among older recipients of managed care, *J Am Geriatr Soc* 45:614-617, 1997.

81. Pearlman DN, Branch LG, Ozminkowski RJ, et al: Transitions in health care use and expenditures among frail older adults by payor/provider type, *J Am Geriatr Soc* 45:550-557, 1997.

82. Phillips PA, Rolls BJ, Ledingham JGG, et al: Reduced thirst after water deprivation in healthy elderly men, *N Engl J Med* 311:753-759, 1984.

83. Philp I, Newton P, McKee K, et al: Geriatric assessment in primary care: formulating best practice, *Br J Community Nurs* 6(6):290-295. 2001.

84. Ragen PB, Mitchell J: The effects of aging on the cardiovascular response to dynamic and static exercise. In Weisfelt ML, ed: *The aging heart*, New York, 1980, Raven Press, pp 269-296.

85. Reed RL, Hepburn KW: Managed care for older people: a primer for the geriatrician, *J Am Geriatr Soc* 47:241-249, 1999.

86. Reuben DB: Organizational interventions to improve health outcomes of older persons, *Med Care* 40:416-428, 2002.

87. Robuschi G, Safran M, Braverman LE: Hypothyroidism in the elderly, *Endocr Rev* 8:142-153, 1987.

88. Roglieri JL, Futterman R, McDonough KL: Disease management interventions to improve outcomes in congestive heart failure, *Am J Managed Care* 3:1831-1839, 1997.

89. Sandholzer H, Hellenbrand W, v Renteln-Kruse W, et al: An evidence-based approach to assess older people in primary care, *Occas Pap R Coll Gen Pract* 82(2):iii-vi, 1-53, 2002.

90. Schaufele M, Bickel H, Weyerer S: Predictors of mortality among demented elderly in primary care, *Int J Geriatr Psychiatr* 14:946-956, 1999.

91. Scherger JE: Challenges and opportunities for primary care in 2002, *Medscape Family Medicine* 2(1), 2002, Medscape Portals.

92. Schiller AL: Bones and joints. In Rubin E, Farber JL, eds: *Pathology*, ed 2, Philadelphia, 1994, JB Lippincott, pp 1273-1347.

93. Schneider EL, Reed JD: Modulations of aging processes. In Finch CE, Schneider EL, eds: *Handbook of the biology of aging*, New York, 1985, Academic Press.

94. Sevush S, Minagar A, Peruyera G: Ventricular dilation on magnetic resonance imaging predicts early onset of urinary incontinence in patients with probable Alzheimer's disease. Program and abstracts of the 125th Annual Meeting of the American Neurological Association, poster 43, Boston, October 15-18, 2000.

95. Shem S: *The house of God*, New York, 1979, Bantam Doubleday Dell Publishing Group.

96. Shepard RJ: *Physical activity and aging*, ed 2, Gaithersburg, MD, 1987, Aspen Publishers.

97. Sloan JP. *Protocols in primary care geriatrics*, New York, 1991, Springer-Verlag.

98. Solomon PR, Hirshcoff A, Kelly B: A 7-minute neurocognitive screening battery highly sensitive to Alzheimer's disease, *Arch Neurol* 55:344-355, 1998.

99. Steen B: Preventive nutrition in old age—a review, *J Nutr Health Aging* 4:114-119, 2000.

100. Stump TE, Callahan CM, Hendrie HC: Cognitive impairment and mortality in older primary care patients, *J Am Geriatr Soc* 49:934-940, 2001.

101. Taxel P: Osteoporosis: detection, prevention, and treatment in primary care, *Geriatrics* 53:22-23, 27-28, 1998.

102. Travis LA, Lyness JM: Minor depression. Diagnosis and management in primary care, *Geriatrics* 57:65-66, 2002.

103. Valcour VG, Masaki KH, Curb JD, et al: The detection of dementia in the primary care setting, *Arch Intern Med* 160:2964-2968, 2000.

104. Vellas B, Guigoz Y, Garry PJ, et al: The mini nutritional assessment (MNA) and its use in grading the nutritional state of elderly patients, *Nutrition* 15:116-122, 1999.

105. Walters K, Iliffe S, Tai SS, et al: Assessing needs from patient, career, and professional perspectives: the Camberwell assessment of need for elderly people in primary care, *Age Ageing* 29:505-510, 2000.

106. Waters CH: *Management of Parkinson's disease*, ed 2, Caddo, OK, 1999, Professional Communications.

107. Winograd CH, Lindenberger EC, Chavez CM, et al: Identifying hospitalized older patients at varying risk for physical performance decline: a new approach, *J Am Geriatr Soc* 45:604-609, 1997.

108. Wolf RS, Li D: Factors affecting the rate of elder abuse reporting to state protective services program, *Gerontologist* 39:222-228, 1999.

109. Woolf SH, Kamerow DB, Lawrence RS: The periodic health examination of older adults: the recommendations of the US Preventive Service Task Force. Part I, *J Am Geriatr Soc* 38:817-823, 1990.

110. Woolf SH, Kamerow DB, Lawrence RS: The periodic health examination of older adults: the recommendations of the US Preventive Service Task Force. Part II, *J Am Geriatr Soc* 38:933-942, 1990.

111. World Health Organization: *Constitution of the World Health Organization*, Geneva, 1964, World Health Organization.

Clinical Medicine

Pharmacologic Considerations for the Physical Therapist

16

William P. Brookfield, RPH, MSc

Objectives

After reading this chapter, the reader will be able to:

1. Describe the principles of pharmacokinetics as they apply to the general population and to the elderly.
2. Explain the principles of pharmacodynamics, including the role of receptors and the modes of action of drugs as they apply to the learning of pharmacology.
3. Apply the principles of patient screening to the subject of pharmacovigilance.
4. Describe clinical considerations germane to physical therapist practice of commonly prescribed medications.
5. Identify valuable clinical sources of drug information.

The role of the pharmacist as a member of the health care team is evolving. The standard academic training (Doctor of Pharmacy degree) now encompasses a 6-year program, with a year of clinical rotations included in the educational process. This training includes emphasis on clinical decision-making and has produced a significant number of pharmacists with improved clinical skills. As a result of this academic evolution, the role of the practicing pharmacist is in transition. The educational experience has produced a practitioner with the ability to effectively monitor drug therapy for side effects and suggest drug therapy to physicians and nurse practitioners.

The physician community has not yet widely accepted the pharmacist as a prescriber of drugs. In the future, certain categories of drugs that fall somewhere between prescription-only and over-the-counter may be prescribed directly by the pharmacist. The future may bring a number of circumstances in which the PT and the clinical pharmacist can interact to improve the care of the patient.

PTs work with patients who are taking medications in virtually every health care setting. Medications are being administered to a large percentage of physical therapy outpatients, and polypharmacy may be pronounced in some. Medication use in many situations will have a significant effect on the health of the patient and may alter the clinical presentation or course of treatment. The PT must have a working knowledge of pharmacology to help the patient, physician, and pharmacist in the management of disease. This knowledge will allow the PT to fully participate in a collaborative medical model within a primary-care environment.

Understanding how drugs work and mastering the vast amount of information about drugs are seemingly insur-

mountable tasks. When the health care practitioner learns pharmacology by regurgitating isolated facts, he or she will have great difficulty applying the information in a practical manner to improve patient care. Only when both teacher and student understand and practice certain principles will the student learn pharmacology and be able to apply it to the treatment of the patient. Some key tips in the study and presentation of pharmacology are shown in Box 16-1.

The presenter of pharmacology information must be able to give the student of pharmacology some guidance to ease the anxiety that often accompanies the learning of pharmacology. This text provides a framework that allows the reader to apply the knowledge that he or she has gained to foster safe and effective patient care while avoiding rote memorization of information. In addition, the PT can learn to apply this knowledge to communicate effectively with pharmacists and physicians.

Pharmacokinetics

Pharmacokinetics should be considered *"what the body does to the drug"*; this definition will allow the PT to keep information about the term in perspective. Pharmacokinetics incorporates all aspects of the transport of a drug to its target site and subsequent removal of the drug and its metabolites from the body. Pharmacokinetics has four primary divisions: absorption at the site of administration, distribution within the body to the tissues, metabolism of the drug to more active or inactive forms, and excretion of the drug and its metabolites.

Absorption

Absorption is the process by which drugs are made available to the body fluids that distribute the drugs to organ systems. A key term within any discussion of absorption is *bioavailability*. Bioavailability is the study and measurement of the completeness of absorption. It is the most important concept within the study of absorption within pharmacokinetics. The two primary factors associated with drug absorption and ultimately bioavailability are the route of administration and the dosage formulation. The primary routes of administration include oral, sublingual, buccal, transdermal, inhalation, subcutaneous, intramuscular, intravenous, rectal, and topical. Examples of drugs and their primary routes of administration are aspirin (oral), nitroglycerin (sublingual), insulin (subcutaneous), meperidine (intramuscular), and hydrocortisone (topical).

Tips in the Study and Presentation of Pharmacology

- Focus on principles relevant to health care professionals in their everyday practice.
- Concepts or principles applied to a particular class of drugs will vary little, if any, among drugs within the class. In the study of pharmacology, a person *cannot* learn everything about all available drugs.
- Knowledge of pharmacology allows one to bring *systematic* order to drug-related information.
- Therapeutic responses vary widely among different drugs.

These examples should help the reader appreciate the variety of choices available for administration of a drug.

This discussion focuses primarily on the oral route of administration because this route is the most common mode of drug delivery. Some drugs cannot be administered orally because of degradation by intestinal enzymes (proteases). Insulin is an example of such a drug, as the insulin product undergoes complete degradation and is not absorbed. For any drug to be effective after oral administration, it must be absorbed through the intestinal epithelium and enter the blood vessels of the intestinal tract. The drug is then carried directly to the liver by the hepatic portal system before it reaches the systemic circulation.

If a drug has properties that allow the liver to rapidly metabolize it, then little if any will actually enter the systemic circulation. The liver extraction is called the *"first-pass effect"* and may render an orally administered drug ineffective. An example of such a drug and its pharmacokinetic application is lidocaine. Lidocaine is not available in an oral formulation but rather is available in topical, subcutaneous, and intravenous forms because of the 100% first-pass effect of the molecule.

Many other molecules exhibit partial first-pass effects and require oral doses that may be significantly larger than those needed for parenteral (injectable) dosing. An example of a partial first-pass effect can be observed with the beta-receptor blocker propranolol. Propranolol intravenous dosing is 1 to 3 mg, while the oral route requires 10 to 80 mg to produce a similar pharmacologic response.

Changes in the formulation may significantly change absorption properties. The first-pass effect can be altered in some situations by changes in the oral formulation. *Timed-release* or *sustained-release* formulations are designed to produce slow, uniform dissolution of the drug and thus allow more drug to reach the systemic circulation. An example of a timed-release medication is nifedipine (Procardia XL and Adalat CC).

Enteric-coated or *delayed-release* formulations may be used with orally administered medications to alter absorption. If a medication is prone to acidic degradation in the stomach, it may be helpful to give the medication an outer coat of a chemical that will resist acid. The outer-coat chemical will dissolve in the alkaline environment of the intestine, and the actual drug may be released effectively from the intestinal location and produce a pharmacologic response. An example of a medication with such a formulation is omeprazole (Prilosec). The granules within the capsule are enteric coated. Enteric coating (delayed release) of a medication also is employed when the medication may be irritating to the stomach to avoid this gastrointestinal side effect. This formulation allows the stomach-irritating drug to be released in the intestine rather than in the stomach. Many aspirin formulations are enteric coated to minimize stomach irritation.

Distribution

The second division of pharmacokinetics is distribution, the movement or transport of a drug to the site of action. Distribution of a drug to the different tissues depends on blood flow. The transportation phase of distribution in the blood is facilitated by the binding of a percentage of the drug molecules to serum protein. The primary protein that binds drug molecules is serum albumin. The "free" drug or "unbound" molecules are the portion that can penetrate capillary walls to reach the site of action. The "bound" drug cannot exert any pharmacologic action.

At times a problem may arise when two or more drugs compete for the same binding site. This competition may create higher levels of "free" drug or unbound drug for one of the competing molecules. For example, the anticoagulant warfarin can potentially compete for protein binding sites with ibuprofen. The nonsteroidal antiinflammatory drug ibuprofen has a much greater affinity for serum albumin than does warfarin. Therefore, if a patient taking warfarin starts taking ibuprofen, the antiinflammatory drug may "bump" the warfarin off the albumin, resulting in higher concentrations of warfarin as *free drug* now available to act upon the body. The concentration of warfarin may then reach toxic levels, putting the patient in danger. The PT may be the practitioner that discovers that the patient has recently started taking ibuprofen for a minor musculoskeletal symptom.

Despite adequate blood flow, all drugs do not gain access to all areas of the body (e.g., the central nervous system [CNS]). When a drug reaches the plasma, it must cross several barriers before it can reach its final site of action. For any drug to have effects in the CNS, it must be able to cross the *blood-brain barrier*. A drug may enter the cerebral circulation yet not be able to enter the cells of the brain. The blood-brain barrier is a "tight" barrier that does not allow the molecules to "squeeze" through or diffuse through the barrier.

The blood-brain barrier was originally postulated from experiments in which dyes were injected into the systemic circulation but were found not to reach the cells of the brain. Later work has shown that although there is such a barrier, it is not an absolute barrier. A more appropriate term may be the blood-brain sieve.

Many drugs that easily penetrate other body organs do not appreciably enter the brain. A practical application of this concept for the orthopedic PT is a comparison of the safety profiles of morphine and ibuprofen. Morphine is prone to cause vivid dreams (nightmares) and hallucinations, while ibuprofen does not have these issues in its safety profile. This is because morphine will readily cross the blood-brain barrier while acting on the CNS, but ibuprofen does not. An important question to ask about a medication is the drug's propensity to cross the blood-brain barrier. The drug's blood-brain barrier profile is information that may assist in the prediction of whether the undesired CNS effect is drug-induced or induced by the disease state.

Lipid-soluble drugs are more likely to penetrate the blood-brain barrier than other drugs because they pass through the cell membrane instead of "squeezing through the openings." In addition, lipid-soluble drugs may be stored in adipose tissue, which acts as a drug repository. This has the potential to cause a lower plasma concentration but a longer duration of action. Storage in fatty tissue is of concern in the obese, in those who have an absolute increase in adipose tissue, and in the elderly when the ratio of body fat to lean body weight increases while the body weight remains the same.

Finally, an important term in distribution is *bioavailability*, just as it was in the absorption phase. Bioavailability from the distribution aspect is defined as the amount of drug that reaches its target of action, and it may be affected by protein binding, gastrointestinal absorption, adipose tissue storage, metabolism to other products, and elimination.

Metabolism

Metabolism is the process of transforming drugs into more water-soluble compounds so they can be excreted by the kidneys. Metabolism occurs primarily within the liver, although other organs such as the kidneys and cardiovascular system may be involved. Most drugs are not excreted unchanged by the body but will undergo a biotransformation after they enter the body. Metabolism usually changes active drugs to inactive metabolites. However, a few drugs are not active until transformed by the liver to an active metabolite. Most drugs are detoxified in the liver, but in some circumstances, metabolites may be more toxic than the parent compound. An example is the seizure potential of meperidine compared with its metabolite normeperidine. Normeperidine has a threefold greater seizure potential than meperidine and therefore has increased toxicity regarding seizures.

Many drugs are metabolized by the microsomal mixed-function oxidase enzyme system in the liver. Most microsomal enzyme reactions degrade a drug to more water-soluble end products, which are then excreted by the kidneys. The cytochrome P-450 enzyme system is the most clinically important system of microsomal enzymes in the liver. Many clinically important drug interactions involve the cytochrome enzyme system. The enzymes are inducible by drugs that may stimulate the metabolism of another drug. For example, carbamazepine (Tegretol) has the ability to stimulate or induce a number of enzymes. This induction may increase the metabolism of drugs such as olanzapine (Zyprexa). In addition, some drugs may reduce the metabolism of another drug, resulting in a plasma level of the drug that is higher than normal. An example of the latter is the elevated levels of terfenadine (Seldane) caused by concomitant administration of erythromycin, leading to ventricular arrhythmias and ultimately withdrawal from the market. The co-administration of terfenadine and erythromycin did not allow the terfenadine to be fully metabolized to a less toxic metabolite.

Some drugs are secreted with the bile into the intestinal tract and can then either be reabsorbed or excreted with the feces. When a drug is reabsorbed by this mechanism involving the intestinal tract and given a second chance to exert its effect, it is considered to have undergone enterohepatic circulation. This process affects a small number of drugs but may have some clinical significance. The presence of liver disease may interfere with the metabolism of a drug so that repeated dosing may result in the development of elevated serum levels that may prove toxic to the body. Therefore the PT should be aware of the patient's liver function and understand the primary route of excretion for the drugs being taken.

Excretion

Excretion of drugs or their metabolites is carried out in the kidney by two processes, glomerular filtration and tubular secretion. Glomerular filtration is the process in which drugs are filtered through the glomerulus and then carried through the tubule into the urine. A drug may be reabsorbed to some extent, depending on the lipid solubility of the drug and pH of the urine, while others are not reabsorbed and are eliminated in the urine. The other process of elimination or excretion is the active secretion of the drug by the tubule into the urine. Drugs also may be excreted in fluids other than urine, and these would include milk, saliva, sweat, and feces. The preceding discussion of metabolism mentioned biliary secretion; this process places drugs in the feces for elimination.

The health care professional must recognize that the patient with reduced kidney function may have problems eliminating certain drugs that are excreted primarily unchanged in the urine. The geriatric patient and the patient with renal disease fit the category of reduced kidney function. Drugs that depend entirely on the kidney for elimination have the highest risk for adverse reactions in the geriatric patient. The elimination aspect of pharmacokinetics is the most clinically significant in alterations of drug response and issues of adverse events or side effects.

The health care professional should be able to estimate the patient's ability to avoid problems with drugs that are excreted by the renal system. One method for estimating the glomerular filtration rate of any patient is the Cockroft and Gault formula. The formula generates an estimate of the creatinine clearance for a given patient. Creatinine clearance measures the elimination capabilities of the patient. The larger the creatinine clearance value in milliliters per minute, the greater the ability of the patient to avoid problems with a drug that employs renal excretion. The formula and key facts are enclosed in Box 16-2.

The normal value for a creatinine clearance would be 90 to 120 mL/min, with the female toward the lower end of the range. The male patient will have a normal creatinine clearance toward the high end of the range. The lower the number, the more compromised the creatinine clearance and degree of change in the handling of renally excreted drugs.

Drug Half-Life

In any discussion of pharmacokinetics and elimination, one must understand the concept of drug half-life ($t^1/_2$). The *elimination half-life* and the *biological half-life* are two terms

---

BOX 16-2

Cockroft and Gault Creatinine Clearance Formula

- Estimates the creatinine clearance in milliliters per minute (mL/min).
- Can assist in determining age-related changes in the ability to handle drugs.
- Determines the value for the male; if patient is a female multiply the results by 0.85.
- Formula:

$$\frac{(140 - \text{age in yr}) \times \text{weight in kg}}{72 \times \text{serum creatinine in mg/dL}}$$

---

that one should understand. The elimination half-life is defined in all books that discuss pharmacokinetics but for some drugs is less practical than the biologic half-life when working with real-world patients.

The elimination half-life of a drug is the time in which the concentration of the drug in the plasma falls to one half of its original amount. The elimination half-life describes a drug's rate of disappearance from the body, whether by metabolism, excretion, or a combination of both. The half-life usually is measured in hours, but for some drugs the half-life is measured in days, and for others, in minutes or even seconds. In contrasting the cardiac drugs amiodarone, propranolol, and adenosine, one can appreciate the great variation in half-life. The elimination half-life for amiodarone is 26 to 107 days because the drug is very lipid soluble. The elimination half-life for propranolol is 3 to 4 hours, while the elimination half-life for adenosine is 10 seconds.

The $t^1/_2$ of a drug is useful information when determining the amount of time the drug will remain in the body and potentially exert a pharmacologic effect. In addition, this information helps determine how often a drug should be administered to the patient.

The biological half-life of the drug is the time in which the duration of action falls to one half of its original duration. This $t^1/_2$ refers to the time of the drug's response rather than the plasma concentration. Several drugs have durations of action that are longer than the plasma levels indicate. This difference may result from interactions of the drug with its receptor that may initiate activity that continues even without the presence of the drug. Therefore, with some drugs, the biological half-life may be more clinically useful than the elimination half-life.

The $t^1/_2$ information can be applied to discussions about the loading dose of a drug, the therapeutic range of a drug, and the *steady-state* level of a drug. One must understand the concept of steady state because this term is used in many articles that discuss drug therapy. Steady-state plasma levels are most important in understanding and interpreting chronic drug therapy rather than acute drug therapy. Drugs tend to accumulate in the body if given on a regular schedule until the amount eliminated is equal to the amount administered. When this happens, the steady-state level is reached.

At the steady-state level, plasma concentrations will oscillate around the mean plasma concentration. The concentration will vary between the peak plasma level after administration of

---

BOX 16-3

Pharmacokinetics: The Geriatric Patient

Pharmacokinetic Functions	Alterations in the Geriatric Patient	Clinical Consequences
A Absorption	Decreased gastrointestinal tract motility Slower gastric emptying Increased gastric pH	Bloating after eating more common. Medication effects may be altered. Less important than M and E.
D Distribution	Decreased cardiac output Increased body fat Decreased lean body mass	Less important than M and E to drug action changes. Cardiac output change when accompanied by decreased renal and liver blood flow can be important.
M Metabolism	Decreased liver mass Decreased liver enzyme activity Decreased liver blood flow	Liver enzyme changes (reduced activity) can increase the intensity of the drug action
E Excretion	Decreased kidney blood flow Decreased glomerular filtration rate	Change in renal function is the single most important pharmacokinetic factor resulting in adverse drug reactions

---

the drug and the minimum plasma level just before the next administered dose. If a drug has been administered on a regular basis, the steady-state level usually will be reached after five half-lives of the drug have passed. Some authors also call the steady-state level the plateau level.

When the patient stops taking the drug, five half-lives usually must pass before the drug is considered to no longer have the ability to affect the patient's system. This is important to the PT because when investigating a patient's use of medication, asking the question, "Have you recently stopped taking any medications?" is very important. A drug with a long half-life stopped only a couple of days ago may account for the presence of symptoms or complications noted by the PT.

Another important consideration in drug response is patient compliance. The patient who is noncompliant may not be allowing the drug to reach steady state. The patient's level of compliance with medications also may indicate his or her compliance with a home exercise program or modifications of body mechanics with daily activities.

Some key facts about pharmacokinetics and the geriatric population are shown in Box 16-3. The examples in this box illustrate some of the challenges of determining proper dosing for the elderly population. See Chapter 15 for further discussion of polypharmacy and the elderly population.

Pharmacodynamics

The pharmacodynamic principles are the heart of pharmacology. The PT should think of pharmacodynamics as "*what the drug does to the body,*" that is, the study of the mechanisms and action created by drugs.

The study of pharmacodynamics includes four areas that the PT should understand: the general mode of action, including secondary modes of action; the indications for use; the safety profile; and rehabilitation considerations. Pharmacodynamics involve both the biochemical and physiological effects of a drug. The site of action of a drug may be a specific organ system, or the drug may cause a more generalized body effect. In general, drugs act by forming a bond, usually reversible, with some cellular constituent (receptor).

Most drugs act on a specific receptor. For a drug to have an action in the body, the drug must bind to a receptor to a sufficient degree to create a pharmacologic response. A *receptor* is defined as a specific macromolecule that recognizes the drug. The receptor may be on the cell membrane or inside the cell. *Affinity* describes the degree of attraction or binding power a given drug has for the receptor. Some degree of affinity must be inherent in the drug for it to bind to a receptor.

A drug that binds to a receptor and produces an action is called an *agonist.* Thus an agonist is a drug with affinity that can elicit a pharmacologic response. A drug that binds to a receptor and does not produce an action is called an *antagonist* or *blocker.* An example of the concepts of agonist activity and antagonist activity is seen in histamine-antihistamine interaction. Diphenhydramine (Benadryl) is an antihistamine that blocks the histamine-1 (H_1) receptor site by binding to the receptor. This binding prevents histamine from binding to the receptor and creating responses such as itching of the skin. The drug diphenhydramine has affinity for the histamine receptor (binds to the receptor) and displays antagonist activity in that the histamine cannot exert a physiological change (increased itching). *Partial agonist* drugs are drugs that bind with a receptor but cannot produce maximal response compared with the agonist.

Potency and Efficacy

Two confusing terms associated with pharmacodynamics are *potency* and *efficacy.* Potency describes the dose of a drug required to produce a given effect relative to a standard. This is usually not important clinically. Efficacy is the capacity to stimulate or produce an effect for a given occupied receptor. Efficacy in everyday terms describes how well the drug works or the maximum response to a drug. This is clinically important. The word *potency* can mislead one into believing that because a drug is more potent, it is more effective. An illustration of this difference is the use of morphine and meperidine (Demerol) in treating pain. If morphine, 10 mg, and meperidine, 75 mg, both alleviate the pain of a patient, one can state that morphine is more potent (10 mg versus 75 mg for meperidine); however, both drugs may display equal efficacy.

Tolerance

Pharmacodynamics may involve the development of *tolerance* to a given drug. The pharmacologic effect of tolerance has developed with a given drug when increasing amounts (more milligrams) are required to produce the same effect or when the same dose on repeated occasions produces lower responses. This may occur with some drugs but not with others. Narcotic analgesics are a class of drugs that are well known to exhibit tolerance, as increasing doses are required to produce the same effect. The other aspect of *tolerance* is classified as *tachyphylaxis.* Tachyphylaxis is considered a rapidly developing tolerance and may be seen after only a few administrations of some drugs. Nasal decongestants for allergic rhinitis have been associated with tachyphylaxis.

Autonomic Nervous System and Pharmacodynamics

An extremely important concept in the understanding of pharmacodynamics for the PT is the autonomic nervous system. The discussion of receptor activity along with agonist and antagonist properties strongly affects one's ability to understand pharmacologic responses of the autonomic nervous system. Terminology regarding the autonomic nervous system and the subsequent pharmacologic changes should be reviewed. The PT must understand the following terms to study pharmacodynamics:

- Parasympathetic (cholinergic) subdivision
- Sympathetic (adrenergic) subdivision
- Parasympathomimetic drug (cholinergic agonist or stimulant)
- Parasympatholytic drug (cholinergic antagonist) (anticholinergic)
- Sympathomimetic drug (adrenergic agonist or stimulant)
- Sympatholytic drug (adrenergic antagonist or blocker)
- Alpha-blocker (specialized adrenergic antagonist)
- Beta-blocker (specialized adrenergic antagonist)
- $Beta_1$-blocking properties only (cardioselective adrenergic antagonist)
- $Beta_1$- plus $beta_2$-blocking properties (nonselective adrenergic antagonist)
- $Beta_2$-agonist properties (bronchoselective adrenergic agonist)
- $Beta_2$-plus $beta_1$-agonist properties (nonselective beta-receptor agonist)

Some examples of prototype drugs within the aforementioned therapeutic categories may help the PT better understand pharmacology. In the study of pharmacology, it is always helpful to apply focused rote memorization to the indications for use and safety profiles of a prototype drug within each major mode-of-action category. This approach offers a more systematic way to learn pharmacology across the wide array of available drugs. Examples of such drugs are:

- Parasympathomimetic drug: Bethanechol (Urecholine) or pilocarpine
- Parasympatholytic drug: Atropine or ipratropium (Atrovent)
- Sympathomimetic drug: Epinephrine (Adrenalin)
- Sympatholytic drug: Must determine alpha-receptor or beta-receptor antagonist
- Alpha antagonist: Prazosin (Minipress) or terazosin (Hytrin)
- Alpha agonist: Norepinephrine (Levophed) or phenylephrine (Neosynephrine)
- Combined $beta_1$ and $beta_2$ antagonist: Propranolol (Inderal)
- $Beta_1$ antagonist: Atenolol (Tenormin) or metoprolol (Lopressor)

TABLE 16-1

TABLE 16-1

Possible Cholinergic Responses: The SLUD Acronym

Mnemonic Letter	Pharmacologic Response	Parasympathetic (Cholinergic) Stimulation	Cholinergic Blockade (Anticholinergic Activity)
S	Salivation	Increased saliva/drooling	Xerostomia (dry mouth)
L	Lacrimation	Increased tearing/watery eyes	Dry eyes/blurred vision/loss of power of accommodation
U	Urination	Increased genitourinary motility (urine flow increased)	Retention of urine
D	Defecation	Increased gastrointestinal motility (diarrhea)	Constipation

- Beta$_2$ agonist: Albuterol (Ventolin)
- Combined beta$_2$ and beta$_1$ agonist: Isoproterenol (Isuprel)

The concept of alpha receptors and beta receptors is associated with the sympathetic subdivision of the autonomic nervous system only.

An understanding of the primary changes that take place with agonist and antagonist activity within these two subdivisions of the autonomic nervous system is extremely useful in learning pharmacology. One should master some key pharmacologic responses within each subdivision. This key information is provided in the following text.

Parasympathetic (Cholinergic) Subdivision: Selected Pharmacologic Responses

Tables 16-1 and 16-2 describe the clinically important aspects of the cholinergic subdivision of the autonomic nervous system. As can be seen from the tables; these pharmacologic changes are *daily functional aspects* and typically are not life-threatening aspects, as can be the case with adrenergic pharmacologic changes.

The mnemonic *SLUD* is helpful in learning the parasympathetic (cholinergic) actions.

Changes in the urinary bladder are an example of how the charts might be used. Urinary incontinence and benign prostatic hypertrophy are common problems in some patient groups. One can develop an understanding of drug-induced bladder function changes regarding urinary flow by reviewing the parasympathetic and sympathetic nervous systems. The accompanying parasym-

pathetic chart (Table 16-2) displays the detrusor muscle surrounding the urinary bladder as innervated by the parasympathetic system. Therefore drugs that are parasympathetic agonists will promote the flow of urine. Any drug that is a parasympathetic antagonist, however, will tend to cause retention of urine. The male patient with benign prostatic hypertrophy (BPH) may notice an exacerbation of urinary retention when taking drugs with parasympathetic antagonist properties. The PT must review drug-therapy regimens for any and all medications with parasympathetic antagonistic (anticholinergic) actions.

Autonomic Nervous System Sympathetic (Adrenergic) Subdivision: Selected Pharmacologic Responses

Table 16-3 describes important clinical pharmacologic parameters of the receptor site that has the ultimate control on the given pharmacologic parameter. Several of the adrenergic responses are critical to the cardiovascular system, and alterations can be *life threatening*.

Pharmacodynamic Considerations in the Elderly

- Orthostatic (postural) hypotension: May be aggravated by some drug therapy. Any drug that has the ability to deplete vascular volume, or has vasodilating activity, or has sympatholytic (adrenergic blocking) activity will be prone to cause clinically significant orthostatic hypotension.
- Confusion and mental fuzziness: The elderly are vulnerable to increased response to agents that have parasympatholytic (anticholinergic) effects. The aging patient has increased sensitivity of the central nervous system (CNS) resulting from decreased cerebral blood flow (20% decreased by the aging process)
- Mobility alteration (prone to falls and gait disturbance): The elderly are profoundly affected by drugs that cause sedation, reduce coordination, and cause tremors. In addition to the previously mentioned effects, their mobility may be affected by orthostatic hypotension and confusion/mental fuzziness.
- Extrapyramidal (EPS) effects: The elderly are more prone to the complex of side effects called extrapyramidal symptoms resulting from a decrease in the activity of dopamine in the CNS. This is due in part to a decreased production of

TABLE 16-2

Cholinergic Actions

Pharmacologic Response	Parasympathetic (Cholinergic) Stimulation	Cholinergic Blockade (Anticholinergic Activity)
Detrusor muscle around urinary bladder	Muscle contraction (increase in urine output)	Muscle relaxation (decrease in urine output)
Pupil size	Miosis (pupil constriction)	Mydriasis (pupil dilation)
Lungs (bronchioles)	Bronchoconstriction	Bronchodilation (slow dilation)
Heart rate (chronotropic)	Decrease in heart rate (bradycardia)	Increase in heart rate (tachycardia)

TABLE 16-3

Adrenergic Responses with Receptor Site

Pharmacologic Parameter	Alpha Receptor Stimulation	Beta₁-Receptor Stimulation	Beta₂-Receptor Stimulation	Dopamine Receptor Stimulation (Non-CNS Receptors)
Heart rate (chronotropic)		Increase in heart rate (positive chronotropic)		
Heart contractility (pumping force) (inotropic)		Increase in pumping force of heart (positive inotropic)		
Peripheral vasculature*	Vasoconstriction		Vasodilation	
Renal vasculature	Vasoconstriction			Vasodilation
Lungs (bronchioles)			Bronchodilation	
Uterine smooth muscle			Relaxation (reduced contractions)	
Urinary bladder internal sphincter muscle tone	Contraction (closure of bladder outlet)			
				Non–central nervous system dopamine

The lack of a comment in any box in this table does not imply that the receptor has no effect on the parameter, *only that the primary influence resides with the receptor that has the comment in the box.*
*Although alpha and beta₂ responses affect the peripheral vasculature parameter, the alpha influence is the stronger of the two. In the normal condition, homeostasis is maintained with input from both aspects.

dopamine in the elderly patient. Altered levels of CNS dopamine will change the frequency and intensity of EPS effects when given medications that block dopamine receptors, such as the neuroleptics.

Extrapyramidal symptoms (EPS) include akathisia, parkinsonism-like symptoms (e.g., tremor, cogwheel rigidity), dystonia, and dyskinesia. In addition, tardive dyskinesia is included in the broad category of EPS symptoms. These symptoms may be very prominent in any patient on antipsychotic medications but can be especially troublesome in the geriatric patient. An imbalance between the neurotransmitters of acetylcholine and dopamine is the basis for the development of EPS symptoms. This imbalance is focused toward the central nervous system rather than the autonomic nervous system.

In the study of pharmacology, one must not only understand the autonomic nervous system but also have a basic understanding of serotonin and dopamine as neurotransmitters. Antipsychotic drugs (neuroleptics) have multiple modes of actions that are used for therapeutic indications and that can produce side effects. Table 16-4 will help the PT learn the pharmacologic profile of drugs for mental disease.

All drugs classified as antipsychotics used to treat schizophrenic symptoms are classified as neuroleptics. One should note that some medications used as ancillary medications in the treatment of schizophrenia may work by other modes of

TABLE 16-4

Neuroleptic Receptor Blockade and Resulting Pharmacodynamics

Receptor Type	Pharmacologic Changes from Blockade	Comments
Dopamine (D₂)	Treatment of schizophrenic positive symptoms. Production of extrapyramidal side effects. Increase in prolactin blood levels.	Prolactin level increase can lead to breast swelling and tenderness along with galactorrhea.
Serotonin (5HT₂ₐ)	Treatment of schizophrenic negative symptoms.	Action seen with some newer neuroleptics that may block serotonin.
Serotonin (5HT₂c)	Anxiolytic properties. Increase in food intake (weight gain).	Reduction of anxiety prompts use in anxiety states and in treating panic attacks.
Histamine (H₁)	Sedation Weight gain	Blockade of histamine is a secondary effect and leads to side effects.
Cholinergic	Peripheral anticholinergic effects (SLUD): dry mouth, blurred vision, retention of urine, and constipation. Central nervous system anticholinergic effects: confusion, delirium, and cognitive deficits.	Central nervous system effects may mimic schizophrenic symptoms and may not be readily recognized as drug-induced side effects.
Alpha-adrenergic (alpha receptors)	Orthostatic (postural) hypotension Syncope from blood pressure changes Nasal congestion Priapism	Most troublesome is the hypotension resulting from the vasodilation, leading to falls.

TABLE 16-5

Selected Adverse Drug Reactions Affecting Mobility in the Elderly

Drug Category	Adverse Reaction(s)	Comments
Tricyclic antidepressants (e.g., amitriptyline [Elavil])	Postural hypotension Tremors Sedation Arrhythmias	May lead to syncope and balance difficulty. Cardiac rhythm changes may cause dizziness and mobility problems.
Benzodiazepines (e.g., diazepam [Valium], alprazolam [Xanax], lorazepam [Ativan])	Sedation Weakness Decreased coordination Confusion	Prone to cause oversedation and morning balance problems. Many hypnotics are in this class, such as flurazepam (Dalmane) and temazepam (Restoril)
Sedative hypnotics (e.g., secobarbital [Seconal], zolpidem [Ambien]	Sedation Weakness Decreased coordination Confusion	May lead to falls. Prone to cause morning hangover.
Antihypertensives, alpha receptor blockers (e.g., prazosin [Minipress], terazosin [Hytrin], doxazosin [Cardura])	Orthostatic (postural) hypotension	May cause significant problems with syncope and lead to falls. Not all classes of drugs for hypertension are prone to postural hypotension.
Narcotic analgesics (e.g., morphine or Vicodin)	Sedation Reduced coordination Confusion	May contribute to clouded thinking and balance problems.
Beta receptor blockers (e.g., propranolol [Inderal], atenolol [Tenormin])	Reduced ability to respond to workload changes	May lead to weakness and lethargy due to a blunting of homeostasis mechanisms. Heart rate and cardiac output may not respond to workload change.
Antipsychotics or neuroleptics (e.g., haloperidol [Haldol], risperidone [Risperdal], olanzapine [Zyprexa], fluphenazine [Prolixin])	Orthostatic hypotension Sedation Extrapyramidal effects	Significant amount of movement disorders and fainting spells. Extrapyramidal effects may take the form of tremors, abnormal gait, or muscle rigidity.

action. Neuroleptics have differing blockade properties and intensities of blockade. The ideal neuroleptic would have strong blockade of the $5HT_{2a}$ receptor and moderate blockade of the D_2 receptor along with no blockade of the H_1, cholinergic, or alpha receptors (no side effects). Such an agent does not exist. Moderate blockade at the D_2 receptor allows control of schizophrenic symptoms and minimal extrapyramidal side effects. Extrapyramidal side effects take place with strong blockade of the D_2 receptor.

In the area of pharmacodynamics, an ideal drug would produce only one effect (desired therapeutic effect), but this is not reality. In addition to the desired action, drugs also have undesired effects called *side effects*. Side effects are responses other than the intended medical effect. *Side effects often are an extension of the known pharmacologic activity of the drug.* Many side effects of medications affect the mobility of the geriatric patient. Table 16-5 presents a few of the many categories of medications that can have a clinically significant effect on the geriatric patient.

In addition to mobility issues in the elderly, medications with anticholinergic activity (cholinergic antagonist) may cause confusion and mentation difficulties. Many therapeutic categories contain drugs that may create undesired anticholinergic effects in the geriatric population. Anticholinergic effects include mental confusion and hallucinations. Table 16-6 lists some of the therapeutic categories that have these anticholinergic properties.

To review the study of pharmacodynamics, see the key facts in Box 16-4.

TABLE 16-6

Drugs with Potential to Cause Confusion in the Elderly

Medication Category	Examples within the Category
Antispasmodics	Dicyclomine (Bentyl), hyoscyamine (Levsin)
Antiparkinsonism	Benztropine (Cogentin), trihexyphenidyl (Artane)
Antihistamines	Diphenhydramine (Benadryl), Chlorpheniramine
Antidepressants	Amitriptyline (Elavil), imipramine (Tofranil)
Antiarrhythmics	Quinidine, disopyramide (Norpace), procainamide
Antipsychotics (neuroleptics)	Thioridazine (Mellaril), chlorpromazine (Thorazine)
Selected hypnotics	Hydroxyzine (Vistaril)
Over-the-counter medications	Antidiarrheals such as Imodium, OTC sleep aids such as doxylamine (Unisom), cold remedies such as Contac

BOX 16-4

Key Concepts in the Study of Pharmacodynamics

- An agonist drug will display affinity and activity at the receptor.
- An antagonist drug will display only affinity and no activity at the receptor.
- Drug efficacy is important clinically, whereas drug potency is not important clinically.
- Most pharmacologic responses (desired as well as undesired) can be predicted when one knows the mechanism of action of the drug (pharmacodynamic activity)

Pharmacovigilance

Pharmacovigilance is the practice of monitoring the safety of a drug-therapy regimen. In addition, it can be defined as *"watchfulness in guarding the safety of drugs,"* and through this function the PT can offer meaningful input as part of a health care team. Adverse events (side effects) caused by drug therapy are best monitored by those who spend the most time with the patient. The physician in many cases does not spend sufficient quality time with the patient to perform good pharmacovigilance. The PT can apply knowledge of pharmacokinetics and pharmacodynamics toward the application of pharmacovigilance and use the examination tools described in Sections Two and Three of the text to screen the patient for such events. See Chapters 5, 6, and 7 for detailed explanations of how to screen patients for medication use and adverse reactions.

The key to understanding pharmacovigilance is to remember that drugs do not do just one thing. Drugs will display the desired effect, if they have efficacy, but also will display undesired effects called adverse events or side effects. Side effects can be divided into two categories, *predictable* and *unpredictable reactions.*

Predictable side effects make up 80% of all drug reactions and in most situations are an extension of the known pharmacology of the compound. Another explanation of a predictable side effect is an increased intensity of a predictable action of the drug. For a key example of a predictable side effect, consider the use of metoprolol (Lopressor) to treat hypertension. Metoprolol is a beta-receptor antagonist drug that lowers blood pressure and heart rate. When metoprolol excessively lowers the heart rate (bradycardia), the patient may experience dizziness, lack of energy, and even fainting spells. The bradycardia would be an increased or unexpected intensity of a predictable action of the drug (lowering of heart rate). This type of side effect may be dose related or the result of comorbidities of a given patient. The dose of the metoprolol may have been excessive for the patient, or the dose may have been low, but this patient might have had a history of myocardial infarction and altered cardiac activity.

The second category of side effects is the unpredictable reactions. Unpredictable side effects may be subdivided into idiosyncratic and allergic reactions. The *idiosyncratic reaction* is an unusual or unexpected reaction that cannot be explained by the pharmacology of the drug. An example of this type of reaction is a patient who becomes hyperexcitable and hyperactive on a sedating drug such as phenobarbital. *Allergic reactions* also are examples of unpredictable side effects caused by medication. These reactions constitute only about 8% of all side effects and also are not related to the pharmacologic profile of the drug. The allergic reaction is unlikely to be dose related and normally is not reproducible across a number of different patients. The reaction is reproducible only in the individual who experienced the reaction.

The PT also should understand the term *anaphylactic reaction.* An *anaphylactic reaction* is considered an unpredictable side effect and is an allergic reaction that may occur quickly and is manifested with the symptoms of bronchospasm, hypotension, shock, and potentially death.

A final concept in pharmacovigilance is the *drug interaction.* A drug interaction is an adverse event involving the interplay between two or more drugs. The more drugs in a therapeutic regimen, the greater the propensity for drug interactions and the greater the need for pharmacovigilance. The single most important contributor to drug interactions is polypharmacy. Polypharmacy is common because of the many patients who have multiple disease states in addition to communication problems. Many clinicians have prescribed drugs over the telephone rather than performing an examination in the office. Therefore unrecognized side effects may be treated with more drugs. The clinician may view the geriatric patient as having problems that are disease-state driven rather than medication driven (side effects). Clinicians often are more thorough in investigating patient symptoms in the younger patient than in the elderly. Indifference to the finer points of medication management appears to contribute to drug interactions.

By strict definition, drug interaction does not have to be adverse, but the common use of the term implies an adverse event. An example of a drug interaction that is not adverse is the use of levodopa and carbidopa in a product named Sinemet to treat Parkinson's disease. The carbidopa creates more efficient use of levodopa and increases the ability of levodopa to penetrate the blood-brain barrier. However, most drug interactions do involve adverse events and should be closely monitored.

Drugs may interact through both pharmacokinetic and pharmacodynamic mechanisms. An extremely important key to predicting drug interactions is the ability to recognize underlying liver or renal disease in the patient. The PT should constantly ask the important question, "Is the drug necessary?" This question alone can prevent drug interactions or at least uncover problems early in a drug regimen.

Often drugs are released on the market while the patient-care team has limited knowledge about its safety profile. From the perspective of the pharmaceutical manufacturers, clinical trials are performed to establish efficacy (to determine whether the drug works), and the development of a safety profile is only a secondary goal in most cases. The patient in clinical trials typically is not treated for a sufficiently long enough time to guarantee the detection of all the adverse effects of the study medication. In addition, the adverse effects may be rare, delayed, or a result of interactions with other drugs. Clinical trials may not have allowed the drug to be tested in a particular subgroup of patients who may be very vulnerable to the pharmacologic actions of the drug. Caregivers who spend the most time with patients must monitor these drugs after they enter the market.

Pharmacovigilance also has an increasingly important role in the risk-benefit assessment of drugs. The risk-benefit assessment continues regardless of whether the drug is new to the market or has been on the market for years. Both the efficacy and the safety of a drug are of equal importance, and the PT can provide information on both. However, the focus of the caregiver regarding pharmacovigilance should be on the safety concerns or hazards of a drug rather than on its benefits. An example of a hazard is the case of the antihistamine terfenadine (Seldane). The safety concern with terfenadine was not discovered until the drug was on the market for more than 10 years. The disturbances in

Key Concepts in the Understanding of Pharmacovigilance

- Drug safety: Drug safety is monitored by watching over therapeutic regimens.
- Side effects: Most side effects are increased intensity of a predictable action of the drug.
- Polypharmacy: The more drugs, the greater the need for pharmacovigilance.
- Listen to the patient symptoms and weigh the risk/benefit ratio of every drug.
- Use of over-the-counter medication must be investigated with direct questions.

cardiac rhythm created by terfenadine resulted from a drug interaction that was not detected in clinical trials or in the early marketing stages of the drug. The discipline of pharmacovigilance requires the PT to ask constantly whether the patient's symptom or problem is drug related or disease-state related.

Box 16-5 lists some key concepts in understanding pharmacovigilance.

Over-the-Counter Medications

The PT, in examining drug regimens, must never overlook the influence of over-the-counter (OTC) medications. The patient often will not consider OTC drugs to be important information to pass along to the health care professional. The patient often assumes the OTC drug is safe and therefore devoid of side effects. The patient may believe that an OTC drug would not have been approved as an OTC medication by the Food and Drug Administration (FDA) unless it was completely safe. Aspirin and oral contraceptives are only two of the many drugs that many patients do not list when questioned about their medication. The PT must ask direct questions and incorporate any mentioned medications into the evaluation plan.

The PT should apply the principles of pharmacovigilance and must incorporate knowledge of OTC medications into the screening plan. Many OTC medications began as prescription-only drugs and are not without safety issues. The nonsteroidal antiinflammatory drugs (NSAIDs), such as naproxen (Aleve), and the histamine-2 receptor antagonists, such as cimetidine (Tagamet), are two of the many therapeutic categories that now appear in the OTC list of medications. The PT must not overlook OTC medications in the patient's drug regimen.

Clinical Considerations of Selected Drug Classes for the Physical Therapist

A list of selected therapeutic categories and their corresponding clinical considerations is found in Appendix 16-1 at the end of this chapter. The considerations noted are associated with commonly prescribed drugs.

Reference Sources for Drug Information

A vast array of information on drugs and the therapeutic application of drugs is available. With the wide use of various computer programs and the Internet, one can find a great deal of information that was not available to the health care professional in past years. Even the brightest of pharmacologists and physicians must consult the literature for drug information. This section discusses some of the most-consulted sources of drug information known to the PT along with some of the more valuable sources not readily known.

The *Physicians' Desk Reference (PDR)* is a drug information source that nurses and physicians often consult. This reference is published once a year in the spring and contains information provided by the manufacturers of drugs (pharmaceutical industry). The information is the same as that found in the package insert or package circular approved by the Food and Drug Administration (FDA).

The *PDR* has some major limitations that the PT should keep in mind. Older, established medications may not be included in the current *PDR* because the pharmaceutical industry uses the *PDR* as a method of promoting newer drugs. For example, try to find some clinical information about aspirin in a *PDR*. Aspirin is not discussed in the current *PDR*. Generic products also are not discussed within the *PDR*. Try to find some information on the generic drug fluoxetine rather than the brand name of Prozac in the current *PDR*.

The *PDR* is tremendously selective in its product information. Many PTs are surprised to learn that the pharmacologist rarely, if ever, consults the *PDR* for drug information. The pharmacologist may consult the *PDR* to help identify a product by looking in the section that contains pictures of dosage formulations.

Many other sources of useful drug information are available to the PT besides the *PDR*. One excellent resource is *Mosby's Drug Consult 2004*, a traditional book reference that also contains a CD-ROM. It provides information on pharmacology, indications for use, available dosage formulations, dosing recommendations, and adverse reactions. The four sections include keyword and international brand indices, complete drug information, monographs on the 50 most commonly used herbal drugs and supplements, and appendices containing comparative drug tables, additional information, and supplier profiles. *Mosby's Drug Consult* lists all medications alphabetically by generic name. The trade name is listed in a shaded summary text box immediately after the generic drug entry name. The detailed information for each drug then follows. In addition, the PT should readily consult with the pharmacist on hand when facing important medication-related clinical questions. See the Suggested Readings for other valuable resources for drug information.

Summary

The medical team is an important element in the monitoring of drug therapy. The pharmacist, nurse, dietitian, respiratory therapist, and PT all can be important in the monitoring of drug therapy, as they may spend extensive time with the patient. An understanding of pharmacology and drug regimens can prove invaluable in assisting the physician in medication management. The practicing physician's training or awareness is not always adequate for the task of pharmacovigilance. Not all prescribers could possibly become experts in the evaluation of the causal relationship between a drug and an adverse clinical event. Assessing the role of a drug is only one aspect of the classic medical diagnostic process, which includes a differential diagnosis and an etiologic diagnosis. The etiologic diagnosis, as far as drugs are concerned, is based on evidence for or against a temporal relationship (the timing of the event) and on the elimination of other principal non–drug-related causes of the observed event. The PT traditionally has not been considered an important source of information about adverse clinical events associated with medication use, nor as having the role of identifying patients at risk for an adverse event. By working closely with pharmacists, nurses, and physicians, however, PTs can improve patient care and educate others about the important role they can play.

SUGGESTED READINGS

American Society of Health-System Pharmacists: *ASHP drug information*, Bethesda, Md, 2004, American Society of Heath-System Pharmacists.
Applegate WB, Blass JP, Williams TF: Instruments for the functional assessment of older patients, *N Engl J Med* 322:107-1214, 1990.
Brawn LA, Castleden CM: Adverse drug reactions: an overview of special considerations in the management of the elderly patient, *Drug Safety* 5: 421-435, 1990.
Ciccone CD: *Pharmacology in rehabilitation*, ed 3, Philadelphia, 2002, FA Davis.
Drug Facts and Comparisons, St Louis, Facts and Comparisons. Available at: www.drugfacts.com.
Gilman AG, Rall TW, Nies AS, et al, eds: *The pharmacological basis of therapeutics*, ed 10, New York, 2000, Pergamon Press.
Keltner NL, Folks DG: *Psychotropic drugs*, ed 4, St Louis, 2001, Mosby.
Lacy CF, Armstrong LL, Goldman MP, et al: *Drug information handbook*, ed 12, Hudson, Ohio, 2004, Lexi-Comp.
Mosby's Drug Consult 2004, St Louis, 2004, Mosby.
Peters NL: Antimuscarinic side effects of medications in the elderly, *Arch Intern Med* 149:2414-2420, 1989.
Pratt WB, Taylor P, eds: *Principles of drug action: the basis of pharmacology*, ed 4, New York, 1995, Churchill Livingstone.
Thomson Corporation: www.micromedex.com (online drug information source).

Appendix 16-1 Clinical Considerations of Pharmacologic Agents in the Rehabilitation Patient

Therapeutic Category	Clinical Considerations	Drug Examples
Sedative/hypnotic/ antianxiety drugs (anxiolytics)	Prevalence of their use is high. Tension and anxiety are major in some patient populations, and these agents may be required to treat these symptoms to assist in rehabilitation. The rationale of these agents can backfire if the drug produces significant sedative effects or morning hangover. Some types of rehabilitation are best accomplished through scheduling the dose of the drug at least 2 hours away from the rehabilitation efforts.	Benzodiazepines: diazepam (Valium), alprazolam (Xanax), lorazepam (Ativan), flurazepam (Dalmane), temazepam (Restoril). Barbiturates: secobarbital (Seconal), pentobarbital (Nembutal). Miscellaneous: buspirone (BuSpar), zolpidem (Ambien).
Antidepressants/ antimanic drugs	May make the patient more optimistic and improve therapy potential. The patient may become more interested in rehabilitation. Certain side effects can be troubling during physical-therapy treatments. Tricyclic antidepressants can produce orthostatic hypotension, causing syncope and subsequent injury from falls. Sedation, lethargy, and muscle weakness may occur.	Tricyclic agents: amitriptyline (Elavil), imipramine (Tofranil), desipramine (Norpramin), nortriptyline (Aventyl). SSRIs: fluoxetine (Prozac), paroxetine (Paxil), sertraline (Zoloft). Antimanic: Lithium.
Antipsychotics (neuroleptic drugs)	These drugs tend to "normalize" patient behavior. Withdrawn patient becomes more active. Agitated patient becomes calmer and more relaxed. Will cause sedation and anticholinergic side effects. Guard against orthostatic hypotension.	Chlorpromazine (Thorazine), fluphenazine (Prolixin), trifluoperazine (Stelazine), perphenazine (Trilafon), prochlorperazine (Compazine), thioridazine (Mellaril), haloperidol (Haldol), clozapine (Clozaril), olanzapine (Zyprexa), risperidone (Risperdal). Some antiemetics are in this category of neuroleptics, such as droperidol (Inapsine).

Continued

Appendix **16-1** Clinical Considerations of Pharmacologic Agents in the Rehabilitation Patient—cont'd

Therapeutic Category	Clinical Considerations	Drug Examples
	Major side effects are EPS. PT always should be alert for motor involvement manifested as balance changes, involuntary movements, and other motor dysfunction.	The promotility drug metoclopramide (Reglan) may cause some EPS.
Anticonvulsants (antiepileptic agents)	PT should be aware of any patient with a history of seizure disorder. Common side effects: headache, dizziness, sedation, and gastrointestinal disturbances may be bothersome during rehabilitation. Cerebellar side effects such as ataxia are the most important to monitor and may impair the rehabilitation ability. All of these drugs have therapeutic serum levels (look for toxic levels). Many of these drugs often are used as mood stabilizers with the antipsychotics.	Phenobarbital, primidone (Mysoline), phenytoin (Dilantin), carbamazepine (Tegretol),valproic acid (Depakote), Gabapentin (Neurontin), lamotrigine (Lamictal).
Antiparkinsonism drugs	PT should coordinate therapy sessions with the peak effect of the drug. In patient on levodopa, the peak usually occurs 1 hr after a dose. Optimal therapy sessions can be achieved by scheduling after the breakfast dose of levodopa (may find maximal drug effect and lower fatigue levels in the patient). PT should monitor blood pressure in patients because most are prone to hypotension. Dizziness with positional changes will at times produce falls.	Levodopa: Sinemet. Anticholinergic agents: benztropine (Cogentin), trihexyphenidyl (Artane), procyclidine (Kemadrin), biperiden (Akineton). Dopamine agonists: pergolide (Permax), bromocriptine (Parlodel), pramipexole (Mirapex), ropinirole (Requip). Miscellaneous: selegiline (Eldepryl), amantadine (Symmetrel).
Skeletal muscle relaxants	By reducing muscle tone in spasticity, these drugs may allow more effective passive range of motion and stretching activities. General muscle weakness may occur with some drugs such as Dantrium. The patients' ability to support themselves during ambulation may be impeded by the drug, which causes overall muscle weakness. The PT should be aware of drug choices and work closely with the patient.	Dantrolene (Dantrium), baclofen (Lioresal), cyclobenzaprine (Flexeril), diazepam (Valium), carisoprodol (Soma).
Analgesics: opiates	Side effects of sedation and gastrointestinal upset may be particularly troublesome. Relief of pain may have a positive effect on rehabilitation. Drugs may tend to blunt the respiratory response to exercise. Respiratory depression usually will not occur unless preceded by mental alteration. Recognize mental change.	Morphine, oxycodone (Percocet and Percodan), hydrocodone (Vicodin), hydromorphone (Dilaudid), meperidine (Demerol), fentanyl (Duragesic), pentazocine (Talwin), buprenorphine (Buprenex), nalbuphine (Nubain).

Appendix **16-1** Clinical Considerations of Pharmacologic Agents in the Rehabilitation Patient—cont'd

Therapeutic Category	Clinical Considerations	Drug Examples
Analgesics: NSAIDs	Overall blunting effect is a descending response, and thus diaphragm usually will follow mental changes. Aspirin and other NSAIDs are among the most common medications used by the patient in rehabilitation. Side effects usually will not interfere with physical therapy. Recognize that gastrointestinal symptoms are the most common problems, but renal symptoms are the most critical issue. Renal problems with a rising potassium level may put the patient at risk for severe problems. The patient often will ask questions about the use of Tylenol versus aspirin; be able to explain the differences.	Salicylate NSAID: aspirin and others. Non-salicylate NSAID: ibuprofen, naproxen, sulindac, ketoprofen, tolmetin, indomethacin. COX-2 inhibitors: rofecoxib (Vioxx), celecoxib (Celebrex), valdecoxib (Bextra).
Antihypertensive drugs	Common medications: antihypertensives; these drugs produce a diverse set of side effects. Be aware of orthostatic hypotension. Activities that will produce widespread vasodilation such as whirlpools: use with caution with patient on a vasodilator drug. Exercise tolerance may be impaired when beta-blockers are used; myocardium will not respond as strongly to sympathetic influences. Be aware of coughing problems when patient is using ACE inhibitor medications.	Beta-blockers: propranolol (Inderal), metoprolol (Lopressor), atenolol (Tenormin). ACE inhibitors: captopril (Capoten), lisinopril (Zestril or Vasotec), ramipril (Altace). Calcium channel blockers: nifedipine (Procardia), diltiazem (Cardizem), verapamil (Isoptin), isradipine (DynaCirc), hydralazine (Apresoline), minoxidil (Loniten). Alpha blockers: doxazosin (Cardura), terazosin (Hytrin), prazosin (Minipress).
Antianginal drugs	Activities in rehabilitation will increase myocardial oxygen demand with subsequent anginal pain. If patient uses sublingual nitroglycerin, have patient bring drug to rehabilitation. Beta-blockers may slow heart rate and reduce myocardial contractility in some situations. Nitrates and calcium channel blockers both produce peripheral vasodilation. Heat and exercise may be additive to the drug's effect, resulting in syncope.	Nitrates: nitroglycerin, Isordil, ISMO (isosorbide mononitrate). Beta-blockers: see above. Calcium channel blockers: see above. Persantine.
Antiarrhythmic drugs	These drugs may produce side effects that can affect rehabilitation. These drugs usually will not alter exercise parameters such as heart rate or blood pressure. PT should monitor for faintness and dizziness, as these may be signs of a rhythm disturbance.	Quinidine, procainamide (Procan SR), disopyramide (Norpace), lidocaine, mexiletine (Mexitil) flecainide (Tambocor), propafenone (Rhythmol), digoxin (Lanoxin), adenosine (Adenocard).

Continued

Appendix **16-1** Clinical Considerations of Pharmacologic Agents in the Rehabilitation Patient—cont'd

Therapeutic Category	Clinical Considerations	Drug Examples
Anticoagulants	Primary outpatient agent is warfarin (Coumadin). PT should be aware of increased tendency to bleed. Any situation that deals with open wounds should be handled with some caution. Be aware of all antiplatelet drugs that may increase bleeding tendency. Antiplatelet drugs: Ticlid, aspirin, Persantine.	Warfarin (Coumadin). Heparin. Low molecular weight heparins, including enoxaparin (Lovenox).
Antibiotics	PT should be aware of gastrointestinal side effects with antibiotics. PT should recognize diarrhea, nausea, vomiting, and GI cramping. Some antibiotics increase the sensitivity to UV light and make the patient more (Cipro) prone to burns.	Sulfa: sulfamethoxazole/trimethoprim (Bactrim). Quinolones: ciprofloxacin ofloxacin (Floxin), tetracycline (Sumycin), doxycycline (Vibramycin), demeclocycline (Declomycin).

ACE Angiotensin-converting enzyme; *COX-2*, cyclooxygenase 2; *EPS*, extrapyramidal symptoms; *NSAIDs*, nonsteroidal anti-inflammatory drugs; *SSRI*, selective serotonin reuptake inhibitors.

Appendix **16-2** Glossary

Affinity: The amount of attraction or binding power a given drug has for its receptor site. Some degree of attraction must be inherent in the drug for it to bind to a receptor.

Agonist: A drug with affinity that can elicit a pharmacologic response. The pharmacologic action generally is stimulation, but inhibition also may be the action.

Antagonist: A drug with affinity (binds to receptor) but that does not produce an inherent action.

Bioavailability: The measure of the completeness of absorption combined with a measure of the amount of drug that will reach the target organ.

Biological half-life ($t^1/_2$): The time in which the pharmacologic response falls to one half of its original effect.

Blood-brain barrier: The sieve through which a drug must pass from the cerebral circulation into the brain cells to exert a pharmacologic effect in the central nervous system.

Efficacy: The capacity to produce an effect for a given occupied receptor. The term describes how well a drug works or the maximum response to a drug.

Elimination half-life ($t^1/_2$): The time in which the plasma concentration of a drug falls to one half of its original amount.

First-pass effect: The rapid extraction and metabolism of a drug by the liver, thereby blocking all of the drug or greatly minimizing the amount of drug available in the systemic circulation.

Pharmacology: The study of the action of any chemical on a living system. The methodology of the field relies heavily on both physiology and biochemistry.

Pharmacotherapeutics: The study of the use of drugs in the treatment, prevention, and diagnosis of disease. This aspect of pharmacology correlates pharmacodynamics with the pathophysiology of the clinical issue and applies rigorous patient-monitoring principles.

Pharmacovigilance: The monitoring of the safety profile (side effects) of medications to protect the patient. It applies the aspect of watchfulness in protecting the patient's safety from untoward conditions with the use of medications.

Potency: The amount of drug required to produce a given effect relative to a standard. The amount of drug usually is not important clinically.

Steady-state level: Condition in which the amount of drug eliminated is equal to the amount administered and the plasma levels oscillate around the mean. This is one of the goals of drug therapy for the clinician.

Tachyphylaxis: A rapidly developing tolerance that prevents the desired pharmacologic effect from being achieved. Rebound congestion that occurs with a nasal decongestant is an example.

Tolerance: The clinical situation in which increasing amounts of drug are required to produce the same pharmacologic effect, or the situation in which the same dose of the drug on repeated occasions produces a less intense pharmacologic effect.

Diagnostic Imaging in Primary Care Physical Therapy

17

Gail Deyle, PT, DPT, OCS, FAAOMPT

Objectives

After reading this chapter, the reader will be able to:

1. Evaluate the details of the patient history, the review of systems, and the tests and measures to determine if the indications for diagnostic imaging are present.
2. Apply the known risks, contraindications, and benefits of diagnostic imaging to recommend diagnostic imaging only when the diagnostic benefits outweigh the disadvantages.
3. Apply the knowledge of the diagnostic utility of the various types of imaging to select or recommend the appropriate modality for a specific patient presentation.

The role of diagnostic imaging in the practice of physical therapy is rapidly evolving. The availability of diagnostic images to physical therapists (PTs) varies greatly depending on the practice setting. PTs in the U.S. Army with primary care physical therapy provider credentials have had privileges for ordering diagnostic imaging procedures since the early 1970s (see Chapter 1).[12] In other settings, PTs often practice without the benefit of being able to order or even routinely view diagnostic images. This inability to order diagnostic imaging tests has probably contributed to PTs learning to depend on their clinical examination skills to formulate a clinical diagnosis. Other providers with ready access to imaging procedures may have learned to depend more on the diagnostic imaging modalities for making a clinical diagnosis rather than fully developing their physical examination skills. A study comparing PTs and orthopedic surgeons in the primary care management of musculoskeletal conditions found that care provided by the PTs was more cost effective, with no difference in patient outcomes. One reason for the cost effectiveness was that the PTs were less reliant on imaging procedures.[7] Other studies have found that the use of PTs in a primary care setting reduced the need for diagnostic imaging by up to 50%.[22]

Regardless of whether PTs can order diagnostic imaging tests in their practice setting, they should be familiar with musculoskeletal diagnostic imaging protocols and standards. PTs may be called on to provide guidance to another provider who will ultimately order the imaging. The type of diagnostic imaging modality or the specific views that will best reveal the suspected pathology, with the least risk to the patient and at a reasonable price, should be recommended. Although most providers who refer to PTs have privileges to order diagnostic imaging, their knowledge and experience associated with musculoskeletal

diagnoses may be limited.[18] The clinical examination findings from PTs can also provide the appropriate relevance to the pathology identified by the diagnostic imaging tests. This is important considering there are many examples in the published literature of pathology found on images of the spine and extremities in asymptomatic populations.[13,29,38]

A strong case can be made for making diagnostic imaging a routine practice privilege for PTs, but only within the context of established comprehensive practice guidelines.[24] A comprehensive examination scheme and a targeted, preferably evidence-based, intervention are essential to determine accurately the need for diagnostic imaging. Practice guidelines, such as the low back pain (LBP) guidelines presented in this chapter, illustrate the importance of PTs integrating findings from the history and physical examination, establishing an accurate prognosis, and determining the patient's goals and the degree of response to physical therapy interventions before making a decision related to the need for diagnostic imaging. If the patient's condition does not improve after the intervention, the next diagnostic step may include a diagnostic imaging modality, but in some circumstances there may not be a need for diagnostic imaging even with a negative response to physical therapy treatment.

When there is little likelihood that imaging will reveal anything that will change the course of treatment, the tests should be considered unnecessary. Although imaging may provide evidence of pathology, the mere presence of the abnormality may not change the course of treatment when there is no successful pathology-based treatment plan. For example, a patient may have clinical findings suggesting that a surgical procedure may be of benefit. However, if the patient is unwilling to undergo the procedure that requires imaging or is not a suitable candidate for the surgery, then there is no reason for diagnostic imaging.

Imaging is normally indicated only when positive findings will change the course of treatment. For example, pubic rami and proximal tibial stress fractures are fairly common in the military population. When appropriately managed, these injuries will rarely require medical or surgical intervention. If the patient history, review of systems, and tests and measures do not suggest infection or neoplasm, treatment for these suspected stress fractures may be initiated without diagnostic imaging. In contrast, high-grade stress fractures of the femoral neck are often treated surgically to prevent the possible catastrophic consequences of a complete femoral neck fracture.

Diagnostic imaging that reveals a femoral neck stress fracture will alter the conservative treatment course and may dictate the need for surgery. Therefore whenever a PT is suspicious of a femoral neck stress reaction or fracture, imaging that is sensitive for the disorder is promptly indicated (Figure 17-1).

The interpretation of diagnostic images is always the responsibility of the radiologist. However, in the clinical setting it is not unusual for primary care providers to have access to the diagnostic images before they are officially read. In some cases in which a quick interpretation is paramount to the disposition of the patient, it may be possible to request a "wet read" or less formal opinion from the radiologist as soon as the imaging is completed. At other times, the PT may be faced with initiating treatment before diagnostic images have been officially read. If the imaging films are available for the PT to review, they should be reviewed while waiting for the official interpretation by a radiologist because the images may provide useful information for patient management or clinical decision making.

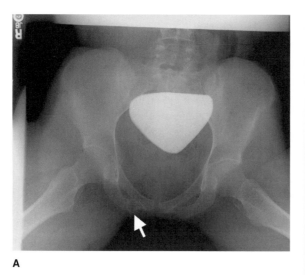

A

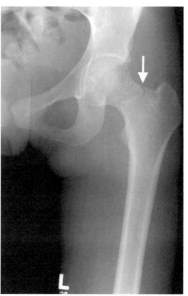

B

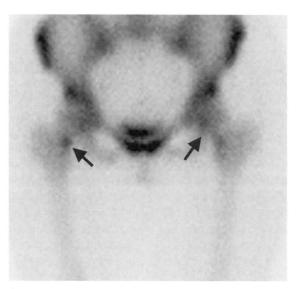

C

FIGURE 17-1 A, Anteroposterior radiograph of the pelvis reveals a pubic ramus stress fracture developing callus after simply reducing the physical activity level of the patient. **B,** This anteroposterior radiograph of the hip reveals a femoral neck stress fracture that requires immediate surgical stabilization to prevent the possible consequences of a completed fracture. Although radionuclide bone scans have a higher sensitivity than plain radiographs for detecting early femoral neck stress fractures, this AP film clearly reveals the extent of the fracture line. **C,** This bone scan of a physically active person reveals multiple areas of increased metabolic activity. Increased radiopharmaceutical uptake in the femoral necks suggests a stress fracture of the right femoral neck and stress-related changes of the left femoral neck. The stress fracture appears to be primarily on the compression, or inferior, side of the femoral neck and is considered to be more stable than a tension, or superior, side femoral neck fracture.

When referring a patient to a radiologist, any provider, including the PT, should provide the important details of the history (e.g., specific location of symptoms, mechanism of injury), physical examination, and tests and measures. Rarely will the radiologist have the opportunity to gather patient information directly. Being able to correlate the clinical information with the diagnostic imaging findings will allow the radiologist to formulate an accurate diagnosis. Guidance on the interpretation of radiographs or other imaging is beyond the scope of this chapter. PTs should become familiar with the wealth of material available in textbooks and through the Internet. A recommended resource list is provided at the end of this chapter.

Diagnostic Imaging as Part of Patient Management

Whenever PTs have privileges for ordering diagnostic imaging or are in a situation in which it is possible to recommend imaging, it is essential that that they do not attempt to substitute diagnostic imaging for the normal procedures of patient management. Only in the context of the clinical examination findings will the diagnostic imaging results have any relevance. The practice patterns of the expert PT have been previously described. The expert PT will use the history and review of systems for early hypothesis formation, which then guides the selection of tests, measures, and treatment. The expert PT will also use cumulative knowledge, clinical experience, and the evaluation of movement dysfunction to help determine the need for diagnostic imaging.[24,28]

Physical examination principles critical to effective clinical decision making regarding the need for diagnostic imaging include palpating all possible injured structures, examining the joint above and below the area of symptoms, and examining the cervical spine for upper extremity symptoms and the lumbar spine for lower extremity symptoms. PTs must remain vigilant for the possibility of referred pain both from proximal structures of the musculoskeletal system and from other systems such as the genitourinary and gastrointestinal systems. Failure to identify the true source of pain may result in images that do not reveal all the associated injuries or the true area of pathology. For example, hip problems commonly refer symptoms to the knee, particularly in the younger patient.[16,35,57] The initial symptoms of slipped capital femoral epiphysis and Legg-Calvé-Perthes disease are frequently pain around the knee. A wide variety of conditions of the cervical spine refer symptoms to the upper extremity, and many conditions of the lumbar spine are known to refer symptoms to the pelvis and lower extremity. The following case overview dramatically underscores the importance of examining proximal structures to determine the true source of distal pain.

An 18-year-old man presented to a military treatment facility with a primary symptom of hip and knee pain for the prior 2 weeks. The patient was uncertain of the origin of his symptoms, although he had been participating in physical training on a daily basis. The initial examination by the primary care physician revealed tenderness over the iliac crest, anterior superior iliac spine, and mid quadriceps. A diagnosis of a quadriceps strain was made and the patient was prescribed anti-inflammatory medication, activity was restricted, and a referral was written to physical therapy.

By the time the patient was seen in physical therapy 1 week later, his primary symptom was knee pain. Over the next few months this patient had a wax and wane of his symptoms with physical therapy and medical treatment. His primary symptom was always knee pain, but the painful areas were variable enough to prompt several different medical and physical therapy diagnoses.

After 4 months, a PT who was not previously involved in the patient's care before the current appointment observed and palpated a large mass protruding from the patient's right iliac wing. After completing his examination, radiographs of the hip and pelvis were obtained. The differential diagnosis based on the radiographic findings was osteogenic sarcoma or chondrosarcoma. Osteogenic sarcoma became the definitive diagnosis. Despite the large size of this primary malignant tumor, the patient and a number of PTs and medical providers were misled into thinking this patient had primary knee pain (Figure 17-2).

Significant disease processes or injuries may be obscured in other ways besides the issue of referred pain. The primary injury in an emergent situation may mask a less symptomatic injury until the primary injury is treated and the acute symptoms are reduced. Injuries associated with alcohol, other drug use, or a loss of consciousness require a particularly thorough review of systems, tests, and measures because the patient will be limited in his or her ability to guide the diagnostic process during the history.

With the advent of evidence-based medicine, the meaning of diagnostic tests must be viewed in the context of the clinical examination combined with the pretest probability.[25,42] For diagnostic imaging, the pretest probability may be determined by a number of factors. Consider the example of an elderly patient with diabetes who exhibits increasing back pain, spasm, fever, and malaise, 2 weeks after a surgical procedure for the lumbar spine. This patient history, as well as the clinical signs, establishes a strong pretest probability of an infection. Normal radiographs viewed in the context of the high pretest likelihood of systemic illness should be regarded with some suspicion. A more sensitive imaging procedure for infection, such as a magnetic resonance imaging (MRI) or bone scan, and the appropriate laboratory tests must be ordered. In comparison, a patient who is not diabetic, has a postoperative transient increase in back pain without constitutional symptoms of fever or malaise (see Chapter 7) may only require a decrease in the intensity of the rehabilitation program. The probability of an infection in the second example is so low that diagnostic imaging in this instance is unlikely to contribute to patient management.

As stated earlier, the PT must initiate treatment in some situations before the results of diagnostic imaging are known. The following case example illustrates this scenario, and it also reinforces the importance of using the pretest probability to guide the pursuit of diagnostic imaging.

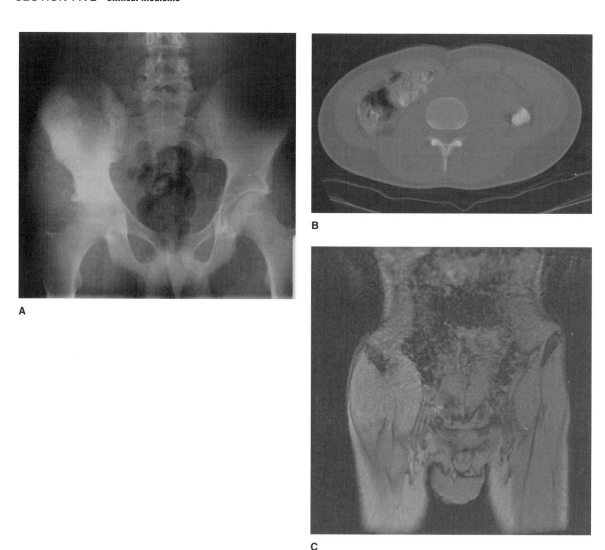

FIGURE 17-2 Despite the significant size of this primary malignant tumor located in the ilium, the patient had a primary symptom of knee pain. This case example highlights the importance of examining the joints and areas proximal to the painful area to rule out referred pain and to image the proper area. **A,** The radiograph initially identified the lesion. **B,** The CT scan reveals the bony structure of the osteogenic sarcoma. **C,** The MRI scan delineates the extent of the soft tissue involvement, including the integrity of the fascial planes.

A 64-year-old woman was referred to physical therapy for treatment of progressively intense hip pain. During the history, the patient related that she had been limited in her ability to squat or move her hip for approximately 8 months. Her pain had reached a peak approximately 3 months earlier; it then lessened somewhat, although her ability to move her hip had correspondingly deteriorated. The patient denied any injury, although she related that she had been active most of her life and that her current occupation was housekeeping for several clients. She had progressively become more limited in her ability to perform her normal cleaning activities, which required squatting, kneeling, and bending. The patient indicated that her primary care physician had ordered radiographs of her hip but she had not been informed of the results.

The tests and measures revealed a grossly antalgic and asymmetrical gait with the patient weight bearing on her forefoot on the affected lower extremity. Active and passive range of motion of the involved hip was dramatically limited in all directions, and there was an apparent total leg shortening of approximately 2 inches.

The patient's radiographs were not available for review and there was no official reading in the system. The patient stated that the imaging studies were performed 2 weeks earlier after her appointment with her physician. The referring physician was contacted and the relevant examination findings were detailed. The physician agreed that it would be appropriate to repeat the studies because it seemed likely that the films were misplaced or lost. The new images revealed severe osteoarthritis of the hip with a collapse of the acetabulum and penetration of the femoral head into the pelvic cavity (acetabular protrusion). The patient was subsequently given a priority referral to orthopedic surgery.

In this example, the diagnostic imaging was repeated because the results of the initial study were unknown. However, even if the original films had been read and the reported results were negative, the strong pretest probability of hip pathology in this case requires careful further investigation, including repeating of the test when the test results are unknown or the test is reportedly negative.[25,42] Other possible sources of diagnostic test error include confusing one set of images with those of another patient or selecting a diagnostic test that is not sensitive for the disorder.

Radiography

Conventional radiographs use ionizing radiation to produce typically high-resolution analog images on specialized film. Radiographs are usually easy to obtain with comparatively minimal associated expense. They provide a means to distinguish air, bone, calcification, fat, soft tissue, and fluids.[31] Radiographs produce superior resolution for fine cortical and trabecular detail in bone. Conventional radiographs are typically used to identify fractures ranging from stress fractures to avulsion fractures and complex fractures. Radiographs are not useful to distinguish differences in soft tissue contrast for the evaluation of muscle, ligament, or tendon injuries.[14,39] Because a film represents a two-dimensional picture of the anatomy, the minimal radiographic examination typically includes two views of the imaged body part at right angles to each other. Specialized views may be required in addition to standard views for adequately assessing the local anatomy and differentiating specific injuries.

Limiting exposure to ionizing radiation is an important aspect of diagnostic radiology. Body parts that will be exposed to radiation but are of no interest regarding the differential diagnosis should be adequately shielded with lead garments. Selection of the appropriate view can also help limit radiation exposure. For example, posterior to anterior (PA) rather than anterior to posterior (AP) views are used to limit radiation exposure of the breasts; breast shields should be used whenever possible.[33] Oblique views of the lumbar spine have traditionally been used to visualize defects of the pars articularis found in spondylolysis and spondylolisthesis. Because of the high levels of gonadal radiation associated with these views and the evolution of CT as the diagnostic standard, oblique views of the lumbar spine are not routinely obtained.

Radiographs may be more specific than MRI in differentiating potential causes of bony lesions because of the proven ability to characterize specific calcification patterns and periosteal reactions. Plain radiographs are not considered sensitive to the early changes associated with tumors, infections, and some fractures.[43] The following case example highlights the lack of sensitivity of plain radiographs for certain types of fractures.

An obese 55-year-old man sought physical therapy care for LBP after slipping and landing on his buttocks in a local department store. The patient had been seen in the emergency department after the fall where AP and lateral radiographs were taken of the lumbar spine. The images were interpreted as normal by one of the hospital radiologists. The PT reviewed the lumbar images from the hospital's networked imaging system, and no pathologic findings other than minor degenerative changes were apparent.

The physical examination by the PT revealed diffuse pain with active range of motion and palpation of the lumbar spine, although the morbid obesity was a limiting factor in performing a typical examination. The neurologic screening examination was unremarkable.

Treatment was initiated consisting of gentle range-of-motion exercises and walking in the therapeutic pool. After 3 weeks, the patient was concerned about his lack of progress and he went to a local Veterans Administration hospital for further evaluation. The same radiographic procedure was repeated, this time revealing a 30% compression fracture of the fifth lumbar vertebrae.

The structural elements of the lumbar vertebrae had probably been disrupted by the fall, although there was no initial radiographic evidence. The patient's size may well have contributed to the extent of the eventual compression and collapse of the vertebral body. Computed tomography (CT), MRI, and a bone scan would have been more sensitive to the bone pathology in this case and should be considered when patients with normal radiographs do not respond to treatment.[14,15] Typical radiographic views, imaged structures, and commonly revealed pathologic findings are provided in Table 17-1.

GUIDELINES FOR THE SELECTIVE USE OF RADIOGRAPHS. Overuse of radiologic studies has become a significant economic problem in the United States. Although radiographic procedures are relatively inexpensive, the economic impact of high-volume, low-cost procedures can be equal to low-volume, high-cost imaging procedures.[55] Because of the overutilization of radiographs, clinical prediction or decision rules indicating a need for radiography for specific types of injuries at certain areas of the body have been developed. A clinical decision rule (CDR) is a clinical tool that can quantify individual contributions from the components of the examination to determine the diagnosis, prognosis, or treatment for a given patient. CDRs attempt to formally test, simplify, and increase the accuracy of clinicians' diagnostic and prognostic assessments. Attempts have been made to categorize a CDR based on the criteria of the method of derivation, the validation of the CDR to ensure that its repeated use leads to consistent results, and its predictive value.[36]

Radiographic images of the knee are frequently ordered, although fractures are present in only 6% of cases and are generally clinically detectable. The Ottawa knee rules and the Pittsburgh decision rules are guidelines for the selective use of radiographs in knee trauma. Application of these rules may lead to a more efficient evaluation of knee injuries and a reduction in health costs without an increase in adverse outcomes.[55] The Ottawa knee CDR summarized in Table 17-2 indicates when radiographic studies are appropriate to consider. Exclusion criteria for these rules are age younger than 18 years; isolated superficial skin injuries; injuries greater than 7 days old; recent injuries being reevaluated; and patients with altered levels of consciousness, paraplegia, or multiple injuries.[44,50] The Ottawa knee rules have been demonstrated to have near 100% sensitivity for knee fractures and reduce the need for knee radiographs by 28% when used by emergency physicians.[50]

TABLE 17-1

Radiographic Views, Structures Imaged, and Typical Pathologic Condition by Body Region

Region	Radiographic View	Structures Imaged	Common Pathologic Condition
Cervical spine	AP open mouth	Odontoid process, body of axis, lateral masses of atlas and atlantoaxial joint	Fractures of the upper cervical spine, asymmetrical location of the dens between the lateral masses indicating ligamentous stretching or injury
	AP	C3 to C7 spinous processes and vertebral bodies	Fractures of C3 to C7; disc space changes and pathology of the uncovertebral joints
	Lateral (standing, seated, or supine cross table)	Occiput to C7	Fractures, dislocations, postural curves and contour lines, alignment changes, spondylitic changes
	Lateral flexion-extension	Occiput to C7 in active flexion and active extension	Unstable joint segments from ligamentous injury
	Obliques	Intervertebral foramina, facet joints, pedicles, and uncovertebral joints	Narrowing and degenerative changes of the intervertebral foramina and apophyseal joint
	Swimmer's view	Best view of C7 to T2, prevents obstruction by shoulders	Fractures of C7 to T2
Shoulder	AP	Proximal humerus, lateral clavicle, A-C joint, superior lateral aspect of the scapula	Fractures of the proximal humerus and glenoid; changes in humeral head position from rotator cuff tears or glenohumeral dislocations; osteoarthritis, calcific tendonitis, or bursitis
	AP standing with arm in internal rotation		Hill-Sachs lesion
	AP standing with arm in external rotation		Compression fracture of the humeral head usually associated with posterior dislocation
	Axillary, oblique	Humeral head in relation to the glenoid	Anterior and posterior glenohumeral dislocations; fractures of the proximal humerus and scapula
	West Point view	Humeral head in relation to the glenoid and the anterior inferior rim of the glenoid	Anterior and posterior glenohumeral dislocations; pathology of the anterior inferior glenoid
A-C joint	AP bilateral with and without weight	Both A-C joints, both sternoclavicular joints, clavicles	Ligamentous instability of the A-C joint or S-C joint; fractures of the clavicle
Scapula	AP, lateral scapula	Entire scapula, body of scapula	Fractures of the scapula
	Transcapular or Y view	Entire scapula; best view for comminuted and displaced fractures of the scapula	Fractures of the scapula
Humerus	AP, lateral humerus	Entire humerus	Fractures of the humerus; myositis ossificans of the anterior compartment
	Transthoracic lateral view	True lateral view of the proximal humerus	Fractures of the proximal humerus
Elbow	AP	Distal humerus, proximal radius and ulna	Fractures of the distal humerus and proximal radius and ulna; dislocations of the elbow; ligamentous avulsions with bony attachments; varus and valgus deformities; heterotopic bone formations
	Lateral	Distal humerus, proximal radius and ulna	Supracondylar fractures of the distal humerus, radial head fractures; fat pad sign; elbow dislocations
	Internal oblique	Best view of coronoid process	Fractures of the coronoid process and medial epicondyle

TABLE 17-1

Radiographic Views, Structures Imaged, and Typical Pathologic Condition by Body Region—cont'd

Region	Radiographic View	Structures Imaged	Common Pathologic Condition
	External oblique	Best view of radial head, neck, and tuberosity	Fractures of the radial head, neck, tuberosity, and lateral epicondyle
	Radial head-capitellum	Best view of radial head, capitellum, and coronoid process	Fractures of radial head, capitellum, coronoid process; joint abnormalities
Forearm	AP, lateral	Entire radius and ulna, wrist, elbow	Fractures of the radius, ulna, wrist, and elbow
Hand	PA or dorsovolar, oblique, lateral	Distal radius and ulna to phalanges	Fractures of the wrist and hand; rheumatoid arthritis and osteoarthritis; avascular necrosis of the lunate or scaphoid; carpal instabilities
Thoracic spine	AP	T1-T12 vertebral end plates, pedicles, and spinous processes; intervertebral disc spaces; costovertebral joints; medial aspect posterior ribs	Fractures of the vertebral bodies, posterior elements, and ribs; pneumothorax
	Lateral	T1-T12 vertebral bodies, pedicles, and spinous processes; intervertebral disc spaces and foramina	Fractures of the vertebral bodies and posterior elements; changes in postural alignment from scoliosis, fractures, and ligamentous disruptions; pedicle obliteration from tumors
	Posterior oblique	Facet joints, pedicles, and the pars interarticularis	Fractures of the lamina and facets
	Anterior oblique (right)	Sternum, axillary portion of the ribs	Fractures of the sternum and ribs; costosternal disruptions
Ribs	AP, PA, AO, PO, PA chest	Anterior and posterior aspects of the ribs	Fractures of the ribs
Lumbar spine	AP	Vertebral bodies and end plates, transverse processes, intervertebral disc spaces, pedicles, and spinous processes	Fractures of the vertebral bodies, end plates, and posterior elements; disc space abnormalities
	Lateral	Vertebral bodies, end plates, and posterior elements; intervertebral disc spaces	Fractures of the vertebral bodies, end plates, and posterior elements; vertebral alignment; disc space abnormalities
	Coned down lateral spot	Vertebral bodies, end plates, and posterior elements of L5 and S1; L5-S1 intervertebral disc space	Fractures of the vertebral bodies, end plates, and posterior elements; vertebral alignment; disc space abnormalities
	Obliques	Facet joints, lamina	Fractures and defects in the pars interarticularis and articular facets
Sacroiliac joint	AP axial, obliques	AP images bilateral S-I joints; obliques image unilateral S-I joint	Degenerative changes, ankylosis
Hip and pelvis	AP unilateral or entire pelvis	Acetabulum, femoral head and neck, greater trochanter, angle of inclination of the femoral neck to the shaft of the femur	Fractures of the proximal femur, acetabulum, pubic rami, and ischial tuberosities; hip joint dislocations; slipped capital femoral epiphysis; Legg-Calvé-Perthes disease; osteoarthritis
	Frog-leg lateral	Femoral head and neck, proximal third of femur, acetabulum	Fractures of the femoral head and neck, greater and lesser trochanters
Knee	AP	Distal femur, proximal tibia, head of the fibula, tibiofemoral joint space	Fractures of the patella, tibial plateau, femoral condyles, distal femur, and proximal fibula; osteochondral fragments; osteoarthritis and rheumatoid arthritis; varus and valgus alignment
	AP with valgus or varus stress	Relation of distal femur to proximal tibia	Ligamentous instability; changes in articular cartilage thickness
	Lateral with AP or PA stress	Relation of distal femur to proximal tibia	Ligamentous instability

Continued

Radiographic Views, Structures Imaged, and Typical Pathologic Condition by Body Region—cont'd

Region	Radiographic View	Structures Imaged	Common Pathologic Condition
	Lateral	Relation of patella to femur; length of patella to patellar ligament	Osteochondral fractures, tibial apophysitis, quadriceps tendon ruptures, patellar ligament tears
	Notch or tunnel	Intercondylar fossa, notch of popliteal tendon, tibial spines, intercondylar eminence, posterior aspects of the distal femur and proximal tibia, intercondylar eminence of tibia	Osteochondral defects and loose bodies, fractures of the tibial spines
	Sunrise axial	Patella, femoral condyles	Relation of patella to femoral condyles, subluxation and dislocation of the patella, patellar fractures
	Merchant axial	Patella, femoral condyles	Preferred view of articular surface of the patella, subtle dislocations
Lower leg	AP, lateral	Shaft of tibia and fibula	Fractures and dislocations of the tibia and fibula
Ankle	AP	Distal tibia and fibula, body of the talus, tibiotalar joint	Fractures of the distal tibia, fibula, and talus; dislocations and subluxations of the tibiotalar joint; osteoarthritis
	AP mortise	Joint space between distal fibula and talus, ankle mortise	Fractures of the distal tibia and fibula; fractures of the talus
	AP with inversion or eversion stress	Ankle mortise	Fractures and subluxations, mortise instability
	Lateral	Distal tibia and fibula, calcaneus, tibiotalar and subtalar articulations	Fractures and dislocations of the distal tibia and fibula, talus, and calcaneus; osteoarthritis
	External oblique	Lateral malleolus, anterior tibial tubercle, distal tibiofibular syndesmosis, talofibular joint	Fractures of the lateral malleolus, talus, and tuberosity of the calcaneus; disruptions of the distal tibiofibular syndesmosis
	Internal oblique	Medial and lateral malleoli, tibial plafond, dome of the talus, tibiotalar joint, tibiofibular syndesmosis	Best view of pathology of the tibial plafond; fractures of the medial malleolus
Foot	AP	Talus, navicular, cuboid, cuneiforms, metatarsals, phalanges	Fractures and dislocations of the foot
	Lateral	Calcaneocuboid and talonavicular articulations, calcaneus, talus, subtalar joint	Fractures and dislocations of the foot, heel spurs, osteoarthritis
	Oblique	Midtarsal joints to the phalanges	Fractures of the foot

A-C, Acromioclavicular; *AO,* anterior oblique; *PO,* posterior oblique; *S-I,* sacroiliac; *S-C,* sternoclavicular.

Ottawa Knee Rules for Radiography

Indications for Radiography, if Any	Exclusion Criteria
Patient older than 55 years	Age younger than 18 years
Tenderness at the head of the fibula	Isolated superficial skin injuries
Isolated tenderness of the patella	Injuries more than 7 days old
Inability to flex to 90 degrees	Recent injuries being reevaluated
Inability to weight bear four steps both immediately after the injury and in the emergency department	Patients with altered levels of consciousness
	Paraplegia or multiple injuries

The rules are 97% sensitive and 27% specific for knee fractures.
From Seaberg D, Yealy M, Lukens T, et al: Multicenter comparison of two clinical decision rules for the use of radiography in acute, high-risk knee injuries, *Ann Emerg Med* 32:8-13, 1998.

The Pittsburgh CDR for the knee indicating the need for radiographic studies is summarized in Table 17-3. The Pittsburgh rules are not applicable in knee injuries sustained more than 6 days before presentation, in patients with only superficial lacerations and abrasions or a history of previous surgeries or fractures on the affected knee, and in those patients being reassessed for the same injury.[44] In a multicenter convenience sample of 934 patients, the Pittsburgh decision rules have been determined to be 99% sensitive and 60% specific for knee fractures. The positive predictive value was 24.1. This positive predictive value indicates that 24.1% of patients actually had a fracture when the rules indicated that a fracture was present. The negative predictive value was 99.8, thereby indicating that 99.8% of the time when the rules indicated that no fracture was present, the patient did not have a fracture. The Ottawa knee rules were 97% sensitive and 27% specific for

TABLE 17-3

Pittsburgh Decision Rules for Radiography

Indications for Radiography if the Mechanism of Injury is Blunt Trauma or a Fall and Either:	Exclusion Criteria
(1) The patient is younger than 12 or older than 50 years	Knee injuries sustained more than 6 days before presentation
(2) The injury causes an inability to walk more than four weight-bearing steps in the emergency department	Patients with only superficial lacerations and abrasions
	History of previous surgeries or fractures on the affected knee
	Patients being reassessed for the same injury

The rules are 99% sensitive and 60% specific for knee fractures.
From Seaberg D, Yealy M, Lukens T, et al: Multicenter comparison of two clinical decision rules for the use of radiography in acute, high-risk knee injuries, *Ann Emerg Med* 32:8-13, 1998.

knee fractures, with three missed fractures.[44] The authors concluded that both rules were equally useful for the diagnosis of knee fractures with no significant difference in sensitivity.

The Ottawa ankle (Box 17-1) and foot (Box 17-2) CDRs were developed to help predict fractures in patients with ankle and foot injuries. The Ottawa ankle rules have been shown to be 100% sensitive and 40% specific and to reduce the need for emergency department ankle radiographs by 36%.[48,49,51] Examples of commonly overlooked foot fractures with ankle sprains are provided in Figure 17-3.

CDRs for the evaluation of cervical spine injuries remain controversial, although consensus exists that cervical radiographic studies are overutilized in the emergency department.[47] Stiell et al prospectively evaluated outcomes from 8924 adults present-

BOX 17-1

Ottawa Ankle Rules for Radiography

INDICATIONS FOR RADIOGRAPHY IF ANY OF THE FOLLOWING ARE PRESENT
Bone tenderness at the posterior edge or tip of the lateral malleolus
Bone tenderness at the posterior edge or tip of the medial malleolus
Inability to bear weight both immediately and in the emergency department

The rules are 100% sensitive and 40% specific for ankle fractures.
From Stiell I, Greenberg G, McKnight R, et al: Decision rules for the use of radiography in acute ankle injuries: refinement and prospective validation, *JAMA* 269:1127-1132, 1993.

BOX 17-2

Ottawa Foot Rules for Radiography

INDICATIONS FOR RADIOGRAPHY IF ANY OF THE FOLLOWING ARE PRESENT
Bone tenderness at the base of the fifth metatarsal
Bone tenderness at the navicular
Inability to bear weight immediately and in the emergency department

From Stiell I, Greenberg G, McKnight R, et al: Decision rules for the use of radiography in acute ankle injuries: refinement and prospective validation, *JAMA* 269:1127-1132, 1993.

ing to the ED with head and neck injuries. A total of 1.7%were found to have important cervical injuries. Analysis of the data resulted in the Canadian C-Spine Rule. The three questions relevant to the Canadian cervical rule and the important responses are described in Box 17-3. By using three questions, the rules had 100% sensitivity and 43% specificity for identifying important cervical spine injuries. The expected radiography ordering rate when using these guidelines is be 58% as opposed to the current ordering rates of more than 90% for cervical injuries.[52]

Besides the aforementioned rules, guidelines exist for the lumbar spine. Because these guidelines are tightly interwoven into decision making regarding the ordering of laboratory tests, they are presented later in this chapter. Besides the cervical spine, knee, ankle, foot, and lumbar spine guidelines, similar CDRs for other frequently injured and imaged areas of the body are notably lacking and will most likely be established with the further development of evidence-based practice.

Scintigraphy

Scintigraphy, or bone scans, reveals pathology through the uptake and subsequent detection of a radiopharmaceutical substance (e.g., radiolabeled phosphate) into areas of reactive bone. Patients who will undergo a bone scan receive an intravenous injection with the radiopharmaceutical substance. Hours after the injection, the skeletal system is scanned by a detector for areas of increased radionuclide uptake. Although all bone will absorb some of the radiopharmaceutical substance, areas of increased osteoclastic and osteoblastic activity will absorb the most and are revealed as black, or *hot*, areas on the scan. Bone scans are considered sensitive for changes in bone associated with fractures (including stress fractures), infections, and tumors.[39] Some types of bony lesions such as those associated with multiple myeloma may not be reactive enough or have enough osteoblastic activity for the bone scan to be positive. These types of lesions are therefore referred to as *cold lesions* and are best revealed by other types of diagnostic imaging such as MRI or CT. Radiographs will also eventually reveal the typical osteopenic and radiolucent areas associated with myelomatosis.

Although bone scans are considered sensitive, they are not specific with many of the mentioned processes producing similar appearances on bone scan. Bone scans are important for evaluating the distribution of lesions (Figure 17-4).[14] Bone scans are commonly used by PTs in the U.S. Army to detect stress fractures among training soldiers. Although radiographs may also eventually reveal stress fractures when gross changes or healing are evident, they are not considered sensitive enough to be a reliable diagnostic tool. Femoral neck stress fractures that result in a complete femoral neck fracture have the potential for resulting in avascular necrosis of the femoral head. Therefore, as previously mentioned, the sensitivity of a bone scan is warranted to evaluate femoral neck stress-related changes.

The radionuclide bone scan is useful in localizing the extent of multifocal bone disease but is less sensitive than MRI in detecting metastases and does not have the spatial resolution to detail the extent and anatomic association of disease processes often necessary for optimal clinical decision

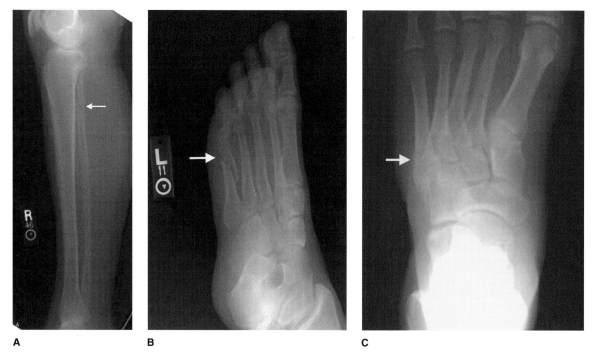

A   B   C

FIGURE 17-3 Radiographs revealing fractures that can be overlooked in the examination of an acute ankle sprain. **A,** Proximal fibula fracture. **B,** Oblique displaced midshaft fifth metatarsal fracture. **C,** Nondisplaced base of the fifth metatarsal fracture.

making.[43] Old and well-healed fractures, degenerative joint disease, open growth plates, and the sacroiliac joints may all have areas of increased uptake and will need to be differentiated for relevance during the patient examination.

Tomography

Tomography is radiography of a body section that permits more accurate visualization of lesions too small (down to 1 mm) to be noted on conventional radiographs. Tomography also demonstrates anatomic detail obscured by overlying structures.[23] Conventional tomograms and computer-assisted tomography (CT scans) use ionizing radiation. Radiation doses to imaged areas may indeed be higher than those of plain radiographs. The dose to areas outside those imaged is,

however, greatly reduced and considered negligible.[39] In plain radiographs, the beam of ionizing radiation and the film cassette are positioned and stationary, whereas the film and the body part are exposed to the radiation. In conventional tomograms, the radiographic film and the tube producing the radiographic image move simultaneously so that only a specific area of the body is not blurred and becomes sharply outlined in a single plane of focus. The radiographer can control the thickness of the imaged area. Images are usually sequentially taken through parallel planes until the desired area has been adequately imaged. Technologic advances have resulted in the ability of the radiographic tube to move in complex angles and arcs, resulting in even greater imaging detail. The advantage of conventional tomography over conventional radiography includes the improved visualization of subtle fractures, fracture lines, and the presence and extent of fracture healing. Conventional tomograms are particularly useful to evaluate small tumors and cystic and sclerotic lesions. Tomograms and radiographs are often interpreted together for the purpose of comparison.[23]

COMPUTED TOMOGRAPHY. CT is a radiologic modality containing a source of ionizing radiation, detectors, and a computer data-processing system. A CT system includes a circular scanning gantry that houses the radiographic tube image sensors, a table for the patient to lie on, an x-ray generator, and a computerized data processing unit. The patient to be imaged lies on the table and is placed inside the gantry. The x-ray tube is rotated 360 degrees around the patient and administers multiple x-ray beams projected at different angles; the computer collects the data and formulates axial cross-sectional images of the body, referred to as *slices.*[23] After determining the relative impedance

---

BOX 17-3

Canadian C-Spine Rules

INDICATIONS FOR RADIOGRAPHY ARE PRESENT IF THE ANSWER TO QUESTION 1 IS POSITIVE, 2 IS NEGATIVE, OR 3 IS NEGATIVE

(1) Is there any high-risk factor present that mandates radiography (e.g., age greater than 65 years, dangerous mechanism of injury, or paresthesias in the extremities)?

(2) Is there any low-risk factor that allows safe assessment of range of motion (e.g., simple rear end motor vehicle accident, normal sitting posture in ED, ambulatory at any time since injury, delayed onset of neck pain, and absence of midline tenderness)?

(3) Is the patient able to actively rotate the neck 45 degrees to the right and to the left?

From Stiell I, Wells G, Vandemheen KL: The Canadian C-spine rule for radiography in alert and stable trauma patients, *JAMA* 286:1841-1848, 2001.

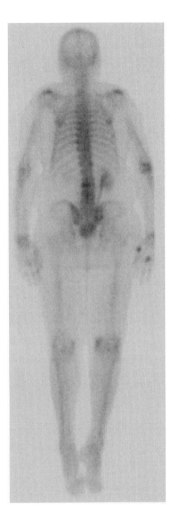

FIGURE 17-4 Although bone scans do not reveal the intricate details of fractures or bony lesions, they are useful to screen for the presence of lesions in the skeletal system. In this case, the areas of relative increased radiopharmaceutical uptake in the fourth and fifth lumbar vertebrae are consistent with metastatic prostate cancer. The other areas of increased uptake in this study, such as the elbows, wrists, hands, and knees, are more consistent with degenerative arthritic changes.

of the body tissues to the X-rays, the computer assigns values of relative density to each point in the body and constructs images in relative shades of gray.[5] The most striking differences are between bone and soft tissue, but differences between the various types of soft tissue are subtle. This accounts for the excellent detail of bone produced by CT, but this modality is much less useful for imaging tendons and ligaments. CT also has the capability to provide images in the transverse plane (axial views) and to produce multiplanar reconstructions.

CT provides excellent cortical and trabecular definition that allows for detection and characterization of the complex geometry of tri-plane fractures as well as those fractures with suspected intra-articular extension.[39] CT is useful to probe further for fractures when radiographic results are normal and the pretest probability strongly suggests fracture (Figure 17-5). High-resolution MR is also considered valuable in evaluating these types of injuries because of the excellent soft tissue detail. The combination of CT and high-definition MR reveals com-

binations of bony and soft tissue injuries such as a tibial plateau fracture and a meniscal tear.

Other uses for CT include investigating suspected visceral organ injuries, spine and extremity imaging, and head injuries. Soft tissue mineral deposition and destructive humeral head amyloidomas associated with end-stage renal disease are well demonstrated by CT. Kinematic CT with slip ring technology has been used to demonstrate patellar tracking in chondromalacia and degenerative joint disease. Slip ring technology allows continuous rotation of the x-ray sources and detectors during patient movement. Depuy et al[8] used slip ring technology and continuous 10-second exposures to demonstrate patellar tracking from 45 degrees of knee flexion to full extension. It is also combined with arthrography to reveal additional joint detail and has been particularly useful in the imaging of articular cartilage.[14] CT is useful to image spinal conditions such as degenerative spondylosis and intervertebral disc disease. MR images are considered more useful in evaluating disc herniations, whereas CT is more useful to provide the details of spinal osteophytes. Greater understanding of spinal fracture patterns ranging from stress fractures of the pars interarticularis to the complex burst fractures of the intervertebral bodies can be gained from CT. CT allows for the reconstruction of thin axial images from the spinal segment into images in the sagittal, coronal, or oblique planes. The use of contrast in the subarachnoid space provides even greater detail and contrast of the nerve roots and subarachnoid spaces to spinal images, although this introduces the additional risk associated with invasive procedures. CT is generally considered to be less complex and expensive than MRI. The main variable in CT is the thickness of the slice. Slices as thin as 1 mm may be required to produce good reformations. Finally, CT accurately analyzes bone mineral content, providing valuable information for the diagnosis and treatment of metabolic bone diseases. Disadvantages of CT include the higher radiation dose and cost when compared with conventional radiography.[39]

Magnetic Resonance Imaging

The ability of MRI to image bone and soft tissue structures and reveal pathologic conditions in three dimensions has made it a powerful and popular form of imaging. MRI is the primary imaging method for detailed evaluation of a broad spectrum of musculoskeletal disease processes.[41,43] MRI scans use magnetic fields to produce computer-generated axial and sagittal cross-sectional images of the body.[4] Numerous texts provide excellent and detailed descriptions of the rather complex physics principles involved in MRI.[30,40]

In brief, MRI uses the magnetic characteristics of the body's tissues rather than ionizing radiation to produce an image. Patients are positioned in the scanner within a strong magnetic field that produces changes in the body's atoms. The ability of MRI to image various parts of the body depends on the intrinsic spin of atoms with an odd number of neutrons or protons, thereby producing a magnetic moment. The atomic nuclei of tissues placed within the field align along the direction of the magnetic field. Stronger magnets are generally associated with better images, although there are some exceptions. Images obtained with these atoms are subjected to the additional

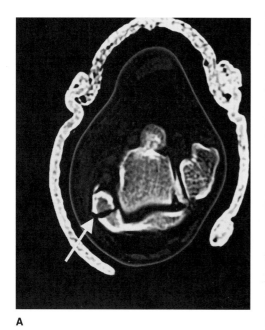

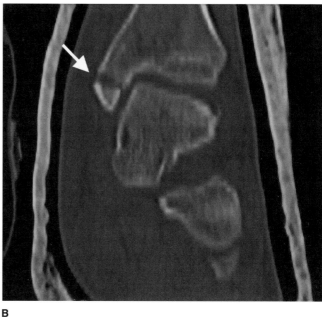

A   B

FIGURE 17-5 CT can reveal fractures that may otherwise not be apparent on plain radiographs. In this case a medial malleolar fracture was not revealed on the plain films but is clearly identified with CT images in the transverse **(A)** and frontal **(B)** planes.

influence of magnetic coils and subsequently register the atomic response. Radiofrequency (RF) pulses from the coils cause the nuclei to absorb energy and produce resonance. When the RF pulse is removed, the energy absorbed is released as an electrical signal from which digital images are derived. The signal intensity refers to the strength of the radio wave that a tissue emits after removal of the RF pulse. The strength of the radio wave produces either bright (high) signal intensity or dark (low) signal intensity images. Signal intensity in a specific tissue will depend on the concentration of hydrogen ions as well as the T1 and T2 relaxation times.[23]

MR images are subsequently referred to as *T1* or *T2 weighted*. T1 images are obtained with RF pulses that have a short repetition time and a short echo time. The T1 image, or longitudinal relaxation, is used to describe the return of protons back to equilibrium after the application and removal of the RF pulse. T2 images are obtained with a long repetition time and a long echo time. The T2 image, or transverse relaxation time, is used to describe the associated loss of coherence or phase between individual protons immediately after the application of the RF pulse. The necessary imaging contrast between tissues is produced by varying the RF pulse sequences to increase the differences in T1 and T2. Repetition time is defined by the recovery time of the transverse and longitudinal orientation of protons after being subjected to the RF pulse. T1 is typically eight to 10 times larger than T2. If T1 is the focus, the RF is kept relatively short, allowing tissues of various composition to recover to distinct levels, and producing tissue contrast.

The rapid application of a second RF pulse produces a spin echo effect. A spin echo is used to cause magnetization vectors to come back into phase and create an echo of the original signal. Conventional spin echo pulse sequences include T1, T2,

and proton density-weighted images. Fast spin echo acquisition of images can reduce the required acquisition time and therefore lessen the potential for patient movement.

T1-weighted images will show subacute hemorrhage and fat as a bright intensity. Fluids contained in abscesses or cysts that contain high levels of protein will also have a bright appearance. Other soft tissues will have characteristic low signal intensity. T1-weighted images are useful for delineating the architecture of soft tissues such as marrow, fascia, and anatomic planes.[30] Bone has a characteristic bright signal in T1-weighted images because of the high fat content. T2-weighted images reveal fluids as high signal intensity images. Kaplan et al suggest using the "two" in water (H_2O) to help remember that fluids are bright in T2-weighted images. Fluid-containing structures such as bursae, inflamed tendons, tumors, and abscesses will have a bright appearance on T2-weighted images.

In certain situations, the high signal intensity of fat will need to be suppressed to reveal the signal differences between fat and fluid. Fast spin echo T2-weighted images produce particularly bright fat images. Therefore fat suppression produces a dull appearance of fat for a better contrast with fluids. Proton density-weighted images combine the properties of T1- and T2-weighted images and produce good anatomic detail with little tissue contrast.

Metal implants, such as cerebral aneurysm clips and pacemakers, or metal foreign bodies, such as the slivers a machinist may have lodged in the eye, may be displaced during the MRI and are contraindications. Advances in technology and design have allowed MRI to produce high-quality images of small joints, fine soft tissue structures, and large joint components such as fibrocartilage, ligaments, capsules, and synovium (Figure 17-6). The ability to provide the appropriate detail

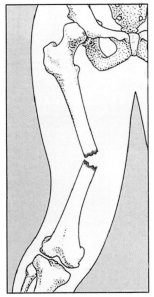

Medial angulation
(or lateral
angulation of
distal fragment—
valgus configuration)

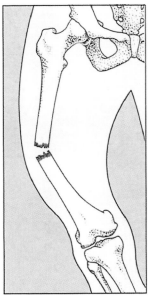

Lateral angulation
(or medial
angulation of
distal fragment—
valgus configuration)

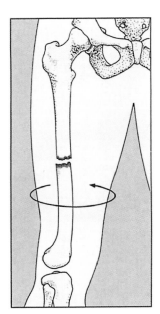

Internal rotation

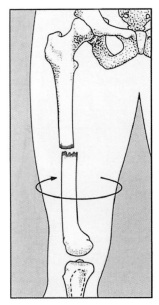

External rotation

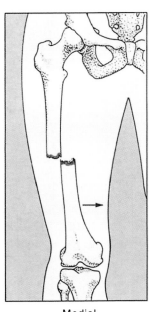

Medial
displacement

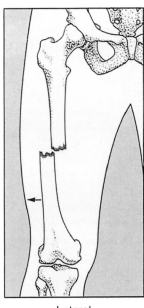

Lateral
displacement

PLATE 17-1 Alignment of fractures. (Plates 17-1 through 17-4 from Greenspan A: *Orthopaedic radiology: a practical approach,* ed 2, Philadelphia, 1996, Lippincott-Raven.)

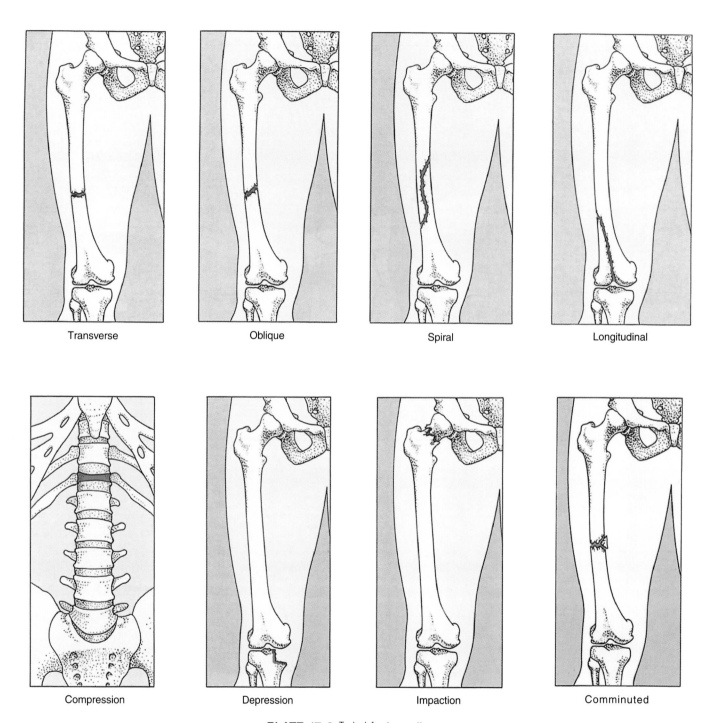

PLATE 17-2 Typical fracture patterns.

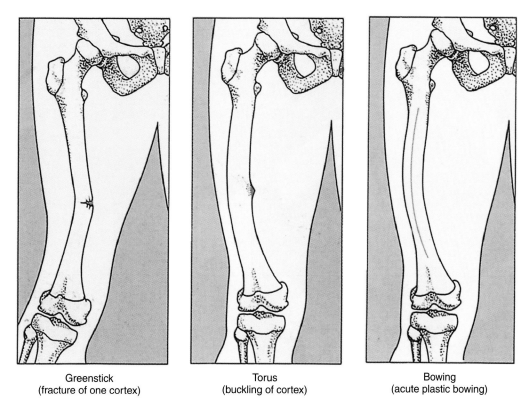

Greenstick
(fracture of one cortex)

Torus
(buckling of cortex)

Bowing
(acute plastic bowing)

PLATE 17-3 Fracture patterns typically seen in younger patients with more flexible bony structure include greenstick fractures.

INVOLVEMENT OF THE GROWTH PLATE

Salter-Harris Classification

I

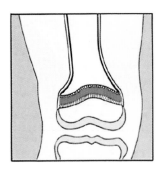

Fracture through
growth plate

II

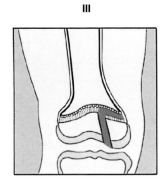

Fracture through
growth plate
and metaphysis

III

Fracture through
growth plate
and epiphysis

IV

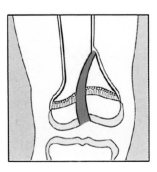

Fracture through
growth plate,
metaphysis,
and epiphysis

V

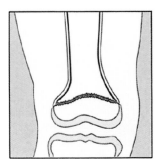

Compression
fracture through
growth plate

PLATE 17-4 Salter-Harris classification of growth plate injuries.

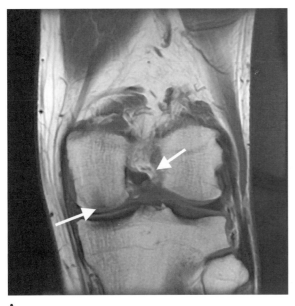 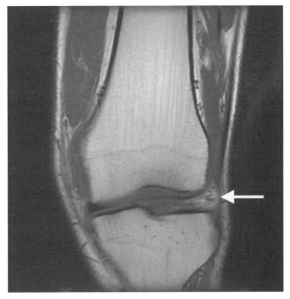

A **B**

FIGURE 17-6 MRI provides excellent detail of soft tissue injuries. **A,** A coronal section reveals a complete anterior cruciate ligament tear with articular cartilage damage to the medial femoral condyle. **B,** A coronal section reveals a complex degenerative lateral meniscus tear.

largely depends on the use of the appropriate coils and pulse sequences. Joints should be imaged in three orthogonal planes, one of which suppresses the characteristic bright signal of fat for better contrast (fat suppressed). One sequence such as fast-spin echo or gradient echo to evaluate articular cartilage should be included in each joint study. Intra-articular contrast may be used to evaluate the shoulder or hip for rotator cuff tears, labral lesions, or articular cartilage injuries (Figure 17-7).

Both CT and MRI are capable of producing high-resolution scans, but the ability of MRI to differentiate the different types of tissue based on their signal intensities (soft tissue contrast) sets it apart. The CT image is based on x-ray attenuation properties of tissues, whereas the soft tissue contrast in MRI is related to the differing proton resonances in the tissues.[30] MRI has proven to be superior to CT in simultaneously delineating multiple soft tissue and osseous insults.[14] The gold standard for the evaluation of anterior cruciate ligament injuries is arthroscopy. Compared with this standard, MRI has a diagnostic accuracy of more than 90%.[55] MRI is considered the imaging of choice to demonstrate both acute and chronic stages of muscle damage caused by infarcts from sickle cell disease, diabetes, primary or metastatic tumors, and trauma.[14] MRI is considered more useful than CT in demonstrating bone marrow abnormalities, and specific types of MR sequences can also distinguish benign from malignant spinal lesions.[14] MRI may be more accurate in defining the extent of tumors and their relation to neighboring tissues, and functional MRI to measure blood flow may aid in the diagnosis of musculoskeletal neoplasms.

Finally, high field strength magnets have provided a level of detail that surpasses arthrography, CT arthrography, and ultrasonography for depicting changes in articular cartilage.[27] MRI, under routine clinical parameters, provides limited detail

within the small tendons and images the coarse detail of muscle. Contrast agents may improve the definition of detail and reveal significant lesions and normal variants.[14,59] Feldman et al[15] described 30 patients with normal radiographs, bone scans, and CT scans but determined that MRI allowed identification of acute fractures in the emergency department as well

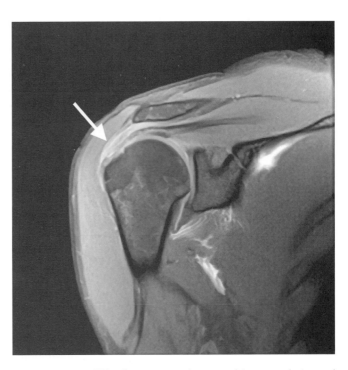

FIGURE 17-7 MR arthrogram reveals a complete supraspinatus and partial infraspinatus tear.

as subtle subacute or chronic fractures in the context of strong clinical suspicions. They also concluded that MRI is the most sensitive way of simultaneously documenting the earliest changes in traumatized osseous and soft tissue structures. They also provided a case example of an elderly person seen in the emergency department after a fall. The initial radiographs and conventional tomograms were normal, but a T1-weighted MRI obtained the same day revealed an intertrochanteric fracture.[14]

Several factors can alter the quality of the MRI. Motion from voluntary movements, restlessness, involuntary spasms, respiratory movements of the ribcage, and peristaltic movements of the bowel can all reduce the quality of the acquired images. Slices that are too thin or that are acquired too close to each other can produce interference. Disadvantages of MRI include intolerance of the procedure by claustrophobic patients, the requirement for patients to be motionless during the procedure, and cost.

ARTHROGRAPHY. Arthrography entails the introduction of a positive contrast agent, such as iodide, or a negative contrast agent, such as air, or a combination of both into the joint space.[23] This procedure is not considered to be technically difficult, and the results are relatively easy to interpret. Arthrography is most often conducted at the wrist, shoulder, elbow, and ankle regions. Plain film radiographs are generally obtained before arthrography because of the possibility of obscuring certain radiographic findings once the contrast agent is applied. In some settings, the role of arthrography has become increasingly limited because of the increased use of MRI. Arthrography is primarily used when MRI is contraindicated or when the details of intra-articular pathologic conditions such as labral and articular cartilage lesions are desired. In addition, arthrography is particularly useful to detect rotator cuff tears of the shoulder and triangular fibrocartilage lesions of the wrist.[23] Finally, the combination of CT and arthrography is frequently used, as previously described.[3,39,60]

MYELOGRAPHY. Plain myelography includes plain film radiographs taken after a nonionic water-soluble contrast medium is injected into the subarachnoid space by a puncture needle to produce images of the borders and contents of the dural sac. The contrast medium mixes with the cerebrospinal fluid and travels up or down the thecal sac as the patient's position is altered by tilting the bed or table. CT myelography uses a CT scan, taken after a contrast medium has been injected into the dural sac, in the same manner as for plain myelography. This modality produces axial cross-sectional images of the spine that enhance the distinction between the dural sac and its surrounding structures. For examination of the lumbar segment an L2-L3 or L3-L4 puncture site is used, whereas for the cervical segment a C1-C2 puncture site is used. Myelographic examination has been almost entirely replaced by high-resolution CT and high-quality MRI.[23]

DISCOGRAPHY. Discography is an imaging procedure that involves injection of contrast material into the nucleus pulposus of the intervertebral disc. It is typically combined with CT. Discography has been used less frequently in recent years, but under certain conditions, such as determining the source of a patient's LBP, it is still of some diagnostic benefit. The symptoms produced with the injection of the contrast material may be of even greater diagnostic value than the images produced.

Discography may be indicated for the evaluation of unremitting spinal pain that is unresponsive to conservative treatment.[23]

ULTRASOUND. Ultrasound imaging is a fast and inexpensive tool for excellent images of the musculoskeletal system. This modality is useful for imaging ligaments, tendon, nerves, muscles, tumors, and foreign bodies. Real-time imaging allows for the imaging of muscles as they contract and tendons as they glide. Ultrasound creates an image by sending sound waves into the tissues under the sound head and then imaging the sound waves as they return. Substances that reflect sound, such as bone and metal, cannot be adequately imaged. It is thought that ultrasonography is of more use in thin than in obese patients. Ultrasound is an excellent modality for imaging the rotator cuff of the shoulder, but it is typically unable to image some aspects of the glenoid labrum and certain structures within the knee such as the menisci, articular cartilage, and cruciate ligaments. Ultrasound has also been shown to be useful in the evaluation of a traumatic hemarthrosis of the knee.[55]

Ultrasound has the advantage of requiring direct operator interaction with the patient. In a fashion, the operator is performing a physical examination and palpating deeply with the aid of the ultrasound as guided by the patient description of their symptom location. Operator skill is a large factor in the diagnostic utility of ultrasound images. Power Doppler ultrasound produces detailed images of intramuscular and intratendinous structures and demonstrates hyperemia in the rotator cuff and biceps tendon as well as other soft tissue shoulder pathologic conditions. Depending on operator skill, power Doppler ultrasound may be as sensitive as MRI and may be particularly useful in distinguishing chronic tendonitis from acute tendonitis and rotator cuff tears. In contrast, MRI performed within routine clinical parameters demonstrates coarse intramuscular structure and poorer detail within small tendons.[58,59] Ultrasound images are currently used in PT practice to study the quality of muscle contraction and to detect the presence of muscle atrophy.

Combined Modalities

As previously noted, in certain situations a combination of diagnostic modalities may be of more value than a single type of imaging. Feldman et al[14] describe the advantages of a combination of imaging modalities in the case of a patient with hyperparathyroidism. MRI or CT demonstrates the extensive detail of the pathologic condition, whereas radiographs effectively demonstrate the classic characteristics of the underlying disease, such as osteopenia, bone resorption, and soft tissue calcification. Radiographs and CT may provide details of a specific lesion, whereas a bone scan may be useful to screen for multiple lesions throughout the skeletal system. The astute PT will keep in mind the diagnostic utility and limitations of each type of imaging modality.

Advances in Diagnostic Imaging

Advances in imaging over the last few decades have had a significant impact on patient care largely because of progress in diagnostic capability. The introduction and evolution of digital cross-sectional imaging with CT and the subsequent development of MRI have forever changed the landscape of diagnostic imaging. Conventional radiology has evolved from analog images on standard radiographic film to digital datasets produced by laser scanning and "dry processed," or sent through wire or fiberoptic cables to computerized workstation displays.[26]

Technology has progressed to the point of allowing computer-assisted interpretation of certain types of images. Because of increasing demands for more timely distribution of radiographic information and space constraints, many departments or practice settings are becoming completely digital. High-speed networks transfer images from acquisition workstation to interpretation workstation. These image transfer systems are called picture archiving and communication systems.

CT and MRI technology are still evolving, and efforts are focused on improving portability, speed of acquisition, and image quality. Medical facilities of the future may have designs that conveniently locate imaging technology within emergency departments, intensive care units, and high-volume outpatient clinics. Beds from the intensive care unit or emergency department may evolve from being merely portable to being integral, with imaging devices for quick and easy docking, thereby reducing the need for patient transfer. Improved facility design may allow transport of the smaller but still significantly sized imaging devices.[26]

Progress in imaging technology and the ease of access to diagnostic imaging will drive many changes in their use. As these changes occur in settings where PTs are contributing to the management of patients with musculoskeletal problems, PTs will want to provide input whenever possible. This will allow for the diagnostic imaging to readily assist with the diagnosis and other aspects of physical therapy patient management.

Risks Associated with Diagnostic Imaging

The risks reported with diagnostic imaging include exposure to ionizing radiation, infection and procedural complications from invasive procedures, reaction to contrast materials, interference with mechanical devices such as pacemakers, and dislodging of embedded or implanted metal objects. The risk to special populations, such as patients with scoliosis, for developing cancer caused by radiation exposure has been formally studied. A retrospective study of patient cohorts with adolescent idiopathic scoliosis was used to determine the cancer risks associated with the typical radiographic studies. The researchers found that an average of 10 to 12 radiographic procedures over the lifespan of a typical scoliosis patient increased the risk of developing cancer of the breast and thyroid gland. Unfortunately, the radiation exposure in patients with scoliosis typically occurs during the highest periods of adolescent growth. Cumulative x-ray doses were also found to be higher in those patients who were diagnosed at a younger age and with more severe curves. PA views reduce radiation exposure to the breast and thyroid by 94% to 96%. By simply ensuring that all radiographs in these patients are PA views rather than AP views, the risks of developing breast cancer are reduced three- to four-fold and the lifetime risk of thyroid cancer is reduced by half.[33]

Ordering Diagnostic Imaging

Whenever the decision is made that diagnostic imaging is necessary, the description of the mechanism of injury, the results of clinical examination with the highest diagnostic utility for the suspected disorders, and the location of significant findings, including palpation tenderness, are essential information for the radiologist. The radiologist will probably not have access to the patient when interpreting the image. Therefore the description of the presentation and key clinical findings becomes critical to accurate and relevant image interpretation.[39] It is also crucial to examine for related injuries and appropriately image all areas that could have sustained significant injury or that could be the source of referred symptoms. Clinical examples of commonly missed injuries from incomplete physical examination and imaging include fifth metatarsal fractures accompanying ankle sprains, proximal fibula fractures accompanying malleolar fractures and ankle sprains, compression fractures at thoracic and upper lumbar levels with symptoms or injury to the lower lumbar levels or the lower extremities, proximal radial injuries accompanying distal radius and wrist injuries, and referred pain to the knee from conditions that exist at the hip and pelvis.[35,39]

Correlations must be made between the results of the diagnostic imaging and the clinical examination. In evidence-based medicine, the clinical examination helps establish the pretest likelihood of the pathologic condition.[42] When the signs and symptoms of a significant injury are present from the clinical examination, a negative diagnostic imaging procedure must be repeated or an imaging procedure with increased sensitivity must be used.

The following case example reinforces the need to proceed with caution when the history indicates potential or a high pretest likelihood for a significant injury but the diagnostic imaging is negative.

A 25-year-old male rugby player was referred to physical therapy for treatment of a cervical sprain after an injury sustained in a rugby match 2 days earlier. The consult requested cervical traction for the injury. During the history and review of systems the patient indicated that he had sustained one of the hardest hits that he had ever received in a sporting event. The patient stated that he attempted to continue to play but the pain was particularly sharp and it was difficult to turn his head. Of particular concern to the patient was his ability to participate in the upcoming championship game. The patient was carrying his radiographs and he stated that they had been read as normal in the emergency department. He denied loss of consciousness, numbness, tingling, or weakness of the extremities. He also denied any previous history of neck injuries despite playing football and rugby for many years.

The tests and measures were carefully performed because the patient was in obvious distress. An upper and lower motor neuron screening examination was normal. Cervical active range of motion was severely restricted in all directions, and gentle palpation performed in the seated position revealed local tenderness and spasm at the level of C5.

On the basis of the examination results, the PT took the films to the radiology reading room and reviewed them with the radiologist on duty. By focusing on the area of the palpation findings, an abnormality in the lamina of C5 was visualized. The patient's neck was immediately immobilized in a collar and a subsequent CT examination clearly revealed a laminar fracture.

Correspondingly, in the absence of any clinical findings imaged pathology may not be significant. Artifacts, overlapping cortices, clothing, and normal variants can all be mistaken for subtle fractures or other pathologic conditions (Figure 17-8). When pathology and symptoms are both present in the same region of the body, a common pitfall is to assume the visualized pathologic condition is the reason that the patient is symptomatic. Careful palpation and precise examination skills are required to determine the correlation between pathology and symptoms. Incorrect conclusions may be particularly dangerous when the pathologic condition would not necessarily require surgical treatment if the patient was not symptomatic. This teaching point is nicely reinforced with the following case example of an active duty soldier with severe LBP.

An 18-year-old soldier was sent to a Regional Army Medical Center for further evaluation of LBP. This soldier's pain was particularly severe whenever he tried to run or perform sit-ups. No relief had been achieved with conservative treatment, including rest, medication, physical therapy modalities, and exercise.

The soldier had a grade II spondylolisthesis at the fifth lumbar level identified on plain radiographs and confirmed by CT. The radiologist and neurosurgeon agreed that the images represented a nonunion of a relatively recent injury, although a specific incident could not be identified. The patient was placed in a body cast to immobilize the "symptomatic" vertebra. The patient's response to this treatment was unanticipated. He had a dramatic

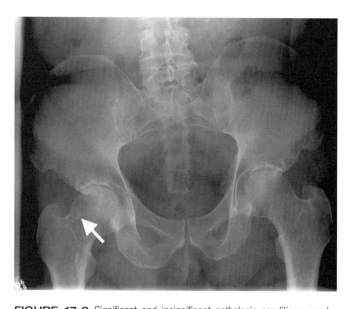

FIGURE 17-8 Significant and insignificant pathologic conditions can be strikingly similar. The radiologist needs the important clinical examination findings to help make the radiographic diagnosis. In this case the differential of the small sclerotic lesions is either benign bone islands or metastatic cancer. Note the arthritic changes in this hip that may produce symptoms and reinforce the importance of a careful clinical examination to distinguish new pathologic conditions such as metastatic cancer from other conditions such as osteoarthritis.

increase in LBP and the cast had to be removed. Surgical fusion of the segment was planned because of the failure of the casting.

Shortly before the planned surgery, the soldier contracted an acute respiratory infection. He went to the outpatient clinic at the medical center for treatment. On hearing the soldier's story about his respiratory ailment and his LBP, the attending physician's assistant referred the patient to a PT with manual therapy expertise at the medical center.

The physical examination by the PT reproduced the soldier's LBP with unilateral segmental palpation at the first and second lumbar levels. After three sessions of joint mobilization reinforced with self range-of-motion exercises, the patient became asymptomatic and was able to return to full duty and physical training.

This brief case example is an excellent illustration of how the results of imaging are only meaningful in the context of the larger comprehensive examination. The temptation is to draw conclusions relative to the identification of specific pathologic conditions on diagnostic imaging. The diagnostic imaging literature provides examples of pathologic conditions in asymptomatic individuals.[29] This evidence places a burden on the clinician and the interpreting radiologist to determine when the condition is relevant to the clinical examination and ultimate treatment.

It has been my clinical experience that radiologists appreciate the quality of the information provided by PTs when diagnostic imaging procedures are ordered. The radiologist will probably not have access to the patient when interpreting the image. They depend on the description of clinical findings provided when the diagnostic imaging is ordered. Remembering that you are essentially the hands, eyes, and ears of the radiologist for the clinical examination will help to guide what information to provide when ordering diagnostic imaging. The following clinical example of a diagnostic imaging order provides insight into the value of information supplied by the ordering provider.

DESIRED STUDY

AP and lateral radiographs of the right elbow.

HISTORY

The patient is a 13-year-old middle-school student who fell directly onto her right elbow while roller-blading 3 days ago at a school retreat. Physical examination reveals moderate ecchymosis and swelling of the proximal lateral forearm and distal upper arm. Pain was present with all active motions of the elbow and forearm, and there was a partial loss of elbow flexion, extension, supination, and pronation. Effusion and tenderness are present over the radial head. The proximal shoulder, distal forearm, wrist, and hand are without significant findings or palpation tenderness.

This brief but comprehensive overview of the clinical presentation helps guide the radiologist to be alert for pathologic conditions from trauma at the elbow. Particular emphasis will be placed on looking for those signs associated with fractures of the elbow. Diagnostic imaging findings not associated with the injury or location of symptoms will be kept in the appropriate perspective in the subsequent radiographic report.

Specialized Areas of Imaging

Osteochondral Injuries

The diagnosis of articular cartilage injuries depends on a careful clinical examination and the appropriate diagnostic imaging modality. Osteochondral injuries require specialized imaging, and although radiographs are typically the standard for imaging joint abnormalities, they are insensitive to early articular cartilage changes.[27] The detection of articular cartilage defects is important to facilitate the timely and appropriate management of the injury and must be differentiated from other common injuries to the involved joint. The PT must be alert for articular cartilage injury in acute injuries and in chronic injuries with persistent pain or mechanical dysfunction. Osteochondral injuries can accompany other acute injuries such as sprains of the cruciate or collateral ligaments of the knee. Acute injuries may produce fragments of pure articular cartilage or cartilage and underlying bone. Standard spin echo MRI and spin echo MRI with fat suppression have proven to be inadequate for evaluating articular cartilage. A spoiled gradient echo sequence MRI with fat suppression is advocated to evaluate articular cartilage changes because it uses the advantages of the reduced imaging time associated with gradient echo pulse sequences and eliminates select frequencies to enhance the contrast of articular cartilage. The technique is useful to evaluate cartilage degeneration, demonstrating signal loss in the superficial bright layer, and can illustrate varying degrees of loss of signal in intermediate and deep layers within the cartilage.[27,34] The water content of these layers of cartilage will vary with fibrillation and inflammation, producing variations in the signal intensity.

A trabecular microfracture or bone bruise is the first stage of an osteochondral fracture. Although the injury may not be revealed by conventional radiography, bone contusions have typical appearances on both T1-weighted and T2-weighted MRI. Osteochondral fractures resulting from significant impaction and shearing forces may also be missed by conventional radiography. MR images may reveal osteochondral fractures as curvilinear fracture lines, irregularities of the cartilage, bone bruises, or loose bodies. MRI with the addition of a contrast agent, conventional arthrography, and computed arthrotomography have all been advocated for imaging the details of lesions associated with osteochondritis dissecans.[34] The lesions of osteochondritis dissecans are commonly found on the capitellum, talus, patella, and femoral condyles.

Advanced articular cartilage degenerative changes may be revealed by a loss of joint space in the weight-bearing compartment in standing radiograph images. Weight-bearing joint spaces may also be altered by meniscus injuries and subsequent surgical procedures. Additional evidence of degenerative changes on standard radiographs includes subchondral sclerosis and cysts, bone eburnation, articular surface collapse, and bony spurs. Stress radiographs have been used to obtain the same information from the non-weight-bearing joint compartment by using mechanically imposed stress.[54]

Osteoarthritis of the knee is a good example of a condition in which conservative treatment should not be based on the results of diagnostic imaging. Clinical diagnostic criteria developed by Altman et al[2] (Box 17-4) have been found to be 89% sensitive and 88% specific for knee osteoarthritis. Physical therapy has been demonstrated to be of benefit to the patient with knee osteoarthritis.[9] Decisions for surgery are typically based on intolerable pain, loss of function, and a progressive varus or valgus deformity that should be clinically obvious.

Sports-Related Injuries

Imaging in the management of sport injuries, as in other types of injuries, should be focused on the situations in which positive findings would alter the course of treatment. Relevant questions for the PT may include: Does the patient's clinical presentation suggest the presence of a fracture, arthritis, sprain, or a strain? Does this patient require rest, immobilization, vigorous rehabilitation, or possibly a surgical consult?[39] The spectrum of sports injuries ranges from those that do not need imaging, to suspected fractures that require imaging, to injuries that do not normally require imaging but do not respond to treatment and therefore eventually require imaging as part of the plan of care process. An example provided by Mintz[39] is the back injury that does not respond to conservative therapy within the normal time frame and therefore requires appropriate imaging to rule out a pars fracture. The types of injuries seen in different athlete populations vary depending where the athlete is in his or her life cycle. For example, pediatric populations are more susceptible to bony avulsion injuries because of their strong ligament support and relatively weaker bone structure. Pain in proximity to a long bone may herald a bone bruise or muscle injury but may also signal the presence of a pathologic fracture from a bone cyst or neoplasm.[39] See Chapters 12, 13, and 15 for more details regarding the adolescent, obstetric, and geriatric populations.

Fractures and Dislocations

The diagnosis of fractures and dislocations is probably the most recognized use of plain radiographs. Fractures and dislocations are the most common traumatic conditions encountered by radiologists. Fractures are classified as either complete or incomplete depending on whether any of the bony trabeculae are left intact. Dislocations are considered complete when the joint surfaces are no longer in contact. Subluxations represent changes in relation of the articular surfaces when the

---

BOX 17-4

Clinical Criteria for the Diagnosis of Osteoarthritis of the Knee

1. Knee pain, age 38 years or younger, and bony enlargement
2. Knee pain, age 39 years or greater, morning stiffness more than 30 minutes, and bony enlargement
3. Knee pain, crepitus on active motion, morning stiffness more than 30 minutes, and bony enlargement
4. Knee pain, crepitus on active motion, morning stiffness 30 minutes or less, and age 38 years or greater.

From Altman R, Bloch D, Bole G Jr, et al: Development of clinical criteria for osteoarthritis, *J Rheumatol* 14:3-6, 1987.

structures are still in contact.[23] Plain radiographs taken in at least two planes are required to rule out fractures, to judge the degree of displacement of fracture, and to rule out joint dislocation (Figure 17-9). The evaluation and description of noted fractures should include the site and extent of the fracture; whether the fracture is complete or incomplete; and the alignment of the fragments regarding distraction, foreshortening, angulation, rotation, and displacement (Plates 17-1 through 17-6). The diagnosis of an open fracture (a fracture segment that communicates directly with the outside environment) is based on the clinical examination. Fractures are also described according to the characteristics of the fracture line, such as longitudinal, spiral, transverse, and oblique (Plates 17-7 through 17-17). Special types of fractures include stress or fatigue fractures and pathologic fractures that are typically caused by metabolic changes in bone or tumors.

FRACTURES IN CHILDREN. Fractures in children may be especially challenging to recognize because of difficulties encountered with carrying out the history, review of systems, and tests and measures as well as the often-subtle presentation both clinically and on imaging. The PT may have to use various strategies of distracting the child and involving him or her in play while observing the child's willingness to use the injured extremity. Initially palpating well away from the injured area may help the examiner distinguish response to palpation. In the older child, allowing the child to point with one finger where it hurts the most may be useful. Additional strategies include asking the child to rate the pain as a "big pain" or "little pain" while palpating. The examiner may be able to differentiate the areas for diagnostic imaging and help guide the radiographic interpretation by asking

the child, "which hurts the most—when I push here on A, or when I push here on B?" Distracting the child and then repalpating areas of suspected fractures may provide insight regarding whether the severity of the pain is consistent with a fracture.

Fractures in children have the potential to interfere with the growth plate and therefore represent a possible danger to the future growth of the involved bone (see Chapter 12). The Salter-Harris Classification System is commonly used to classify growth plate injuries (Plates 17-18 through 17-22). Comparison views of the uninvolved extremity or repeating the radiographs after allowing time for cortical reaction may be necessary to reveal the injury in children.

STRESS FRACTURES. Stress fractures are common injuries in a population of athletes or training military populations. Stress fractures are multifactorial injuries with contributing factors of gender, hormonal influences, diet, training regimen, footwear, and running surfaces. Stress fractures are thought to comprise as many as 10% of all sports injuries. They have been described in tennis, football, basketball, and hockey players; aerobic and ballet dancers; runners; gymnasts; kayakers; golfers; and throwing athletes.[40] Stress fractures are thought to be the result of cyclic overloading of bone that exceeds the ability of bony tissue to strengthen and repair itself. Both high-repetition, low-load cyclic stress and low-repetition, high-load stress may result in the development of stress fractures.

Initial radiographs of early-stage stress fractures may be read as normal. Plain film diagnosis of stress fractures depends on a number of factors. The site of injury and the timing of the films related to the stage of the osteoclastic resorption, the osteoblastic repair, periosteal reaction, and new bone formation

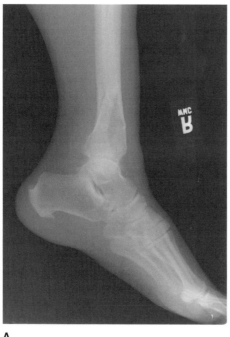
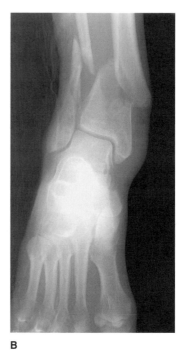

A   B

FIGURE 17-9 Two views at 90 degrees to each other are the minimum to reveal the characteristics of a fracture or dislocation. **A,** The lateral view radiograph of this distal tibia and fibula fracture suggests that it is oblique and minimally displaced. **B,** The anteroposterior view radiograph reveals the true degree of displacement and angulation.

will all have an impact on the appearance of the injury on plain films. In general, there must be significant bone response to the imposed stresses before the changes become apparent on plain films. Plain films typically require 2 to 3 weeks to reveal new stress fractures and may be normal for up to 3 months after the onset of symptoms.

Bone scintigraphy is considered a more sensitive but non-specific modality for diagnosing stress fractures. Bone scans can become positive within 6 to 72 hours of the initial onset of the fracture. The differential diagnosis process in the presence of a positive bone scan must include ruling out benign and malignant neoplasms and osteomyelitis. A system for grading stress fractures based on the bone scan images is described by Zwas et al.[61] Grade 1 is described as mildly increased activity in a small ill-defined area. Grade 2 is a larger, more defined, and elongated cortical area. Grade 3 fractures have highly increased activity in a fusiform corticomedullary pattern. Grade 4 lesions have intensely increased transcortical activity.[40,61] Typical appearances of stress fractures on both MRI and bone scans are summarized in Table 17-4.

More recently, other authors have proposed that MR images are preferred for grading stress fractures because of the risk associated with the ionizing radiation exposure from bone scans, the excellent MRI anatomic detail not available through bone scan imaging, and the reduced time to complete an MRI.[17] Although bone scans remain the gold standard for detecting stress fractures, T1-weighted and T2-weighted MRI reveals the tissue damage associated with a stress fracture. Typical tissue changes seen on MRI include periosteal and bone marrow edema. Therefore the MR images may be more useful than bone scans as an aid in designing rehabilitation programs based on the extent of the injury.[40]

Shoulder/Rotator Cuff Tears

Ultrasound has been demonstrated to be a sensitive and specific diagnostic tool for imaging complete and partial rotator cuff tears.[56,58] The primary difficulty reported with using ultrasound for shoulder imaging is the apparent long learning curve for mastery of the technique. Sonography can detect abnormal amounts of fluid or synovial changes and can provide dynamic assessment of the shoulder region, thereby revealing acromial impingement on subacromial

structures. Van Holsbeeck et al[58] studied the diagnostic utility of ultrasound used by a single trained examiner for partial bursal side rotator cuff tears compared with arthroscopic findings. Ultrasound was found to be to 93% sensitive and 94% specific, with a positive predictive value of 82% and a negative predictive value of 98%, although the surgeons were not blinded to the preoperative ultrasound results.

MRI has a similar diagnostic utility as CT arthrography in the shoulder, and both have the primary advantage of being noninvasive. Reported sensitivity for detection of labral tears with high-resolution MRI has ranged from 74% to 100%, with specificity of 95% to 100%.[3] MR arthrography is considered by some authors to be superior to other imaging techniques in evaluating the glenohumeral joint.[3] Pathologic conditions associated with instability and anterior inferior dislocation of the glenohumeral joint are readily identified with MR arthrography. These pathologic conditions include anteroinferior labral tears, classic and osseous Bankart lesions, fracture and sclerosis of the glenoid, Hill-Sachs lesions, and superior labral AP lesions. Some of the normal variants reported to cause diagnostic difficulty are the anterosuperior sublabral foramen, the Burford complex, and hyaline cartilage under the labrum.[3] MR arthrography has been found to have a moderate to good correlation to anatomic dissection for determining the size and morphologic features of the glenohumeral ligaments.[60]

Spinal Injuries

Imaging in the event of spinal trauma must be fully evaluated regarding the forces involved as well as the metabolic bone health of the patient. Less force is required to produce fractures in the presence of osteoporosis and advanced age. Symptoms that are not relieved by rest or changes in position, symptoms that sharply increase with movement, unremitting paraspinous musculature spasm, and an unwillingness to move the spine all suggest a spinal fracture. Facet and intervertebral disc pathologic conditions are best revealed with CT scans and MR imaging. Plain radiographs can adequately reveal spinal fractures, but a CT scan remains the imaging modality of choice to reveal the intricate details of spinal fractures (Figure 17-10).

Conventional radiographs are the initial imaging of choice for most cervical spine injuries. A typical cervical radiographic series would include AP, lateral, and open-mouth

---

TABLE 17-4

Grading of Stress Fractures from Typical Appearance on Bone Scan and MRI

Grade of Stress Fracture	Bone Scan Appearance	MRI Appearance
Grade 1	Relatively small, poorly defined cortical area of moderately increased activity	Mild to moderate periosteal edema on T2-weighted images
Grade 2	More defined area of moderately increased cortical activity	Moderate to severe periosteal edema with marrow edema on T2-weighted images
Grade 3	Wide to spindle-shaped area of highly increased cortical-medullary activity	Moderate to severe periosteal edema with marrow edema on T2- and T1-weighted images
Grade 4	Transcortical area of intensely increased activity	Moderate to severe periosteal edema with marrow edema on T2- and T1-weighted images; fracture line obvious

Adapted from Frederichson M, Bergman A, Hoffman K, et al: Tibial stress reaction in runners: correlation of clinical symptoms and scintigraphy with a new MRI grading system, *Am J Sports Med* 23:472-481, 1995.

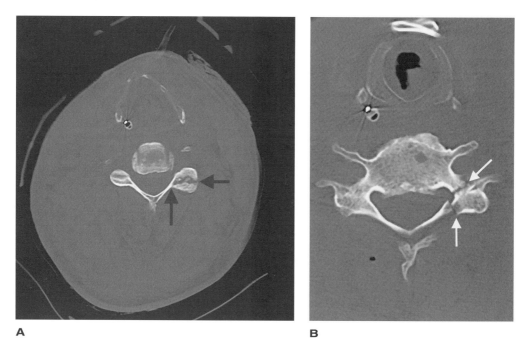

FIGURE 17-10 CT can reveal subtle fractures not apparent on plain films. These two fractures were found in the cervical spine of a patient after a motor vehicle accident. The presence of fractures at different spinal levels underscores the importance of the complete examination. **A,** Facet fracture at C4-C5 level. **B,** C6 pedicle and lamina fracture.

odontoid views. Flexion and extension views may aid in the evaluation of suspected cervical instability. It has been reported that up to 20% of cervical fractures are undetected on plain radiographs. Although some missed cervical fractures and dislocations are the result of misinterpretation, the most frequent cause of an overlooked injury is an inadequate film series. It is critical for the lateral view to include all seven cervical vertebrae as well as the interspace between the last cervical and first thoracic vertebrae.[21]

Significant cervical injury is unlikely in adults with normal mental status; not under the influence of drugs or alcohol; and in the absence of findings such as neck pain, palpation tenderness, loss of consciousness, concurrent distracting injury, or neurologic signs such as numbness or weakness of the upper extremities. Children may have spinal cord injury without radiographic evidence of damage to the cervical spine. Careful examination for neurologic findings is required after any head and neck trauma in these patients. Emergent spinal cord treatment is indicated in the presence of positive neurologic findings. Cervical spinal stenosis can be initially evaluated by plain radiographs with the examination for adequate AP diameter. Normal AP diameter of the cervical spine spinal canal is 13 mm. Suspected cases can be further evaluated with myelography, MRI, or CT.

The following brief case example highlights a situation in which the clinical examination and initial radiographs suggest a possible significant injury. Guided by the pretest probability and the inconclusive radiographs, a more sensitive study is ultimately performed with a subsequent diagnosis.

A 21-year-old man was referred to physical therapy for treatment of neck and upper trapezius pain. During the his-

tory portion of the examination, the patient related passing out while sitting at his desk and striking his head on the desk. The injury had occurred approximately 2 weeks before the physical therapy appointment. The patient also related that shortly after the event it was very difficult for him to move his head, but this symptom had subsequently improved. Immediately after the injury there had been numbness and tingling on the top of his head, but that had also resolved. He had also been having difficulty swallowing since his injury because of activity-related neck pain. He denied any significant medical history, including seizures, but stated that he had been out late drinking the night before he passed out at his desk. No diagnostic imaging had been performed before seeing the PT. On the basis of the history findings the PT was not comfortable performing a physical examination before a radiographic examination was obtained. A cervical series was ordered and the radiologist was contacted to review the study. The radiologist noted obliquity of the dens and an abnormal position of C1 in relation to C2. The radiologist also thought there was a subtle lucency across the base of the dens. The radiologist recommended an immediate CT. The patient's neck was immobilized and he was transported by ambulance to the hospital for the CT scan. The CT confirmed the radiologist's suspicions. There was an oblique comminuted dens fracture, with a fracture line involving the right lateral mass of C2. The fracture line extended into the foramen transversarium on the right side. Minimal to mild anterior displacement of C1 was also noted. The patient was subsequently taken to the operating room and stabilized with a halo collar (Figure 17-11). The patient's report of difficulty

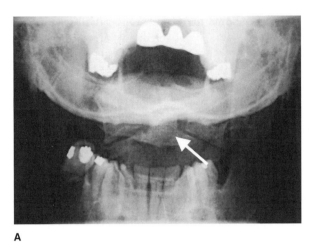
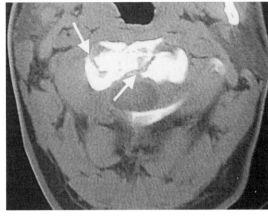

A   B

FIGURE 17-11 A, The open-mouth anteroposterior radiograph suggests abnormality of the position of the dens with subtle fracture line at the base. **B,** The fracture of the lateral mass and dens of C2 is confirmed by a computed tomographic scan.

with chewing was probably related to retropharyngeal bleeding from the upper cervical fracture.

LOW BACK PAIN. Categoric classification of LBP derived from the Agency for Health Care Policy and Research (ACHPR) guidelines has been proposed: (1) LBP from potentially serious underlying conditions, including infections, fractures, neoplasms, aortic abdominal aneurysms, inflammatory conditions of the kidneys, and cauda equina syndrome, (2) LBP with sciatica from irritation or impingement of lumbosacral nerve roots, and (3) LBP with nonspecific symptoms thought to be from the spectrum of musculoligamentous and degenerative conditions. Most LBP falls into the third category and can improve significantly with proper treatment within 4 weeks and therefore does not require diagnostic imaging.[46] Although patients may occasionally request imaging to satisfy their fears regarding the source of LBP, those who receive an adequate explanation for their symptoms are less likely to want additional diagnostic tests.[10,46]

For persons younger than 45 years, low back problems are the most frequent cause of disability.[4] The use of diagnostic imaging in the management of acute LBP is controversial. Overuse of lumbar spine films can result in increased cost, excessive gonadal radiation exposure, and irrelevant findings that lead to inappropriate diagnoses and treatment.[46] For example, pathologic conditions demonstrated on diagnostic imaging may not be relevant to the patient's symptoms. Studies have shown degenerative changes, bulging disc, and herniated disc in 25% to 50% of the asymptomatic population.[29]

Lower back radiographs are frequently described as the single most overprescribed diagnostic imaging procedure.[1] Specific guidelines have been developed to help reduce the ordering of lumbar plain films that are of minimal diagnostic value.[1,4] The Agency for Health Care Policy and Research (AHCPR) (now the AHRQ) published guidelines on the management of acute LBP in adults in 1994.[4] Although these guidelines are now officially archived and not considered to be

the current standard for evidence-based practice, the imaging recommendations for acute LBP remain pertinent. Primary care provider education regarding the evidence for the management of LBP has been shown to reduce the use of diagnostic imaging, specialty referrals, and surgery.[32]

Before considering the relevance of diagnostic imaging, first-contact providers should complete a thorough history and then select the tests and measures with the highest diagnostic utility for patients with acute LBP. PTs must be particularly vigilant for the presence of any clinical manifestations that would demand special consideration beyond the ordinarily administered plan of care for patients with routine lower back symptoms. Key findings include medical history responses or physical examination findings that suggest the presence of a serious underlying spinal condition such as fracture, tumor, infection, or cauda equina syndrome (see Chapters 5 to 8). These responses or findings are commonly referred to as red flags. Certain diagnoses can be effectively ruled out by using combinations of screening questions. For example, in the absence of age greater than 50 years, personal history of a primary cancer, unexplained loss of weight, or failure to respond to conservative therapy, cancer can be ruled out in LBP patients with 100% sensitivity.[10,11] After 4 weeks, basic laboratory studies, including a complete blood cell count and sedimentation rate, help identify patients with conditions such as osteomyelitis and occult neoplasms.[10] The combination of radiographs and an erythrocyte sedimentation rate is a very sensitive method to screen for occult neoplasms. Deyo and Diehl[10] reported that all cases of occult neoplasms in 1975 that screened patients with back pain had either an abnormal film or an elevated erythrocyte sedimentation rate. Unfortunately, equally sensitive combinations of questions for spinal infections and fractures have not yet been determined.[11] The physical therapy examination should also assess for red flags of nonspinal conditions such as vascular, abdominal, urinary, or pelvic pathologic conditions capable of referring symptoms to the lower back (see Chapter 6). If multiple red flags are present, radiographs and laboratory studies are indicated at the initial visit. Clinical judgment is necessary to determine if plain radiographs or laboratory tests are required at the initial visit because of the presence of a single red flag.

According to the 1994 ACHPR guidelines, routine testing such as laboratory tests, radiographs, and other imaging studies is not recommended during the first month of acute LBP management. Most patients, even with symptoms of nerve root impingement, improve within 4 to 6 weeks and do not require diagnostic imaging.[1] The exception is when the aforementioned red flags are noted during the examination that raise suspicions of a dangerous low back or nonspinal condition.[1,4,10] Plain radiographs are not effective for diagnosing lumbar nerve root impingement from a herniated disc or spinal stenosis or for ruling out cancer or infection. Only one in 2500 radiographs detects something not suspected on the medical history and examination that has an impact on patient care.[46]

When diagnostic imaging is indicated, the initial radiographs should be limited to AP and lateral views. The additional diagnostic value of coned lateral views (for a close-up view of the lumbosacral junction region) and oblique radiographs is generally not worth the additional radiation exposure, particularly to women. Oblique lumbar radiographs, usually taken to screen for spondylolysis, rarely add useful clinical information in adults and double the x-ray dose to the patient. Patients with spondylolisthesis can be safely treated in the same fashion as those with other types of acute low back problems. Therefore radiographs performed specifically to screen for spondylolisthesis are not necessary for the first 3 months of symptoms. Although oblique radiographs do provide visualization of the pars interarticularis in the case of suspected spondylolisthesis, CT will best provide the details of a suspected acute pars fracture. Flexion/extension films are useful to identify spondylolisthesis with associated instability.[53]

In the rare case in which a condition may be clinically significant, such as sudden onset or progression of neurologic findings, the need for more extensive diagnostic evaluation such as bone scans, MRI, and CT is often in order even if the initial radiographic findings are negative. In the event of red flags suggesting cauda equina syndrome or progressive major motor weakness MRI, CT, myelography, or CT myelography is recommended. Facet and intervertebral disc pathology are best revealed with CT scans and MRI. Although spinal fractures may be adequately revealed by plain radiographs, a CT scan remains the imaging modality of choice to reveal the intricate details of spinal fractures. Bone scans are considered to be more sensitive than plain films for detecting infections or neoplasms of the spine. MRI provides more anatomic detail and greater sensitivity and specificity at approximately twice the cost of a bone scan. In patients with a history of a malignant process, metastatic disease must be ruled out as a cause of LBP. The lumbar spine is the most common site for metastasis to musculoskeletal tissues from primary cancers. Common primary cancers that metastasize to the axial skeleton are breast, lung, kidney, and prostate. The presence of constitutional symptoms, unexplained weight loss, age greater than 50 years, and symptoms that are not relieved with the typical changes in posture or position are causes for concern and must be determined during the history. Plain films have the least sensitivity for detecting metastasis, whereas bone scans are 77% sensitive and MRI is 96% sensitive.[6]

Spinal infections are associated with intravenous drug use, recent urinary tract infections, pelvic inflammatory conditions, and surgery. Plain films have poor sensitivity in detecting spinal infections because radiographic abnormalities may not be apparent for 2 to 8 weeks.[45] MRI has a 96% sensitivity and 92% specificity in the diagnosis of spinal infection and has been found to be equally sensitive to spinal infections such as CT myelography. In addition, MRI provides better imaging of the vertebral bodies, intervertebral discs, and paravertebral tissues. T1-weighted MR images provide more details of the anatomic limits of the abscess, the degree of cord compression, and paraspinal and vertebral involvement than CT myelography.[45,46]

For patients limited by sciatica for more than 4 weeks without clear evidence on physical examination of nerve root compromise, electromyography and H-reflex tests of the lower limb may provide evidence of suspected neurologic dysfunction. The clinical examination for patients with sciatica should include straight leg raising and neurologic testing. A positive straight leg raise at less than 60 degrees is 80% sensitive but not specific for disc herniation. A neurologic baseline established by the examination in the first clinical visit can reveal neurologic conditions that require immediate referral as well as those that do not respond to treatment over time. Sensory evoked potentials may be a useful adjunct for assessment of suspected spinal stenosis or spinal cord myelopathy. For patients limited by sciatica for more than 4 weeks with physiological evidence of neurologic dysfunction, MRI or CT is an appropriate consideration to provide anatomic detail of a possible herniated disc before surgery.

Most PTs are familiar with the clinical presentation and typical intolerance to upright activities associated with spinal stenosis.[19,20] In most cases, conservative therapy is appropriate for the first few months before surgical consideration, and additional imaging such as MRI and CT are warranted. A referral for surgical consultation is reasonable for patients with sciatic symptoms who have activity limitations for more than 1 month without improvement, clear clinical or electrophysiological evidence of nerve root compromise, or corroborative findings on imaging studies. A history of neurogenic claudication and clinical findings of spinal stenosis with severe symptoms may prompt early surgical referral. Prompt emergency consultation is reserved for patients with findings of bowel or bladder dysfunction or progressive or severe neurologic impairment. Table 17-5 provides a summary of the red flags indicating a need for diagnostic imaging as well as the imaging modality considered to have the greatest diagnostic utility for each condition.

TABLE 17-5

Summary of LBP Red Flags and the Appropriate Diagnostic Imaging

Potentially Serious Conditions	History and Review of Systems Red Flags	Diagnostic Testing Indicated
Possible tumor	Age greater than 50 years or less than 20 years; history of cancer; pain that increases when supine or at night	AP and lateral radiographs; CBC, ESR, UA; if radiographs are negative or laboratory tests are positive, then bone scan, MRI or CT
Possible infection	Fevers, chills, or unexplained weight loss; recent bacterial infection; intravenous drug use; immunosuppressed from HIV, steroids, or transplantation	Bone scan, MRI, or CT; CBC, ESR, UA
Possible cauda equina syndrome	Saddle anesthesia; recent onset bladder dysfunction such as urinary retention, overflow, and incontinence; symptoms of severe or progressive neurologic deficit	Emergent surgical consultation when supported by physical findings of unexpected laxity of the anal sphincter; perianal/perineal sensory loss; major motor weakness of knee extensors, ankle plantar flexors, ankle dorsiflexors, or ankle evertors; appropriate imaging is MRI or CT or myelography or CT myelography
Possible spinal fracture	History of significant trauma such as a fall from a height, motor vehicle accident, or direct blow to the back for a young adult; a minor fall or moderate lift in an elderly or osteoporotic individual; prolonged use of steroids; age greater than 70 years	AP and lateral radiographs; if negative then MRI or CT

From Staiger T, Paauw D, Deyo R, et al: Imaging studies for acute low back pain: when and when not to order them, *Imaging* 105:161-172, 1999.
CBC, Complete blood count: *ESR,* erythrocyte sedimentation rate; *UA,* urinalysis.

Summary

Available Resources for Physical Therapists

Several excellent resources exist for this material that are particularly useful in daily practice. The recommended resource list follows the reference list at the end of this chapter, and the complete reference list may be found on each text within the bibliography. There is a wealth of information on diagnostic imaging of the musculoskeletal system available on the Internet. The key words of "diagnostic imaging of the musculoskeletal system" produce a large number of sites. The sites range from single case teaching examples, to university-based diagnostic image libraries, to central listings of radiology sites with teaching libraries. Focusing on the sites intended for PTs and other primary care providers may initially be more clinically useful for the practicing PT.

PTs have been shown to be valuable and cost-effective members of primary care teams for musculoskeletal injuries and conditions. They have demonstrated under formal research conditions that they appropriately use diagnostic imaging. For maximal patient benefit, PTs should have ready access to the results of diagnostic imaging ordered by other providers. Assuming the appropriate training, PT privileges for ordering the diagnostic imaging modalities based on the patient presentation and the diagnostic benefit of the study could facilitate quality patient management. Both patients and health care organizations benefit from the timely treatment provided by PTs in the primary care of musculoskeletal conditions and injuries. The judicious and evidence-based ordering of diagnostic imaging by PTs will be an important aspect of that care. Currently, patients must often undergo one or more examinations before finally arriving at the PT who provides the definitive treatment for the condition. If it becomes apparent during the physical therapy examination or treatment that diagnostic imaging is required, the patient is forced to repeat the same time-consuming and costly path to obtain the necessary imaging.

Whenever providers not trained in musculoskeletal medicine are making decisions on diagnostic imaging, the patient may be exposed to the documented risks of unnecessary ionizing radiation, and the treatment facility incurs unnecessary cost. All PTs must be ready to articulate the research that supports their role in primary care and demonstrates their appropriate and sparing use of diagnostic imaging. A streamlined and user-friendly process that directly connects evidence-based diagnosis with expert treatment is the goal.

Over the next few decades, PTs will undoubtedly continue to establish themselves as a doctoring profession and providers of choice for the conservative care of neuromusculoskeletal conditions. PTs may soon apply for the privilege of ordering diagnostic imaging outside the military health care system. It seems logical that with such compelling evidence from both quality of care and cost of care perspectives, PTs will achieve wider privileges to the diagnostic imaging, laboratory tests, and medications that will enable them to care for their patients efficiently and effectively within an interdisciplinary health care delivery model.

REFERENCES

1. Acute Low Back Problems Guideline Panel: Acute low back problems in adults: assessment and treatment, *Am Fam Phys* 51:469-484, 1995.
2. Altman R, Bloch D, Bole G Jr, et al: Development of clinical criteria for osteoarthritis, *J Rheumatol* 14:3-6, 1987.
3. Beltran J, Rosenberg Z, Chandnani V, et al: Glenohumeral instability: evaluation with MR arthrography, *Radiographics* 17:657-673, 1997.
4. Bigos SJ: *Acute low back problems in adults,* Clinical Practice Guideline no. 14, ACHPR publication no. 95-0642, Rockville, Md, 1994, U.S. Dept. of Health and Human Services, Public Health Service, Agency for Health Care Policy and Research.
5. Bushberg J, Siebert J, Leidholt E Jr, et al: The essential physics of medical imaging, Baltimore, 1994, Williams & Wilkins.

6. Colleti P, Dang H, Deseran M, et al: Spinal MR imaging in suspected metastases: correlation with skeletal scintigraphy, *Magn Reson Imaging* 9:349-355, 1991.

7. Daker-White G, Carr A, Harvey I, et al: A randomised controlled trial: shifting boundaries of doctors and physiotherapists in orthopaedic outpatient departments, *J Epidemiol Community Health* 53:643-650,1999.

8. Depuy D, Hangen D, Zachazewski J, et al: Kinematic CT of the patellofemoral joint, *AJR* 169:211-215, 1997.

9. Deyle G, Henderson N, Matekel R, et al: Effectiveness of manual physical therapy and exercise in osteoarthritis of the knee: a randomized, controlled trial, *Ann Intern Med* 132:173-181, 2000.

10. Deyo R, Diehl A: Cancer as a cause of back pain: frequency, clinical presentation, diagnostic strategies, *J Gen Intern Med* 3:231-240, 1988.

11. Deyo R, Rainville J, Kent D: What can the history and physical examination tell us about low back pain? *JAMA* 268:760-765, 1992.

12. Dininny P: More than a uniform, the military model of physical therapy, *PT Magazine* March:40-51, 1995.

13. Ebenbichler GR, Erdogmus CB, Resch KL, et al: Ultrasound therapy for calcific tendinitis of the shoulder, *N Engl J Med* 340:1533-1538, 1999.

14. Feldman F: Musculoskeletal radiology: then and now, *Radiology* 216: 309-316, 2000.

15. Feldman F, Staron R, Rubin S, et al: MR imaging: its role in detecting occult fractures, *Skeletal Radiol* 23:439-444, 1994.

16. Flatman J: Hip disease with referred pain to the knee, *JAMA* 234:967-968, 1975.

17. Frederichson M, Bergman A, Hoffman K, et al: Tibial stress reaction in runners: correlation of clinical symptoms and scintigraphy with a new MRI grading system, *Am J Sports Med* 23:472-481, 1995.

18. Freedman K, Bernstein J: Educational deficiencies in musculoskeletal medicine, *J Bone Joint Surg Am* 84-A:604-608, 2002.

19. Fritz JM, Delitto A, Welch WC, et al: Lumbar spinal stenosis: a review of current concepts in evaluation, management, and outcome measurements, *Arch Phys Med Rehabil* 79:700-708, 1998.

20. Fritz JM, Erhard RE, Delitto A, et al: Preliminary results of the use of a two-stage treadmill test as a clinical diagnostic tool in the differential diagnosis of lumbar spinal stenosis, *J Spinal Disord* 10:410-416, 1997.

21. Graber M, Kathol M: Cervical spine radiographs in the trauma patient, *Am Fam Physician* 59:331-342, 1999.

22. Greathouse D, Schreck R, Benson C: The United States Army physical therapy experience: evaluation and treatment of patients with neuromusculoskeletal disorders, *J Orthop Sports Phys Ther* 19:261-266, 1994.

23. Greenspan A: *Orthopaedic radiology, a practical approach,* ed 3, Philadelphia, 2000, Lippincott Williams & Wilkins.

24. Guide to physical therapist practice, ed 2, *Phys Ther* 81:39-724, 2001.

25. Guyatt G, Drummond R: *Users' guides to the medical literature: a manual for evidence-based clinical practice,* New York, 2002, American Medical Association, pp 101-141.

26. Henry D: Imaging in the new millennium, *Crit Care Clin* 16:579-598, 2000.

27. Hodler J, Resnick D: Current status of imaging of articular cartilage, *Skeletal Radiol* 25:703-709, 1996.

28. Jensen G, Gwyer J, Shepard K, et al: Expert practice in physical therapy, *Phys Ther* 80:28-43, 2000.

29. Jensen M, Brant-Zawadzki M, Obuchowski N, et al: Magnetic resonance imaging of the lumbar spine in people without back pain, *N Engl J Med* 331:69-73, 1994.

30. Kaplan P, Helms C, Dussault R, et al: *Musculoskeletal MRI,* Philadelphia, 2001, WB Saunders, p 1-22.

31. Keats T: *Atlas of normal roentgen variants that may simulate disease,* ed 6, St Louis, 1996, Mosby.

32. Klein B, Radecki R, Foris M, et al: Bridging the gap between science and practice in managing low back pain, *Spine* 25:738-740, 2000.

33. Levy A, Goldberg M, Mayo N, et al: Reducing the lifetime risk of cancer from spinal radiographs, *Spine* 21:1540-1548, 1996.

34. Loredo R, Sanders T: Imaging of osteochondral injuries, *Clin Sports Med* 20:249-287, 2001.

35. Matava M, Patton X, Luhmann S, et al: Knee pain as the initial symptom of slipped capital femoral epiphysis: an analysis of initial presentation and treatment, *J Pediatr Orthop* 19:455-460, 1999.

36. McGinn T, Guyatt G, Wyer P, et al: Users' guides to the medical literature XXII: how to use articles about clinical decision rules, *JAMA* 284:79-84, 2000.

37. McKinnis L: *Fundamentals of orthopaedic radiology,* Philadelphia, 1997, FA Davis.

38. Milgrom C, Schaffler M, Gilbert S, et al: Rotator-cuff changes in asymptomatic adults: the effect of age, hand dominance and gender, *J Bone Joint Surg Br* 77:296-298, 1995.

39. Mintz D: Imaging of sports injuries, *Phys Med Rehab Clin North Am* 11:435-469, 2000.

40. Reeder M, Dick B, Atkins J, et al: Stress fractures: current concepts in diagnosis and treatment, *Sports Med* 22:198-212, 1996.

41. Resnik D, Kang H: *Internal derangement of joints, emphasis on MR imaging,* Philadelphia, 1997, WB Saunders, pp 3-24.

42. Sackett D, Straus S, Richardson S, et al: *Evidence-based medicine,* Philadelphia, 2000, Churchill Livingstone, pp 67-93.

43. Sartoris D: *Musculoskeletal imaging, the requisites,* St Louis, 1996, Mosby.

44. Seaberg D, Yealy M, Lukens T, et al: Multicenter comparison of two clinical decision rules for the use of radiography in acute, high-risk knee injuries, *Ann Emerg Med* 32:8-13, 1998.

45. Smith A, Blaser S: Infectious and inflammatory processes of the spine, *Radiol Clin North Am* 29:809-827, 1991.

46. Staiger T, Paauw D, Deyo R, et al: Imaging studies for acute low back pain: when and when not to order them, *Imaging* 105:161-172, 1999.

47. Stiell I: Clinical decision rules in the emergency department, *Can Med Assoc J* 163:1465-1466, 2000.

48. Stiell I, Greenberg G, McKnight R, et al: Decision rules for the use of radiography in acute ankle injuries: refinement and prospective validation, *JAMA* 269:1127-1132, 1993.

49. Stiell I, Greenberg G, McKnight R, et al: A study to develop clinical decision rules for the use of radiography in acute ankle injuries, *Ann Emerg Med* 21:384-390, 1992.

50. Stiell I, Greenberg G, Wells G, et al: Prospective validation of a decision rule for the use of radiography in acute knee injuries, *JAMA* 275:611-615, 1996.

51. Stiell I, McKnight R, Greenberg G, et al: Implementation of the Ottawa ankle rules, *JAMA* 271:827-832, 1994.

52. Stiell I, Wells G, Vandemheen KL: The Canadian C-spine rule for radiography in alert and stable trauma patients, *JAMA* 286:1841-1848, 2001.

53. Stillerman C, Schneider J, Gruen J: Evaluation and management of spondylolysis and spondylolisthesis, *Clin Neurosurg* 40:384-415, 1993.

54. Tallroth K, Lindhollm S: Stress radiographs in the evaluation of degenerative femorotibial joint disease, *Skeletal Radiol* 16:617-620, 1987.

55. Tandeter H, Shvartzman P, Stevens M: Acute knee injuries: use of decision rules for selective radiograph ordering, *Am Fam Physician* 60:2599-2608, 1999.

56. Thain L, Adler R: Sonography of the rotator cuff and biceps tendon, *J Clin Ultrasound* 27:446-458, 1999.

57. Tippet S: Referred knee pain in a young athlete: a case study, *J Orthop Sports Phys Ther* 19:117-120, 1994.

58. van Holsbeeck M, Kolowich P, Eyler W, et al: US depiction of partial thickness tear of the rotator cuff, *Radiology* 197:443-446, 1995.

59. Verstraete K, Van der Woude H, Hogendoorn P, et al: Dynamic contrast-enhanced MR imaging of musculoskeletal tumors: basic principles and clinical applications, *J Magn Reson Imaging* 6:311-321, 1996.

60. Yeh L, Kwak S, Kim YS, et al: Anterior labroligamentous structures of the glenohumeral joint: correlation of MR arthrography and anatomic dissection in cadavers, *AJR Am Roentgenol* 171:122-136, 1998.

61. Zwas ST, Elkanovitch R, Frank G: Interpretation and classification of bone scintigraphic findings in stress fractures, *J Nucl Med* 28:452-457, 1987.

SUGGESTED READINGS

Bullough PG: *Orthopaedic pathology,* ed 3, London, 1997, Mosby-Wolfe.

Greenspan A: Orthopaedic radiology, ed 3, Philadelphia, 2000, Lippincott Williams & Wilkins.

Kaplan P: *Musculoskeletal MRI,* Philadelphia, 2001, WB Saunders.

Keats T: *Atlas of normal roentgen variants that may simulate disease,* St Louis, 2001, Mosby.

Manaster BJ: *Musculoskeletal imaging: the requisites,* ed 2, Philadelphia, 2002, Mosby.

McKinnis LN: *Fundamentals of orthopaedic radiology,* Philadelphia, 1997, FA Davis.

Stoeller D: *Magnetic resonance imaging in orthopaedics and sports medicine,* Philadelphia, 1997, Lippincott Raven.

Web Resources

http://www.skeletalrad.org/teachingfiles.htm
Radiology Teaching Files on the Internet With Musculoskeletal Cases, Amilcare Gentili, MD, Society of Skeletal Radiology

http://www.ptcentral.com/radiology/
Diagnostic Imaging for the Physical Therapist, Darryl Hosford and Ken Hurd

http://www.rad.washington.edu/mskbook/
Approaches to Differential Diagnosis in Musculoskeletal Imaging, Michael L. Richardson, MD, University of Washington School of Medicine

http://chorus.rad.mcw.edu/
CHORUS: Collaborative Hypertext of Radiology, Medical College of Wisconsin

http://brighamrad.harvard.edu/education/online/ftp/FTP.html
Finding-the-Path: A Problem-Based Guide to Diagnostic Imaging Strategies in the Emergency Room, Leyla Azmoun, MD, Piran Aliabadi MD, B. Leonard Holman, MD, Brigham and Women's Hospital, Harvard Medical School

http://www.radsci.ucla.edu:8000/ms/y1/
Standardized Guidelines for Reporting of Musculoskeletal Imaging Studies, Lawrence Yao, MD, Amilcare Gentili, MD, UCLA Department of Radiological Sciences

Laboratory Tests and Values

18

Lucy J. Wall, MT (ASCP), MA

Objectives

After reading this chapter, the reader will be able to:

1. Describe the personnel and setting of a clinical laboratory.
2. Provide an overview of the role laboratory tests and reported values play in patient management.
3. Describe the clinical practice implications of values associated with commonly used laboratory tests.

Laboratory testing is a part of diagnostic testing and commonly refers to procedures that provide insight into the physiological status of human beings as reflected by body fluids and tissues, especially blood and urine. Hundreds of analyses can be performed to gain insight into human biochemical processes. Laboratory tests are used as an adjunct to the patient history and physical examination. Laboratory testing is objective and usually quantitative. These characteristics add an additional fact-finding dimension to the patient history and physical examination. Test results have little meaning in isolation.

The clinical laboratory has evolved as an essential partner in providing patient information for diagnosis and treatment. As the principles of infectious disease became known in the 1890s, laboratory tests evolved as applications of the principles. The American College of Surgeons created a plan to ensure minimum standards for hospital care in 1919, including establishing clinical laboratories. More and more tests gradually became available, improved methods brought more reliable results, and physicians increasingly realized the value of the information.[15] This pattern has repeated itself throughout the twentieth century—new basic science, new applications and standards, leading to increasingly reliable information produced and incorporated into health care. In the twenty-first century, it is taken for granted that the clinical laboratory will meet the challenge to provide increasing levels of test sophistication and information pertaining to patient care.

The overall objectives of this chapter are to familiarize the physical therapist (PT) with the clinical laboratory personnel, setting, and the roles that laboratory tests play in the overall management of patients. In addition, the information presented provides examples of how laboratory test results may affect clinical decision-making on the part of the PT.

Specifically, this chapter discusses personnel who perform tests, uses of laboratory tests, regulations and standards, and costs for tests. Additionally, tests, values, and clinical significance are provided for many body systems addressed in primary care.

Information provided by the examination of body tissues and cells with histology and cytology is not within the scope of this discussion.

Laboratory Personnel

The people who perform or assist with clinical laboratory tests are often unseen caregivers and unsung heroes. These personnel include laboratory scientists, technicians, and phlebotomists.

Laboratory scientists typically have the title of clinical laboratory scientist (CLS) or medical technologist (MT). Laboratory scientists are certified by either the American Society for Clinical Pathology (ASCP) or the National Credentialing Agency for Laboratory Personnel (NCA). The benchmark for the laboratory scientist is a bachelor's degree awarded by a regionally accredited college or university as well as successful completion of a clinical laboratory scientist program accredited by an agency recognized by the U.S. Department of Education.[1]

Laboratory technicians usually have the title of clinical laboratory technician (CLT) or medical laboratory technician (MLT). Technicians are certified by the same credentialing agencies as laboratory scientists. The benchmark for the technician is an associate's degree awarded by a regionally accredited college or university as well as successful completion of a clinical laboratory science technician program accredited by an agency recognized by the U.S. Department of Education.[15]

All laboratory technical personnel are trained and skilled in sample collection. However, the phlebotomist performs most of the sample collection. Phlebotomists often develop a high level of expertise in venous and capillary collection and establish working relationships with patients. The benchmark for the phlebotomist is successful completion of a formal education program that includes a clinical component in phlebotomy (e.g., phlebotomy, medical assistant, laboratory assistant, or certified nurse assistant).

Laboratory scientists and technicians are currently licensed in 11 states. Other laboratory personnel are certified, although some may be neither licensed nor certified. Licensure of laboratory personnel has been a recent effort by laboratory professionals. Licensure is a governmental activity taken on behalf of the public to protect the community from potential harm. Certification is a private sector activity. A major difference between the two involves the consequences of engaging in practice without each credential. If a license is required to practice a profession in a particular state, engaging in the work without one is illegal and the consequences of doing so are very serious. Not being certified may make it more difficult to get a job, but it is not illegal to work without it.

The *Code of Ethics* of the American Society for Clinical Laboratory Science (ASCLS), which appears below, sets forth the principles and standards by which clinical laboratory professionals practice their profession.[1]

DUTY TO THE PATIENT. Clinical laboratory professionals are accountable for the quality and integrity of the laboratory services they provide. This obligation includes maintaining individual competence in judgment and performance and striving to safeguard the patient from incompetent or illegal practice by others.

Clinical laboratory professionals maintain high standards of practice. They exercise sound judgment in establishing, performing, and evaluating laboratory testing.

Clinical laboratory professionals maintain strict confidentiality of patient information and test results. They safeguard the dignity and privacy of patients and provide accurate information to other health care professionals about the services they provide.

DUTY TO COLLEAGUES AND THE PROFESSION. Clinical laboratory professionals uphold and maintain the dignity and respect of their profession and strive to maintain a reputation of honesty, integrity, and reliability. They contribute to the advancement of the profession by expanding the body of knowledge, adopting scientific advances that benefit the patient, maintaining high standards of practice and education, and seeking fair socioeconomic working conditions for members of the profession.

Clinical laboratory professionals actively strive to establish cooperative and respectful working relationships with other health care professionals. Their primary objective is ensuring a high standard of care for patients.

DUTY TO SOCIETY. As practitioners of an autonomous profession, clinical laboratory professionals have the responsibility to contribute from their sphere of professional competence to the general well-being of the community.

Clinical laboratory professionals comply with relevant laws and regulations pertaining to the practice of clinical laboratory science and actively seek, within the dictates of their consciences, to change those [laws and regulations] that do not meet the high standards of care and practice to which the profession is committed.

Clinical Uses of Laboratory Tests

Physicians order and use laboratory tests as additional tools for screening, diagnosing, and managing patient health and disease. Screening tests are usually relatively inexpensive, easily performed, and designed to discern the possibility of disease that has gone unnoticed. Examples of screening tests commonly used today are prostate specific antigen (PSA) to assess the possibility of prostatic cancer, or cholesterol to shed light on cardiac disease risk. The PSA is not specific for cancer of the prostate, but elevated levels may indicate the presence of prostate cancer. Additional diagnostic work needs to be performed when PSA levels are elevated. Similarly, an elevated

Patient history ↔ Physical findings ↔ Laboratory screening
Test results
↓
Hypothesis—wellness
Possibility of disease
↓
Laboratory diagnostic test results exclude confirm
↓
Laboratory monitoring test results—provide diagnostic information
Stage disease severity
Monitor disease
Manage therapy

FIGURE 18-1 Algorithm for test use. (Modified from The medical decision-making model as a framework for laboratory testing. In Speicher CE: *The right test: a physician's guide to laboratory medicine*, ed 2, Philadelphia, 1993, WB Saunders, p 3.)

cholesterol level signifies the possibility of a lipid disorder or increased risk of coronary artery disease, signaling the need for additional diagnostic considerations.

Diagnostic tests are designed to be specific in the information they provide and are used to confirm a clinical impression or rule out a disease. Examples are tests for human immunodeficiency virus, thyroid function, and anemia.

Other laboratory tests are performed to assist the physician in managing the patient's condition. Drug assays help manage therapeutic drug levels to prevent toxicity and ensure efficacy. Liver function tests help monitor side effects of drugs intended to lower lipid levels. Some tests provide a prognostic guide; for example, the prothrombin time test provides a guide regarding the anticoagulation effect of warfarin drugs (Figure 18-1).

Regulation of Laboratory Tests

The Centers for Medicare and Medicaid Services (CMS) of the Department of Health and Human Services regulates all laboratory testing (except research) performed on human beings in the United States through the Clinical Laboratory Improvement Amendments (CLIA). Congress passed CLIA in 1988 to establish quality standards for all laboratory testing ensuring reliability and timeliness of test results wherever the test was performed. The CMS is charged with the implementation of CLIA and ensuring compliance with the requirements.

A laboratory is defined as any facility that performs testing on specimens derived from human beings for the purpose of providing information on the diagnosis, prevention, or treatment of disease or the impairment or assessment of health.

The final CLIA regulations were published on February 28, 1992, and are based on the complexity of the test method; thus the more complicated the test, the more stringent the requirements. Three categories of tests have been established: waived complexity, moderate complexity (including the subcategory of provider-performed microscopy), and high complexity.[6]

Personnel requirements under the CLIA regulations vary with test complexity. Except for waived testing, personnel must demonstrate ongoing competency once trained. As the complexity of testing increases, so does the need for independent judgment and interpretation by the personnel.

Testing Standards

It has been said that quality clinical laboratory testing is performing the correct test on the right patient at the right time and producing accurate test results with the best outcome in the most cost-effective manner.[15] The practice of clinical laboratory science requires the development and implementation of a comprehensive quality management system that includes quality control and quality assurance of testing services. The system must also include competency assessment of personnel and continuous process improvement to maximize human resources. Appropriate use of clinical laboratory testing services is ensured through integration with other aspects of health care delivery.

Quality assurance in testing includes internal and external programs. Internal systems include the use of standards, calibrators, controls, and blind samples coupled with statistical analysis of the findings. External efforts include participation in proficiency testing programs, accreditation of laboratories, laboratory inspections, and compliance with CLIA regulations. Proficiency testing consists of periodic samples received as a subscription. The analytes in the sample are of unknown concentration. The job of the clinical laboratory is to assay the samples, report concentrations, and demonstrate proficiency in performance by reporting the correct results.

CLIA specifies quality standards for proficiency testing, patient test management, quality control, personnel qualifications, and quality assurance for laboratories performing moderate- or high-complexity tests. Patient test management includes sample integrity and positive patient identification throughout the testing process. Waived complexity testing, such as glucose measured with glucose monitors, requires that testing personnel follow the manufacturers' instructions for performing the tests.

To enroll in the CLIA program, laboratories must first register by completing an application, paying fees, being surveyed (if applicable), and becoming certified. CLIA fees are based on the certificate requested by the laboratory (waived, provider-performed microscopy (PPM), accreditation, or compliance) and, for moderate- and high-complexity laboratories, the annual volume and types of testing performed. Tests in waived and PPM laboratories are performed by physicians, physician assistants, nurse-midwives, and nurse practitioners as part of their practice of medicine. Waived and PPM laboratories may

apply directly for their certificate because they are not subject to routine inspections. Laboratories that must be routinely surveyed are those performing moderate- or high-complexity testing; they can choose whether they wish to be surveyed by CMS or by a private accrediting organization. The CMS survey process is outcome oriented and uses a quality assurance focus and an educational approach to assess compliance.

Laboratory Testing Considerations

The goal of laboratory testing is to provide the most accurate results possible. This can best be achieved through knowledge of and attention to factors that influence test results. These factors are categorized into three areas: preanalytical, analytical, and postanalytical. Many of the preanalytical factors are outside the laboratory. There is an attempt to control these factors through the use of procedure manuals for health care team members regarding patient preparation, sample collection, and specimen transport for specific tests. Analytical factors relate to the actual analysis of samples and are addressed within the laboratory. Postanalytical factors occur after analysis is completed and are largely controlled through the use of computer applications and interpretation of results by clinicians (Table 18-1).

Testing Sites

Laboratory tests are performed in the home by patients, at the point of care, in physician office laboratories, and in centralized laboratories. Instruments and methods of detection have been designed specifically for use in different settings by operators with varying levels of expertise. The reliability of test results tends to increase with the use of moderate to highly complex methods, increased analyst expertise, and the use of quality assurance plans. Centralized laboratories have traditionally provided the highest level of reliability.

Home, point-of-care, and physician office tests provide greater access and shorter turnaround times. The challenge at these sites is to have methods that provide useful and reliable information. Recent advances in technology address many of these concerns. Additionally, clinical laboratory personnel now commonly organize, implement, and oversee point-of-care quality programs in health care settings.

Some examples of the tests performed at each site are listed in Table 18-2. Blood glucose levels may be performed at all

---

TABLE 18-1

Factors Influencing Test Results

Preanalytical Factors: Biological and Methodologic	Analytical Factors	Postanalytical Factors
Appropriate test ordered	Instrument performance	Recording data
Patient status regarding nutrition, drugs, smoking, stress, sleep, posture	Reagent quality and status	Transmitting and storing data
Specimen collection, labeling, transport, preparation, storage	Standards, calibrators, controls	Providing interpretive information
	Analyst expertise	Clinician interpretation

TABLE 18-2

Testing Sites and Examples of Tests Performed at Each Site

Home	Point of Care	Physician Office	Centralized Laboratory
Blood glucose	Blood glucose	Blood glucose	Blood glucose
Pregnancy status	Electrolytes	Blood counts	Transfusion services
Urine protein	Clotting times	Strep detection	Therapeutic drug assays
Drug screens		Urinalysis	Toxicologic studies
Prothrombin times		Sedimentation rates	Enzyme assays

sites of testing, but different methods of determining the glucose level are used at different sites. Other analytes may be assayed at one or many sites as well.

Methodologies

Many test methods and detection systems are used in clinical laboratory assays, including the following:

- Color detection by spectrophotometry
- Particle counting by laser detection
- Color comparison to a colored chart
- Microscopic identification of morphology
- Compound separation by chromatography
- Chemiluminescence
- Ion selective electrodes
- Radioisotopes
- Immunochemistry
- Nucleic acid techniques
- Cell sizing by flow cytometry

Methods that are selected for use in clinical laboratories depend on what has been researched and developed for possible use, technical information about the methods, and managerial aspects of the methods. Information about methods is collected from manufacturers, sales representatives, colleagues, scientific presentations, and scientific literature. The managerial aspects for consideration are costs, including cost per test, test throughput, sample volume and type, personnel requirements, space, environment, and utility requirements. The technical aspects include the following:

- Analytical sensitivity—the smallest concentration that can be accurately measured
- Analytical specificity—the ability to measure only the analyte of interest
- Linear range—the concentration range over which the measured concentration is equal to the actual concentration
- Interfering substances as they relate to analytical specificity
- Estimates of imprecision and inaccuracy

Once a method for a specific assay is selected and implemented, it is continuously monitored by the quality assurance program.[3]

Billing and Payment for Laboratory Tests

Charges for laboratory tests range from several dollars to hundreds of dollars. Charges reflect the cost of performing the tests. Most laboratory procedures are billed separately, but some batteries of tests are billed together.

Medicare billing regulations require that all laboratory tests have International Classification of Disease (ICD) codes and that the medical necessity of the test be documented. If Medicare does not pay for a test, the cost for such a test is the responsibility of the patient. Regulations require that the patient must be informed of the costs and agree to pay before the specimen is obtained.

Payment comes from the same sources as payment for other health care costs: Medicare, third-party payers, and private payers. Laboratory test payment policies of Medicare Part B and managed care organizations have created a shift from laboratories being "profit centers" to being "cost centers." This financial shift and the requirement of documenting the medical necessity of laboratory tests have changed the utilization of laboratory tests.[12]

Having some sense of the cost of laboratory tests is important for clinicians. As with many health care costs, we know that in general the cost is high. PTs typically do not know what laboratory charges run because providers are removed from billing. Cost is seldom a specific topic of discussion between providers and patients; when a physician suggests that a patient have a blood count, urinalysis, and lipid profile as part of an annual physical, the physician likely does not know what costs will be incurred for the testing.

An example of a bill for laboratory tests ordered as part of an annual physical could include the following:

- Blood sample collection: $18.00
- Serum glucose: $28.00
- Cholesterol: $28.00
- Complete blood count: $56.00
- PSA: $103.00
- Fecal blood: $21.00
- Thyroid-stimulating hormone: $100

Total charges for the above tests are $354. These tests provide significant screening information about the potential for diabetes, cardiac risk, oxygen carrying capacity and immune response of the blood cells, disease of the prostate, intestinal bleeding, and thyroid function.

Reported Values and Interpretation

Each laboratory test ordered by a physician and performed by the laboratory is reported and becomes a part of the medical record for the given individual. The report identifies the patient, the test, the findings of the test, and information to use in the interpretation of the test findings. Test findings are most often quantities. In the United States, mass per unit volume, expressed in milligrams per deciliter, is the typical expression of quantity. Much of the rest of the world uses Systeme Internationale (SI) units, or moles per unit of volume (the gram molecular weight of a substance per liter of solution).

Mass per mole varies with the gram molecular weight of the analyte, making conversion from one system to the other cumbersome. Some test results are expressed in units of activity per unit of volume.

The interpretation of laboratory test results is a comparative decision-making process. The result of a test for a given individual is compared with a reference range to make a medical diagnosis, manage therapy, or provide other physiological assessment.[23] The reference range is the interval between and including the lower and upper reference limits. The interval is determined statistically by the assay of the analyte of interest in a selected population. The range reflects the selected population only. The traditional reference range for quantitative tests is the range of values of the central 95% of the healthy population.

Reference ranges are commonly established for adult populations but also are studied for individuals by age, by sex, and in specific populations (e.g., hemoglobin variants in persons of Mediterranean descent).

Reference values from birth into adulthood with hemoglobin as the analyte are shown in Table 18-3.[19]

When physicians, PTs, or other members of the health care team see laboratory results as part of a patient's medical record, they see the result of the test as well as the reference range appropriate for the age and sex of the patient, the methods used, and any other considerations essential to help make an interpretation in light of the patient's history and physical findings. If additional information is desired, contact the laboratory performing the test. Clinical laboratories have medical directors, usually pathologists, who also consult about the selection and interpretation of test values.

An example of a laboratory report is shown in Table 18-4.

Today, some reference limits may be based on the risk of disease as determined from outcome studies.[7] Cholesterol reference limits are an example of the application of outcome studies. Additionally, reference ranges are specific to the sex and age of the population. Other considerations reported may include ethnic origin, pregnancy, height, weight, body surface area, nutritional status, time of day, time of last dose and type of drug administered, time of last meal, and smoking status.

Reference ranges are reported in the same units as the test result and depend on the method used. There can be multiple reference ranges for the same analyte because there are multiple

methods to assay the same analyte. With experience, clinicians develop a working knowledge of commonly assayed analytes and their reference ranges. However, because of reference range variations caused by methods used, it is important to note the reference range information that accompanies test results. It is also important to add a caution to this interpretive information: a given specimen from a healthy individual is unlikely to have all analytes within the reference range. Laboratory test findings need clinical correlates to substantiate their significance.[26]

Additional statistical concepts related to test interpretation are sensitivity, specificity, and predictive value. There is overlap between test results in healthy and diseased individuals. Evaluating the test results in terms of sensitivity, specificity, and the likelihood of disease is a pragmatic approach in discerning overlap. Sensitivity is the ability of a test to detect disease; results are positive when the disease is present. Specificity is the ability of a test to give normal results in patients without a particular disease. The mathematical likelihood that a test result correctly identifies a patient as normal or abnormal is the predictive value.[8]

Other interpretive assistance is available. Abnormal results are often flagged in the reporting process, drawing special attention to the finding. Laboratories may add statements to test reports that are interpretive statements or provide considerations for interpretation. Flowcharts and pathways exist for reference. Centralized laboratories may offer online reporting of current and past test results. Some services provide secure electronic clinical laboratory reporting systems for physicians. Such laboratory services focus on providing patient-centered diagnostic testing.

Critical Values for Laboratory Tests

Critical values for laboratory tests indicate that a patient may be in a life-threatening situation. Critical values for selected

---

TABLE 18-4

Sample Laboratory Report

Laboratory Name Location	
Patient Name: Smith, Joe	Current date & time:
Patient ID#: 1247	02/10/02/13:15
Specimen ID#: 0038	Date & time collected:
Age: 37 years	02/10/02/6:55
Sex: male	Specimen drawn by: WL
Patient Location: Med/surg	Physician: N Delson

Test Name	Results	Units	Flag	Reference Range
Total protein	9.0	g/dL	HIGH	6.0-8.5
Glucose	82	mg/dL		70-106
Sodium	151	mmol/L	HIGH	135-145
Potassium	4.1	mmol/L		3.5-4.8
Chloride	84	mmol/L	LOW	95-103
Phosphorus	3.7	mg/dL		2.4-4.7
Triglycerides	235	mg/dL	HIGH	35-160

TABLE 18-3

An Example of Reference Values for Hemoglobin from Birth to Adulthood

Age	Hemoglobin (g/dL)
Birth (cord blood)	3.5-19.5
1-3 days (capillary)	14.5-22.5
6-24 months	10.5-13.5
2-12 years	11.5-15.5
12-18 years (male)	13.0-16.0
12-18 years (female)	12.0-16.0
18-49 years (male)	13.5-17.5
18-49 years (female)	12.0-16.0

See reference 19 for more complete information on hemoglobin values.

TABLE 18-5

Some Critical Values that Must Be Immediately Reported

Test	Result
Acid-fast culture or smears	All positive
Blood culture	All positive
Bone marrow culture	All positive
Cryptococcal antigen detection	All positive
Cerebrospinal fluid culture or Gram stain	All positive
Group A streptococci (other than throat cultures)	All positive
Group B streptococci (children <1 year of age)	All positive
Herpes culture	All positive

analytes reflect medical decision making and are not related to reference ranges. They are often established by consensus of the medical staff of critical care and emergency care units of hospitals and may be related to specific medical conditions. When a critical value is identified in the clinical laboratory, the laboratory should immediately contact the physician or patient care area with the test results.

A partial list of critical values for which all positive results must be brought to the immediate attention of the physician is shown in Table 18-5.

Laboratory Tests

There are hundreds of tests that can be performed on human blood and urine specimens. The tables that follow are intended *to provide basic insight only* regarding tests that are commonly performed in clinical laboratories, their basic role in reflecting physiologic processes, some of the conditions in which abnormal results occur, and an example of the reference ranges for adults. All tests are performed on venous blood samples unless otherwise stated.

Indications of how they are used clinically are also shown, such as screening, diagnostic, or monitoring tests. Their purpose is based on medical necessity for a given patient in his or her particular health or disease status. One size does not fit all when it comes to laboratory tests.

Kidney Function

Tests commonly associated with kidney function are shown in Table 18-6.

IMPLICATIONS FOR THE PHYSICAL THERAPIST. Changes in blood urea nitrogen (BUN) and creatinine levels do not usually contraindicate physical therapy intervention. Physical therapy treatment considerations may need to be made because of the renal disease symptoms of anemia, hypertension, decreased endurance, and general deconditioning.[28] The most common reason for increased creatinine levels is decreased kidney function. Beyond that, rising levels of creatinine may indicate muscle wasting from increased corticosteroid dosage or exercise beyond the person's physiological limits. Increased BUN levels can be caused by dehydration, in which symptoms of light-headedness or dizziness during exercise may occur. Patients with burns are especially likely to have elevated BUN levels.[10]

Urinalysis

Urinalysis is a reflection of concentration-dependent excretion and abnormal renal function. Testing is used to screen for, diagnose, and monitor patients with certain conditions (Table 18-7).

INTERPRETATION OF URINALYSIS FINDINGS. It is essential to correlate the physical, chemical, and microscopic findings of urinalysis reports. A working knowledge of kidney function is essential to correlating the findings. A pale, clear urine with a low specific gravity, pH of 6.0, an essentially negative dipstick, and an occasional epithelial cell in the microscopic examination describes a random specimen from a healthy male (unless it is a catheterized specimen) individual. Conversely, a cloudy, smelly urine specimen with protein, white blood cells both on the chemical tests and microscopic exam, and some cellular casts may indicate some type of renal disease.

If there were no casts present in the microscopic exam of the above specimen, contamination on voiding and the time of the specimen collection would have to be considered. When interpreting urinalysis results, considerations must be made for the possibility of false-positive and false-negative results. When urinalysis findings are not supported by other clinical observations, consult the laboratory for possible sources of false results.[5]

TABLE 18-6

Kidney Function Tests

Test	Related Physiology	Increased Values in:	Decreased Values in:	Reference Range Example
Blood urea nitrogen (BUN)	Amino acid metabolism in the liver produces urea as waste; urea is filtered by the kidney with the portion passively reabsorbed being measured in the plasma	Excessive protein intake, kidney damage, certain drugs, low fluid intake, intestinal bleeding, exercise, heart failure	Poor diet, malabsorption, liver damage, low nitrogen intake	Adult range: 8-22 mg/dL
Creatinine	Muscle creatine degradation produces creatinine, which in turn is excreted by the kidneys	Kidney disease, muscle degeneration, kidney impairment from drugs	Kidney damage, protein starvation, liver disease, pregnancy	Adult range: 0.7-1.4 mg/dL
BUN/creatinine ratio	Assessment of kidney and liver function	Dehydration, acute obstruction, acute glomerulonephritis	Renal dialysis, severe skeletal muscle injury, liver disease, malnutrition	Adult range: 6-25 mg/dL

TABLE 18-7
Urinalysis

Test	Related Physiology	Increased Values in:	Decreased Values in:	Reference Range Example
PHYSICAL OBSERVATIONS				
Color	From presence of urochrome; color reflects concentration of urine	Bilirubin, hemoglobin, RBCs, homogentisic acid, dyes, medications	Increased fluid intake; polyuria	Varying shades of yellow
Clarity	Depends on amount of suspended particulate matter	Cloudy/turbid: degree depends on amount and type of pathologic (WBCs, RBCs, bacteria, yeast, renal epithelial cells, fat, abnormal crystals) or nonpathologic elements (urates, phosphates, other crystals), spermatozoa, mucus, contaminants	NA	Clear
Odor	From organic and inorganic byproducts of metabolism	Sweet: ketones; fetid: microorganisms; ammoniacal: improperly stored, "old"; unusual: amino acid disorders (e.g., "mousy" in phenylketonuria)	Bleach: adulteration or contamination	Aromatic
Osmolality	Reflects the solute particles or substances secreted by the renal tubules	Water deprivation (antidiuretic hormone–driven)	Excess water intake	275-900 mOsm/kg; varies with diet, health, physical activity
Volume	Reflects diet, health, exercise, environmental conditions, such as increased sweat and decreased urine output; kidneys excrete any excess fluid ingested but have limited ability to compensate for lack of adequate fluid intake	Polyuria/diuresis (>3 L/day): compulsive water intake, diabetes insipidus, renal disease, drugs, diabetes mellitus, diuretic therapy	Oliguria (<400 ml/day): water deprivation, excess sweating, diarrhea, vomiting; anuria: no urine excreted; acute renal failure; renal obstruction; hemolytic transfusion reactions	600-1800 mL/day
CHEMICAL TESTS				
Specific gravity	Expresses ability of renal tubules to concentrate ultrafiltrate	Excessive sweating, dehydration, fluid restriction, excretion of radiographic contrast media or mannitol	Not physiologically possible; verify that specimen is urine	1.002-1.025
pH	Kidneys selectively excrete acid or alkali to help regulate acid-base balance	Values greater than 8.0 not physiologically possible	Values less than 4.5 or more than 8.0 not physiologically possible	5.0-8.0
Blood	Blood entering urinary tract from glomeruli to urethra	Urinary tract disease or specimen contamination during collection	NA	Negative
Leukocyte esterase	Detects granulocytic leukocytes present in urine as a result of kidney damage or urinary tract leakage	Commonly indicates bacterial infection of kidneys or urinary tract	NA	0-8 per high-power field
Nitrite	Detects the reduction of urinary bacterial nitrates to nitrites	Helps detect asymptomatic bacterial urinary tract infection	NA	Negative
Protein	Indicates increased amounts of protein being filtered and not reabsorbed or reduced tubular reabsorption ability	Dubbed "first indicator of renal disease"; caused by prerenal, renal, or postrenal conditions	NA	Negative
Glucose	Blood level of glucose exceeds renal tubular reabsorption capacity	Diabetes mellitus, hormonal disorders, liver and pancreatic disease, central nervous system damage, drugs	NA	Negative
Ketones	In starvation or when carbohydrates are unavailable, fatty acids are mobilized from triglyceride stores to provide energy; ketones result from ketogenesis and ketonemia	Inability to use available carbohydrates (e.g., uncontrolled diabetes mellitus), insufficient carbohydrate consumption (e.g., severe exercise), loss of carbohydrates (e.g., vomiting)	NA	Negative

TABLE 18-7

Urinalysis—cont'd

Test	Related Physiology	Increased Values in:	Decreased Values in:	Reference Range Example
Bilirubin	Results from the degradation of red blood cells (heme) and may abnormally occur in urine in the water-soluble form instead of being converted to urobilinogen	Hepatic disease, posthepatic disease (obstruction)	NA	Negative
Urobilinogen	Formed in the conversion of water-insoluble bilirubin in the intestinal tract; a portion is reabsorbed into the blood and a smaller portion remains in the blood and is excreted by the kidneys	Prehepatic and hepatic disease	Posthepatic disease (obstruction)	<1.0 mg/dL

FORMED ELEMENTS

Test	Related Physiology	Increased Values in:	Decreased Values in:	Reference Range Example
RBCs	Damaged vascular barrier in kidneys or urinary tract allows leakage into the urine	Renal disease including trauma, drugs that are toxic, inflammatory processes, contamination from vaginal secretions, hemorrhoids	NA	0-3 per high power field; smoking and exercise may cause increases
WBCs	Damaged vascular barrier in kidneys or urinary tract allows leakage into the urine	Renal disease, inflammatory conditions, vaginal contaminants	NA	0-8 per high-power field
Epithelial cells: squamous, transitional, renal tubular	Some from turnover of aging cells, others from renal disease, inflammatory processes with the cell type indicating the location of the disease	Renal disease, inflammatory conditions, contamination during specimen collection	NA	A few per low-power field of all types
Casts: hyaline, granular, cellular, waxy	Tubular formations from mucoproteins and other elements that may be present; reflect status of renal tubules with the number indicating the extent and severity of disease	Renal disease, inflammatory conditions, urinary stasis, conditions characterized by increased plasma proteins	NA	0-2 per high-power field; hyaline; strenuous exercise may cause increased casts in the urine of healthy individuals
Crystals: urates, uric acid, calcium oxalate (common in acidic urine); urine phosphates, triple phosphate, ammonium biurate, calcium carbonate (common in alkaline urine)	From precipitation of urinary solutes		NA	Not present in fresh urine; most not clinically significant when present; radiographic contrast media may precipitate on excretion
Abnormal crystals:			NA	Not present in fresh urine; most not clinically significant when present; radiographic contrast media may precipitate on excretion
Bilirubin	Large amount of bilirubin excreted			
Tyrosine and leucine	Result of aminoacidemia			
Cystine	In disease (congenital cystinosis, cystinuria)			
Cholesterol	Nephrotic syndrome, rupture of lymphatic vessels into renal tubules			
Those from medications	Sulfonamides, ampicillin			

Continued

TABLE 18-7

Urinalysis—cont'd

Test	Related Physiology	Increased Values in:	Decreased Values in:	Reference Range Example
MISCELLANEOUS				
Mucus threads	Fibrillar protein	No clinical significance		Frequently noted
Bacteria	Normal urine is sterile	Urinary tract infection		None in catheterized specimens; contaminant in other types of specimens
Yeast	Usually a contaminant	Vaginal infection		None
Fat	From renal tissue damage	Renal disease (nephrotic syndrome), severe crushing injury		None
Hemosiderin	Hemoglobin metabolized to ferritin and denatured to hemosiderin	Severe hemolytic episode		None
Spermatozoa	Indicates recent intercourse or ejaculation	No clinical significance		None
Parasites	E.g., pinworms	Contaminant in urine; indicates parasitic infection		None

NA, Not applicable; RBC, red blood cells; WBC, white blood cells.

Fluid and Electrolyte Balance

Tests commonly associated with the assessment of fluid and electrolyte balance are shown in Table 18-8.[18]

IMPLICATIONS FOR THE PHYSICAL THERAPIST. Potassium levels less than 3.2 or more than 5.1 mmol/L contraindicate physical therapy intervention because of the possibility of arrhythmia and tetany. Exceptions to this guideline are patients with chronic renal failure and those receiving potassium supplementation (e.g., fast-acting oral medication). Usually patients with chronic renal failure can tolerate potassium levels as high as 5.5 mmol/L. People receiving potassium supplements are usually taking diuretics and may be cleared for treatment with close monitoring of the electrocardiogram during activity. There are other critical values for potassium levels, but the PT bases intervention decisions on these guidelines.[10]

Acid-Base Status

Tests commonly associated with acid-base status are listed in Table 18-9. Table 18-10 lists acid-base disturbances.

IMPLICATIONS FOR THE PHYSICAL THERAPIST. Supplemental oxygen should be continued when the patient demonstrates impaired oxygenation status. If that is not possible, treatment plans should be modified and overexertion prevented. Keep in mind that increased physical activity requires increased oxygen. Oxygen administration is contraindicated in persons with chronic obstructive pulmonary disease because it can further depress the respiratory drive, causing death.

Any indication of hyperventilation (i.e., decreased carbon dioxide level or increased respiratory rate) should be addressed during therapy. Relaxation techniques and breathing exercises, such as pursed-lip or diaphragmatic breathing, can be incorporated into the treatment plan.

Hypoventilation (increased carbon dioxide level), as noted by shallow breathing, can be addressed by deep-breathing activities and upright positioning to improve carbon dioxide removal and optimize oxygenation.

Changes in metabolic aspects of arterial blood gases may affect other organ systems and therefore affect a patient's tolerance for physical activity. The PT must always monitor the patient's vital signs and tolerance for activity and observe for associated signs and symptoms. In general, therapy interventions are usually not carried out when arterial blood gas results reflect the critical value range.[10]

Liver Function

Tests commonly associated with liver function that are primarily used to diagnose and monitor hepatic conditions are listed in Table 18-11.[16,25]

IMPLICATIONS FOR THE PHYSICAL THERAPIST. When liver dysfunction is indicated, monitor the patient for signs and symptoms of hepatic disease such as altered behavior or mental status, fluctuating levels of consciousness, edema or ascites, right upper abdominal pain, and musculoskeletal pain. The patient with liver dysfunction is at increased risk of infection and requires careful practice of standard precautions.

The heart tries to compensate for fluid shifts and alterations in vascular status as a result of liver dysfunction, necessitating the monitoring of vital signs. Heart failure can occur when collateral circulation can no longer support body systems.

When liver dysfunction results in increased blood ammonia and urea levels, peripheral nerve function can also be impaired. Asterixis and numbness or tingling (misinterpreted as carpal or tarsal tunnel syndrome) can occur as a result of this ammonia abnormality, causing intrinsic nerve pathology.

Albumin, glucose, hemoglobin, and hematocrit levels can help assess nutritional status and monitor wound healing. Guidelines for impaired nutrition and wound healing from the Agency for Health Care Policy and Research specify an albumin level of less than 3.5 mg/dL and total lymphocyte count of 1800/mm^3. These considerations must be taken into account in planning interventions.[2,10]

TABLE 18-8

Fluid and Electrolyte Tests

Test	Related Physiology	Increased Values in:	Decreased Values in:	Reference Range Example
Sodium	Major extracellular cation: serves to regulate serum osmolality, fluid, and acid-base balance; maintains transmembrane electric potential for neuromuscular functioning	Excessive sweating, hypothalamic disease, diabetes insipidus, hyperadrenalism, excess sodium intake	Diuretic medication, kidney disease, congestive heart failure, diabetic ketoacidosis, sweating, severe vomiting and diarrhea	136-145 mmol/L
Potassium	Major intracellular cation: maintains normal hydration and osmotic pressure	Tissue damage, urinary obstruction, primary adrenal insufficiency, diabetes mellitus	Prolonged vomiting and diarrhea, diuretic medication, corticosteroid excess	3.5-5.5 mmol/L
Chloride	Extracellular anion: maintains electrical neutrality of extracellular fluid	Hyperventilation, drugs, dehydration	Hypoventilation, prolonged vomiting, chronic diarrhea, diabetic ketoacidosis, lactic acidosis, adrenal disease, renal failure	96-106 mmol/L
Carbon dioxide	Reflects body's ability to control pH; important in bicarbonate-carbonic acid blood buffer system	Increased bicarbonate and elevated pH: increased intake of sodium bicarbonate, excess loss of acid stomach contents; increased bicarbonate and decreased pH: lung disease impeding excretion of carbon dioxide (e.g., emphysema)	Decreased bicarbonate and elevated pH: hyperventilation syndrome, toxicity; decreased bicarbonate and decreased pH: diabetic coma, shock	24-30 mmol/L
Anion gap (sodium minus the sum of chloride and carbon dioxide)	Calculated value helpful in evaluating metabolic acidosis	Increase in weak acids, presence of additional anions, antibiotic drugs	Multiple myeloma, high lipids, low albumin, lithium intoxication	3-11 mmol/L
Calcium	Transmission of nerve impulses, muscle contractility; cofactor in enzyme reactions and blood coagulation	Hyperparathyroidism, carcinoma metastatic to bone, multiple myeloma; loss of neuromuscular excitability and muscle weakness may be seen	Vitamin D deficiency, malabsorption, kidney disease, hypoparathyroidism; muscle tetany may be observed	8.5-10.8 mg/dL; inversely related to phosphorus level
Phosphorus	Integral to structure of nucleic acids, in adenosine triphosphate energy transfer, and in phospholipid function	Kidney disease, hypoparathyroidism, hyperthyroidism	Malabsorption, hyperparathyroidism	2.6-4.5 mg/dL; inversely related to calcium level

See reference 18 for more complete information.

TABLE 18-9

Acid-Base Status Tests

Test	Related Physiology	Reference Range Example
Arterial PO_2	Reflects the dissolved oxygen level based on the pressure it exerts on the bloodstream	80-100 mm Hg
Arterial PCO_2	Reflects the dissolved carbon dioxide level based on the pressure it exerts on the bloodstream	36-44 mm Hg
Arterial pH	Reflects the free hydrogen ion concentration; collectively this test and the arterial PO_2 and arterial PCO_2 tests help reveal the acid-base status and how well oxygen is being delivered to the body	7.35-7.45
Oxygen saturation	Usually a bedside technique (pulse oximetry) to indicate the level of oxygen transport	95%-100%

TABLE 18-10

Acid-Base Disturbances

Type	Cause
Metabolic acidosis	Excess hydrogen production
Metabolic alkalosis	Excess hydrogen loss or excess alkali intake
Respiratory acidosis	Excess carbon dioxide accumulation
Respiratory alkalosis	Excess carbon dioxide loss
Hormonal causes	Antidiuretic hormone, aldosterone, renin
Renal causes	Tubular reabsorption and secretion abnormalities
Cystic fibrosis	Lung obstruction

Hemostatic Mechanisms

Tests commonly associated with hemostatic mechanisms that are used to screen, diagnose, and monitor bleeding and clotting conditions are listed in Table 18-12.[13]

IMPLICATIONS FOR THE PHYSICAL THERAPIST. It is desirable for the international normalized ratio (INR) to be less than 2. A value of 2 to 3 may be considered "therapeutic" for someone being treated with coumadin or warfarin. When the INR exceeds 2 and the patient is not receiving coumadin therapy, the PT should check with the physician to find out whether the patient is at an increased risk of bleeding. An exception to this is in patients with mechanical heart valves, who should have a target INR of 2.5 to 3.5. INR values exceeding 3 may place the patient at risk of hemarthrosis, which requires care during therapy and exercise.[25]

In the presence of liver disease, there is an increased chance of bleeding disorders. Bleeding under the skin and easy bruising in response to slight trauma may occur because of impaired production of coagulation factors by the liver as well as by decreased platelet production or function. Caution is necessary in interventions requiring manual therapy or equipment such as gait training belts, physical therapy modalities, and weight training devices. Patients with end-stage liver disease may also have decreased and dysfunctional platelets, placing them at additional risk for easy bleeding. INRs, activated partial thromboplastin time, and platelet levels may be within reference range margins but collectively put the patient at risk for bleeding.[10]

Myocardial Infarction

Tests commonly associated with myocardial infarction (MI) include assessing values of total creatine kinase, creatine kinase-MB isoenzyme, troponin, and myoglobin (Table 18-13).

Total creatine kinase (CK) commonly has a value less than 230 U/L and is normally composed of:
- CK-MM (skeletal muscle) >95%
- CK-MB (myocardial) <5%
- CK-BB (brain) 0%

Increased total CK is not specific for MI. Increased levels of CK are also seen in skeletal muscle trauma, myositis, dystrophy, electrical cardioversion, cardiac catheterization, hypothyroidism, and convulsions.

Creatine kinase-MB isoenzyme (CK-MB) levels are highest in cardiac muscle (up to 25%) and low in other muscles. Cardiac surgery, myocarditis, and electrical cardioversion may all cause a rise in CK-MB. Reperfusion of necrotic cardiac tissues by "clot-busting therapy" may show a dramatic rise in

TABLE 18-11

Liver Function Tests

Test	Related Physiology	Increased Values in:	Decreased Values in:	Reference Range Example
Alanine aminotransferase (ALT)	Enzyme released in cytolysis and necrosis of liver cells	Most important test for recognition of acute and chronic hepatic injury	Vitamin B deficiency	1-21 Units/L
Aspartate aminotransferase (AST)	Enzyme released in cytolysis and necrosis of liver cells; also in heart and skeletal muscle tissues	Hepatic injury	Vitamin B deficiency	7-27 Units/L
Alkaline phosphatase (ALP)	Enzyme released in cytolysis and necrosis of liver cells; also in bone	Cholestasis, metastatic liver disease, pregnancy		13-39 Units/L
γ-Glutamyltransferase (GGT)	Enzyme released in cytolysis and necrosis of liver cells; also in kidney tissue	Cholestasis, marker for immoderate alcohol intake		5-38 Units/L
Albumin	Index of liver synthetic capacity	Dehydration	Proteinuria, inflammatory states, severe malnutrition, pregnancy	3.5-5.0 g/dL
Bilirubin, total	Results from enzymatic breakdown of heme	Hepatic disease, obstructive jaundice, hemolytic anemia, neonatal jaundice		0.2-1.0 mg/dL; direct: 0-0.2 mg/dL; indirect: 0.2-1.0 mg/dL
Ammonia	Liver converts ammonia from blood to urea	Liver failure		12-55 μmol/L

See references 16 and 25 for more complete information on liver function tests.

TABLE 18-12

Hemostatic Mechanisms Tests

Test	Related Physiology	Prolonged times/results in:	Decreased Values in:	Reference Range Example
COAGULATION ASSESSMENT				
Prothrombin time (PT); now referred to as the INR	Reflects liver synthesis of factors II, VII, IX, X	Acute liver failure, vitamin K deficiency, coumadin therapy	$INR = \dfrac{(Patient\ PT)^{ISI}}{(Control\ PT)}$	A patient adequately controlled on coumadin will have an INR in the range of 2-3
Partial thromboplastin time (PTT)	Reflects on level and function of factors II, V, X, VIII, IX, XI	Heparin therapy, lupus anticoagulant		22-33 sec
Bleeding time	Reflects function of platelets and blood vessels	Thrombocytopenia, platelet function disorders	NA	8-10 min
Thrombin time	Evaluates the conversion of fibrinogen to fibrin	Fibrinogen deficiency, dysfibrinogenemia, presence of antithrombins		9-15 sec
FIBRINOLYTIC ASSESSMENT				
D-dimer*	Plasmin lysis of cross-linked fibrin (a clot) generates the D-dimer fragment	Deep vein thrombosis, pulmonary embolism, arteriole thromboembolism, DIC	NA	Negative
Fibrin split products (FDP)	Products of primary or secondary clot lysis	DIC, primary or secondary fibrinolysis, myocardial infarction, pulmonary embolism, malignancy, liver disease, infection or inflammation	NA	<10 μg/ml

INR, International normalized ratio; *ISI*, International Sensitivity Index of the reagent used; *DIC*, disseminated intravascular coagulation; *NA*, not applicable.
*See reference 13 for more complete information on D-dimer assays.

CK-MB after an MI. A relative index (RI) of more than 5% is highly suggestive of MI.

$$CK\text{-}MB/CK_{Total} \times 100 = RI$$

Troponin is the gold standard cardiac marker. It has excellent specificity and sensitivity for acute and subacute MI.

Myoglobin is the only heme protein in cardiac myocytes. It is rapidly excreted in urine but is nonspecific for myocardial damage (skeletal muscle also contains high quantities).

IMPLICATIONS FOR THE PHYSICAL THERAPIST. Physical activity is limited for patients known to have recently incurred an MI (detected by increased CK-MB, troponin, and/or myoglobin). Vital signs are monitored, as is oxygenation with pulse oximetry. Chest physical therapy treatments should continue according to the individual's tolerance, with frequent rest periods provided throughout the session. Anyone with significant arrhythmia or myocardial dysfunction such as angina, hypotension, or congestive heart failure may be excluded from therapy. Activity may be increased according to the cardiac rehabilitation protocol in use. Always monitor the patient for bradycardia or tachycardia, arrhythmias, and associated signs and symptoms of MI (chest pain, unexplained perspiration, nausea, vomiting, shortness of breath, feeling of impending doom).[10]

Infectious Disease

Tests commonly associated with screening and diagnosing infectious disease are listed in Table 18-14.

IMPLICATIONS FOR THE PHYSICAL THERAPIST. Notify the physician when pus from a deep wound, incision, or abscess is observed, especially when it is accompanied by a foul odor. Culture specimens are taken from the suppurative material rather than the skin edge. Pathogens may be characterized by color and consistency:

- Streptococcal pus is thin and serous
- Staphylococcal pus is gelatinous
- *Pseudomonas* pus is blue-green and putrid smelling

When skin lesions are present the PT must follow standard precautions carefully to prevent the spread of infection to the patient and to avoid self-inoculation and subsequent infection.[10]

TABLE 18-13

Serum Cardiac Markers

Marker	Rise	Peak	Return	Reference Range Example
CK	3-8 hours	10-24 hours	3-4 days	<230 Units/L
CK-MB	3-8 hours	10-24 hours	3-4 days	<4 ng/mL
Troponin	3-8 hours	24-48 hours	7-10 days	<2 ng/mL
Myoglobin	1-3 hours	6-9 hours	24 hours	<76 ng/mL

Pancreatic Function

Tests commonly used to diagnose pancreatic conditions are listed in Table 18-15.

Immune Function

Tests used primarily for screening and diagnosis of immune function are listed in Table 18-16.[30]

Skeletal Muscle Pathology

Tests commonly associated with skeletal muscle pathology diagnosis are listed in Table 18-17. All the proteins listed are found in cardiac and skeletal muscle. Differentiating the source of increased levels of each in the blood is important.

IMPLICATIONS FOR THE PHYSICAL THERAPIST. It is not common to assess skeletal muscle injury with blood tests. These tests are

---

TABLE 18-14

Tests for Infectious Diseases

Test	Related Physiology	Testing Approaches	Reference Range Example
Bacterial studies	Pathologic bacteria invade and damage tissue	A sample of the tissue of interest is obtained, including bacteria that may be present	
Direct stain		Screening procedure to get an indication of the presence or absence of bacteria	Negative
Culture		Conditions designed to promote growth and identification of bacteria or viruses	No growth, or normal flora only
Antibiotic susceptibility		Bacteria identified by culture are tested to determine which antibiotics are able to inhibit bacterial growth	Treatment is anticipated to be effective by using study outcomes
Immunologic procedures	Detect antibodies produced by microorganisms, or antigens and nucleic acids of organisms (e.g., β-streptococcus, viral hepatitis, human immunodeficiency virus, Epstein-Barr virus, sexually transmitted diseases, Lyme disease)		Negative

---

TABLE 18-15

Pancreatic Function Tests

Test	Related Physiology	Increased Values in:	Decreased Values in:	Reference Range Example
Amylase	Digestive enzyme secreted by pancreas	Acute pancreatitis, gastrointestinal obstruction, pancreatic carcinoma, intestinal infarct, obstruction or perforation, pancreatic trauma, acute ethanol ingestion, mumps, parotitis	Marked pancreatic destruction	53-123 Units/L
Lipase	Digestive enzyme secreted by pancreas	Acute pancreatitis; same as amylase but not in mumps, parotitis		4-24 Units/dL

TABLE 18-16

Immune Function Tests

Test	Related Physiology	Increased Values in:	Decreased Values in:	Reference Range Example
Rheumatoid factor (RF)	Immunoglobulin M molecule that binds other immunoglobulins as antigens	Rheumatoid arthritis, other inflammatory conditions, acute illness, smoking	NA	Negative
C-reactive protein (CRP)	Acute phase reactant; activates complement; level rises quickly	Nonspecific indicator of inflammation or infection	NA	0.3-20 mg/dL
High-sensitivity CRP*	As above; method detects lower level of CRP	Associated with increased cardiovascular disease risk	NA	Lower level detection at 0.01 mg/dL
α₁-Antitrypsin	A protease inhibitor; limits damage from WBC products	NA	Congenital deficiencies associated with emphysema, hepatitis; can also occur with protein loss, malnutrition, cirrhosis	85-213 mg/dL
Antinuclear antibodies (ANA)	Detects autoantibodies present from systemic rheumatic disease	Autoimmune diseases (e.g., systemic lupus erythematosus, viral hepatitis, mononucleosis, renal failure, leprosy)	NA	Negative at 1:8 dilution of serum

NA, Not applicable; *WBC*, white blood cell count.
*See reference 30 for more complete information on C-reactive protein.

TABLE 18-17

Skeletal Muscle Tests

Test	Related Physiology	Increased Values in:	Reference Range Example
CK	Major skeletal muscle enzyme; 5-8 times as much as in cardiac muscle	Muscle injury, strenuous activity (can be 10 times baseline)	Level related to muscle mass and muscle activity
CK isoenzymes (MM, MB, BB)		Muscle injury	CK-MB normally <2% of total CK; may be 5%-10% in chronic muscle injury, <3% in muscle injury; Higher levels occur in cardiac muscle injury
Lactate dehydrogenase	High concentration in muscle cells	Muscle injury	Increase in isoenzymes 4 and 5 at 4-6 hours after injury
Aspartate aminotransferase (AST)	Released by injured muscle cells	Muscle injury	CK/AST ratio >20 is indicative of skeletal muscle injury
Myoglobin	Muscle oxygen-binding protein	Muscle injury	Rapid rise after injury in 2-4 hours, peak at 8-12 hours, return to normal in 24-30 hours
Troponin-T	Small protein that activates muscle contraction in skeletal and cardiac muscle	Produced by regenerating skeletal muscle, renal failure, myocardial injury	

performed most often to assess cardiac muscle injury. There is no group of laboratory tests used clinically that provides cost-effective information to assess skeletal muscle directly. The history and symptoms of the patient are usually the most significant sources of information assisting the PT in the evaluation.

Hormone Function

Tests used to analyze hormone function are listed in Table 18-18.[21]

IMPLICATIONS FOR THE PHYSICAL THERAPIST. Hypothyroidism was reported by 7% and hyperthyroidism reported by 1% of women surveyed in an outpatient orthopedic setting.[4] The percentages for the overall therapy population are probably equal or even higher. With adequate replacement therapy, these people will be euthyroid and present no particular problem to the PT. Replacement needs vary over time, however, and these patients may become hyperthyroid or hypothyroid. Signs and symptoms of these conditions include myalgia, arthralgia, and numbness, all symptoms for which the person may seek out a physical or occupational PT.

The fact that many women develop carpal tunnel syndrome at or near menopause suggests that the soft tissues around the wrist may be affected in some way by hormones.[9,11,24,29]

Hormone testing to determine a woman's menopausal status (premenopausal, perimenopausal, postmenopausal) can be performed. This information is also helpful when the woman is considering hormone replacement therapy and can be used by the PT to facilitate patient education regarding prevention of osteoporosis.[10]

Some forms of fibromyalgia present a "hypothyroid tendency" (symptoms with thyroid function tests within the reference ranges). Compromised conversion of T_4 to T_3 may lead to neuromuscular molecular abnormality demonstrated

TABLE 18-18

Hormone Function Tests

Test	Related Physiology	Values Reflect:	Reference Range Example
Thyroid-stimulating hormone (TSH)	Assesses the hypothalamic-pituitary-thyroid axis	In general, abnormal values of thyroid tests indicate conditions of hypothyroidism and hyperthyroidism.	0.3-4.0 μIU/mL
Total T_4	Assesses concentration of hormone secreted by the thyroid	Contact the physician for the interpretation of thyroid test values in light of clinical findings.*	4-12 μg/dL
T_3	Assesses concentration of hormone secreted by the thyroid		75-195 ng/dL
Free T_4	Hormone not bound to protein		0.7-1.8 ng/dL
Human chorionic gonadotropin (HCG)	Recognizes trophoblastic tissue	Trophoblast cells of the placenta produce HCG and indicate pregnancy; hydatidiform moles, choriocarcinoma, and tumors also produce HCG	<5 mU/mL

An informative website regarding thyroid testing and test interpretation is The National Academy of Clinical Biochemistry Laboratory Medicine Practice Guidelines: Thyroid Disease, available at http://www.nacb.org/lmpg/thyroid_LMPG_Word.stm.
*See reference 21 for more complete information on thyroid testing.

by stiffness, aching, decreased basal body temperature, constipation, and dry skin.[10,14,20]

Tumors/Malignancies

Tests commonly associated with the screening and monitoring of tumors and malignancies are listed in Table 18-19.[17]

Therapeutic Drug Management/Monitoring

Tests for therapeutic drug management are listed in Table 18-20.

Cerebrospinal Fluid

Tests associated with cerebrospinal fluid and used in diagnosis are listed in Table 18-21.

TABLE 18-19
Tests for Tumors and Malignancies

Test	Related Physiology	Increased Values in:	Decreased Values in:	Reference Range Example
Prostate-specific antigen (PSA), free PSA (FPSA)*	Normal prostatic secretion; enters blood in cancerous or abnormal prostate conditions	Prostatic cancer	NA	PSA <4 ng/mL; FPSA/PSA <25%
Carcinoembryonic antigen (CEA)	Cell surface glycoproteins produced in small amounts in adults	Carcinomas of gastrointestinal tract, lung, breast, bladder, ovary, uterus; liver disease	NA	Up to 3 ng/mL

Many other laboratory procedures are performed to detect markers of malignant tumors of multiple types.
*See reference 17 for more complete information.

TABLE 18-20
Tests for Therapeutic Drug Management

Drug Assayed	Use	Considerations in Interpretation of Levels	Therapeutic Range
Digoxin	Treatment of congestive heart failure, cardiac arrhythmias	Other metabolic factors and conditions of the patient	Therapeutic drugs are assayed to ensure efficacy of treatment and avoid toxicity; there are levels known to be in the therapeutic range; results of drug assays need to be interpreted in light of the multiple considerations
Theophylline	Treatment of obstructive lung disease	Route of excretion of each drug (e.g., kidney, liver) and the health of the excretory organ/tissue. Time of drug administration	
Primidone	Antiepileptic barbiturate	Time required for drug to reach equilibrium	
Methotrexate	Treatment of malignant tumors	Time that the sample is obtained. Presence of other interfering drugs or metabolites of drugs	
Cyclosporine	Immunosuppressant after organ transplantation	Formulation of a drug and variance in absorption rate	

TABLE 18-21
Tests Associated With Cerebrospinal Fluid

Test	Related Physiology	Increased Values in:	Decreased Values in:	Reference Range Example
Glucose	Glucose level in CSF from filtration and active transport	Reflect hyperglycemia; not clinically informative	Increased cells are in contact with CSF (e.g., acute inflammation, meningeal carcinoma)	60%-70% of blood glucose level over past 4-6 hours
Lactate	Product of anaerobic glycolysis; increases with increased numbers of cells present	Tumors, bacterial infections, granulocyte WBCs (e.g., meningitis)		10-22 mg/dL
Total protein	Ultrafiltrate of plasma	Inflammation, tumor, degenerative disease; traumatic tap	Loss of CSF by lumbar puncture, decreased dialysis from plasma	15-40 mg/dL
Microorganisms (direct stains, cultures, antigen tests may be performed)	Blood-brain barrier normally prevents microorganisms from entering CSF	Infection	NA	None
Cells: WBCs, RBCs	Blood-brain barrier normally prevents cells from entering CSF	Inflammation, infection, bleeding; traumatic tap must be ruled out	NA	<5/mm³; normally none

CSF, Cerebrospinal fluid; *WBCs*, white blood cell counts; *RBCs*, red blood cell counts; *NA*, not applicable.

IMPLICATIONS FOR THE PHYSICAL THERAPIST. If a spinal headache occurs after lumbar puncture, the patient may be instructed to stay flat in bed for several hours. However, most adults and children who receive a lumbar puncture in an outpatient setting are allowed to go home without position restrictions. Any report of numbness or tingling in the lower extremities or drainage of blood or cerebrospinal fluid at the puncture site must be reported.[10]

Cellular Elements of Blood

The complete blood cell count (CBC) is a commonly ordered and performed group of tests (Table 18-22). It consists of the white blood cell count, red blood cell count, hemoglobin, hematocrit, red cell indexes (mean cell volume, mean corpuscular hemoglobin, mean corpuscular hemoglobin concentration), red cell distribution width, platelet count, mean platelet volume, and white cell differential (including percentage and absolute numbers of neutrophils, lymphocytes, monocytes, eosinophils, and basophils). The CBC provides much information regarding the level of production of blood cells, the relative maturity of cells in the peripheral blood, and insight into cellular immune response according to the relative numbers of blood cells. Individual tests may also be ordered separately and tailored to the specific information desired.

IMPLICATIONS FOR THE PHYSICAL THERAPIST. Low hemoglobin values (8 to 10 g/dL) typically result in decreased exercise tolerance, increased fatigue, and tachycardia, conditions that may contraindicate aggressive therapeutic measures, including strength and endurance training. Exercise tolerance in anyone with hemoglobin values of less than 8 g/dL is poor, and therapeutic intervention is contraindicated.

White Blood Cell Count. It is important for the PT to be aware of the patient's most recent white blood cell count before and during the course of intervention. If the count is low, the patient may be extremely susceptible to opportunistic infections and severe complications. The importance of good handwashing and hygiene practices cannot be overemphasized when treating these patients. Some centers recommend that people with a count of less than 1000/mm³ or a neutrophil count of less than 500/mm³ should wear a protective mask. PTs should ensure that all equipment is disinfected according to standard precautions when working with this population.

Platelets. Platelets initiate the clotting sequence to plug damaged blood vessels. Exercise guidelines for the patient with reduced platelet counts (thrombocytopenia) or elevated platelet counts (thrombocytosis) exist in each institution. The PT needs to check the guidelines for the institution and patient population.[10]

Carbohydrate Metabolism

Tests associated with carbohydrate metabolism are listed in Table 18-23.

IMPLICATIONS FOR THE PHYSICAL THERAPIST. Although "safe" blood glucose levels are between 80 and 250 mg/dL, the ideal range is between 80 and 120 mg/dL. The PT should be aware of the goal of medical management for each person. For example, a young person with insulin-dependent diabetes may be working toward tighter control (e.g., 80 to 120 mg/dL), whereas an older adult with non-insulin-dependent diabetes may be looking for more moderate control (e.g., up to 150 mg/dL). Insulin therapy can result in hypoglycemia (low blood sugar, also called an insulin reaction). Symptoms can occur when the blood glucose level drops to 70 mg/dL or less. In diabetes, an overdose of insulin, illness, late or skipped meals, or overexertion in exercise may cause hypoglycemic reactions. The clinical picture may vary from a report of headache and weakness, to irritability and lack of muscular coordination (much like someone who is drunk), to apprehension, inability to respond to verbal commands, and psychosis.

Patients can exhibit signs and symptoms of hypoglycemia when their elevated blood glucose level drops rapidly but to a level that is still elevated (e.g., 400 to 200 mg/dL). The rapidity of the drop is the stimulus for sympathetic activity-based symptoms; even though a blood glucose level appears elevated, affected persons may still have hypoglycemia. Usually people become symptomatic at blood glucose levels of 60 mg/dL or less.[30]

Glucose levels should be monitored before and after exercise (or therapy activities), remembering that the effect of exercise can be felt up to 12 to 24 hours later. Monitoring is not as crucial for the person who has an established pattern of activity or exercise. When a new activity is introduced, as occurs in an exercise or rehabilitation program, monitoring blood glucose levels is recommended until the patient's response to the change is known and predictable in maintaining stable blood glucose levels.

The PT must always be alert for signs of diabetic ketoacidosis (e.g., blood glucose levels 250 mg/dL or greater), a condition that can occur when complications develop from severe insulin deficiency. Observe for symptoms of breath smelling like acetone, dehydration, weak and rapid pulse, and very deep gasping (Kussmaul's) respirations. Most episodes of diabetic ketoacidosis occur in people with previously diagnosed insulin-dependent diabetes mellitus. Immediate medical care is essential. If uncertain whether the patient is hypoglycemic or hyperglycemic, the health care worker is advised to administer fruit juice or honey. This procedure will not harm the hyperglycemic patient and may potentially save the hypoglycemic patient.[10]

Lipid Metabolism

The Third Report of the National Cholesterol Education Program (NCEP) Expert Panel on Detection, Evaluation, and Treatment of High Blood Cholesterol in Adults (Adult Treatment Panel III [ATP III]) presents the NCEP's current clinical guidelines for cholesterol testing and management. The ATP III full set of guidelines is an evidence-based, extensively referenced report that is the basis for several related products and tools.

The ATP III guidelines provide detailed information on topic areas such as classification of lipids and lipoproteins, coronary heart disease (CHD) risk assessment, lifestyle interventions, drug treatment, specific dyslipidemias, and adherence issues. Recommendations for special populations such as patients with CHD, patients at high risk for developing CHD, patients with diabetes, women, older Americans, young adults, and racial and ethnic groups are provided.[22]

TABLE 18-22

Tests of Cellular Blood Elements

Test	Related Physiology	Increased Values in:	Decreased Values in:	Reference Range Example
WBC count	Produced in bone marrow; provide defense against foreign agents/organisms	Infection, inflammation, leukemias, stress, overall stimulation of bone marrow	Chemotherapy, bone marrow failure, viral infections, malaria, alcoholism, AIDS	4,000-10,000 WBCs/μL
Platelet count	Reflects potential to address injury to vessel walls, thus regulating hemostasis	Severe bleeding, infection, strenuous exercise, pregnancy, splenectomy, iron deficiency, rheumatoid arthritis, leukemia	Infection, vitamin B_{12} or folic acid deficiency, severe internal bleeding, cancers, autoimmune conditions	140,000-450,000/μL
WBC differential	Differentiation of white blood cell types by relative percentages			All components totaled equal 100%
Segmented neutrophils	Phagocytizes	Infection (especially bacterial) heart attack, burns, severe stress, use of steroids	Exposure to radiation, some infections (e.g., HIV), vitamin B_{12} or folic acid deficiency, autoimmune diseases	~37%-77%
Band neutrophils	Phagocytizes; less mature neutrophil	Acute response to severe infection, especially from bacteria		~0%-11%
Lymphocytes	B cells produce immuno-globulins; T cells provide regulatory and effector functions in immunity	Viral infections, immune system disease, some types of leukemia	Steroid medications, immune system conditions (e.g., HIV), malnutrition, severe chronic illness	~10%-44%
Monocytes	Phagocytize and contribute to cellular and humoral immunity in association with T lymphocytes	Viral or fungal infection, some cancers and leukemias, tuberculosis		~2%-10%
Eosinophils	Also function as phagocytes, somewhat less effectively than neutrophils	Allergies, parasitic infections, skin diseases, medications	Severe stress, Cushing's syndrome	~0%-7%
Basophils	Also function as phagocytes; synthesize and store histamine	Some leukemia, cancers, or poorly functioning thyroid	Pregnancy, stress, overactive thyroid	~0%-2%
Red blood cell count	Produced in bone marrow, carry oxygen to tissues	Lack of oxygen, smoking, exposure to carbon monoxide, long-term lung disease, diseases of kidney, heart, bone marrow; dehydration, vomiting, diarrhea, sweating, severe burns, diuretics	Anemia from blood loss (colon cancer), decrease in RBC production (tumor, medication, lack of nutrients), increased RBC destruction (sickle cell disease)	4.2-6.2 $\times$ 10^6/μl
Hemoglobin	Reflects concentration of hemoglobin in blood	See RBCs	See RBCs	12-16 g/dL
Hematocrit	Reflects packed cell volume of blood	See RBCs	See RBCs	36%-54% (approximately three times hemoglobin)
Mean cell volume (MCV)	Measure of average size of RBCs	Alcoholism, liver disease, folic acid, and B_{12} deficiencies; bone marrow disorders	Iron deficiency anemia, thalassemia, lead poisoning, long-term infection, chronic disease	80-100 fl
Mean cell hemoglobin concentration (MCHC)	Indicates average concentration of hemoglobin of RBCs	NA	Same as MCV	32-36 g/dL; cannot exceed 37 g/dL
Mean cell hemoglobin (MCH)	Indicates average weight of hemoglobin per RBC	Should correlate with MCV and MCHC	Should correlate with MCV and MCHC	28-32 pg
RBC distribution width	Standard deviation of MCV; measure of degree of uniformity in size of RBCs	Increased values not specific	Iron-deficiency anemia	11.7%-14.2%
Erythrocyte sedimentation rate (ESR)	Nonspecific indicator of inflammation or tissue damage	Inflammatory conditions, infections, pregnancy, menstruation	NA	0-20 mm/1 hr

WBC, White blood cells; *RBC,* red blood cells.
From Lotspeich-Steininger CA, Stiene-Martin AE, Koepke JA: Clinical hematology; principles, procedures, correlations, Philadelphia, 1992, JB Lippincott.

TABLE 18-23
Tests of Carbohydrate Metabolism

Test	Related Physiology	Increased Values in:	Decreased Values in:	Reference Range Example
Glucose: used to screen, diagnose, monitor	Reflects status of carbohydrate metabolism	Diabetes mellitus	Diabetic coma	80-100 mg/dL
Hemoglobin (A1c-HbA1c): used to monitor diabetes	Glucose-modified proteins reflect long-term blood glucose levels	Uncontrolled diabetes mellitus		<7.25%

TABLE 18-24
Tests Associated with Lipid Metabolism

Test	Related Physiology	Increased Values in:	Decreased Values in:	Reference Range Example
Cholesterol, total	Required for steroid synthesis and cell membranes			See Table 18-25
HDL cholesterol	Converts cholesterol to cholesterol esters; returns cholesterol to liver	Vigorous exercise, increased triglyceride clearance (VLDL), ethanol consumption, insulin, estrogens	Starvation, obesity, smoking, diabetes mellitus, hypothyroidism, liver disease, nephrosis, uremia	See Table 18-26
LDL cholesterol: primary target of cholesterol-lowering therapy to reduce CHD	Delivers cholesterol from liver synthesis to cells; inhibits further synthesis when binding to receptors	CHD		See Table 18-25
Triglycerides	Component of lipoproteins that become an energy source for tissues	Dietary excess, nephrosis, cholestasis, pancreatitis, cirrhosis, diabetes mellitus, hepatitis, heredity	Malnutrition	10-190 mg/dL

Tests associated with lipid metabolism are listed in Table 18-24. Cholesterol levels are shown in Tables 18-25, 18-26, and 18-27 .

Laboratory Test Panels

As automation and multichannel analyzers became widely used, it was convenient and cost effective to group laboratory tests together to assess multiple parameters of organ function or perform comprehensive metabolic screens. The configuration of test panels changes and evolves as new assays are implemented and as the practice of medicine evolves. Some examples of panels are seen in Table 18-28.

TABLE 18-26
ATP III Classification of HDL Cholesterol

Serum HDL Cholesterol (mg/dL)	
<40	Low HDL cholesterol
≥60	High HDL cholesterol

TABLE 18-25
ATP III Classification of Total Cholesterol and LDL Cholesterol

Total Cholesterol (mg/dL)		LDL Cholesterol (mg/dL)	
		<100	Optimal
<200	Desirable	100-129	Near optimal/above optimal
200-239	Borderline high	130-159	Borderline high
≥240	High	160-189	High
		≥190	Very high

TABLE 18-27
Classification of Serum Triglycerides

Triglyceride Category	ATP II Levels (mg/dL)	ATP III Levels (mg/dL)
Normal	<200	<150
Borderline high	200-399	150-199
High	400-1000	200-499
Very high	<1000	≥500

TABLE 18-28

Laboratory Test Panels

Comprehensive Metabolic	Basic Metabolic	Renal	Hepatic	Lipid/Cardiac Risk	Acute Hepatitis	Arthritis	CBC
Sodium	Sodium	Sodium	Total protein	Cholesterol	Hepatitis A IgM	Erythrocyte sedimentation rate	Red blood cell count
Potassium	Potassium	Potassium	Albumin	Triglycerides	Hepatitis B$_s$ Ag	Rheumatoid arthritis factor	White blood cell count
Chloride	Chloride	Chloride	Total bilirubin	HDL	Hepatitis B core Ab IgM	Antinucleic acid	Hemoglobin
Carbon dioxide	Carbon dioxide	Carbon dioxide	Direct bilirubin	LDL	Hepatitis C virus	Uric acid	Hematocrit
BUN	BUN	BUN	AST	C-reactive protein			Mean cell hemoglobin concentration
Creatinine	Creatinine	Creatinine	ALT				Mean cell volume
Calcium	Calcium	Calcium	Alkaline phosphatase				Mean cell hemoglobin
Phosphorus	Phosphorus	Phosphorus					White cell differential
Glucose	Glucose						Platelet count
Total protein							Red cell distribution width
Albumin							
Total bilirubin							
AST							
ALT							
Alkaline phosphatase							

AST, Aspartate aminotransferase; *ALT*, alanine aminotransferase; *BUN*, blood urea nitrogen; *HDL*, high-density lipoprotein; *LDL*, low-density lipoprotein; *IgM*, immunoglobulin M.

Summary

In the practice of clinical medicine, laboratory tests are used to provide insight into the physiological processes of the human body. This insight is used in conjunction with physical findings and patient history. The interpretation of laboratory test values is aided by understanding the training of those who perform the tests and the high value placed on reliable test results by laboratory professionals. This chapter has not discussed all the considerations made by laboratory professionals in achieving reliable results. That discussion is pertinent to the study of clinical laboratory science.

The tests noted in the tables are by no means an exhaustive list of tests available. Those noted are some of the more commonly performed clinical laboratory assays. The medical necessity of laboratory tests must be documented to obtain Medicare and managed care payment.

The PT is likely to note many areas of common knowledge between physical therapy and clinical laboratory science. Where overlap does not exist, learning and consultation are encouraged. Consult laboratory personnel, attending physicians, and pathologists about which tests provide needed information in a cost-effective manner. Also contact the laboratory for a copy of the handbook that provides information about tests. Similar information may also be on a website.

Remember that in today's world, laboratory test reports provide the results and reference ranges as well as other information that will assist in interpreting what the results mean. That complete report, along with the history and physical findings, assists with clinical decision making.

As a PT, you may observe symptoms in your patient that alert you to the need for additional medical attention. For example, you may observe shortness of breath in your elderly patient. You would then consult with your patient's primary care physician about your observation, suggesting that it would be helpful to know the patient's blood oxygen saturation level from a pulse oximeter attached to a finger. The physician concurs, asks to have your patient referred to the physician, and will inform you of any laboratory findings based on medical necessity of the tests. In this example, you begin your conversation by asking for an oxygen saturation level by pulse oximetry rather than information generated by performing blood gases. You know that blood gases require an arterial sample and are much more costly to perform.

Having some knowledge of laboratory tests helps PTs think about additional care for patients and helps them talk with physicians. Ultimately, PTs will provide better, more cost-effective care for patients.

Glossary

Terms to review to facilitate understanding the content of this chapter:

Analyte
The substance of interest within a sample

Assay
A method of testing or detection

Blind sample
A sample with no identifiers or characteristics differentiating it from other samples assayed for the purpose of ensuring test performance

Reliability
Reflects the accuracy and precision of a test method

Thrombocytopenia
A decrease in the number of platelets from the reference range

Throughput
Number of samples that can be analyzed per unit of time in an automated analyzer

Urine casts
Cylindrical bodies that form in the renal tubules containing mucoprotein and chemical or formed elements present in the tubule, such as cells, bacteria, or fat

Urine Volume

Anuria
Absence of urine excretion

Diuresis
Increase in urine excretion

Oliguria
Significant decrease in the volume of urine excreted (e.g., less than 400 ml/day)

Polyuria
Excretion of large volumes of urine (e.g., greater than 3 L/day)

REFERENCES

1. American Society for Clinical Laboratory Science: Scope of practice position paper. Available at: http://www.ascls.org/position/scope_of_practice.htm. Accessed Sept 11, 2002.
2. Bergstrom N: *Treatment of pressure ulcers: clinical practice guideline no. 15*, Bethesda, Md, 1994, Agency for Health Care Policy and Research.
3. Bishop ML, Duben-Engelkirk JL, Fody EP: *Clinical chemistry: principles, procedures, correlations*. Philadelphia, 2000, JB Lippincott, pp 58-75.
4. Boissonnault WG: Prevalence of co-morbid conditions, surgeries and medication use in a physical therapy outpatient population: a multi-centered study. *J Orthop Sports Phys Ther* 29:506-519, 1999.
5. Brunzel NA: *Fundamentals of urine and body fluid analysis*, Philadelphia, 1994, WB Saunders, pp 119-263, 365-381.
6. Centers for Medicare & Medicaid Services: General program description. Available at: http://www.cms.hhs.gov/clia/progdesc.asp/ Accessed Sept. 10, 2002.
7. Dufour DR: Tips from the clinical experts, *Medical Laboratory Observer*, August 2002, p 20.
8. Dufour DR: *Clinical use of laboratory data: a practical guide*, Baltimore, 1998, Williams & Wilkins, pp 3-13.
9. Ferry S, Hannaford P, Warskyj M, et al: Carpal tunnel syndrome: a nested case-control study of risk factors in women, *Am J Epidemiol* 151:566-574, 2000.
10. Goodman CC, Boissonnault WG, Fuller KS: *Pathology: implications for the physical therapist*, ed 2, Philadelphia, 2003, WB Saunders, pp 1174-1197.
11. Grossman LA, Kaplan HJ, Ownby FD, et al: Carpal tunnel syndrome: initial manifestations of systemic disease, *JAMA* 176:259-261, 1961.
12. Hanson K, Lavantry D: Payment for laboratory services, *Clin Lab Sci* 15:66, 2002.
13. Hassett AC: D-Dimer testing and acute venous thromboembolism, *Transfus Med Update*, February 2000. Available at: http://www.itxm.org/TMU2000/tmu2-2000.htm. Accessed Sept 19, 2002.
14. Hulme JA: *Fibromyalgia: a handbook for self care & treatment*, ed 3, Missoula, Mt, 2000, Phoenix Publishing.
15. Kotlarz V: Tracing our roots: origins of clinical laboratory science, *Clin Lab Sci* 11:5-7, 1998.
16. Johnston DE: Special considerations in interpreting liver function tests, *Am Fam Physician* 59:2223-2232, 1999.
17. Lamb DJ: The clinical and economic benefits of PSA and fPSA, *Testing, Medical Laboratory Observer* 3:32-38, 2001.
18. Larson FC, Traver M: *Clinical significance of tests available from Dupont*, Wilmington, DE, 1991, DuPont Company.
19. Lotspeich-Steininger CA, Stiene-Martin AE, Koepke JA: *Clinical hematology: principles, procedures, correlations*, Philadelphia, 1992, JB Lippincott. pp 57-72, 303-346, 635-649, 650-656.
20. Lowe J, Reichman A, Yellin J: A case-control study of metabolic therapy for fibromyalgia: long-term follow-up comparison of treated and untreated patients, *Clin Bull Myofascial Ther* 3:65-79, 1998.
21. Mitchem K: NACB releases updated thyroid testing guidelines, *Clinical Laboratory News*, November 2002, p 18.
22. National Institutes of Health: The Third Report of the National Cholesterol Education Program (NCEP) Expert Panel on Detection, Evaluation, and Treatment of High Blood Cholesterol in Adults (Adult Treatment Panel III, or ATP III) presents the NCEP's updated clinical guidelines for cholesterol testing and management. Available at: http://www.nhlbi.nih.gov/guidelines/cholesterol/atp3_rpt.htm. Accessed Sept. 10, 2002.
23. NCCLS: *how to define and determine reference intervals in the clinical laboratory: approved guideline*, ed 2, Wayne, Pa, 2000, Author.
24. Phalen GS: The carpal tunnel syndrome: seventeen years, experience in diagnosis and treatment of six hundred and fifty-four hands, *J Bone Joint Surg Am* 48:211-228, 1966.
25. Pratt DS, Kaplan MM: Laboratory tests. In Schiff ER, Sorrell MF, Maddrey WC, editors: *Schiff's diseases of the liver*, ed 9,. Philadelphia, 2003, JB Lippincott, pp 221-256.
26. Stein PD: Antithrombotic therapy in patients with mechanical and biological prosthetic heart valves, *Chest* 119:220S-227S, 2001.
27. Uthman E: Interpretation of lab test profiles, *American Board of Pathology*. Available at: http://web2.airmail.net/uthman/lab_test.html. Accessed June 28, 2004.
28. Valentine V: The patient with diabetes mellitus. In Lewis S, Heitkemper M, Dirksen S, editors: *Medical-surgical nursing: assessment and management of clinical problems*, ed 5, St Louis, 2000, Mosby, pp 1367-1405.
29. Watnick S, Morrison G: Kidney. In Tierney L, McPhee S, Papadakis M, editors: *Current medical diagnosis and treatment*, ed 39, New York, 2000, McGraw-Hill, pp 886-916.
30. Woodhouse S: C-reactive protein: from acute phase reactant to cardiovascular disease risk factor, *Medical Laboratory Observer* 34:12-20, 2002.

Index